NEW COMPREH
HOEOEOPATHIC MATERIA MEDICA

OF

MIND

By
Dr. H. L. CHITKARA

assisted by
ASHOK GUPTA

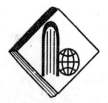

B. JAIN PUBLISHERS PVT. LTD.
NEW DELHI (INDIA)

First Edition : 1994
Second Edition : 1995
Third Edition : 1998

Price : **Rs. 225/-**

© H. L. Chitkara

Jacket design adopted from illustrations in the
fly leaf of *Picture Dictionary for Children*
By Aloke Kashyap, Holy Faith International.

Published by :
B. Jain Publishers Pvt. Ltd.
7, Wazirpur Printing Press Complex,
Ring Road, Delhi-110052 (INDIA)

Printed in India by :
J.J. Offset Printers
7, Wazirpur, Delhi - 110052

ISBN 81-7021-446-7

BOOK CODE : BC 3657

List of Contents

Dedication

For upward of three generations of homoeoapths, Kent's Repertory has been a bulwark of the homoeopathic practice. Comprising as it does thoroughly proven and verified rubrics, it has been looked upon as sacrosanct. The other more enthusiastic and knowledgeable group has been trying to rectify the entries, because according to one scholar there are upto 10,000 printing mistakes in the text. This exercise is still going on. ·

No one however ventured to improve or add more rubrics or medicines to the Repertory even though the source material, the materia medica has been enlarged greatly since after the death of Dr. Kent. Till, the authors of the Synthetic Repertory attempted to do something about it. Guided by the experience of the practitioners all over the world, they decided to retain and enlarge the core - Mind, Generalities, Sleep, Dreams and Sexuality - and off-load the particulars. This commendable work has come to be accepted by the profession as a useful successor to the Kent's Repertory for the last 20 years.

This New Comprehensive Homoeopathic Materia Medica of Mind, is dedicated to the authors of Synthetic Repertory, Barthel and Klunker, who dared touch the sacred cow.

Preface and Acknowledgements

Soon after the publication of the *Word Index of the Expanded Repertory of Mind* in 1989, work was taken up to compile a comprehensive Materia Medica compatible with the Synthetic Repertory Vol. I. Dr Ashwani Singh and Dr Ravinder Singh of our clinic laboured for months to prepare cards for the manuscript. Their efforts were, however, completely thwarted by the ineptitude and bungling of the programmer who fed the data into the computer for the purpose of printing. His equivocation and prevarication put the schedule behind by two years. He had dispersed the cards of mss beyond redemption. There was no other way except to write the mss all over again. This task was taken up by Dr Ashok Gupta of the Group Promisalone.* Additional rubrics for inclusion in the new compilation were taken from the *Additions to the Repertory of Mind* (fully referenced) prepared separately. The work was thoroughly screened to exclude non-authentic material and bring about conformity in the compilation. The most difficult part of the project was the task of proof-corrections with reference not only to the correctness of spelling, etc. but also to ensuring the proper arrangements of the rubrics, sub-rubrics and sub-rubrics of sub-rubrics in print. Besides Dr Ashok Gupta others who did their bit in this behalf were Dr Nitin Khadse and Ms Susan Gimbel Niekamp working in the clinic and our good friend Dr. BP Rao.

Thanks for due to all those named above and to M/s B Jain Publishers for their cooperation in bringing out this work.

Dr H L Chitkara
BA (Hons); DHS (Hons)

May 7, 1994
B-1/24, Malviya Nagar
New Delhi - 110 017

* The word **Promisalone** in the title of the series *Technique Promisalone Homoeopathique* is an acronym for **PR**escribing **O**n **MI**nd Symptoms **ALONE.**

Preface to the Second Edition

As a result of using this compilation in the clinic in practice and on hearing from colleagues by correspondence, it was found that this compilation contained a number of errors, most of which have been corrected now. This second edition of the New Comprehensive Homoeopathic Materia Medica of Mind has therefore undergone considerable revision :

Mistakes in denoting the singular (•) and additions (★) have been corrected. Additional rubrics from out of authentic sources have been added.

The alignment of printing of the 2nd line of some rubrics has been corrected, to avoid possible confusion in reading.

The sequence of medicines described in this Materia Medica is not in accordance with strict alphabetical order. For instance, Phosphoric Acid precedes Pheliandrium, Phaseolus, Phenobarbitalum. Then comes Phosphorus. This odd arrangement is in fact the result of following the alphabetical order of the abbreviations as prefixed to the Synthetic Repertory. *In this revised edition, while it has not been possible to rearrange the text, the list of remedies given in the introductory pages now provides their abbreviations also and hence the existing order of the text of the medicines described. Readers are requested to locate the correct page numbers of the medicines by referring to this list.*

Thanks are due to the following colleagues for assistance in correctting the mistakes :
1. Dr. Horst Barthel, Switzerland, the author of the Synthetic Repertory Volume 1.
2. Dr. G.M. Deshpande, Betual, (M.P.)
3. Dr. Mohd Imam Azam, Sitarampur (W.B.)
4. Dr. M.L. Sehgal, New Delhi.
5. Dr. Peter Kubis, Czechoslovakia.
6. Dr. S.M. Gunavante, Bombay.
7. Dr. Nitin Khadse of our clinic who saw this print through the press.

Dr H.L. Chitkara

Feb 8, 1995.

Preface to the Third Edition

This third edition of the New Comprehensive Homoeopathic Materia Medica of Mind has undergone further revision. Some more mistakes have been corrected and many omissions have been retrieved. Out of the 892 medicines in the Materia Medica, one of them has been deleted and one has been clubbed with another, thus reducing the number to 890. There was a controversy in our mind regarding the rubric, **Embarrassed, after ailments,** and **Ailments from embarrassment;** we had opted for the former in place of the latter. However, on reconsoderation and in consultation with colleagues, we have now opted for the second rubric. Necessary corrections have therefore been carried out accordingly. Some more printing anamolies have been corrected.

Although more comprehensive and allegedly more complete Repertories and Materia Medicas of the Mind have since been published, this publication still remains more handy and more authentic. The arrangement of the medicines in the text still remains the same, and a need for retaining the **List of Remedies** prefixed to the text is still there.

Thanks are due to the following colleagues in revising this editions:

1. Dr. Ravdeep Arora of our clinic
2. Dr. Mohd. Imam Azam of Sitarampur (West Bengal).

Readers are welcome to point out any omissions and mistakes which will be gratefully received for consideration while bringing out the new edition.

Dr H.L. Chitkara

B-1/24, Malviya Nagar,
New Delhi-110017

Feb. 24, 1998.

Ground Plan
Objective, Format, Construction, Revision and Scope

The Synthetic Repertory Vol I dealing with Mind symptoms provides a delightful gamut of mind rubrics most gratifying and welcome in homoeopathic practice. But there is a snag. After a case is repertorised pointing maybe to two or more remedies, there is no "court of appeal", a materia medica reflecting other rubrics of the remedy/remedies selected, to enable clinching of the issue. The present work is meant to be the answer. It fulfils an acutely felt need particularly of the elite group that swears by Mind symptoms alone.

It was decided to build up the materia medica by reduction of the rubrics from the Synthetic Repertory and putting them into remedy slots. The adoption of this procedure restricted the format of the work. Each remedy is therefore presented in the form of repertory and as a corollary, also retains by and large the other features of the Synthetic Repertory, namely,

(1) Only three gradations of the rubrics have been made as in Kent's Repertory, instead of four of the Synthetic Repertory. The distinguishing type-faces also conform to the Kent's model.

(2) Spelling of some of the words such as *labor, honor, behavior* has been retained inthe American style as in the Synthetic Repertory.

(3) The word *am.* (which also means *forenoon*) used in the sense of amelioration has been changed to *amel.* to remove the confusion.

(4) The specific times have been shown in hours such as *6 hours, 19 hours* instead of the prevalent 6 am, 7 pm to conform to the style in the Synthetic Repertory.

(5) In the Repertory some rubrics are repeated under different key-words such as *Delusion, Driving sheep* and *Delusion, Sheep, driving.* This duplication has been retained in the compilation.

(6) The names of the remedies are the same as in the Synthetic Repertory and mostly follow the spellings and style of the German Pharmacopoeia. However, the more common usage in English works has also been mentioned for purposes of elucidation. It may be noted that the remedy Bacillus Dysenterie appears under the alphabet 'D' and not under 'B'. This also applies to the names of other Bowel Nosodes.

Revision

In the process of transferring the rubrics to the remedy slots, each rubric was given a once-over and in this way numerous errors of print and diction were noticed and corrected, e.g.

Page No.	Original Text	Corrected
175 of SR	Confusion, scratching behind the ear, on	Confusion, scratching behind the ear, in
676 of SR	Jealousy, saying and making what he would not say and make	Jealousy, saying and doing what he would not say and do
1078 of SR	Weeping, emotion, after light slight	Weeping, emotion, after slight

A few rubrics were suspect and required a more thorough examination. This necessitated reference to the original sources, e.g.

Page No.	Original Text	Corrected
324 of SR	Delusion, move hears things that are high up near him out of sight (Kent, Kunzli and SR)	Delusion, move, hears invisible things (Boger-Boenninghausen)

An important deviation from the SR is the shifting of "Embarrassment" from under the main rubric, "Ailments from" to an independent position in the rubrics, as "Embarrassed, ailments after."

Scope

This compilation lists all the 890 remedies referred to in the Synthetic Repertory. But many new additions to the rubrics have been included. Particular care has been taken to exclude all doubtful and non-authentic rubrics, as was done by Kent himself and to some extent by Barthel and Klunker. *It may be noted that the additions to the rubrics are marked by asterisk (★) and the singular symptoms by dots (•).*

As it is, this compilation is *more comprehensive, more authentic, more accurate* and *more elucidated* than any other work of this kind extant today. Also, *easy to refer and use.*

Review.....

The first edition of the (New Comprehensive Materia Medica of Mind) is followed after a year by the second edition, which proves that the work is wanted not only by the followers of the "Promisalone Technique" (Prescribing on mind symptoms alone). On the contrary, the reviewer finds it of use in many respects. With the difficulties now-a-days with the patients, on the one side, the psychology subject to contradiction, on the other side; with no direct connection to their being mentally ill, I find it as practical in cases, because it is possible with the help of this Materia Medica to differentiate the remedies which contain the remaining symptoms by indirectly aimed questions especially of the singular mental symptoms.... The recommendation of this reliable and well-get-up work for practical work can be re-emphasised.

Klunker

(From ZKH 40, 4/1996, a German Journal)

Chitkara, H.L.: New Comprehensive Homoeopathie Materia Medica of Mind, 2 improved edition 692 pp., B. Jain Publishers; New Delhi 1995 Rs. 200/-.

The first edition (see Review ZKH, 39, 1995 p. 81) is followed after an year by the second, which proves that the work is wanted not only by the followers of the "Promisalon. technique" (Prescribing on Mind Symptoms Alone). On the contrary the reviewer finds it of use in many respects. With the difficulties now-a-days with the patients, on one side the psychology subject to contradiction, on one side the spychology subject to contradiction, on the other side with no direct connection to their being mentally ill, I find it as practical in cases, because it is possible with the help of this Materia Medica to differentiate the remedies which contain the remaining symptoms by indirectly aimed questions especially of the singular mental symptoms. It deserves to be stressed that in this new edition errors and structural orders have been corrected. And it is understandable that the corrections of small deviations of alphabets in the order of the the medicines and in the remedy index would have been corrected in this. Above all the use of remedy abbreviations which does not all the same appear in a Materia Medica, as a principle of arrangement becomes an unnecessary problem. The recommendation of this reliable and well-got-up work for practical work can be reemphasised.

Klunker.

(From ZKH 40 4/1996, German Journal)

List of Remedies

ABELMOSCHUS

Anxiety, night, children, in
Delusions, imaginations, hallucinations,
        illusions
    assaulted, is going to be
Fear, animals, of
        night, of venomous •
    apoplexy, of
    flies, of •
    insects, of •
    scorpions, of •
    snakes, of
    spiders, of •
Indifference, surroundings, to the

ABIES CANADENSIS

Heedless
Irritability
Morose, cross, fretful, ill-humor, peevish
Quiet disposition
Restlessness
        night

ABIES NIGRA

Dullness, sluggishness, difficulty of
        thinking and comprehending,
        torpor.
            daytime
Hypochondriasis
Restlessness
        night
*Sadness, despondency, dejection, men-
        tal depression, gloom, mel-
        ancholy*
Work, mental, impossible

ABROTANUM

Anger, irascibility
Anxiety
    stomach, in ★
Cheerful, gay, mirthful
    alternating with sadness

Contrary
Cruelty, inhumanity
Delusions, brain, has softening of
    voices, hears
        cease when listening intently
        in bed •
Dullness, sluggishness, difficulty of
        thinking and comprehending,
        torpor
    children, in
Excitement, excitable
Exertion, agg. from mental
Fear, apprehension, dread
    brain, of softening of
    tremulous
    waking from a dream, on
Forgetful
Frightened, easily
    waking from a dream, on
Hysteria
Indolence, aversion to work
Irritability
        children, in
Loquacity
Malicious, spiteful, vindictive
Memory, weakness of
Mood, agreeable
Moral feeling, want of
Morose, cross, fretful, ill-humor, peevish
Obstinate, headstrong
    children
Prostration of mind, mental exhaus-
        tion, brain-fag
Restlessness
        night
Sadness, despondency, dejection, men-
        tal depression, gloom, mel-
        ancholy
    children, in
Starting, sleep, from
Talk, indisposed to, desire to be silent,
        taciturn
Violent, vehement
Work, mental, fatigues
    impossible

1

ABSINTHIUM

Aversion, persons, to all
Brutality
Busy, fruitlessly
Confusion of mind
Cruelty, inhumanity
Death, desires, during convalescence
Delirium
    convulsions, after
Delusions, imaginations, hallucinations,
    illusions animals, of
        grotesque •
    cats, sees
    hearing, illusions of
    murdered, he will be
    pursued by enemies
        he was
            soldiers, by
    rats, colors, of all •
    visions, has
    horrible
Dipsomania, alcoholism
Dream, as if in a
    beautiful •
Dullness, sluggishness, difficulty of
    thinking and comprehending,
    torpor
Excitement, excitable
Fancies, exaltation of
Fear, apprehension, dread
    killing, of
    murdered, of being
Foolish, behavior
Forgetful, epilepsy, of what happened
    before •
Hysteria
    attacks, in
Idiocy
Imbecility
Indifference, apathy
    life, to
Insanity, madness
    brutal ★
Irritability
Kleptomania
Mania

Memory, loss of
    epileptic fits, after
Memory, weakness of
    done, for what has just
Restlessness
    children, in
Shrieking, screaming, shouting
Speech, hesitating
    incoherent
Stupefaction, as if intoxicated
    alternating with violence •
Unconsciousness, coma, stupor
    alternating with dangerous vio-
        lence •
    sudden
Violent, vehement
    alternating with stupor
Weeping, convulsions, during
    epileptic

ACALYPHA INDICA

Sadness, despondency, dejection, men-
    tal depression, gloom, mel-
    ancholy

ACETICUM ACIDUM

Ailments from :
    excitement, emotional
Anger, irascibility
Anguish
Anxiety
    children, about his
    family, about his
    health, about
Borrows trouble ★
Carried, desires to be
Complaining
Confusion of mind
Crawling on floor
    rolling on the floor
Delirium
    alternating with sopor
    distension of abdomen and consti-
        pation, with ★

Delusions, imaginations, hallucinations,
    illusions
       stomach, has corrosion of, an
        ulcer
Dullness, sluggishness, difficulty of
    thinking and comprehending,
    torpor
Excitement, excitable
Fear, apprehension, dread
    approaching him, of others
    everything, constant of
    happen, something will
    people, of
    water, of
Forgetful
Grief
Hydrophobia
Hysteria
Ideas, deficiency of
Indifference, apathy
    everything, to
Irritability
    headache, during
Lamenting, bemoaning, wailing
Memory, weakness of
    expressing oneself, for
    occurrences of the day, for
    persons, for
Mistakes
    speaking, in
    work, in
Morose, cross, fretful, ill-humor, peevish
Prostration of mind, mental exhaustion, brain fag
    injuries, from
Recognize, relatives, does not, his
Rolling on the floor
Sadness, despondency, dejection, mental depression, gloom, melancholy
    sleeplessness from sadness
Stupefaction, as if intoxicated
    morning
    alternating with delirium •
Unconsciousness, coma, stupor
Weeping, tearful mood
Work, mental, aversion to

ACETANILIDUM

Moral feeling, want of

ACHYRANTHES CALEA

Answers, monosyllable
Anxiety
    conscience, as if guilty of a crime
Company, aversion to; presence of
    other people agg. the symptoms; desire for solitude
Company desires,
    spoken to, but averse to being •
Darkness, desire for •
Exertion, agg. from mental
Fear, suffering, of
Light, aversion to
Moral feeling, want of
Religious
    preoccupations •
Remorse
Sadness, despondency, dejection, mental depression, gloom, melancholy
Sensitive, noise, to
Unconsciousness, wakes often, but only for a short time
Work, mental, fatigues

ACONITUM NAPELLUS

Absent-minded, unobserving
Absorbed, buried in thought
Abusive, insulting
Activity, mental
    morning •
    alternating with dullness •
Affectionate
Affections, in general ★
Ailments from:
    anger, vexation
      anxiety, with
      fright, with
      silent grief, with
    anticipation, foreboding, presentiment
    excitement, emotional
      moral ★

Ailments from:

fear
fright
    accident, from sight of an
hurry
indignation
joy, excessive
mortification ★
scorn, being scorned
shock, mental
Ambition
Anger, irascibility
children, in
cough from a.
trembling, with
trifles, at
violent
Anguish
cardiac
driving, restlessness, with
stool, before
tossing about, with
Answers, monosyllable ★
slowly
Anxiety
    forenoon
    evening
    night
    midnight, after
air, in open
breathing deeply, on
children, infants, in
chill, during
climacteric period, during
cold drinks amel.
company, when in
crowd, in a
drinking, cold water amel.
fear, with
fever, during
fright, after
future, about
head, with congestion to
headache, with
health, about
hypochondriacal

Anxiety,
    menses, before
      during
        anger and a.
    mental exertion, from
    motion, from
      amel.
    pains, from the
    paroxysms, in ★
    perspiration, with cold
    pregnancy, in
    pressure on the chest, from
    sleep, on going to
      during
    stool, before
      during
      after
    urination, during
    vexation, after
    waking, on
    walking, while
Audacity
Aversion :
    affection for anybody during
      pregnancy, has none   ●
Bed, aversion to, shuns bed
Beside oneself, being
    anxiety, from
Bite, desire to
    fist ★
    himself, bites
Busy
Capriciousness
Carried, desires to be
    caressed and, desires to be
    desires to be, fast ★
Cautious
Censorious, critical
Chaotic, confused·behaviour
Cheerful, gay, mirthful
    alternating with bursts of passion
      moroseness
      sadness
      weeping
    foolish, and
    heat, during
    menses, before

Childbed, mental symptoms, during, agg.
Childish behavior
Clairvoyance
Climacteric period agg.
Communicative, expansive
Company, aversion to; presence of other people agg. the symptoms; desire for solitude
   alternating with desire for company ●
avoids the sight of people
Company, desire for; aversion to solitude, company amel.
Complaining
Concentration, difficult
   studying, reading etc., while
   writing, while
Confusion of mind
      morning
         waking, on
     air, in open, amel.
     chill, during
     intoxicated, as if
       as after being
     motion, from
     paroxysms of pain, during
     waking, on
     walking, air, in open
     warm room, in
Contradiction, is intolerant of
Contradictory to speech, intentions are
Contrary
Conversation agg.
Courageous
Cowardice
Dancing
Darkness agg.
Death:
   desires ★
   dying, feels as if
   presentiment of
     predicts the time
   thoughts of
Defiant
Delirium
     night
   alternating with consciousness
   anxious

Delirium,
   bed and escapes, springs up suddenly from
   convulsions, during
   crying, with
   death, talks about ●
   encephalitis
   fever, during
   foolish, silly
   frightful
   gay, cheerful
   headache, during
   jerking, with ●
   jumping, with
   laughing
   look fixed on one point, staring
   maniacal
   menses, during
   pains, with the
   pupils, with dilated
   raging, raving
   restless
   sad
   sleep, during
     comatose, during
   sleeplessness, with
   sorrowful
   trembling, with
   violent
Delirium tremens, mania-a-potu
Delusions, imaginations, hallucinations, illusions,
     night
   anxious
   assembled things, swarms, crowds etc.
   body: deformed, some part is ●
   die, he was about to
   disease, incurable, has
   doomed, being
   driving, sheep ●
   engaged in some occupation, is
   enlarged
     body, part of
     distances are
     head is
     objects are

Delusions,
    faces, larger, grow
    fancy, illusions of
    figures, sees
    floating in air ★
    head, large, seems too
    hearing, illusions of
    home, away from, is
    imagess, phantoms, sees
      night
    insane, she will become
    large, parts of body seem too
    sheep, driving •
    sleeping, while awake, that he
      was, insists
    small; smaller, of being
    spectres, ghosts, spirits, sees
    swollen, is
    voices, hears
    weeping, with
Dementia
    epileptics, of
Despair
    alternating with hope
    chill, during
    heat, during
    pain, with the
    recovery, of
Dipsomania, alcoholism
Discontented, displeased, dissatisfied
Discouraged
    anxiety, with
Disobedience
Doubtful, recovery, of
Dream, as if in a
Dullness, sluggishness, difficulty of thinking and comprehending, torpor
    evening, 22h., after ★
    emotions, from
    reading, while
    smoking, from •
    warm room, on entering a
    wine, after
    writing, while
Ecstasy
Escape, attempts to

Excitement, excitable
    agg.
    chill,.during
    nervous
    perspiration, during
    pregnancy, during
    suppression of excretions, from
Exhilaration
Fancies
    exaltation of
      capricious
    vivid, lively
Fear, apprehension, dread
    night
    accident, of
    bed, of the
    busy streets ★
    crowd, in a
      public place, of; agoraphobia
    dark, of
    death, of
      heart symptoms, during
      heat, during ★
      impending death, of
      labor, during
      menses, before
        during
      predicts the time
      pregnancy, during •
    diarrhoea with
    disease, of impending
      incurable, of being
    evil, of
    falling, of
    ghosts, of
      night
    heat, during
    imaginary things, of
    insanity, losing his reasion, of
    labor, during
    long-lasting ★
    men, dread, fear of
    menses, before
      during
      suppressed from f.
    misfortune, of
    music, from

Fear,
> narrow places, in; claustrophobia
> noise, from
> overpowering
> *palpitation, with*
> *people, of*
> *pregnancy, during*
> restlessness from f.
> sleep, before
> **suffocation, of**
> *touch, of*
> tremulous
> *walking across busy street* •

Foolish behavior
> fever, during •

Forgetful
> *emotions, from*

Fright, menses, during ★
Frightened easily
Gestures, confused ★
> convulsive
> grasping
>> genitals, delirium, during
>> picks at bed clothes
> hands, motions of the, involuntary★
> wild
> uncertain

Grief
Hatred
Haughty
Homesickness
Hopeful
> alternating with despair
> sadness

Howling
Hurry, haste
> movements, in
> occupation
> walking, while

Hypochondriasis
Hysteria
> *fainting, hysterical*
> menses, during
> *plethoric subjects, in*

Ideas abundant, clearness of mind
> *deficiency of*

Imbecility
Impatience
> *tossing about* •

Impertinence ★
Impetuous
> perspiration, with

Inconsolable
Inconstancy
Indifference, apathy
> *anxiety, after* •
> *everything, to*
> *loved ones, to*
> relations, to
> sleepiness, with

Indignation
Indiscretion
Indolence, aversion to work
> sleepiness, with

Industrious, mania for work
Insanity, madness
> menses, during
> **pain, from intolerable**

Introspection
Irritability
> chill, during
> headache, during
> heat, during

Jesting, aversion to
> *joke, cannot take a*

Jumping, bed, out of
Lamenting, bemoaning, wailing
Lascivious, lustful
Laughing, agg. ★
> alternating with rage, frenzy
> spasmodic ★

Light, desire for
Loathing, general
Loquacity
> hasty

Magnetized, desire to be, mesmerism
> amel.

Malicious, spiteful, vindictive
Mania
Meditation
Memory, active
> alternating with weakness of memory

Memory, weakness of
    dates, for
    done, for what has just
    labor, for mental
    thought, for what has just
Menses, mental symptoms agg.
    at beginning of
    during
Mildness
Misanthropy
Mistakes :
    time, in
Moaning, groaning, whining
    anxious
    heat, during
    perspiration, during
Mocking
    ridicule, passion to
Monomania
Mood, alternating
    changeable, variable
    repulsive
Morose, cross, fretful, ill-humor, peevish
    fever, during
Music agg.
    aversion to
    headache from m.
Obstinate, headstrong
    fever, during ●
    tossing about impatiently ●
Offended, easily; takes everything in
    bad part
Perseverance
Prophesying
    predicts the time of death
Prostration of mind, mental exhaus-
    tion, brain fag
Quarrelsome, scolding
Rage, fury
    evening
    night
    alternating with cheerfulness
        consciousness ●
        laughing ●
    menses, at beginning of ●
        during
    pain, from
    paroxysms, in

Reading, aversion to read
Reflecting
    unable to reflect
Reproaches himself
    others
Restlessness
    forenoon
    evening
    night
    anxious
    bed, tossing about in
    busy
    chill, during
    driving about
    heat, during
    internal
        forenoon, on walking ●
    menses, before
        during
    metrorrhagia, during
    pain, during
    parturition, during
    pregnancy, during
    sleep, before
    walking, while
Rocking amel.
Runs about
Sadness, despondency, dejection,
        mental depression, gloom,
        melancholy
    anxious
    chill, during
    health, about
    heat, during
    menses, before
    music, from
    perspiration, during
    walking, while and after
Self-torture
Senses, acute
    dull, blunted
Sensitive, oversensitive
    children
    light, to
    music, to
    noise, to
        slightest, to

Sensitive,
    pain, to
    puberty, in
    touch, to
Sentimental
Shrieking, screaming, shouting
    children, in
    genitals, grasping, with ★
    pain, with the
    touched, when
    urinating, before ★
Sighing
    heat, during
    perspiration, during
Singing,
    alternating with weeping
    trilling
Sit
    inclination to
Slowness
    eating, while ●
Somnambulism
Speech
    childish
    hasty
    nonsensical
    prattling
    unintelligible
    wandering
Starting, startled
    from a dream
    fright, from and as from
    noise, from
    sleep, during
        from
Stupefaction, as if intoxicated
    smoking, from ●
    vertigo, during
Suicidal
    knife, razor, with a
Suspicious, mistrustful
Talk, indisposed to, desire to be silent,
    taciturn
    others agg., talk of
Talking, sleep, in
Terror ★

Thoughts, as if from stomach ●
    intrude and crowd around each
      other
    persistent
      unpleasant subjects, on waking
    rapid, quick
    rush, flow of
    thoughtful ●
    tormenting
    wandering
Throws things away
Timidity
    evening, going to bed, about
    fright, after ●
Torments himself
Touched, aversion to being
Touchy ★
Unbearable, pains ★
Unconsciousness, coma, stupor
    evening
    alternating with restlessness
    apoplexy, in
    emotion, after
    fever, during
    menses, suppression of
    vertigo, during
    vomiting amel.
    warm room, in
Undertakes many things, perseveres in
    nothing
Violent, vehement
    beats the head ★
Wearisome
Weeping, tearful mood
    evening
    aloud, sobbing
    alternating with cheerfulness.
      laughter
      rage
      singing
    anxiety, after
    causeless
    chill, during
    convulsions, during
    coughing, from ★
    heat, during
    music, from
    pains, with the
    perspiration, during

Wildness
Will, contradiction of
Work, mental, impossible
fatigues

ACONITUM CAMMARUM

Anxiety
Concentration, difficult
Memory, weakness of
Rage, fury
Restlessness
    night

ACONITUM FEROX

Activity, mental
Anxiety
Confusion of mind
Memory, active
Restlessness
    painful •
Sadness, despondency, dejection, mental
    depression, gloom, melancholy

ACONITUM LYCOCTONUM

Abstraction of mind
Business, averse to
Concentration, difficult
Inconstancy
Indolence, aversion to work
Laughing
    agg.
    alternating with rage, frenzy
    spasmodic
Mania
Mood, changeable, variable
Restlessness
    heat, during
Wildness
Will, contradiction of
Work, aversion to mental
    fatigues
    impossible

ACONITINUM

Dullness, sluggishness, difficulty of thinking and comprehending, torpor
Hydrophobia

ACTAEA SPICATA

Absent-minded, unobserving
Ailments from :
    fright
Anger, irascibility
Anxiety
    motion amel.
    rest, during
Capriciousness
Company, desire for; aversion to solitude, company amel.
Confusion of mind
Delirium
    fever, during
    raging, raving
Delusions, fail, everything will
Egotism, self-esteem
Fear, apprehension, dread
    alone, of being
    death, of
        night
    menses suppressed from fear
Impatience
Inconstancy
Irresolution, indecision
Irritability
Lamenting, bemoaning, wailing
Libertinism
Loathing, life, at
Memory, weakness of
Obstinate, headstrong
Restlessness
Sadness, despondency, dejection, mental depression, gloom, melancholy
Self-deception
Sighing
    heat, during
    perspiration, during

Singing
alternating with weeping
trilling
Sit, inclination to
Somnambulism
Stupefaction, as if intoxicated
Thinking, aversion to
Unconsciousness, coma, stupor
Weary of life despair about trifles,
with •

ADELHEID AQUA

Restlessness
night
Unconsciousness, coma, stupor

ADLUMIA FUNGOSA

Absent-minded, unobserving
Irritability
Mistakes, writing, in
Sadness, despondency, dejection, mental
depression, gloom, melancholy

ADONIS VERNALIS

Dipsomania, alcoholism
Fear, stomach, arising from
Morose, cross, fretful, ill-humor, pee-
vish
Restlessness
anxious
Sadness, despondency, dejection, mental
depression, gloom, melancholy
Stupefaction, as if intoxicated

AESCULUS HIPPOCASTANUM

Absent-minded, unobserving
Ailments from:
anticipation, foreboding, presentiment
Anger, irascibility
contradiction, from
easily

Cheerful, gay, mirthful
Comprehension, easy
Concentration, difficult
attention, cannot fix ★
Confusion of mind
morning, waking, on
knows not where she is nor when-
ever came to objects around her
waking, on
Death, sensation of
Delirium
Delusions, lost, she is (salvation), wak-
ing, on •
Despair
Dullness, sluggishness, difficulty of think-
ing and comprehending, torpor
morning
waking, on
night on waking
Eccentricity
Escape, attempts to
window, from
Fear, night, waking, after
Ideas abundant, clearness of mind
Indolence, aversion to work
Irritability
evening
Memory, weakness of
Mistakes, localities, in
Morose, cross, fretful, ill-humor, peevish
Recognize anyone, does not
Rest, desire for
Sadness, despondency, dejection, mental
depression, gloom, melancholy
heat, during
Sensitive, oversensitive
Starting, sleep, from
Stupefaction, as if intoxicated
Thoughts, rapid, quick
Tranquillity, serenity, calmness
Unconsciousness, coma, stupor
sitting, while
waking, on
Violent, vehement
Work, aversion to mental

AESCULUS GLABRA

Confusion of mind
Dullness, sluggishness, difficulty of think-
     ing and comprehending, torpor
Stupefaction, as if intoxicated
Unconsciousness, coma, stupor

AETHUSA CYNAPIUM

Ailments from:
     anticipation, foreboding, presen-
        timent
Anger, irascibility
Anguish
     vomiting, with
Anticipation, examination, before
Anxiety
     afternoon
     dark, in
     future, about
     headache, with
Cheerful, gay, mirthful
     forenoon
Company, desire for; aversion to soli-
     tude, company amel.
     alone agg., while
Concentration, difficult
     children, in
     studying, reading etc., while
Confusion of mind
Conversation amel. ★
Darkness agg.
Delirium
     night
     chill, during
     convulsions, during
     delusions, with
     fever, during
     foolish, silly
     maniacal
     perspiration amel. d. ●
     raging, raving
Delusions, imaginations, hallucina-
     tions, illusions
     day and night
     night

Delusions,
     animals, of
        persons are rats, mice, insects
     etc.
     cats, sees
     clothes are beautiful
     dogs, sees
     faces, sees, closing eyes, on
     fancy, illusions of
     great person, is a
     mice, sees
        mouse running from under a
        chair
     rats, sees
        running across the room
     tongue, long, too ●
Discontented, displeased, dissatisfied
Dullness, sluggishness, difficulty of think-
     ing and comprehending, torpor
Excitement, excitable
     morning
      . forenoon
Fear, apprehension, dread
     afternoon
     closing eyes, on
     dark, of
     diarrhoea with f.
     examination before
     sleep, before, close the eyes, lest
        he should never wake, fear to
Forgetful
Gestures, convulsive, sleep, during ●
Idiocy
Imbecility
Impatience
Industrious, mania for work
Insanity, madness
Irritability
     forenoon
     afternoon
     air, in open
     eating, after
     headache, during
     menses, during
     sitting, while
Jesting
Loquacity
Loves, animals ★
     cats ★
     dogs ★

Mania
Memory, weakness of
Morose, cross, fretful, ill-humor, peevish
       afternoon
   air, in open
   heat, in head, with •
Nibble, desire to ★
Prostration of mind, mental exhaustion, brain-fag
Rage, fury
Reading
   unable to read
Reserved
Restlessness
   anxious
   chill, during
Sadness, despondency, dejection, mental depression, gloom, melancholy
       afternoon
       evening
   air, in open
   alone, when
Sensitive, oversensitive
Serious, earnest
      noon, amel. •
Shrieking, screaming, shouting
   children, in
Speech, slow
   wandering
Spit, desire to
Starting, sleep, falling, on
Stupefaction, as if intoxicated
   vertigo, during
   vomiting (in a child), after •
Suicidal, throwing himself, window, from
Talk, indisposed to, desire to be silent, taciturn
       forenoon
Thoughts, persistent
   garment made the previous day, about a •
Timidity, appearing in public, about
Tranquillity, serenity, calmness, forenoon •

Unconsciousness, coma, stupor
   eyes, with fixed
   fever, during
   lying, stretched out while •
   vertigo, during
Wearisome
   air, in open
Weeping, tearful mood
   noise, at
   self discontent, with ★
   stool, during
Witty
Work, aversion to mental
   impossible

AETHER

Anxiety
Cheerful, gay, mirthful
Confusion of mind
Dancing
Death, sensation of
      evening •
Delirium
     night
   raging, raving
Delirium tremens, mania-a-potu
Delusions
   angels, seeing
   bells, hears ringing of, funeral, his•
   companions: is with companions of his youth •
   eternity, lived an, he has •
   God, sees •
   music, he hears unearthly
   mystic hallucinations •
   travelling, worlds, through •
   vivid
Dullness, sluggishness, difficulty of thinking and comprehending, torpor •
Ecstasy
Excitement, excitable
Exhilaration
Fear, apprehension, dread
   danger, of impending
     night •
   disease, of impending
   suffocation, of, evening •

Foolish behavior
Frightened easily
Gestures, convulsive
Helplessness, feeling of
Hysteria
> evening
Ideas abundant, clearness of mind
Insanity, madness
Jesting
Laughing
> evening
> *barking dog, as a* •
> silly
> spasmodic
Loquacity
Mania
Moaning, groaning, whining
Muttering
Pleasure
Restlessness
> evening
Sadness, despondency, dejection, mental depression, gloom, melancholy
Sighing
Speech, extravagant
> incoherent
> merry
> nonsensical
> rapturous •
> strange
Stupefaction, as if intoxicated
Talk, indisposed to, desire to be silent, taciturn
Tranquillity, serenity, calmness
Unconciousness, coma, stupor
Weeping, tearful mood

AGARICUS MUSCARIUS

Absent-minded, unobserving
Activity
Ailments from:
> anger, vexation
> dipsomania
> excitement, emotional

Ailments from:
> fright
> reproaches
> sexual excesses
> work, mental
Amorous
Anger, irascibility
Answer
> *aversion to answer*
> > sings, talks, but will not answer questions •
> *refuses to answer*
Anxiety
> evening
> night
> breathing deeply, amel.
> future, about
> health, about
> *menses, after*
> > which prevents sleep •
> noise, from
> perspiration, amel.
> sleep, during
> > menses, after
> waking, on
Audacity
Awkward, drops things
Battles
> war, talks of
Business, averse to
Capriciousness
Chaotic, confused behavior
Cheerful, gay, mirthful
> evening
> alternating with sadness
> foolish, and
Childish behavior
Company, aversion to; presence of other people agg. the symptoms; desire for solitude
Company, desire for; aversion to solitude, company amel.
> alone agg., while
Concentration, difficult
> studying, reading etc., while
> *learns with difficulty*

Confusion of mind
> morning
>> waking, on
> afternoon
> air, in open
> carrying heavy loads, when •
> eating, after
>> amel.
> headache, with
> intoxicated, as if
>> as after being
> reading, while
> waking, on
> walking, while
>> amel.
>> air, in open

Courageous
Cowardice
Dancing
> grotesque

Deceitful, sly

Delirium
> *bed and escapes, springs up sud-*
>> *denly from*
> *crying, with*
> easy ★
> *exaltation of strength, with*
> exhaustion, with
> fever, during
> fierce
> foolish, silly
> gay, cheerful
>> alternating with melancholy •
> headache, during
> *intoxicated, as if*
> know his relatives, throws wine
>> and medicines at nurse, does
>> not •
> loquacious
> muttering
> noisy
> **raging, raving**
> recognizes no one
> religious
> romping with children •
> silent
> singing
> violent

Delirium tremens, mania-a-potu
Delusions, imaginations, hallucinations,
> illusions
> arms, belong to her, do not
> dead sister, corpse of •
>> persons, sees
> diminished, whole body is •
> enlarged, distances are
>> objects are
> fancy, illusions of
> figures, sees
> great person, is a
> hearing, illusions of
> hell, gate of, obliged to confess his
>> sins at •
> hole appears like a frightful
> chasm,   a small •
> *legs don't belong to her*
> light, incorporeal, he is
> mushroom, he is commanded to
>> fall on his knees and confess
>> his sins and rip up his bowels
>> by a •
> officer, he is an
> people, converses with absent
> small: smaller, of being
>> things grow smaller
> spectres, ghosts, spirits, sees
> superhuman control, is under
> vindictive •
> voices, hears
> water, spoonful, seems like a
>> lake, a •

Dementia
Despair
> *rage, bordering on •*

Destructiveness
Development of children arrested
Dipsomania, alcoholism
Discomfort
> forenoon

Discontented, displeased, dissatisfied
Discouraged
Distances, inaccurate judgement of
Dream, as if in a

Dullness, sluggishness, difficulty of think-
ing and comprehending, torpor
      morning
      evening, amel.
        night, amel. •
   children, in
   chill, during
   . mental exertion, from
Eccentricity, fancies, in
Ecstasy
Egotism, reciting their exploits •
Embraces, companions, his
Escape, attempts to
Excitement, excitable
      evening
      alternating with delirium •
Exertion, agg. from mental
Exhilaration
   exaltation
      bed, in
         night
      sleeplessness, with
Fancies, exaltation of
      evening, bed, in
      night
      sleeplessness, with
Fear, apprehension, dread
      evening, bed, in
   disease, of impending
      cancer, of ↔
   disturbed, of being •
   evil, of
   fit, of having a
   insanity, losing his reason, of
   misfortune, of
   suffocation, of, night
Foolish behavior
Forgetful
   words while speaking, of; word
      hunting
Frivolous
Gestures
   grasping or reaching at some
      thing, at flocks; carphologia
   hands, motions, involuntary, wind-
      ing a ball, as if
   strange attitudes and positions
      head, of
   violent

Grief
Grimaces
Hatred
   revenge, and
Haughty
Heedless
Hydrophobia
Hysteria
   sexual excesses, after
Ideas abundant, clearness of mind
   evening, bed, in
Idiocy
Imbecility
Inconstancy
Indifference, apathy
   business affairs, to
   everything, to
   work, with aversion to
Indolence, aversion to work
      evening
   dinner, after
   eating, after
Industrious, mania for work
Injure himself
   frenzy causing him to injure him-
      self
Inquisitive
Insanity, madness
   malicious, malignant
   shy •
   strength increased, with
Irresolution, indecision
Irritability
      morning, waking, on
   coition, after
   waking, on
Jesting
   trifles with everything
Jumping
Kill, desire to
Kisses, hands, his companions'
Lascivious, lustful
Laughing
   bed, in •
   chill, during
   involuntarily
   loudly

Loquacity
   answers no questions but ●
   changing quickly from one sub-
      ject to another
Malicious, spiteful, vindictive
Mania
   rage, with
Memory, active
   evening
Memory, weakness of
   done, for what has just
   expressing oneself, for
   heard, for what has
   persons, for
   thought, for what has just
   words, of
Mischievous
Mistakes, speaking, in
      agg. after exertion ●
      sleeplessness, after
      spelling, in
      words, using wrong
   writing, in
Mood, changeable, variable
Morose, cross, fretful, ill-humor, peevish
   morning, waking, on
Morphinism
Multilating his body
Nymphomania
Obstinate, headstrong
Occupation, diversion amel.
Offended, easily; takes everything in
      bad part
Pities herself
Plans
   bold ●
   revengeful ●
Prophesying
Proportion, sense of, disturbed ★
Prostration of mind, mental exhaus-
      tion, brain-fag
Quarrelsome, scolding
Rage, fury
   alternating with religious excite-
      ment ●
   constant
   drunkenness, during ●
   mischievous
   strength increased
   violent

Recognize:
   relatives, does not recognize his
Resignation
Restlessness
   evening
   midnight, after, 3h.
   internal
   night, in dream ●
Reveals secrets
Revelry, feasting
Rhythmic ★
Runs about
   dangerous places, in most ●
Sadness, despondency, dejection, men-
      tal depression,
   gloom, melancholy
   morning
   afternoon, amel.
   evening
   coition, after
   exertion, after
   headache, during
   masturbation, from
   pollutions, from
   sexual excesses, from
   trifles, about
Selfishness
Senses, dull, blunted
Sensitive to,
   noise, talking, of
Shrieking, screaming, shouting
   sleep, during
Sighing
Singing
   alternating with vexation
   hilarious, joyously
Sit, inclination to
Size, incorrect judge of
Sociability
Somnambulism
Speech, hesitating
   incoherent
   jerks, by
   merry
   respectful ●
   wandering
Spoken to, averse to being
Squanders

Starting, startled
  jerking or twitching, ceasing on
    falling asleep
  electric, as if
  sleep, falling, on
Stupefaction, as if intoxicated
    morning
      amel. •
    air, in open, amel.
    vertigo, during
    waking, on
Sulky
Talk, indisposed to, desire to be silent,
    taciturn
  others agg., talk of
  slow learning to
Tears things
Temerity
Thinking, aversion to
  complaints agg., of
Thoughts, rush, flow of
    evening, bed, in
    night
    sleeplessness, from
Threatening
Throws things, persons, at
Touched, aversion to being
Unconsciousness, coma, stupor
    morning
    alternating with convulsions
    coition, after
    fever, during
    pain, from
    vertigo, during
Verses, makes
Violent, vehement
  deeds of violence, rage leading to
Whistling
Work, aversion to mental
  impossible
    morning

AGARICUS CITRINUS

Indolence, aversion to work
Unconsciousness, coma, stupor

AGARICUS CAMPESTRIS

Delirium

AGARICUS EMETICUS

Anxiety
  cold drinks amel.

AGARICUS PANTHERINUS

Answers, monosyllable
Delirium
  raging, raving
Unconsciousness, coma, stupor

AGARICUS PHALLOIDES

Answers, slowly
Anxiety
Delirium
Gestures, strange attitudes and posi-
    tions
Impatience
Restlessness
  bed, tossing about in
Speech,
  slow
Unconsciousness, coma, stupor

AGARICUS PROCERUS

Delirium, crying, with
  refuses to take the medicine •
Delirium tremens, mania-a-potu
Unconsciousness, coma, stupor

AGARICUS SEMIGLOBATUS

Exhilaration
Unconsciousness, coma, stupor

AGARICUS STERCORARIUS

Escape, attempts to
Excitement, excitable
  convulsions, after •
Restlessness
Unconsciousness, coma, stupor
Wildness, convulsions, before

AGAVE AMERICANA

Hydrophobia

AGAVE TEQUILANA

Desires, full of
Dipsomania, alcoholism
Excitement, excitable
        amnesia, followed by transient •
Jesting
Sadness, despondency, dejection, mental
        depression, gloom, melancholy
Shrieking, screaming, shouting
Violent, vehement
Pessimist
Unconsciousness, coma, stupor

AGNUS CASTUS

Absent-minded, unobserving
Abstraction of mind
Ailments from:
        anticipation, foreboding, presenti-
        ment
        sexual excesses
Amativeness
Amorous
Anger, irascibility
Anxiety   ⸱
        health, about ↔
        hypochondriacal ↔
Business, incapacity for
Concentration, difficult
        studying, reading etc., while
                learns with difficulty
Confidence, want of self
Confusion of mind
        reading, while
Contemptuous
        self, of
                alternating with eccentricity •
Cowardice
Death, desires
        presentiment of
                soon, believes that she will die,
                and that she cannot be helped •
        sensation of
        thoughts of

Delirium
Delusions, existence, doubt if anything
                had •
        smell, of
        wealth, of
Dementia, senilis
Despair
Discontented, displeased, dissatisfied
        himself, with
Discouraged
        alternating with haughtiness •
Disobedience
Doubtful, recovery, of
Dullness, sluggishness, difficulty of
                thinking and comprehending,
                torpor
        reading, while
Eccentricity
Ecstasy
Excitement, excitable
Exertion, agg. from mental
Exhilaration
        alternating with sadness
Fancies, exaltation of
Fear, apprehension, dread
        death, of
                soon, that she will die
        waking, on
Forgetful
        purchases, of; goes off and leaves
                them
Heedless
Hypochondriasis
Hysteria
        lascivious
Ideas, deficiency of
Imbecility
Indifference, apathy
        alternating with cheerfulness
        external things, to
Insanity, puerperal
Loathing, life at
Loquacity
Memory, weakness of
        business, for
        do, for what was about to
Mood, alternating
        changeable, variable

Morose, cross, fretful, ill-humor, peevish
Obscene, lewd
Prostration of mind, mental exhaustion, brain fag
Rage, fury
    amorous, morning when rising •
Reading, difficult, is
Resignation
Sadness, despondency, dejection, mental depression, gloom, melancholy
    daytime
    headache, during
    milk disappearing, after •
    puerperal
Senses, dull, blunted
Speech, hesitating
Starting
    sleep, during
      from
Suicidal, thoughts
Unconsciousness, coma, stupor
Weary of life
Work, aversion to mental
    impossible

AGREMONE OCHROLEUCA

Anxiety
    night, children, in
Fear, blind, of going
    poisoned, of being
Mania, demoniac
Memory, weakness of

AGROSTEMA GITHAGO

Unconsciousness, coma, stupor

AILANTHUS GLANDULOSA

Anguish
    nausea, with
Answers, incorrectly
Anxiety
    morning
Calculating, inability for geometry
Concentration, difficult
    calculating, while

Confusion of mind
    dream, as if in
Delirium
    exhaustion, with
    face, with red
    fever, during
    headache, during
    maniacal
    muttering
    raging, raving
    recognizes no one
    restless
Delusions, rats; running, a rat, up the leg,
    rat running across the room
    running up the leg a rat
    snakes, crawling up leg, feels a •
    unreal, everything seems
Dream, as if in a
Dullness, sluggishness, difficulty of thinking and comprehending, torpor
Fancies, confused
Forgetful
Frightened easily
Grief
Heedless
Indifference, apathy
    everything, to
    fever, during
    stoical to what happens •
    typhoid, in
Indolence, aversion to work
Insanity, madness
Irritability
Mania
Memory, weakness of:
    facts, for past
    persons, for
    said, for what has
Mistakes, calculating, in
Moaning, sleep, during
Muttering
Prostration of mind, mental exhaustion, brain-fag
Restlessness
    morning
Sadness, despondency, dejection, mental depression, gloom, melancholy
Senses, dull, blunted
Shrieking, children, in

Sighing

Stupefaction, as if intoxicated

Talking, sleep, in

Thinking, aversion to

Unconsciousness, coma, stupor
>> diphtheria, in
>> fever, during
>> *scarlatina, in*
>> vomiting, with

Weeping, tearful mood
>> desire to weep all the time

ALCOHOLUS

Abusive, insulting

Affability, enemy, to an •

Anxiety, alone, when
>> bed, in
>> disguises, which he vainly •

Boaster, braggart

Brutality

Cheerful, gay, mirthful

Childish, behavior

Complaining

Concentration, difficult

Confusion of mind

Courageous

Cowardice

Cursing, swearing

Delirium
>> bed and escapes, springs up sud-
>>> denly from
>> raging, raving
>> religious

Delirium tremens, mania-a-potu

Delusions, imaginations, hallucination,
>> illusions
>> abyss, fear of falling down an •
>> enemy, wait for an, lying in •
>> hydrothorax, he has
>> insulted, he is
>> pursued, murderers, robbers, by •
>>> police, by
>> ship in a storm, they are on board
>>> of •
>> sleeping, while awake, insists that
>>> he was
>> wealth, of

Dementia

Desires, uncontrollable •

Dullness, sluggishness, difficulty of think-
>> ing and comprehending, torpor

Eccentricity

Escape, attempts to

Exhilaration

Fancies, absurd
>> vivid, lively

Fear, misfortune, of
>> unaccountable, vague

Fire, wants to set things on

Friendship, sweet outpourings of •

Gestures, convulsive
>> grasping or reaching,
>>> picks at bed clothes, rest,
>> during •
>> lively

Heedless

Imbecility

Impatience
>> contradiction, at slightest

Indolence, aversion to work
>> physical

Insanity, madness
>> injuries to the head, from

Irritability

Jesting, licentious •

Jumping, bed, out of

Kill, desire to

Laughing

Liar
>> lies, never speaks the truth, does
>> not know what she is saying

Loquacity

Malicious, spiteful, vindictive

Mania

Memory, weakness of

Mistakes,
>> persons, in

Mocking, friends, at his •

Mood, changeable, variable

Morose, cross, fretful, ill-humor, peevish

Obscene, lewdsongs

Obstinate, headstrong

Passionate

Prostration of mind, mental exhaustion
      brain-fag
Quarrelsome, scolding
Rage, fury
Reserved
Restlessness
      bed, tossing about in
      disguise, vainly seeks to •
Reveals secrets
Sadness, despondency, dejection, mental
      depression, gloom, melancholy
      drunkards, in
Senses, acute
      dull, blunted
Sensitive, oversensitive
Sentimental
Shameless
Shrieking, screaming, shouting
Singing, boisterous •
Smiling   •
Sociability
Speech, confused
      hasty
      incoherent
      inconsiderate
Starting, sleep, from
Suicidal disposition
Sympathy, compassion
Talk, indisposed to, desire to be silent,
      taciturn
Thoughts, rapid, quick
      rush, flow of
      thoughtful
      wandering
Tranquillity, serenity, calmness
Unconsciousness, coma, stupor
Undignified •
Unfeeling, hard hearted
Violent, vehement
Witty

ALETRIS FARINOSA

Concentration, difficult
Discontented, displeased, dissatisfied
Unconsciousness, coma, stupor

ALFALFA

Hypochondriasis
Morose, cross, fretful, ill-humor, peevish
Prostration of mind, mental exhaus-
      tion, brain-fag
Sadness, despondency, dejection, mental
      depression, gloom, melancholy

ALLIUM CEPA

Absent-minded, unobserving
      afternoon, coffee or wine, after •
Anger, irascibility
Anxiety
Concentration, difficult
Confusion of mind
      coffee, after
      wine, after
Despair
Discontented, displeased, dissatisfied
Dullness, afternoon, wine, after
Fear, apprehension, dread
      *pain, during, becoming unbear-
        able* ★
Foolish behaviour
Indifference, morning
      on waking
Indolence, morning
Insanity, madness
Misanthropy
Mistakes, speaking, in
      misplacing words
      spelling, in
      work, in
Restlessness
Sadness, despondency, dejection, mental
      depression, gloom, melancholy
Senses, dull, blunted

ALLIUM SATIVUM

Anxiety
Company, desire for; aversion to soli-
      tude,
      company amel.
Escape, attempts to

Fear, alone, of being
    death, of
    medicines, of not being able to bear
        any kind of ●
    taking too much, fear of
    poisoned, of being
    recover, he will not
Gluttony
Ideas, deficiency of
Impatience
Impulse, run, to; dromomania
Memory, weakness of
Restlessness
    alone, when
Sadness, despondency, dejection, mental
      depression, gloom, melancholy
    alone, when
Sensitive, oversensitive
    moral impressions, to
Thoughts, wandering
Weeping, sleep, in

ALLOXANUM

Anger, irascibility
Anxiety
    future, about
Company, aversion to; presence of
    other people agg. the symp
    toms; desire for solitude
    alone, amel. when
Concentration, difficult
Confusion, identity,
    head separated from body, as if
Dictatorial, domineering, dogmatical,
    despotic
Exhilaration
Forsaken feeling
Impatience
Indifference, apathy
    loved ones, to
    surroundings, to the
    work, with aversion to
Industrious, mania for work
Irritability
    noise, from
Memory, weakness of
    do, for what was about to
    done, for what has just

Memory, weakness of,
    facts, for recent
    happened, for what has just ● .
    heard, for what has just
    names, for proper
    places, for
    read, for what has
    say, for what is about to
    words, of
Mistakes, speaking, in
    spelling, in
    writing, in
Sadness, despondency, dejection, mental
    depression gloom, melancholy
    alone, when
      amel. ●
Sensitive, noise, to
Weeping, tearful mood
    alone amel., when ●

ALOE SOCOTRINA

Absorbed, buried in thought
    eating, after ●
Activity
    alternating with exhaustion ●
    mental, alternating with exhaus-
      tion ●
        indolence ●
Anger, irascibility
    contradiction, from
Anguish
Anxiety
    eating, after
    manual labor, during
    motion, from
    paroxysms, in
    standing, while
    walking, while
Cheerful, gay, mirthful
    morning, waking, on
    evening
Company, aversion to: presence of other
    people agg. the symptoms;
    desire for solitude
Complaining
Concentration, difficult

Confusion of mind
     morning
     evening
    chill, during
Contemptuous
Contented
Contradiction, is intolerant of
    restrain himself to keep away from
     violence, has to
Cursing, swearing
Death, presentiment of
    predicts the time
    thoughts of
Despair
Discontented, displeased, dissatisfied
     evening amel.
    himself, with
    rainy weather, during ●
Discouraged
Disgust
Dullness, sluggishness, difficulty of think-
     ing and comprehending, torpor
Excitement, afternoon
    face, heat of, with ●
    urination, during ●
Exertion, agg. from mental
Fear, apprehension, dread
    crowd, in a
    death, of
    men, dread, fear of
    noise, from
    people, of anthrophobia
    pollutions, after
Fraternized with the whole world ●
Frightened, pollutions, after ●
Hatred
    revenge, and
Hurry, haste
    work, afternoon in ●
Hypochondriasis
Hysteria
Ideas abundant, night ★
Imbecility
Indifference, apathy
     evening
    eating, after ●

Indolence, aversion to work
     morning
     noon
     afternoon
     evening amel.
     waking, on
Industrious, mania for work
Introspection, eating, after
Irritability
     afternoon
     evening
      amel.
    pain, during
    stool, before
    weather, in rainy or cloudy
Jesting
Lascivious, lustful
Laughing
    children, in
Loathing, general, pain, during ●
Loquacity
Malicious, spiteful, vindictive
Memory, active
    alternating with lassitude ●
Memory, weakness of,
    labor, for mental
Mischievous
Moaning, sleep, during
Mood, changeable, variable
     dinner, after ●
     repulsive, repels everyone ●
Morose, cross, fretful, ill-humor, pee-
    vish
     evening
    causeless
    cloudy weather, from
Music agg.
    trembling from
Obstinate, headstrong
Playful
Quarrelsome, scolding
Quiet disposition
Rage, suffering, from
Restlessness
Sadness, despondency, dejection, men-
    tal
    depression, gloom, melancholy
     morning
     evening amel.

Sensitive, oversensitive
    music, to
    noise, to
        slightest, to
Shrieking, calls someone ★
Speech, prattling
Starting, anxious
    noise, from
Stupefaction, as if intoxicated
Talk, indisposed to, desire to be silent,
    taciturn
        eating, after
Thoughts intrude, sexual
    rush, flow of, night
    thoughtful
        eating, after ●
        cold wet weather, in ●
    wandering
Time passes too slowly, appears longer
Timidity
    bashful
Tranquillity, serenity, calmness
    reconciled to fate
Unconsciousness, alternating with rage ●
    stool, during
Violent
Vivacious
Weary of life
Work, aversion to mental
    desire for

ALUMINA

Absent-minded, unobserving
    alternating with animation ●
    inadvertence
Absorbed, buried in thought
Abstraction of mind
Affectation
Affectionate
Ailments from :
    anger, vexation
        anxiety, with
        silent grief, with
    anticipation, foreboding, presen
        timent
    disappointments

Ailments from :
    mortification ★
    scorn, being scorned
    sexual excesses
Ambition
Anger, irascibility
    trembling, with
Anguish
    morning
    night
        4h.
Answer, aversion to
Anxiety
    morning
        waking, on
    forenoon
    evening
    night
        waking, on
    midnight, after
        4h.
    air amel., in open
    **conscience, as if guilty of a
        crime**
    conversation, from
    epilepsy, threatened with a fit of ●
    fear, with
    fever, during
    fits, with
    future, about
    health, about
    house, in
        on entering
    hypochondriacal
    noise, from
    paroxysms, in ★
    room, on entering a ●
    sleep, before
    speaking, when
    thinking about it, from
    urination, before
    waking, on
Ardent
Audacity
Avarice
Barking
    growling like a dog
Bed, remain in, desire to

Blood or a knife, cannot look at •
Brooding
Calculating, inability for
    geometry
Capriciousness
Cares, worries, full of,
    morning, bed, in
    waking, on •
Censorious, critical
Cheerful, gay, mirthful
    evening
        bed, in
    night
    alternating with absence of mind
    weeping
    sleep, during
    walking in open air and after, on
Childish, behavior
Color, red, aversion to •
Communicative, expansive
Company, aversion to; presence of
    other people agg. the symp-
    toms; desire for solitude
    morning •
    forenoon •
Complaining
Concentration, active
Concentration, difficult
    studying, reading etc., while
Confidence, want of self
Confusion of mind
    morning,
        rising, after, amel.
        waking, on
    heat, during
    identity, as to his
        duality, sense of
    reading, while
    rising, after
    smoking, after
    spirituous liquor, from
    talking, if someone else ↔
    wine, after
Contemptuous
Contented
Contradict, disposition to
Contradiction, is intolerant of
Contradictory to speech, intentions are
Contrary

Conversation agg.
Courageous
    alternating with fear •
Cowardice
Death, agony before
    desires
    prestiment of
        predicts the time
Defiant
Delirium
    violent
Delusions, imaginations, hallucinations,
    illusions
        evening, bed, in
    animals, of
    consciousness belongs to another •
    crime, committed a, he had
    criminals, about
    dead persons, sees
    disease, has incurable
    double, of being
    enlarged
        body, parts of
    fancy, illusions of
    fire, visions of
    great person, is a
    head belongs to another
    identity, errors of personal
    images, phantoms, sees
        sleep, preventing
    insane, she will become
    large, parts of body seem too
    melancholy
    money, he is counting
    numb, being ↔
    outside his body, some one else
    saw or spoke •
    pains during sleep, he has •
    says something, it seems to him
    as though somebody else has said
    it, when he •
    sees something, when he, it seems
    as though he saw through some-
    body else's eyes •
    smooth, being ↔
    spectres, ghosts, spirits, sees
    talking, someone else is talking,
    when he
        speaks

Delusions,
  thieves, sees
  time, exaggeration of, passes too
    slowly
  unpleasant
  unreal, everything seems
  vermin, sees, crawl about
  visions, has
  water, of
  wedding, of a
  worms, creeping of
Despair
  recovery, of
Dipsomania, alcoholism
Discontented, displeased, dissatisfied
  everything, with
Discouraged
  alternating with confidence •
    hope
Discrimination, lack of
Doubtful, recovery, of
Dream, as if in a
Dullness, sluggishness, difficulty of think-
    ing and comprehending, torpor
  reading, while
  waking, on
Duty, no sense of
Ennui, tedium
    forenoon •
  homesickness, with ★
Excitement, excitable
  heat, during
  palpitation, with violent
  walking in open air, on
Exhilaration
Fancies, exaltation of
    evening, bed, in
    sleeplessness, with
Fastidious
Fear, apprehension, dread
    morning
    evening
  apoplexy, of
  blood, of ★
  death, of
    morning
    dream, from
    waking, on

Fear,
  disease, of impending
    incurable, of being
  epilepsy, of
    morning •
  evil, of
    evening
  falling, of   .
  fit, of having a
  happen, something will
  impulse, of his own •
  insanity, losing his reason, of
  knaves, of
  knives, of ★
  misfortune, of
  noise, from
  palpitation, with
  people, of
  pins, pointed sharp things, of
  red, everything ★
  robbers, of
  room, on entering
  struck, walking behind him, by
  those •
  suicide, of
  waking, on
    dream, from a
    walking, while
  walking, of,
    dark, in the, people behind
    him, might hit him ★
  water, of ★
  wet his bed, he will; incontinence
  in bed •
Foolish behavior
Forgetful
  heat, during •
  name, his own
  words while speaking, of; word
  hunting
Forsaken, feeling
  friendless, feels •
Frightened easily
  blood, at sight of •
  urinating, before •
Grief
    morning
    waking, on

Haughty
Heedless
Howling
Hurry, haste
    awkward from
Hypochondriasis
    morning
    night
    suicide, driving to
    waking, on
Hysteria
Ideas abundant, clearness of mind
    deficiency of
Idiocy
Imbecility
Improvident
Impulse, morbid
    fears his i. ★
Inconstancy
    thoughts, of
Indifference, apathy
    forenoon
    ennui, with
    pleasure, to
Indiscretion
Indolence, aversion to work
    morning
    forenoon
    intelligent, although very
Injure himself, fears to be left alone,
    lest he should
Insanity, madness
Introspection
Irresolution, indecision
Irritability
    afternoon
    chill, during
    talking, while
Jesting, trifles with everything
Kill, desire to
    injure with a knife, impulse to
    knife, with a
        at sight of a
            of a knife or a gun ●
Lamenting, bemoaning, wailing
    asleep, while
    involuntary ●

Laughing
    night
    alternating with spasms ●
    aversion to ★
    contemptuous ●
    convulsions, before, during or after
    dream, during
    sleep, during
    spasmodic
Libertinism
Loathing, general
    evening
Loathing, life, at
Mania
Mathematics, inapt for algebra
    geometry
Meddlesome, importunate
Memory, active
Memory, weakness of
    names, for proper
    thought, for what has just
    words, of
Menses, mental symptoms agg. after
Mental symptoms alternating with
    physical
Mildness
Mistakes, speaking, in
    intend, what he does not
    misplacing words
    words, using wrong
    time, in
    writing, in
Moaning, groaning, whining
    anxious
    ear lobes, with hot ●
    involuntary
    sleep, during
Mocking
Mood, alternating
    changeable, variable
    repulsive
Morose, cross, fretful, ill-humor, peevish
    afternoon
    ear lobes, with hot ●
Music, aversion to

Muttering
    sleep, in
Narrow-minded
Neglects, important things
Objective, reasonable
Obscene, lewd
Obstinate, headstrong
    resists wishes of others
Occupation, diversion amel.
Offended, easily; takes everything in
    bad part
Persevere, cannot ↔
Praying
    fervent
Prostration of mind, mental exhaus-
    tion, brain-fag
    menses, after •
Quarrelsome, scolding
    afternoon
    sleep, in
Quiet disposition
Reading: aversion to read
    unable, read, to, in children
Religious affections
Remorse
Reproaches others
Reserved
Resignation ↔
Rest, desire for
Restlessness
        evening
        night
        midnight, before
    anxious
    bed, tossing about in
    lying, while
    sitting, while
Sadness, despondency, dejection, mental
    depression, gloom, melancholy
        morning
        waking, on
        forenoon
        afternoon
        evening
        night
    company, aversion to; desire for
    solitude

Sadness,
    disease, about
    eating, after
    menses, after
    suicidal disposition, with
    waking, on
Senses, dull, blunted
    vanishing of ↔
Sensitive, oversensitive
    noise, to
Serious, earnest
Shrieking, screaming, shouting
    pain, lumbar region
    sleep, during
    waking, on
Sighing
Sit, inclination to
Sits, still
Smiling, never
Somnambulism
Speech, anxious, in sleep
Squanders
Starting, startled
      night
      midnight in sleep, before
    fall, on hearing anything •
    fright, from and as from
    noise, from
    sleep, before •
        falling, on
        during
        from
    urinate, on beginning to •
Striking
    desires to strike
Stupefaction, as if intoxicated
Suicidal disposition
    courage, but lacks
    fear of death, with
    hypochondriasis, by
    knife, with
      razor, with a
    perspiration, during
    run over, to be
    sadness, from

Suicidal disposition

> *seeing blood or a knife, she has horrid*
>> *thoughts of killing herself, though she*
>>> *abhors the idea* •
>
> shooting, by
> thoughts

Suspicious (doubting people) ★

Talk, indisposed to, desire to be silent, taciturn
> others agg., talk of

Talking agg. all complaints
> sleep, in
>> anxious
>> excited

Thinking, complaints agg., of

Thoughts, disagreeable
> disconnected
> disease, of
> *frightful, seeing blood or a knife, on* •
> perpsistent
> *rush, flow of*
> thoughtful
> tormenting

Time passes too slowly, appears longer

Timidity
> *alternating with assurance* •

Truth, tell the plain

Unconsciousness, coma, stupor
> dream, waking, on

Undertakes, many things, persevers in nothing

Violent, vehement

Vivacious
> alternating with absent-mindedness •

Wearisome

Weary of life
> perspiration, during
> sight of blood or a knife, at •

Weeping, tearful mood
> daytime
> morning, waking, on
> evening
> night
>> sleep, in
> aloud, wobbing

Weeping,
> alternating with cheerfulness
>> laughter
> *convulsions, during*
> easily
> *involuntary*
> menses, after
> sad thoughts, at
> *sleep, in*
> spadmodic
> waking, on
> whimpering, sleep, during

Will, weakness of

Work, aversion to mental
> impossible

ALUMINA PHOSPHORICA

Absent-minded, unobserving

Ailments from:
> grief
> *sexual excesses*
> *work, mental*

Answers, aversion to

Anxiety
> morning, waking, on
> evening
> night
> conscience, as if guilty of a crime
> fear, with
> future, about
> health, about

Company, aversion to; presence of other people agg. the symptoms; desire for solitude

Concentration, difficult

Confusion of mind,
> morning
> waking, on

Contrary

Death, conviction of

Discontented, displeased, dissatisfied

Discouraged

Dullness, sluggishness, difficulty of thinking and comprehending, torpor

Excitement, excitable
> alternating with dullness

Exuberance

Fear, evening
    death, of
    happen, something will
    insanity, losing his reason, of
    misfortune, of
    people, of
    waking, on
Forgetful
Heedless
Hurry, haste
Ideas abundant, clearness of mind
        alternating with deficiency of •
    deficiency of
Imbecility
Indifference, apathy
    alternating with excitement
Indolence, aversion to work
Insanity, madness
Irresolution, indecision
Irritability
    bemoais, wailing
Lamenting, imaginary misfortune, over
      his •
Laughing, spasmodic
Loathing, life, at
Mania
Mood, alternating
    changeable, variable
Obstinate, headstrong
Prostration of mind, mental exhaus-
    tion, brain-fag
Reserved
Sadness,
      morning, waking, on
      afternoon
Senses, dull, blunted
Sensitive, noise, to
Serious, earnest
Sits, still
Starting, sleep, falling, on
Stupefaction, as if intoxicated
Suicidal, thoughts
Talk, indisposed to, desire to be silent,
    taciturn
Talking, sleep, in
Thinking, complaints agg., of
Timidity
Unconsciousness, periodical

Weeping, morning, waking, on
    night
    alternating with laughter
    involuntary
    sleep, in
Work, aversion to mental

ALUMINA SILICATA

Absent-minded, unobserving
Ailments from:
      work, mental
Anger, agg.
Anxiety
    evening
    night
    conscience, as if guilty of a crime
    health, about
    waking, on
Capriciousness
Censorious, critical
Company, aversion to; presence of other
      people agg. the symptoms; de-
      sire for solitude
    alone, amel. when
    but agg. when alone and amel. in
    company •
Concentration, difficult
Confusion of mind
    morning
    waking, on
Contradiction, is intolerant of
Contrary
Cowardice
Death, desires
Delusions
    falling forward, she is
    he is
    small, of being smaller
    visions, has
Despair
Discontented, displeased, dissatisfied
    everything, with
Discouraged
Dullness, sluggishness, difficulty of think-
    ing and comprehending, torpor
    waking, on

Excitement, excitable
    menses, before
Fancies, exaltation of
Fear, apprehension, dread
    insanity, losing his reason, of
    waking, on
Forgetful
Frightened easily
Hysteria
Ideas, deficiency of
Imbecility
Indifference, apathy
Indolence, aversion to work
Insanity, madness
Irresolution, indecision
Laughing, hysterical
Loathing, life, at
Memory, weakness of
Mistakes,
        speaking, in
            words, using wrong
        writing, in
Mood, changeable, variable
Morose, cross, fretful, ill-humor, peevish
Obstinate, headstrong
Prostration of mind, mental exhaustion, brain-fag
Religious affections
Remorse
Restlessness, night
    anxious
*Sadness, despondency, dejection, mental
    depression, gloom, melancholy*
    telling it to somebody, amel. after ●
Senses, dull, blunted
Sensitive, noise, to
Sits, still
Somnambulism
Starting, sleep, on falling
Suicidal, thoughts
Talk, indisposed to, desire to be silent,
    taciturn
Talking, sleep, in
Timidity
Weeping, sleep, in
Will, weakness of

ALUMEN

Ailments from:
    bad news
Anxiety
        forenoon
        night
Aversion
    everything, to
Bed, remain in, desire to
Company, aversion to; presence of
        other people agg. the symptoms; desire for solitude
Confusion of mind, afternoon
Delusions, blood rushed through like
    roar of many waters
Doubtful, recovery, of, medicine is
    useless
Ennui, tedium
Excitement, excitable
Fear, apprehension, dread
    falling, of
    insanity, losing his reason, of
    killing, of
    misfortune, of
    unconsciousness, of ●
Frightened, easily
Gestures, hands, involuntary motion,
    of the
Indifference, apathy
    everything, to
Indolence, forenoon
Irresolution, indecision
Laughing, spasmodic
Loathing, general, evening
Memory, weakness of
Mildness
Morose, cross, fretful, ill-humor, peevish
Obstinate, headstrong
Rage, fury
Restlessness
    bed, tossing about in
Sadness, despondency, dejection, mental
    depression, gloom, melancholy
        morning
            forenoon, 9-12h. ●
Stupefaction, walking, when

Thinking, complaints agg., of
Timidity
Torments those about him
Weeping, morning
        alternating with laughter
Work, aversion to mental

AMBRA GRISEA

Absent-minded, unobserving
    spoken to, when
Absorbed, buried in thought
Ailments from:
    bereavement
    business failure
    cares, worries
    grief
    reverses of fortune
    shock, mental
    work, mental
Anger, irascibility
    alternating with sadness
    trembling, with
    violent
Anguish
        evening
        night
    persiration, during
        night •
Answers, aversion to
  • refuses to
    repeats the question first
Anxiety
        daytime
        evening
            twilight, in the
            bed, in
        night
        midnight, before
    bed, in
    company, when in
    conversation, from
    crowd, in a
    dinner, after
    eating, after
    fever, during
    flushes of heat, during

Anxiety
    sleep, before
    speaking, when
    stool, before
        ineffectual desire for, from
    thinking about it, from
Calculating, inability for, geometry
Cares, worries, full of
    daily cares, affected by
Chaotic, confused behavior
Company, aversion to; presence of other
        people agg. the symptoms; de-
        sire for solitude
    alone, amel. when
    embarassed in ★
    presence of strangers, aver
        sion to
    people intolerable to her dur-
        ing stool,
    presence of •
    smiling faces, aversion to •
Company, desire for; aversion to soli-
        tude, company amel.
    alone agg., while
Complaining
Comprehension, easy
Concentration, difficult
    studying, reading etc., while
Confidence, want of self
Confusion of mind
        morning
    bed, while in
    eating, after
    motion, from
    reading, while
    sleeping, after
    waking, on
Contrary
Conversation agg.
    aversion to
Cowardice ★
Death, desires
Delirium, morning
        waking, on
Delusions, imaginations, hallucinations,
    illusions
        morning, bed, in
        evening, bed, in

Delusions,
>absurd figures are present
>assembled things, swarms, crowds, etc.
>clear, everything is too •
>depressive ★
>devils, sees
>*faces, sees*
>>*diabolical, crowd upon him*
>>>get side of them, cannot •
>>distorted on lying down, day time
>>*hideous*
>*fancy, illusions of*
>*floating in air* ★
>grimaces, sees
>*images, phantoms, sees*
>>night
>>*frightful*
>insane, she will become
>lascivious
>light, there is too much in room (on falling to sleep) •
>spectres, ghosts, spirits, sees
>time, exaggeration of, passes too slowly
>visions, has

Despair
Discouraged
Disgust, laughing of others, at •
Dream, as if in a
Dullness, sluggishness, difficulty of think-ing and comprehending, torpor
>>morning
>**old people, of**
>reading, while
>understands questions only after repetition

Duty, no sense of
Dwells on past disagreeable occurrences
>night
Eccentricity
Embarrassed, company, in ★
Embittered, exasperated

Excitement, excitable
>night
>agg.
>children, in
>*nervous*
>palpitation, with violent
>pregnancy, during
>talking, while
>wine, after
Exertion, agg. from mental
Fancies, exaltation of
>day and night
>evening, bed, in
>>sleeplessness, with
>*lascivious*
>>dreaming, even when •
Fear, apprehension, dread
>*approaching him, of others*
>evil, of
>insanity, losing his reason, of
>men, dread, fear of
>*music, from*
>narrow places in; claustrophobia ★
>people, of
>poverty, of
>strangers, of
>tremulous
Forgetfulness
>*old people, of*
Frightened, waking, on
Grief
Heedless
Hurry, haste
>awkward from
>mental work, in
Hypochondriasis
Hysteria
Ideas abundant, clearness of mind
>deficiency of
Imbecility
Impatience
Inconsolable
Inconstancy
Indifference, apathy
>agreeable things, to
>everything, to
>excitement, after •
>irritating, disagreeable things, to
>joy, to
>>and suffering, to

Indignation

Indolence, aversion to work

        morning ★

Insanity, madness

    erotic

Irritability

    alternating with sadness

    conversation, from

    eating, after

    talking, while

Jumping, bed, out of

Lamenting, bemoaning, wailing

Lascivious, lustful

Laughing

       night

    aversion to

Light, shuns

Loathing, life, at

Looked at, cannot bear to be

Loquacity

    changing quicking from one subject to another

    rambling ★

    sleep, during

Malicious, spiteful, vindictive

Mathematics, inapt for geometry

Memory, weakness of

    forms, for

    persons, for

    read, for what has

Mildness

Misanthropy

Moaning, groaning, whining

Mood, changeable, variable

    repulsive

Morose, cross, fretful, ill-humor, peevish

Music agg.

    cough, music agg.

        piano, cough when playing

    ear-ache from

    headache from

    palpitation when listening to

    trembling with

Nymphomania

Prostration of mind, mental exhaustion,

    brain-fag

Quarrelsome, scolding

    without waiting for answers ★

Questions, speaks continually in

Reading, understand, does not

Reflect, unable to in old age •

Restlessness

      daytime

      night

      midnight 2h

    anxious

    children, in

    conversation, from •

    pregnancy, during

    talking, after

    waking, on

    walking, while

Revelry, feasting

Rudeness

Sadness, despondency, dejection, mental

        depression, gloom, melancholy

    alternating with irritability

      vehemence •

    excitement, after •

    music, from

Senses, acute

    dull, blunted

Sensitive, oversensitive

    music, to

    noise, to

Sentimental

Serious, earnest

Sits, weeping

    wrapped in deep, sad thoughts and

    notices

      nothing, as if

Society, shun, girls, modern ★

Speech, hasty

    wandering

Starting, startled

      evening, asleep, on falling

    sleep, falling, on

Strangers, presence of agg.

    child coughs at sight of strangers

Stupefaction, as if intoxicated

Suicidal disposition

    despair, from

Suspicious, mistrustful
    fear of company
Talk, indisposed to, desire to be silent,
    taciturn
    others agg., talk of
Talking agg. all complaints
    sleep, in
        children, in
Thinking, complaints agg., of
Thoughts, disagreeable
    disconnected
    persistent
     unpleasant subjects, haunted by
    rush, flow of
        day and night
    sexual
    vanishing of
        company, in •
    wandering
Time, passes too slowly, appears longer
Timidity
    appearing in public, about
    awkward, and
    bashful
    company, in
Unconsciousness, coma, stupor
    crowded room, in a
    dream, as in a
Unusual things, from any, agg. ★
Violent, vehement
Weary of life
Weeping, tearful mood
    anger, after
    desire to weep all the time
    music, from
Will, weakness of
Work, mental, impossible
    old age, in •

AMMONIUM BROMATUM

Confusion of mind
Discouraged
Fear, apprehension, dread
    restlessness from fear
Forgetful, words while speaking, of;
    word hunting

Mistakes,
    speaking, in
        words, using wrong
    writing, in
Sadness, despondency, dejection, mental
    depression, gloom, melancholy

AMMONIUM CARBONICUM

Absent-minded, unobserving
    inadvertence
    old age, in
    spoken to, when
Absorbed, buried in thought
Abstraction of mind
Abusive, insulting
    evening •
Ailments from:
    anger, vexation
    anticipation, foreboding, presen-
        timent
    hurry
    love, disappointed
Anger, irascibility
    evening
    contradiction, from
    face, red spots in, with •
    menses, during
Anguish, afternoon
Answers, aversion to
Anxiety
        morning
        forenoon
        afternoon
            17-18h •
        evening
            19h.
            19-20 h.
            amel.
        bed, in
        night
        midnight, before
    bed, in
    conscience, as if guilty of a crime
        afternoon •
    fear, with

Anxiety,
>   fever, during
>   health, about
>   hypochondriacal
>   menses, before
>   perspiration, with cold
>   waking, on

Aversion sex, to opposite
>   water, to •
>   woman, to

Beside oneself bad weather, from •

Business, averse to

Capriciousness

Cautious, anxiously

Censorious, critical

Chaotic, confused behavior

Cheerful, gay, mirthful
>   evening

Concentration, difficult
>   children, in

Confidence, want of self

Confusion of mind
>   evening
>   menses, during
>   sitting, while

Contradiction, is intolerant of

Contradictory to speech, intentions are

Conversation agg.

Cowardice

Cursing, swearing

Death, thoughts of

Defiant

Delirium
>   exhaustion, with
>   intoxicated, as if

Delusions:
>   animals, of
>   criminals, about
>   dead persons, sees
>   hearing, illusions of
>   spectres, ghosts, spirits, sees
>   vermin, sees crawl about
>   worms, creeping of

Despair

Dirtiness
>   dirtying everything
>   skin, dirty, with ★

Discontented, displeased, dissatisfied
>   everything, with

Discouraged, walking, while

Disobedience

Dullness, sluggishness, difficulty of think-
>   ing and comprehending, torpor
>   morning
>   speaking, while

Dwells on past disagreeable occurrences
>   recalls disagreeable memories ★
>   thinks of everything that others
>   have done to displease her;
>   lying awake thinking of it, in
>   the morning she has forgot-
>   ten about it. •

Eccentricity

Ecstasy

Elegance, want of

Envy
>   hate, and

Escape, family, children, from her

Estranged from her family

Excitement, excitable
>   evening
>   thinking of the things others
>   have done to displease
>   her, in bed •
>   night
>   talking, while

Exertion, agg. from mental

Exhilaration

Extravagaence

Exuberance

Fancies, exaltation, evening
>   lascivious
>   evening

Fear, apprehension, dread
>   forenoon
>   afternoon
>   *evening*
>   night
>   death, of
>   night
>   disease, of impending
>   evil, of
>   life long
>   misfortune, of
>   morning
>   forenoon •
>   waking, on

Forgetfulness
    old people, of
Frightened easily
    trifles, at
Gestures
    covers mouth with hands ★
Going out, aversion to
Grief
Hatred
    revenge, and
Heedless
Hurry, haste
Hypochondriasis, weeping, with
Hysteria
    fainting, hysterical
Ideas abundant, clearness of mind
    deficiency of
Imbecility
Inconstancy
    thoughts, of
Indifference, apathy
    external things, to
    morose
Indolence, aversion to work
    morning
    intelligent, although very
Insanity, madness
Intolerance, noise, of
Irresolution, indecision
Irritability
    daytime
    morning
    forenoon
    evening
      amel.
    air, in open
    dinner, after
    eating, after
    amel.
    headache, during
    heat, after
    menses, during
    taciturn
    walking, when
    weather, in rainy or cloudy
Jesting, aversion to
Lamenting, bemoaning, wailing

Laughing
    immoderately
    never
    spasmodic
    trifles, at
Loathing, life, at
Malicious, spiteful, vindictive
Memory, loss of
    injuries, after
    of head, after
Memory, weakness of
    pains, from, suddenly ★
    expressing oneself, for
    say, for what is about to
Menses, mental symptoms agg. before
    during
Mistakes
    calculating, in
    speaking, in
    misplacing words
    old age, in ●
    spelling, in
    words, using wrong
    name of object seen instead of
    one desired
    names, calls things by wrong
    writing, in
    old age, in
    wrong letters, figures
Moaning, groaning, whining
    sleep, during
    waking, on
Mood, changeable, variable
    supper, after
Moral feeling, want of
Morose, cross, fretful, ill-humor, peevish
    morning
    forenoon
    evening
    cloudy weather, from
    eating, after
    fever, after
    menses, during
    rainy weather, from ●

Morose,
> storm, during •
> thunderstorm, from •
> weather, from bad •

Narrow-minded

Neglects everything

Obstinate, headstrong
> children

Prostration of mind, mental exhaustion, brain-fag

Quarrelsome, scolding
> evening
> menses, during •

Quiet disposition
> menses, during

Religious affections

Remorse
> afternoon

Reserved
> menses, during

Restlessness
> *evening*
> > 19 hr. •
> > bed, in
> *anxious*
> *driving about*
> heat, during
> menses, during
> waking, on

Reveals secrets, sleep, in

Sadness, despondency, dejection, mental depression, gloom, melancholy
> morning
> forenoon
> evening
> > amel.
> night
> > amel.
> chill during
> cloudy, weather •
> eating amel., after
> menses, before
> > during
> supper amel.

Senses, dull, blunted

Sensitive, oversensitive
> menses, during
> mental impressions, to
> noise, to
> > painful, sensitiveness to
> > talking, of
> *sensual impressions, to*

Serious, earnest

Shrieking, sleep, during

Sighing

Sit, inclination to

Slander, disposition to

Spineless

Spoiled children

Spoken to, averse to being

Starting, night
> easily
> fright, from and as from
> sleep, on falling
> > *during*
> > *from*

Stupefaction, as if intoxicated
> morning, waking, on
> waking, on

Succeeds, never

Suicidal disposition

Susceptible

Sympathy, compassion

Talk, indisposed to, desire to be silent, taciturn
> *menses, during*
> others agg., talk of

Talking agg. all complaints
> sleep, in
> > reveals secrets
> > thought when awake, what he •

Thinking, complaints agg., of

Thoughts, disconnected
> persistent
> tormenting
> > past disagreeable events, about
> vanishing of
> wandering

Timidity

Travel, desire to

Unconsciousness, coma, stupor
    emotions, after
    scarlatina, in
Verses, makes
Violent, vehement
Wearisome, morning •
Weary of life
Weeping, tearful mood
    morning
    evening
      amel.
    night
    anxiety, after
    anxious
    rising, after •
    waking, on
Will, loss of
    weakness of
Work, mental, impossible

AMMONIUM CAUSTICUM

Anguish
Frightened easily
Irritability
Restlessness, night
Timidity
Unconsciousness, coma, stupor

AMMONIUM MURIATICUM

Absent-minded, unobserving
    spoken to, when
Absorbed, buried in thought
    evening
Abusive, insulting
    children, insulting parents
Ailments from:
    anger, vexation
      silent grief, with
    grief
Ambition, loss of
Anger, irascibility
    morning
    noon
    eating, amel. after •
    talk, indisposed to
Answers, aversion to

Anxiety
    night
    fear, with
    paralysed, as if
    sleep, on starting from
    waking, on
Aversion
    everything, to
    members of family, to
    persons, to certain
Blasphemy, cursing, and
Concentration, difficult
    evening
Confidence, want of self
Confusion of mind
    morning
    air, amel. in open
    intoxicated, as if
Darkness agg.
Delirium, epilepsy, after
Delusions
    animals, of
    bed, under, someone is
    enemy, under the bed, is •
    fire, visions of
      head is surrounded by •
    murdered, he will be
    sword hanging over head •
    water, of
Despair
Dipsomania, alcoholism
Discontented, displeased, dissatisfied
Disobedience
Dullness, sluggishness, difficulty of think-
    ing and comprehending, torpor
    waking, on
Elegance, want of
Envy, hate, and
Excitement, talking, while
Fear, apprehension, dread
    evening, twilight
    crowd, in a
    dark, of
    grief, as from
    killing, of
    life long
    people, of

Frightened easily
    trifles, at
    waking, on
Grief
    cry, cannot
Hatred
    revenge, h. and
Heedless
Indifference, apathy
    external things, to
    sleepiness, with
Indolence, aversion to work
      morning
    sleepiness, with
Introspection
Irritability
      morning
      forenoon
      noon
      evening
    eating, after
    eating, amel. after
    headache, during
Laughing, never
Light, desire for
Malicious, spiteful, vindictive
Meditation
Memory, weakness of
Misanthropy
Mistakes, speaking, in
Morose, cross, fretful, ill-humor, peevish
      morning
      forenoon
      afternoon, twilight, in
Music amel.
Prostration of mind, evening
Reserved, evening •
Restlessness, forenoon
      night
    dinner, after
    eating, after
    waking, on
Sadness, despondency, dejection, mental
      depression, gloom, melancholy
      afternoon, twilight, in
    darkness, in
    eating, amel. after
    grief, after

Sensitive, certain persons, to
Serious, earnest
Sit, inclination to
Starting
      evening, asleep, on falling
    dream, from a
    easily
    sleep, on falling
      during
      from
Stupefaction, as if intoxicated
Talk, indisposed to, desire to be silent,
    taciturn
      evening
Thoughts, thoughtful
Timidity
Travel, desire to
Unconsciousness, coma, stupor
Wearisome
Weeping, tearful mood
      evening
    anxiety, after
    desire to weep
    waking, on
Will, loss of
    weakness of

AMMONIUM NITRICUM

Confusion of mind

AMMONIUM VALERIANICUM

Hysteria

AMYGDALUS PERSICA

Confusion of mind, wine, after

AMYLENUM NITROSUM

Abstraction of mind
Anxiety
    air amel., in open
    climacteric period, during
Climacteric period agg.
Confusion of mind
Delusions, unreal, everything seems
Dream, as if in a

Excitement, excitable
Exertion, agg. from mental
Fear, apprehension, dread
    happen, something will
        still, cannot sit •
    misfortune, of
    restlessness from f.
Hysteria
Ideas abundant, clearness of mind
Insecurity, mental
Restlessness
Sadness, despondency, dejection, mental
        depression, gloom, melancholy
Shrieking, brain cry
    convulsions, before
        during epileptic
Sighing
Starting, sleep, during
Stupefaction, as if intoxicated
Unconsciousness, coma, stupor

AMMONIACUM GUMMI

Discomfort
Discontented, displeased, dissatisfied
    everything, with
Dullness, sluggishness, difficulty of think-
    ing and comprehending, torpor
Excitement
    night
    talking, while
Indifference, sleepiness, with
Indolence, aversion to work
    morning
    sleepiness, with
Morose, cross, fretful, ill-humor, pee-
    vish
Restlessness
    night
Sadness, despondency, dejection, mental
    depression, gloom, melancholy
        night
Slowness
Torpor
Work, impossible, mental

AMNII LIQUOR

Activity
Irritability
Restlessness
    . bed, in
    menses, before

AMORPHOPHALLUS RIVIERI

Anxiety, fear, with
Dullness, sluggishness, difficulty of think-
    ing and comprehending, torpor
Indifference, apathy
Unconsciousness, semi-consciousness

AMPHISBAENA VERMICULARIS

Ennui, tedium
Mildness
Sadness, despondency, dejection, men-
    tal depression,
    gloom, melancholy
        morning

AMYGDALAE AMARAE AQUA

Anxiety
Confusion of mind
    intoxicated, as if
Delirium
    convulsions, during
    muttering
Dullness, sluggishness, difficulty of think-
    ing and comprehending, torpor
Excitement, champagne, as after, followed
    by sudden unconsciousness •
Fear, suffocation, of
Speech, hesitating
    incoherent
    intoxicated, as if
    unintelligible
Stupefaction, as if intoxicated
Unconsciousness, coma, stupor
    excitement, after
    snoring, involuntary urination and
        stool, with
Weeping, tearful mood

ANACARDIUM ORIENTALE

Absent-minded, unobserving
Abusive, insulting
    husband insulting wife before chil-
    dren or vice versa
Affectionate
Ailments from :
    anger, vexation
    anticipation, foreboding, presenti-
        ment
    contradiction
    excitement, emotional
    fright
    grief
    mortification
    work, mental
Anger, irascibility
    contradiction, from
    stabbed anyone, so that he could have
    trifles, at
    violent
Anguish
Answers, averse to
    imperfect
    reflects long
    slowly
Antagonism with herself
Anticipation, examination, before
    stage - fright
Anxiety
        morning
            waking, on
        evening
            bed, in
    air, in open
    bed, in
    business, about
    conscience, as if guilty of a crime
    fear, with
    fever, during
    future, about
    hypochondriacal
    manual labor, during
    pursued, as if, when walking •
    standing, while
    trifles, about
    waking, on
    walking, while
        air, in open

Automatism
Aversion, society, to ★
Beside oneself, being
Blasphemy, cursing, and
Business, averse to
Busy
Cares, worries, full of
Caress :
    caressing husband and child, then
        pushes away •
Chaotic, confused behavior
Cheerful, gay, mirthful
        day time
        afternoon
        evening
    eating, while
    foolish, and
Children, impatient with ★
Childish behavior
Clairvoyance
Company, aversion to; presence of
        other people agg. the symp-
        toms, desire for solitude
Complaining
    sleep, in comatose
Comprehension, easy
Concentration, active
Concentration, difficult
    morning
    studying,
        learns with difficulty
Confidence, want of self
Confusion of mind
    morning
        rising and after, on
        waking, on
    night
    identity: duality, sense of
    intoxicated, as after being
    sleeping, after
    waking, on
Contradict, disposition to
Contradiction, is intolerant of
Contrary
Cowardice

Cruelty, inhumanity
Cursing, swearing
   rage, in
Death, presentiment of
Deceitful, sly
Defiant
Delirium
   anxious
   delusions, with
   eating amel.
   frightful
   nonsense, with eyes open
   raging, raving
Delirium tremens, mania-a-potu
Delusions, imaginations, hallucinations,
   illusions
   accidents, sees
   anxious
   assembled things, swarms, crowds etc.
   bed, someone is in, with him
   bier, is lying on a
   calls, someone
      with name, the absent mother
      or sister •
   child, is not hers •
   churchyard, visits a
   crime, committed a, he had
   cursing, with
   dead, corpse on a bier
      he himself was
      persons, sees
   demoniacal, thinks he is ★
   devils, sees
      blasphemous words, devil
      whispers •
      he is a devil
      present, are
      sits in his neck, devil •
      speaking in one ear, angel in
        the other, prompting to
        murder, or acts of benevo-
        lence, devil •
   double, of being
   dream, as if in a
   enemy, surrounded by enemies
   fancy, illusions of
   figures, sees

Delusions, figures,
      strange f. accompanying him,
        one on his right, the other
        on his left •
   fire, visions of
   grave, he is in his
   hearing, illusions of
   husband, he is not her •
   images, frightful, sees
   mind and body are separated
   people, sees
      behind him, some one is
      beside him, are
   persecuted, he is
   person is in the room, another
   possessed, being
   pursued by enemies
      he was
      horrible things, by some •
   religious
   right, does nothing
   separated from the world, he is
   sight and hearing, of
   smell, of
   soul, body was too small for soul, or
      separated from
   strange, everything is
   strangers, he sees
   succeed, he cannot; does everything
      wrong
   superhuman control, is under
   tactile hallucinations
   three persons, he is
   unreal, everything seems
   visions, has
   voices, hears
      calling his name •
      hears, that he must follow
   walks behind him, someone
   whispering blasphemy •
   wills, possessed of two
Dementia
   senilis
Depravity •
Despair
   work, over his •
Dipsomania, alcoholism

**Discontented, displeased, dissatis
fied**
  everything, with
Discouraged
Distances, inaccurate judgement of
  exaggerated, are
Dream, as if in a
Duality, sense of ★
*Dullness, sluggishness, difficulty of think-
ing and comprehending, torpor*
       morning
         waking, on
      forenoon
      afternoon
        amel. •
      evening
  mental exertion, from
  think long, unable to
  waking, on
Duty, no sense of
Egotism, self-esteem
Estranged from her family
  society, from •
Excitement, excitable
      evening
    alternating with dullness
Exertion, agg. from mental
Exhilaration, evening
Fancies, exaltation of
      afternoon
      evening
    lascivious
      evening
Fastidious
Fear, apprehension, dread
      morning
      evening
  air, in open
  approaching him, of others
  behind him, someone is
  death, of
  devil, of being taken by the
  enemies, of
  evil, of
  examination, before
  men, dread, fear of
  misfortune, of

Fear,
  paralysis, of
  people, of
  poisoned, of being   •
  robbers, of
  walking, while
    air, in open
Foolish behavior
Forgetfulness
      morning
      afternoon
      amel. •
  mental exertion, from
  old people, of
  purchases, of; goes off and leaves
    them
Forsaken, isolation, sensation of
Frightened easily
Gestures, automatic
  childish •
  perseverance, with great •
Godless, want of religious feeling
Grief
Hatred
  revenge, and
Haughty
Heedless
Helplessness, feeling of
Hesitates ★
Honor: sense of honor, no
Hypochondriasis
      morning
  eating, after
  pollutions, after
Hysteria
  pollutions, after
  sexual excesses, after
Ideas, abundant, clearness of mind
      evening
  deficiency of
  fixed ★
  vanish ★
Idiocy
Imbecility
  rage, stamps the feet
Impatience
  playing of children, by •

Impetuous
Impulse, morbid
    contradictory ★
Indifference, apathy
       daytime
     agreeable things, to
     everything, to
     irritating, disagreeable, things, to
     joy and suffering, to
     pleasure, to
     religion, to his
Indolence, aversion to work
       morning
       forenoon
       afternoon
     eating, after
     siesta, after
Insanity, madness
     religious
Insolence
Irresolution, indecision
Irritability
       daytime
       afternoon
       night
     air, amel. in open
     chill, during
     headache, during
     heat, during
     music, during
       piano, of
     waking, on
     warm room, in
Jealousy
Jumping, height, from a, impulse to j. ★
Kill, desire to
Kisses, hands, his companion's
Lamenting, bemoaning, wailing
Lascivious, lustful
Laughing
     immoderately
     serious matters, over
     spasmodic
Learns, poorly ★
Loathing, speaking, at
Loquacity
Malicious, spiteful, vindictive

    anger, with
Mania
    demoniac
Memory, active
     afternoon
Memory-confused
Memory, loss of:
     apoplexy, after
     fear, from •
     imbecility, in •
     sunstroke, after
Memory, weakness of
     names, for proper
     persons, for
     read, for what has
     seen, for everything he has •
     thought, for what has just
     words, of
Mildness
Misanthropy
Mischievous
Mistakes,
     time, in
       confounds future with past
         present with future •
         present with past
Moaning, sleep, during
Monomania .
Mood, alternating
     changeable, variable
Moral feeling, want of
Morose, cross, fretful, ill-humor,
    peevish
       afternoon
       night
     chill, during
     forgetfulness, from •
     sleep, in
     waking, on
Music agg.
     piano playing, from
     weariness, playing piano, from •
Muttering
Obscene, lewd
Obstinate, headstrong
Offended, easily; takes everything in
    bad part

Passionate
Philosophy, ability for
Plans, making many
Profanity ★
*Prostration of mind, mental exhaustion,
        brain-fag*
    afternoon
    eating, after
    fever, in
Quarrelsome, scolding
Quiet, disposition, sleep, after •
Rage, fury
      evening
    cursing, with
    shrieking, with
    violent
Recognize: relatives, does not recognize his
Religious affections;
      feeling, want of
Remorse
Reproaches himself
Reserved, afternoon
    sleep, after •
Rest, desire for
*Rest when things are not in their proper
      place, cannot*
Restlessness
      forenoon
      afternoon
      night
    anxious
    chill, during
    feverish
    headache, during
    heat, during
    periodical, every third day •
Reverence, lack of
Rudeness
*Sadness, despondency, dejection, mental
      depression, gloom, melancholy*
      morning
          waking, after
    amenorrhoea, in
    climaxis, during
    eating, after
    puerperal
    quarrel with husband, after •
    typhus, after

Satyriasis
Self, odd at with ★
Senses, acute
    dull, blunted
    vanishing of
Sensitive, oversensitive
    music, to
        piano, to
    noise, to
Serious, earnest
    absurdities, over •
    ludricous things, when seeing •
Shameless
Shrieking, screaming, shouting
    children, in
    must shriek, feels as though she
    sleep, during
Sighing
    sleep, in
Sit, inclination to
Slander, disposition to
Slowness
    motion, in
Somnambulism
Speech, firmer, surer in afternoon than
      in forenoon •
    hasty
    incoherent
    nonsensical
    prattling
    wandering
Starting
      evening, asleep, on falling
    bed, while lying awake in
    fright, from and as from
    sleep, during
      from
    waking, on
Strange, everything seems
Stupefaction, as if intoxicated
    anxiety, with •
Suicidal disposition
    shooting, by
    throwing himself from a height
Sulky

Suppressed or receding skin diseases or
haemorrhoids, mental symptoms
agg. after
Suspicious, mistrustful
walking, while •
Talk, indisposed to, desire to be silent,
taciturn
headache, during
waking, on
Talking agg. all complaints
Thoughts persistent
separated, mind and body are
rapid, quick
rush, flow of
afternoon
evening
two trains of thought
vanishing of
wandering
Timidity
bashful
Unconsciousness, coma, stupor
morning
conduct, automatic
dream, as in a
pain, from
Unfeeling, hard hearted
Unfriendly humor ★
Unsocial ★
Unsympathetic, unscrupulous
Violent, vehement
deeds of violence, rage leading to
Walk: walking in open air agg. mental
symptoms
Wearisome
Weeping, night
amel.
heat, during
sleep, in
whimpering, sleep, during
comatose
Will, contradiction of
loss of, apoplexy, after •
two wills, feels as if he had
weakness of
Work, aversion to mental
impossible

ANACARDIUM OCCIDENTALE

Confusion of mind
Imbecility
aphasia, with
Indifference, apathy
Memory, weakness of
Muttering, unintelligible

ANAGALLIS ARVENSIS

Cheerful, gay, mirthful
Delirium
fever, during
Excitement, excitable
Exhilaration
Hydrophobia
Hypochondriasis
Hysteria
Ideas abundant, clearness of mind
Insanity, madness
syphilis, in •
Mania
Strength increased, mental

ANANTHERUM MURICATUM

Cheerful, gay, mirthful
Company, aversion to; presence of other
people agg. the symptoms; de-
sire for solitude
Confidence, want of self
Confusion of mind, intoxicated, as if
Contrary
Delirium
Delusions, imaginations, hallucinations,
illusions
Destructiveness
Dullness, sluggishness, difficulty of think-
ing and comprehending, torpor
Egotism, self-esteem
Excitement, excitable
Fear, death, of
Foolish behavior
Hurry, haste
Hydrophobia

Hypochondriasis
Idiocy
Insanity, madness
    masturbation, from
    sexual excesses, from
Irritability
Jealousy
Laughing
Mania
Memory, weakness of
Monomania
    grotesque manner, to appear in a
    public place in a •
Quarrelsome, scolding
Restlessness
Sadness, despondency, dejection, mental
        depression, gloom, melancholy
Singing
Stupefaction, as if intoxicated
Suicidal disposition
Suspicious, mistrustful
Travel, desire to
Weeping, tearful mood

ANGUSTURA VERA

Absent-minded, unobserving
        afternoon •
    dreamy
    reading, while
        on going to sleep •
Abstraction of mind
Activity, mental
Anger, irascibility
Anxiety
        night
    sleep, during
    sudden
Cheerful, gay, mirthful
        afternoon
        evening, bed, in
    air, in open
    manual labor, during •
    walking in open air and after, on
Comprehension, easy
Concentration, difficult
        afternoon
    studying, reading, etc., while

Confidence, want of self
Confusion of mind
    intoxicated, as after being
    mental exertion, from
    reading, while
    walking, while
Conscientious about trifles
Cowardice
Delusions, fancy, illusions of
Discomfort, morning
Discontented, displeased, dissatisfied
        surroundings, with
Discouraged
Dream, as if in a
Dullness, sluggishness, difficulty of think-
        ing and comprehending, torpor
        afternoon
Eccentricity
Ecstasy
Embittered, exasperated
    offences, from slight •
Excitement, excitable
        afternoon
        evening, bed, in
Exertion, agg. from mental
Exhilaration
Fancies, exaltation of
        afternoon
    working, while
Fear, apprehension, dread
        death, during heart symptoms, of
        sleep, before, close the eyes lest he
            should never wake, fear to
        touch, of
Frightened easily
    trifles, at
Hatred, bitter feelings for slight offences,
        has •
Ideas abundant, clearness of mind
    deficiency of
Indolence, morning
Industrious, mania for work
Irresolution, indecision
Irritability
    perspiration, during
    trifles, from

Jesting, aversion to
    joke, cannot take a
Laughing agg.
Loathing, general
Memory, active
        afternoon
Moaning, groaning, whining
Mood, changeable, variable
Morose, cross, fretful, ill-humor, peevish
        coition, after
Offended, easily; takes everything in
        bad part
Plans, making many
Pleasure
Prostration of mind, mental exhaustion,
        brain-fag
Quarrelsome, scolding
Reading, mental symptoms agg. from
Restlessness
        afternoon
        night
    internal
    menses, before
Revelry, feasting
Sadness, despondency, dejection, mental
    depression, gloom, melancholy
Sensitive, oversensitive
    noise, to
Serious, earnest
Sighing
Starting, startled
    noise, from ★
    sleep, during
    sleepiness, with
Stupefaction, as if intoxicated
Suspicious, mistrustful
Theorizing
Thoughts persistent
    rapid, quick
    rush, flow of
        afternoon
        working, during
    wandering
        afternoon
Timidity
Unconsciousness, coma', stupor
        morning
Violent, vehement

Vivacious
Weeping, tearful mood
    sleep, in

ANGELICA ATROPURPUREA

Dipsomania, alcoholism

(RADIX) ANGELICAE SINENSIS

Concentration, difficult
Discouraged
Restlessness

ANHALONIUM LEWINII

Absorbed, buried in thought
Adaptability, loss of ●
Anguish
Anxiety
    chill, during
Automatism
Awareness of body heightened ●
Beside oneself, being
Brooding
Clairvoyance
Company, aversion to; presence of other
        people agg. the symptoms; de-
        sire for solitude
Comprehension, easy
Concentration, active   ·
Concentration, difficult
Confidence, want of self
Confusion of mind
    identity, as to his
        depersonalization, loss of self-
        knowledge and self-control, dis-
        sociation from or self-identifi-
        cation with environment, per
        sonal disruption ●
        duality, sense of
    situations, of ●
Conscientious about trifles
Death, desires
Decomposition of shape ●
    space, of ●
Deformation of all objects ●

Delirium

Delusions, imaginations, hallucinations, illusions

   answers to any delusion

   beautiful

   body, immaterial, is ●

   dead, he himself was

   double, of being

     objects are

   enlarged, objects are   ·

     diminished and ●

      letters are ●

   faces, sees, on closing eyes

     mask-like

     scheming ●

   fancy, illusions of

   figures, sees

   floating in air

   hearing, illusions of

   images, closing eyes, on

   immortality, of ●

   music, he hears

   noise, hears

   objects, delusions from bright

     brilliantly colored

     motion, in

   separated from the world, he is

   small objects appear, in motion ●

   snakes in and around her

   standing by oneself ●

   strange, everything is

   time, exaggeration of, passes too slowly

   transparent, everything is ●

     he is

   unreal, everything seems

   visions, has

     closing the eyes, on

     colourful ●

   voices, hears

Doubtful

Dreams, escape in a world of dreams ●

Dullness, sluggishness, difficulty of thinking and comprehending, torpor

Ecstasy

Environmental orientation increased ●

Euphoria

Excitement, excitable

Execution lost as the result of overpowering visual sensations ●

Express oneself, desires to ●

Fancies, exaltation

   sleeplessness, with

Fear, death, of

   people, of

Forgetful

   words while speaking, of; word hunting

Forsaken, isolation, sensation of

Hysteria

Ideas abundant, clearness of mind

   deficiency of

Inconstancy

Indifference, apathy

Initiative, lack of

Insecurity, mental

Introspection

Irony ●

Irresolution, indecision

Irritability

Light, fullness of, sees ●

Loquacity

   open hearted

Love with one of the own sex, homosexuality, tribadism

Mania

Memory, active

   past events, for

Memory, weakness of

   words, of

Merging of self with one's environment ●

Mistakes

   localities, in

   space and time, in

   time, in

     present merged with eternity ●

Mocking

Mood, alternating

Music, amel.

   carried by, sensation of being ●

   drums produce euphoria ●

Nymphomania

Optimistic

Prophesying

Prostration of mind, mental exhaustion, brain-fag

Quarrelsome, scolding
Reality, flight from •
Resignation
Restlessness
          night
Sadness, despondency, dejection, mental
          depression, gloom, melancholy
Schizophrenia
          hebephrenia
Self-control, loss of
Selfishness, express oneself, desires to •
Selflessness
Sensitive, oversensitive
          noise, to
Speech, hasty
          incoherent
Spoken to, averse to being
Stereotypes •
Stupefaction, as if intoxicated
Suicidal, disposition
Summing-up difficult
Suspicious, mistrustful
Talk, indisposed to, desire to be silent,
          taciturn
Thoughts, monotony of
          persistent, separated,
                    will, thought separated from •
          rapid, quick
          vanishing of
Time passes too slowly, appears longer
          passes too quickly, appears shorter
Unconsciousness, conduct, automatic
Unreliable •
Vivacious
Weeping, tearful mood
Will, loss of
          increased insight, self-aware-
          ness with •
          two wills, feels as if he had
          weakness of
Withdrawal from reality •
Work, mental, impossible   •

ANILINUM

Imbecility
Restlessness, night
Unconsciousness, coma, stupor

ANISUM STELLATUM

Dipsomania, alcoholism

ANTIMONIUM ARSENICOSUM

Anguish
Anxiety
Restlessness
          anxious

ANTIMONIUM CRUDUM

Absorbed, buried in thought
Affectionate
Ailments from :
          debauchery ★
          grief
          love, disappointed
Amativeness
Amorous
Anger, irascibility
          touched, when
Anxiety
                    daytime
                    evening, bed, in
                    night
                    midnight, after
                              3-5 h.
          air, in open
          bed, in
          fear, with
          fever, intermittent, during
          future, about
          knows not, what to do with
                    himself,
          sexual desire, with ★
          stool, before
          touched, anxiety to being
          vomiting, on
          walking, while
          weariness of life, with
Asks for nothing
Aversion
          everything, to
Bed, remain in, desire to
Busy, forgets everything when
Capriciousness

52

Carried, desire to be
Cheerful, gay, mirthful
    evening, bed, in
Company, aversion to; presence of other
        people agg. the symptoms;
        desire for solitude
Concentration, difficult
Confusion of mind
    identity, as to his
    intoxicated, as if
Contradiction, is intolerant of
Contrary
Cross, crossness (anger) ★
Death, desires
Delirium
    maniacal
    sleep, during
        comatose, during
    sleepiness, with
Delirium tremens, mania-a-potu
Delusions, imaginations, hallucinations,
    illusions
    calls, someone
        waking, someone calls on
    dead, mutilated corpse
    fancy, illusions of
    identity, errors of personal
    mutilated bodies, sees
    noise, knocking at the door, hears •
Dementia
    senilis
Desires, woman, ideal •
Despair, pains, stomach, in the
Dipsomania, alcoholism
Discontented, displeased, dissatisfied
Discouraged
Dream, as if in a
Dullness, sluggishness, difficulty of think-
        ing and comprehending, torpor
Ecstasy, night
    walking in moonlight •
Excitement, excitable
    evening, bed, in
    walking, air, on w. in open
Exhilaration
Fancies, exaltation of
        walking in open air

Fear, apprehension, dread
    death, of
    evil, of
    misfortune, of
    noise, from
    touch, of
    tremulous
Foolish behavior
Frightened easily
    waking, on
Gestures,
    grasping or reaching, picks at bed
    clothes
    stamps the feet
Gluttony
Grief
Hydrophobia
Hysteria, puberty, at
Ideas abundant, clearness of mind
Idiocy
    idiotic actions •
    pulling feathers out of bed •
Imbecility
Impatience
Impressionable
Indolence, aversion to work
    dinner, after
    eating, after
Insanity, madness
    stamps the feet
Irritability
    daytime
    morning
    forenoon
    evening
    children, in
    headache, during
    sadness, with
    touch, by
    trifles, from
Loathing, general
Loathing, puberty, in •
Loathing, life, at
Looked at, cannot bear to be
    agg. mental symptoms
Love exalted (love) ★
    love-sick
Mania
Meditation

Memory, active
Misanthropy
Mood, changeable, variable
    repulsive
Moonlight, mental symptoms from
Morose, cross, fretful, ill-humor,
        peevish
    afternoon
    evening
    children, in
        cry, when touched ●
Nymphomania
    menses, suppressed, after
Obstinate, headstrong
    children
Prostration of mind, mental exhaustion,
    brain-fag
Puberty, mental affections in
Quarrelsome, evening
Repugnance, to everything ★
Restlessness
Revelry, feasting
Rudeness, naughty children, of
Sadness, despondency, dejection, mental
    depression, gloom, melancholy
    daytime
    morning
        waking, after
    forenoon
    evening
    chill, before ●
    heat, during
    noise, from
    puberty, in
    respiration, with impeded
    walking, while and after, air, in
    open
Sensitive, oversensitive
    children
    noise, to
        slightest, to
Sentimental
    diarrhoea, during ●
    menses, before ●
    moonlight, in ●
Serious, earnest
Shrieking, screaming, shouting
    sleep, during
    touched, when

Sighing, afternoon ●
Sit, inclination to
Somnambulism
Speech, slow
Spoken to, averse to being
Starting, startled
    dreams, in
    noise, from
    sleep, during
        from
Stupefaction, as if intoxicated
Suicidal disposition
    night
        bed, in ●
    despair, from
    drowning, by
    shooting, by
    thoughts
        drive him out of bed ●
Sulky
Suppressed or receding skin diseases or
    haemorrhoids, mental symp-
    toms agg. after
Suspicious, mistrustful
Talk, indisposed to, desire to be silent,
    taciturn
Thoughts persistent, night
    rush, walking in open air, on
    tormenting
    night
Touched, aversion to being
Touchy ★
Unconsciousness, coma, stupor
Verses, makes
Walk, walking in open air agg. mental
    symptoms
Wearisome
Weary of life
    night
Weeping, tearful-mood
    bell, sound of, from
    heat, during
    looked at, when
    music of bells, from
    touched, when
    trifles, at
    washed in cold water, when ●
Will, weakness of

ANTIMONIUM MURIATICUM

Unconsciousness, coma, stupor

ANTIMONIUM OXYDATUM

Irritability
Restlessness, night
Sensitive, oversensitive
Starting, sleep, during

ANTIMONIUM SULPHURATUM AURATUM

Delirium raging, raving
Excitement, night
Fear, apprehension, dread
Restlessness
    waking, on
Sensitive,
    children
    puberty, in

ANTIMONIUM TARTARICUM

Ailments from :
    anger, vexation
Anger, irascibility
    evening
    alternating with cheerfulness
        exuberance •
    cough from a.
    pains, agg. •
Anguish
Anxiety
        evening
    fear, with
    fever, intermittent, during
    future, about
    pregnancy, in
    sitting, while
Audacity
Beside oneself, being
Bite, desire to
Capriciousness
Carried, desires to be
    sitting up •
Chaotic, confused behavior

Cheerful, gay, mirthful
    day time
    afternoon
    alternating with anxiety
    irritability
    moroseness
    vexation
Company, aversion to; presence of other
    people agg. the symptoms; de-
    sire for solitude
Company, desire for; aversion to soli-
    tude, company amel.
    alone agg., while
Complaining, disease, of
Confusion of mind
    morning
        rising, after, amel.
        waking, on
    air, amel. in open
    mental exertion, from
    waking, on
Contrary
Courageous
Cowardice
Cross, crossness (anger) ★
Delirium
    answers correctly when spoken to,
        but delirium and unconscious
        ness return at once
    fever, during
    gay, cheerful
    muttering
    sleep, in
    raging, raving
Delirium tremens, mania-a-potu
Delusions, imaginations, hallucinations,
    illusions
    fancy, illusions of
    fire, visions of
    spectres, ghosts, spirits, sees
    water, of
        wades in, he •
Despair
    chill, during
    heat, during
    waking, in intermittent fever •
Dipsomania, alcoholism
Discomfort, morning, on waking
Discontented, displeased, dissatisfied

Discouraged
    evening
  alternating with anxiety
Dullness, sluggishness, difficulty of thinking and comprehending, torpor
Excitement, excitable
  feverish
Exuberance, alternating with moroseness •
Fancies, exaltation, sleeplessness, with
Fear, apprehension, dread
    afternoon
    evening
  alone, of being
  death, of
  disease, of impending
  menses, menstrual colic, during •
  recover, he will not
  suffocation, of, night
  touch, of
  waking, on
Fire, wants to set things on
Frightened easily
  trifles, at
Gestures, convulsive
  stamps the feet
Hypochondriasis
Imbecility
Indifference, apathy
  alternating with anxiety and restlessness
  sleepiness, with
Indolence, aversion to work
    morning
  sleepiness, with
Insanity, madness
Irritability
    morning
      waking, on
    forenoon
    afternoon
    evening
    night ⋆
  alternating with cheerfulness
  children, in
    shriek by touch •
  noise, from
  waking, on

Jumping, bed, out of
Lamenting, bemoaning, wailing waking, on
Laughing, spasmodic
Loathing, general
Loathing, life, at
Looked at, can't bear to be
  agg. mental symptoms ⋆
Loquacity
Mania
  rage, with
Memory, weakness of
Moaning, groaning, whining
  sleep, during
  touch, on •
Mood, agreeable
  alternating
  changeable, variable
Morose, cross, fretful, ill-humor, peevish
    morning
    forenoon
    night
  alternating with cheerfulness
    exuberance •
  children, in
  cough, before fits of
  waking, on
Obstinate, headstrong
Quarrelsome, scolding
Rage, fury
  suicidal disposition, with
Restlessness
    night
  anxious
  bed, tossing about in
  children, in
    carried about, relieved by being
  heat, during
  menses, during
Sadness, afternoon
    evening
Senses, dull, blunted
  vanishing of
Sensitive, oversensitive
  children
  noise, to
  puberty, in

Shrieking, screaming, shouting
　　night
　　children, touched, when ●
　　sleep, during
　　　　eyes fixed and trembling, with ★
　　touched, when
Sit, inclination to
Spoken to, averse to being
　　alone, wants to be let
Starting, startled
　　　　midnight in sleep, before
　　easily
　　sleep, during
　　　　from
　　　　　　comatose sleep, from
　　sleepiness with
Stupefaction, as if intoxicated
Suicidal disposition
Talk, indisposed to, desire to be silent,
　　　　taciturn
Talking, sleep, in
Talks, himself, to
Thoughts, vanishing of
Touched, aversion to being
Touchy ★
Unconsciousness, coma, stupor
　　　　morning
　　　　answers correctly when spoken to,
　　　　　　but delirium and unconscious-
　　　　　　ness return at once
　　　　asphyxia, with ●
　　　　cough, between attacks of
　　　　meningitis, in
　　　　standing, while
Violent, vehement
　　pain, from
Weary of life
Weeping, tearful mood
　　night
　　　　agg.
　　anger, with ★
　　attacks, before ★
　　convulsions, during
　　coughing, before
　　　　during
　　　　whooping, cough in
　　sleep, in
　　touched, when

Weeping, tearful mood
　　waking, on
　　whining whimpering, ★
　　　　attacks of sickness, before ★
　　　　whooping cough, in
Wildness
Will, contradiction of

ANTHEMIS NOBILIS

Cheerful, gay, mirthful
Fear
　　approaching vehicles, of
　　happen, something will
　　out of doors, to go ●
　　run over, of being (on going out)
Going out, aversion to
Indolence, aversion to work
Reading, desires to be read to
Restlessness, night
Thoughts, wandering
Work, aversion to mental
　　desire for

ANTHRACINUM

Bite, desire to
Confusion of mind
Death, presentiment of
Delirium
　　fever, during
Excitement, excitable
Irritability, night
Restlessness
　　night
Unconsciousness, coma, stupor

ANTHRACOKALI

Excitement, heat, during
Morose, cross, fretful, ill-humor, peevish
Restlessness
Sadness, despondency, dejection, mental
　　　　depression, gloom, melancholy
　　chill, during

ANTIPYRINUM

Delusions, imaginations, hallucinations,
 illusions
hearing, illusions of
 visions, has ★
Fear, insanity, of ★

APIUM GRAVEOLENS

Irritability
Thoughts persistent

APIS MELLIFICA

Absent-minded, unobserving
Activity, fruitless ★
 mental ★
Affability
Ailments from :
 anger, vexation
 anticipation, foreboding, presentiment
 bad news
 fright
 grief
 jealousy
 rage, fury
 sexual excesses
 shock, mental
Amorous
Anger, irascibility
 violent
Anguish
Antics, plays
Anxiety
Awkward ★
Beside oneself, being
Borrows trouble ★
Break things, desire to
Busy
 fruitlessly
Censorious, critical
Cheerful, gay, mirthful
 perspiration, during
 simulates hilarity, while he feels
  wretched ●
Childish, behavior
 parturition, after ★

Company, desire for; aversion to solitude,
  company amel.
 alone agg., while
Concentration, difficult
Confusion of mind
 eating, after
  amel.
 mental exertion, from
 reading, while
Conscientious about trifles
Contradict, disposition to
Dancing
Death, desires
 forenoon
 presentiment of
 sensation of
 thoughts of
  fear, without
Delirium
 night
  midnight, after ●
 anxious
 congestion, with
 crying, with
 fever, during
 ● laughing
 loquacious, indistinct
 maniacal
 meningitis, cerebrospinalis
 menses, during
  menstrual difficulties, with ●
 mild
 muttering
 raging, raving
 sleep, during
 trembling, with
 violent
 well, declares she is
Delusions, imaginations, hallucinations,
  illusions
 bed, someone is in, with him
 dead, he himself was
 dying, he is
 faces, sees
 fancy, illusions of
 images, phantoms, sees

58

Delusions,
    people, beside him, are
    pregnant, she is
    spectres, sees, on closing eyes
    tongue made of wood ●   ●
    visions, closing the eyes, on
    walk, cannot, run or hop, must
    well, he is
Destructiveness
Dictatorial, domineering, dogmatical,
    despotic
Discontented, displeased, dissatisfied
    everything, with
Discouraged
Dream, as if in a
Dullness, sluggishness, difficulty of think-
    ing and comprehending, torpor
Ecstasy
Excitement, excitable
    night
    bad news, after
    heat, during
    hydrocephalus, in
Fear, apprehension, dread
    alone, of being
    apoplexy, of
    death, of
    heart disease, organic, of
    pins, pointed things, of
    poisoned, of being
    suffocation, of
    touch, of
Foolish behavior
Forgetful
    headache, during
Frivolous
Fussy ★
Gestures, convulsive
Heedless
Hurry, haste
    awkward from
Hysteria
Idiocy
Imbecility
Impatience
Inconstancy

Indifference, apathy
    fever, during
    joyless
    typhoid, in
Indolence, aversion to work
Industrious, mania for work
Insanity, madness
    busy
    erotic
Irresolution, indecision
Irritability
    haemorrhoids, with
    questioned, when
    sends the doctor home, says he is not
    sick
Jealousy
    women, in ●
Jesting, aversion to
Lascivious, lustful
Laughing
    misfortune, at ●
    serious matters, over
    silly
    spasmodic
    stupid expression, with
Loquacity
    insane
Mania
    rage, with
    sexual mania in men
    women, in
Memory, weakness of
Moaning, groaning, whining
    sleep, during
Mood, changeable, variable
Morose, cross, fretful, ill-humor, pee-
    vish
Muttering
    sleep, in
Nymphomania
Obscene, lewd
Obstinate, headstrong
Occupation, diversion amel.
Offended, easily; takes everything in bad
    part

Postponing everything to next day
Prostration of mind, mental exhaustion,
        brain-fag
Rage, fury, night
Restlessness
        afternoon
        night
        alternating with sadness •
        bed, tossing about in
        heat, during
        menses, during
        metrorrhagia, during
        move, must constantly
Sadness despondency, dejection, mental
        depression, gloom, melancholy
            morning
            forenoon
        anger, after
        chill, during
        diarrhoea, during
        heat, during
        perspiration, during
        weep, cannot
Sensitive, oversensitive
        noise, to
        steel points directed toward her
Shrieking, screaming, shouting
        brain cry
        children, in
            sleep, during
        convulsions, before
            during epileptic
        dentition, during
        hydrocephalus, in
        must shriek, feels as though she
        pains, with the ★
        sleep, during
        waking, on
Singing
Speech, incoherent
Starting, startled
        anxious
        fright, from and as from
        noise, from
        sleep, during
            from
Striking,
        knocking his head against wall and
            things

Stupefaction, as if intoxicated
        heat, during
Suspicious, mistrustful
Talking, sleep, in
Talks, himself, to
Theorizing
Thoughts, persistent
        vanishing of
Torpor
Tranquillity, serenity, calmness
Unconsciousness, coma, stupor
        fever, during
        hydrocephalus, in
        meningitis, in
        menses, during
        scarlatina, in
        screaming, interrupted by
Undertakes, many things, perseveres in
        nothing
Violent, vehement
Weary of life
        forenoon •
Weeping, tearful mood
        day and night •
        causeless
        everything, about •
        heat, during
        pregnancy, during
        sleep, in ★
Well, says he is, when very sick
Will, control, has no control over his will,
        does not know what to do; feels so
        dull in the head •

APISINUM

Dementia

APOCYNUM CANNABINUM

Ambition, loss of
Cheerful, gay, mirthful
Confusion of mind
        paroxysms of pain, during
Dipsomania, alcoholism
Eccentricity, fancies, in
Fancies, exaltation of
Indolence, aversion to work

Restlessness
>> night
>> bed, in

Sadness, despondency, dejection, mental
>> depression, gloom, melancholy

Sighing

Talk, indisposed to, desire to be silent,
>> taciturn

Thoughts,, vanishing of
>> wandering

Unconsciousness, coma, stupor
>> *hydrocephalus, in*
>> meningitis, in

Weeping, tearful mood

Work, mental, impossible

APOMORPHINUM

Answers, aversion to

Dipsomania, alcoholism

Dullness, sluggishness, difficulty of think-
>> ing and comprehending, torpor

Morphinism

Restlessness

Unconsciousness, coma, stupor

AQUA MARINA

Absent-minded, unobserving

Anxiety
>> afternoon, 14-16 h. •
>> company agg. •
>> ice-cold drinks agg. •
>> perspiration agg. •
>> salvation, about
>> speaking agg. •
>> waking agg. •

Concentration, difficult

Delusions, watched, she is being

Fear, insanity, losing his reason, of

Indifference, apathy

Restlessness
>> anxious

Sensitive, oversensitive

Slowness

Thoughts, tormenting, sexual

Unconsciousness, coma, stupor

AQUILEGIA VULGARIS

Hysteria

ARAGALLUS LAMBERTI

Absent-minded, unobserving

Company, aversion to; presence of other
>> people agg. the symptoms; de-
>> sire for solitude

Concentration, difficult

Confusion of mind ★

Home, desire to leave

Indifference, apathy ★

Memory, weakness of
>> words, of

Restlessness

ARALIA RACEMOSA

Fear, apprehension, dread
>> *disease, of impending,*
>> *lungs, of* ★

Impatience

ARANEA DIADEMA

Anguish

Anxiety

Cheerful, alternating with sadness

Confusion of mind
>> evening
>> eating, after
>> mental exertion, after

Death, desires

Delusions, imaginations, hallucinations,
>> illusions
>> enlarged, forearm is •
>> hearing: talk seems distant •
>> large, parts of body seem too
>> *swollen, is*
>> unreal, everything seems

Fear, death, of
>> narrow places, in; claustrophobia

Indifference, fever, during

Irritability
>> heat, during
>> menses, during

Morose, cross, fretful, ill humor, peevish
    fever, during
Restlessness
Sadness, despondency, dejection, mental
      depression, gloom, melancholy
    bed, will not leave •
    heat, during

ARANEA IXOBOLA

Absent-minded, unobserving
Anguish
Concentration, difficult
Confusion of mind
Delusions, imaginations, hallucinations,
    illusions
    smell, of
Euphoria
Exertion, agg. from mental
Hurry, haste
Irresolution, indecision
Irritability
Loquacity
Restlessness
    air, amel. in open
Rudeness
Sadness, despondency, dejection, mental
      depression, gloom, melancholy
    loquacity, after •
Sensitive, oversensitive
    noise, to
    odors, to
Snappish
Teasing
Weary of life
Witty

ARANEA SCINENCIA

Anxiety
Prostration of mind, mental exhaustion,
    brain-fag
Speech, heavy •

ARGENTUM METALLICUM

Absent-minded, unobserving

Ailments from :
    anger, vexation
    fear
    fright
Anger, irascibility
    cough from a.
Anguish
    clothes too tight when walking in
    open   air, as if •
    walking in open air
Anxiety
      night
        children, in
    air, in open
    clothes, as if clothing too tight,
      walking out of doors •
    fever, during
    health, about
    waking, on
    walking, while
      air, in open
Cheerful, gay, mirthful
    daytime
    afternoon
    alternating with sadness
      weeping
Concentration, difficult
Confusion of mind
    heat, during
    intoxicated, as if
      as after being
Deceitful, sly ★
Delirium
    epilepsy, after
    pains, with the
    raging, raving
Delusions, imaginations, hallucinations,
    illusions
    absurd, figures are present
    apoplexy, he will have •
    floating in air ★
Dementia, senillis
Desire, uncontrollable, itching of/for ★
Dipsomania, alcoholism
Discomfort, walking, after
Discouraged

Dullness, sluggishness, difficulty of think-
ing and comprehending, torpor
Excitement, excitable
Exertion, agg. from mental
Exhilaration
Fear, apprehension, dread
    apoplexy, of
        palpitation, with •
    crowd, public places, of ★
    happen, something will
    health, own, one's ★
    places, buildings etc ★
    speak, to
Forgetful   •
Gestures, covers mouth with hands ★
Hurry, haste
Hypochondriasis
Ideas, abundant, clearness of mind
    deficiency of
Imbecility
Indolence, aversion to work
Insanity, madness
Irritability
        forenoon
    trifles, from
Jesting
Jumping
    epilepsy, after ★
Laughing
    agg.
Liar ★
Loathing, general
Loquacity
        daytime •
    alternating with sadness •
    changing quickly from one subject
        to another
Mania
    alternating with depression
Memory, weakness of
    said, for what has
    say, for what is about to
Mood, changeable, variable
Morose, cross, fretful, ill-humor, pee-
    vish
Peace, sense of heavenly •

Prostration of mind, mental exhaus-
tion, brain-fag
Rage, fury
    epilepsy, rage after
    pain, from
Restlessness
        night
    bed, driving out of
Sadness, despondency, dejection, mental
    depression, gloom, melancholy
        morning
        forenoon
Sensitive, oversensitive
Serious, earnest
Shrieking, screaming, shouting
    sleep, during
Sit, inclination to
Somnambulism
Speech, nonsensical
Starting, startled
    electric shocks, through the body,
        during sleep, wakening her
Striking
Stupefaction, as if intoxicated
Sympathy, bars, against friend ★
Talk, desire to, to someone
Talk, indisposed to, desire to be silent,
    taciturn
        company, in •
Talking agg. all complaints
Thinking, complaints agg., of
Thoughts, control of thoughts lost, sit-
    ting and reflecting, while •
Tranquillity, serenity, calmness
Unconsciousness, coma, stupor
Vivacious
Weeping, tearful mood
    alternating with cheerfulness
    easily
    trifles, at
Work, mental, impossible

ARGENTUM MURIATICUM

Talk, indisposed to, desire to be silent,
    taciturn

ARGENTUM NITRICUM

Absorbed, buried in thought
    alternating with frivolity •
Activity, fruitless ★
Ailments from
    anger, vexation
    **anticipation, foreboding, pre-
        sentiment**
    debauchery
    excitement, emotional
    fear
    fright
    mortification
    sexual excesses
    work, mental
Air, castles (plans), builds, in ★
Ambition, loss of, disappointment from ★
Anger, irascibility
        forenoon, 11h.
    cough from a.
    easily
    trembling, with
Anguish
    walking in open air
Anticipation, stage-fright
Anxiety
        morning, rising, on and after
        forenoon, 11 h. •
        afternoon
        night
            waking, on
    anticipation, an engagement, of
    eating, after
    faintness, with
    future, about
    health, about
    hypochondriacal
    others, for ★
    rail road, when about to journey
    by, amel. while   in train
    riding, while
    rising, after
    time is set, if a
    waking, on
    walking, while
        air, in open
        **rapidly, which makes him
        walk faster**
Bed, remain in, desire to

Busy, fruitlessly
Childish behavior
Climacteric period agg.
*Company, aversion to; presence of other
        people agg. the symptoms;
        desire for solitude*
**Company, desire for; aversion to
        solitude, company amel.**
Concentration, difficult
    on attempting to concentrates it
    becomes dark before the eyes •
Confidence, want of self
Confusion of mind •
    morning
        rising and after, on
        waking, on
    night
    coffee, after
    dinner, after
    eating, after
    identity, duality, sense of
    motion, amel.
    waking, on
    walking, while
    writing, while
Contrary
Cowardice
*Death, presentiment of
        predicts the time*
Deceitful, sly
Delirium
    pains, with the
    raging, raving
**Delusions, imaginations, hallucina-
        tions, illusions**
    brain, has softening of
    changed, everything is
    clouds, heavy black, enveloped her
    *corners of houses project so that he
        fears he will run against them
        while walking in the street* •
    dead persons, sees
    deserted, forsaken, is
    despised, is
    *die, he was about to
        while walking thinks he will
        have a fit or die, which
        makes him walk faster* •

Delusions,
disease, has incurable
double, of being
enlarged, distances are
objects are
faces, sees
closing eyes, on
distorted on lying down, daytime
fail, everything will
falling out of bed
walls
fit and walks faster, she will have a •
heart stops beating when sitting •
home, changed, everything at, has
houses on each side would approach
and crush him •
images, phantoms, sees
night
closing eyes, on
frightful
sleep, preventing
neglected, he is
place, he cannot pass a certain
repudiated by relatives, he is
right, does nothing
room, walls will crush him •
sick, being
snakes in and around her
soda water, being a bottle of
spectres, closing eyes, sees, on
strange, familiar things seem
succeed, he cannot; does everything
wrong
swollen, is
time, exaggeration of, passes too
slowly
visions, has
closing the eyes, on
walls, falling
work, harm, will do him •
world, he is lost to, beyond hope •
Despair
hypochondriasis, in •
others, oneself, and
religious despair of salvation

Dipsomania, alcoholism
Distance, inaccurate judgement of
Dream, as if in a
Dullness, sluggishness, difficulty of
thinking and comprehend-
ing, torpor
afternoon
children, in
heat, during
writing, while
Dwells on past disagreeable occurrences
Eccentricity
fancies, in
Excitement, excitable
night
agg.
anticipating events, when
climacteric period, during
nervous
Exertion, agg. from mental
Exhilaration, afternoon •
Faces, strange
Fancies, exaltation of
sleeplessness, with
sleep, preventing
falling asleep, on
Fear, apprehension, dread
morning
rising, on •
alone, of being
lest he die
apoplexy, of
church or opera, when ready to
go to
corners, to walk past certain
crossing a bridge or place, of
crowd, in a
public places, of; agoraphobia
death, of
alone, when
predicts the time
diarrhoea, from
disease, of impending
incurable, of being
epilepsy, of
evil, of
failure, of
fainting, of

Fear,
> *fall upon him, high walls and buildings*
> falling, of
> *fit, of having a*
> *high places, of*
> insanity, losing his reason, of
> **late, of being** ★
> *narrow places, in; claustrophobia*
> *ordeals, of*
> *robbers, of*
> *self-control, of losing*
> sleep, before
> suicide, of
> *undertaking anything*
> work, dread of
>> *afternoon* ●

Feigning sick
Foolish behavior
Forgetful
> *words while speaking, of; word*
> *hunting*
Forsaken feeling
> *isolation, sensation of*
> *waking, on*
Frightened easily
Gestures, ridiculous or foolish
> shy ●
Ground gives way ★
Helplessness ★
Hesitates ★
High places agg.
Hurry, haste
> eating, while
> everybody must hurry
> **time, hurry to arrive for the ap-**
> **pointed** ●
> **walking, while**
Hydrophobia
Hypochondriasis
Hysteria
Ideas abundant, clearness of mind
> evening
> deficiency of
> imaginary disease, of ★
> strange ★
Imbecility

Impatience
Impulse, morbid ★
Impulsive
Indifference, apathy
> *business affairs, to*
> **company, society, while in**
> lies with eyes closed
> *pleasure, to*
Indolence, aversion to work
> *work will do him harm, he thinks*
> *the (hypochondriasis)* ●
Injure himself, fear to be left alone, lest
> he should
Insanity, madness
Irresolution, indecision
Irritability
>> morning, rising, after
>>> waking, on
> excited, when
> waking, on
Jumping, bed, out of
> impulse to j. into the river ★
>> height, from a ★
> *tendency to, bridge, crossing, when* ★
Lamenting, bemoaning, wailing
> sickness, about his
Laughing agg.
> serious matters, over
Liar
> lies, never speaks the truth, does
> not know what she is saying
Loathing, general
Loathing, work, at
Loquacity, changing quickly from one
> subject to another
> rambling ★
Mania, periodical
Memory, weakness of
> pains, from, suddenly ★
> expressing oneself, for
> *say, for what is about to*
> *words, of*
Mistakes
> localities, in
> speaking, in
> *words, using wrong*

Mood, changeable, variable
Morose, cross, fretful, ill-humor, peevish
Muttering, night
Obstinate, headstrong
   queerest objection against whatever was proposed, he had the •
Plans, making many
Prophesying, predicts the time of death
Prostration of mind, mental exhaustion,
   brain-fag
   trembling, with
Rage, fury
Recognize: streets, does not recognize
   well known
Religious affections
Reserved
Restlessness
   night
   anxious
      compelling rapid walking
      epilepsy, during intervals of •
   bed, tossing about in
   convulsions, before
   headache, during
Sadness, despondency, dejection, mental
   depression gloom, melancholy
   morning
   air, amel. in open
   climaxis, during
   eating, after
   heat, during
   slight, from an undeserved •
   talk, indisposed to
Senses, confused
   dull, blunted
Sensitive, oversensitive
   noise, to
      slightest, to
Sighing
   dinner, after •
Sit, inclination to
Speech, childish
   hesitating
   incoherent
   slow
Starting, pain agg.

Strange things, impulse to do
Stupefaction, as if intoxicated
   night
   writing, while •
Suicidal, disposition
   drowning, by
   fear of an open window or a knife,
      with.
   thoughts
   throwing himself from a height
   window, from
Susperstitious ★
Suspense agg. ★
Sympathy, compassion ★
Talk, desire to talk to someone
Talk, indisposed to, desire to be silent,
   taciturn
      eating, after
      sadness, in
Talking, agg. all complaints
   sleep, in
Talks anxious about his condition,
   wakes wife and child (in hypo-
   chondriasis) •
   himself, of his suffering constantly •
   one subject, of nothing but
   troubles, of her ★
Theorizing
Thinking, complaints agg., of
Thoughts
   disconnected
   persistent
   strange
   tormenting
   night
Time passes too slowly, appears longer
Timidity
   bashful
Unconsciousness, coma, stupor
   night
   vertigo, during
Undertakes nothing, lest he fail
Wearisome
Weeping, tearful mood
   eating, after
   hopelessness, from ★

Will, loss of, melancholia, from
Work, mental, impossible

ARISTOLOCHIA CLEMATITIS

Anxiety, future, about
Company, aversion to; presence of other
    people agg. the symptoms; de-
    sire for solitude
Fear, apprehension, dread
   alone, of being
   people, of
Forsaken, isolation, sensation of
Industrious, mania for work
Restlessness
   bed, in
   menses, before
*Sadness, despondency, dejection, mental
    depression, gloom, melancholy*
   air, amel. in open
   climaxis, during
   menses amel., during
Weeping, tearful mood

ARNICA MONTANA

Absent-minded, unobserving
   dreamy
Absorbed, buried in thought
Abstraction of mind
Ailments from:
   anger, vexation
   bad news
   excitement, emotional
   fright
   grief
   hurry
   pecuniary loss
   rage, fury
   sexual excesses
   shock, mental
   work, mental
Anger, irascibility
   answer, when obliged to
   cough from anger

Anguish
   night
   cardiac
   chill, during ●
   heat, during
   perspiratin, during
Answers, aversion to
   refuses to answer
   stupor returns quickly after answer
Anxiety
   night
   chill, during
   conscience, as if guilty of a crime
   fever, during
   flushes of heat, during
   future, about
   health, about
   hypochondriacal
   periodical
   sleep, during
   touched, anxiety to being
   waking, on
Audacity
Beside oneself, being
Boaster, braggart
Brooding
Business, averse to
Busy
Capriciousness
Cares, worries, full of
Censorious, critical
Cheerful, gay, mirthful
   evening, bed, in
   thoughtless ●
Clairvoyance
Company, aversion to; presence of other
    people agg. the symptoms; de-
    sire for solitude
Complaining
Concentration, difficult
Confusion of mind
   morning
   dream, as if in a
Consolation, kind words agg.
Contemptuous
Contradict, disposition to
Contradiction, is intolerant of

Contrary
Cursing, swearing
   rage, after •
Death, presentiment of
   thoughts of
Defiant
Delirium
      night
   answers correctly when spoken to,
      but delirium and unconscious-
      ness return at once
   chill, during
   haemorrhage, after
   murmuring
   muttering
   sleep, comatose, during
   sleepiness, with
   well, declares she is
Delirium tremens, mania-a-potu
Delusions, imaginations, hallucinations,
      illusions
      night
   animals, of
   arrested, is about to be
   bed, hard, too
   cats, sees
   church yard, visits a
   council, holding a
   dead, mutilated corpse
      persons, sees
   die, he was about to
   disease, he has incurable
   dogs, sees
   fancy, illusions of
   heart disease, is going to have, and
      die
   images, phantoms, sees, night
      black
      dwells upon
      frightful
   mutilated bodies, sees
   spectres, black forms, when dreaming
   thieves, sees
   visions, has
      fantastic
   well, he is
Desires, scratch, to
Despair

Dictatorial, domineering, dogmatical,
      despotic
   command, talking with air of
Dipsomania, alcoholism
Discontented, displeased, dissatisfied
   everything, with
Discouraged
Disgust
   everything, with
Disobedience
Doubtful, recovery, of
Dream, as if in a
Dullness, sluggishness, difficulty of
      thinking and
      comprehending, torpor
   morning
      waking, on
   dreams, after
   injuries of head, after
   says nothing
   sleepiness, with
   waking, on
Ecstasy
Egotism, self-esteem
Excitement, excitable
      evening, bed, in
Exertion, agg. from mental
Fancies, absorbed in
   exaltation of
Fear, apprehension, dread
      night
   apoplexy, of
      waking, on
   approaching him, of others
   touched, lest he be
   crowd, in a
      public places, of; agoraphobia
   death, of
      night
      alone, when
      heart symptoms, during
      sudden d. of
   disease, of impending
      incurable, of being
   doctors, of ★
   evil, of
   failure, of
   fall upon him, high walls and buildings

Fear,
> happen, something will
>> *night*
> *heart, of disease of* ★
> *hurt, of being*
> misfortune, of
> ordeals, of
> paralysis, of
> physician, of ★
> recurrent
> **struck by those coming towards**
> **him, of being** ●
> suffocation, of, night
> *touch, of*

Flatterer
Foolish behavior
Forgetful
> *heat, during*
> **words while speaking, of; word**
> **hunting**

Frightened easily
> trifles, at

Frivolous
Gestures, grasping or reaching at some-
> *thing, at flocks; carphologia*
> *picks at bed clothes*

Grief
Haughty
Heedless
Howling
> anger, with ★

Hypochondriasis
Hysteria
> fainting, hysterical

Ideas, deficiency of
Impatience, complaints, from ★
Inconstancy
Indifference, apathy
> business affairs, to
> chill, during
> **concussion of brain, after**
> everything, to
> *fever, during*
> pain, to
> *typhoid, in*

Indiscretion
Indolence, aversion to work
> air, in open ●
> walking, while

Industrious, mania for work
Insanity, madness
Introspection
Irresolution, indecision
Irritability
> air, in open
> chill, during
> eating, after
> *questioned, when*
> **sends the doctor home, says she**
> **is not sick**
> supper, after

Lamenting, bemoaning, wailing
> alternating with anger ●
> asleep, while

Laughing
> causeless
> spasmodic

Loathing, general
Loathing, work, at
Loquacity
> speeches, makes

Malicious, spiteful, vindictive
Mania
Memory, active
Memory, loss of
> **injuries of head, after**

Memory, weakness of
> read, for what has
> **for what has just**
> *said, for what has*
> *say, for what is about to*
> *words, of*

Mental, symptoms alternating with
> physical

Mildness
Mischievous
Mistakes
> *speaking, in*
>> *misplacing words*
>> *words, using wrong*

Moaning, groaning, whining
> chill, during
> *heat, during*
> sleep, during

Mood, alternating
> changeable, variable
> repulsive

Morose, cross, fretful, ill-humor, peevish
    eating, after
Muttering
    apoplexy, in
Nothing ails him, says ★
Obstinate, headstrong
Offended easily; takes everythig in bad
    part
Praying
    quietly
Presumptuous
Prostration of mind, mental exhaustion,
    brain-fag
Quarrelsome, scolding
Quiet, repose and tranquillity, desires,
    walking in open air, on
Rage, fury
Refuses to take the medicine
Remorse, complaints, from ★
Reserved
    walking, after
Rest, desire for
Restlessness
    anxious
    bed, tossing about in
    heat, during
    tremulous
Rudeness
Sadness, despondency, dejection, mental
    depression, gloom, melancholy
    night
    injuries, head, of the
Scratches, lime off the walls, the
Senses, acute
    dull, blunted
Sensitive, oversensitive
    external impressions, to all
    noise, to
        painful sensitiveness to
    pain, to
Shrieking, screaming, shouting
    brain cry
    children, sleep, during
    cough agg.
    sleep, during
    waking, on
Sighing, heat, during
Sit, inclination to
Sits, still

Speech, hasty
    loud
        sleep, in
    unintelligible, sleep, in
    wandering
Spoken to, averse to being
Starting, startled
        evening, asleep, on falling
    fright, from and as from
    sleep, on falling
        during
        from
    trifles, at
Stupefaction, as if intoxicated
    injury to head, after
Stupefaction
    vertigo, during
Sulky
Suppressed or receding skin diseases or
        haemorrhoids, mental symp-
        toms agg. after
Suspicious, mistrustful
Sympathy, aversion to ●
Talk, indisposed to, desire to be silent,
    taciturn
        walking in open air, after ●
Talking agg. all complaints
    sleep, in
        loud
Temerity
Teasing
Thinking, afternoon, after walking in
    open air ●
    complaints agg., of
Thoughts, thoughtful
    wandering ●
Timidity
Touched, aversion to being
Tranquillity, serenity, calmness
Traumata, mental ●
Unconsciousness, coma, stupor
    answers correctly when spoken to, but
        delirium and u. return at once
    concussion of brain, from ●
    fever, during
    lies as if dead
    rising up, on
    shock from injury, in
    vertigo, during

Violent, vehement
Wearisome
Weeping, tearful mood
　　　night
　　　agg.
　　　anger, after
　　　coughing, before
　　　　　during
　　　　　after
　　　　　whooping cough, in
　　　eating, after
　　　perspiration, during
　　　sleep, in
　　　supper, after •
　　　waking, on
　　　whimpering, sleep, during
Well, says he is, when very sick
Work, aversion to mental
　　　desire for
　　　impossible

ARSENICUM ALBUM

Abrupt, harsh
Absent-minded, unobserving
Abusive, insulting
　　　husband insulting wife before chil-
　　　　　dren or vice versa
Affections, in general ★
Affectionate
Ailments from:
　　　anger, vexation
　　　　　anxiety, with
　　　　　indignation, with
　　　　　silent grief, with
　　　anticipation, foreboding, pre-
　　　　　sentiment
　　　cares, worries
　　　dipsomania
　　　discords between, parents, friends
　　　　　servants ★
　　　fright
　　　grief
　　　mortification
　　　sexual excesses
　　　work, mental
Ambition, loss of

Anger, irascibility
　　　morning, waking, on
　　　answer, when obliged to
　　　consoled, when
　　　contradiction, from
　　　easily
　　　eat, when obliged to •
　　　face, with pale, livid
　　　himself, with
　　　mistakes, about his
　　　pains, about
　　　trifles, at
　　　violent
　　　waking, on ★
Anguish
　　　evening
　　　cardiac
　　　constricted, as if everything became •
　　　driving from place to place
　　　　　restlessness, with
　　　nausea, with
　　　palpitation, with
　　　respiration, preventing •
　　　tossing about, with
　　　vomiting, with
Anorexia mentalis
Answers abruptly, shortly, curtly
　　　aversion to answer
　　　foolish
　　　hastily
　　　refuses to answer
　　　slowly
　　　unable to answer
Anticipation, complaints from
Anxiety
　　　morning
　　　afternoon
　　　evening
　　　　　twilight, in the
　　　　　bed, in
　　　night
　　　　　children, in
　　　　　waking, on
　　　midnight, before
　　　midnight, after
　　　　　3h.
　　　　　　　after
　　　alone, when

Anxiety,
> *anticipation, from, an engagement* ★
> **bed, in**
>> **driving out of**
>> tossing about, with
> chill, before
>> **during**
>> *after*
> climacteric period, during
> **conscience, as if guilty of a crime**
> cough, before
> *dreams, on waking from frightful*
> driving from place to place
> duty, as if he had not done his •
> *expected of him, when anything is* •
> faintness, with
> **fear, with**
> **fever, during**
>> prodrome of, during
> fits, with
> future, about
> head,
>> perspiration on forehead, with
> *headache, with*
> health, about
> house, in
> hypochondriacal
> lying, while
> mental exertion, from
> *motion amel.*
> *others, for*
> pains, from the
> paroxysms, in
> *periodical*
> perspiration, with cold
> rail road, when about to journey by,
>> amel. while in train
> **salvation, about**
> scruples, excessive religious
> *sedentary employment, from*
> **sleep, during**
> *stool, before*
>> during
> *trifles, about*
> **waking, on**
Asks for nothing
Avarice

Aversion
> everything, to
> those around him •
> wife, to his ★
Bed: aversion to, shuns b.
Begging, entreating supplicating
Beside oneself, being
Bilious disposition
Bite:
> spoon etc., bites
> tumbler, bites his •
Boaster, braggart
Business, averse to
> desires for
> talks of
Busy
> fruitlessly
Capriciousness
Carefulness
Cares, worries, full of
> eveni.ng, bed, in
> others, about
> relatives, about
> *trifles, about*
Carried, desires to be
> **fast**
Cautious
Censorious, critical
Chaotic, confused behavior
Cheerful, gay, mirthful
> alternating with moroseness
> perspiration, during
Childish behavior
Climacteric period agg.
Clinging
> grasps at others
> held, wants to be
> amel., being
Company, aversion to; presence of other
> people agg. the symptoms; de-
> sire for solitude
> avoids the sight of people
> fear of being alone, yet
> meeting of friends, whom he imag-
> ines he has offended, to •
> perspiration, during

Company, desire for; aversion to solitude, company amel.
  alone agg., while
    yet fear of people
Complaining
  pitiful •
Concentration, difficult
  studying
    learns with difficulty
Confusion of mind
    morning
      waking, on
    evening
    air amel., in open
    bed, jump out of, makes him
    room, in
    sleeping, after
    waking, on
    washing the face amel.
Conscientious about trifles
  trifles, occupied with
Consolation, kind words agg.
Contemptuous
Contradict, disposition to
Contradiction, is intolerant of
Contrary
Conversation, aversion to
  desire for
Corrupt, venal
Crawling, rolling on the floor
Cruelty, inhumanity
  loves to makes people and animals suffer ★
Cursing, swearing
  convulsions, during •
Darkness agg.
Death, agony before
  desires
  presentiment of
  sensation of
  thoughts of
Deceitful, sly
Delirium
    night
    anxious
    bed and escapes, springs up suddenly from

Delirium
  chill, during
  convulsions, during
  delusions, with
  fever, during
  headache, during
  haemorrhage, after
  maniacal
  menses, before
  muttering
    sleep, in
  nonsense, with eyes open
  persecution in delirium, delusions of
  raging, raving
  sleep, during
  trembling, with
  violent
  well, declares she is
Delirium tremens, mania-a-potu
Delusions, imaginations, hallucinations, illusions
  day and night
  night
  accidents, sees
  animals, of
    bed, on
    beetles, worms etc
  arrested, is about to be
  assembled things, swarms, crowds etc.
  bed, under it, someone is
  bells, hears ringing of
  body, putrefy, will
    three fold, has a
  business, ordinary, they are persuing
  calls, waking, someone calls, on
  conspiracies against him, there are
  contaminates everything she touches •
  crime, committed a, he had
  criminals, about •
  dead, acquaintance, on sofa and has dread, corpse of absent •
  persons, seees
  devils, sees
  die, time has come to
  doomed, being
  engaged in some occupations, is

Delusions,
ordinary occupation, in
faces, sees
closing eyes, on
falling out of bed
fancy, illusions of
fire, visions of
friend, accident, met with an •
offended, has •
hang himself, wants to •
hanging, sees persons •
happy in his own house, he will
never be •
head, standing on ⋆
hearing, illusions of
house is full of people
images, phantoms, sees
black
frightful
injury, is about to receive
insane, she will become
insects, sees
lost, she is (salvation)
man does all the things he does •
hung himself, saw, who •
murder him, others conspire to
someone, he has to
murdered someone, he had (all
night)
objects, tries to seize
offended, people, he has
people, sees
beside him, are
doing as he does •
closing eyes, sees people on
persecuted, he is
pursued by enemies
he was
police, by
rats, sees
running across the room
religious
scream, obliging to
sick, being
smell, of
spectres, ghosts, spirits, sees
day and night •
black forms when dreaming

Delusions,
starve, family will
suicide, driving to
thieves, sees
night •
house, in
and space under bed are
full of thieves •
vermin, sees, crawl about
his bed is covered with •
visions, has
closing the eyes, on
fantastic
watched, she is being
water, of
well, he is
worms are in bed •
creeping of
wrong, he has done
Dementia
Desires more than she needs
Despair
chill, during
heat, during
life, of
pains, with
periodical
perspiration, during
recovery, of
religious despair of salvation
Dipsomania, alcoholism
weakness of character, from
Discomfort
chill, during •
Discontented, displeased, dissatisfied
daytime
everything, with
himself, with
Discouraged
Disgust
Dishonest
Doubtful, recovery, of
medicine is useless
soul's welfare, of
Dream, as if in a
daytime
Drinks more as she should •

Dullness, sluggishness, difficulty of think-
    ing and comprehending, torpor
        forenoon
        noon
        afternoon
        coryza, during •
        perspiration, during
Duty, no sense of duty
Eat, refuses to
Eats more as she should •
Eccentricity political
Envy
    avidity, and
    qualities of others, at
Escape, attempts to
    springs up suddenly from bed
        change beds, to
        visit her daughter, wants to •
Estranged from her family
    wife, from his
Excitement, excitable
        morning
        chill, during
        palpitation, with violent
Exertion, agg. from mental
Faces, made strange
Fancies, exaltation of
        night
        alone, when •
        periodically returning •
Fastidious
Fear, apprehension, dread
        day and night •
        morning
        evening, bed, in
        night
        midnight, after, 3h.
    alone, of being
        lest he die
            injure himself •
    bed, of the
    cholera, of
    crowd, in a
    dark, of
    death, of
        night 1-3h.

Fear, **death**
    alone, when
        evening in bed
        impending death, of
        sudden death, of
        vexation, after •
        vomiting
        waking, on
    disease, of impending
    cancer, of ★
    evil, of
    falling, of
    friend has met with accident, that a •
    ghost, of
        night
    happen, something, will
    heat, during
    imaginary things, of
    insanity, losing his reason, of
        if he wants to repose, must al-
        ways move
    jumps out of bed, from f.
        window, out of the •
    killing, of
        knife, with a
    knaves, of
    knives, of
    labor, during
    misfortune, of
    narrow places, vaults, churches and
        cellars, of
    over-powering
    people, of
    pins, pointed things, sharp things, of
    recurrent
    restlessness from fear
    robbers, of
    solitude, of
    suffocation, of
        night
    suicide, of
    tremulous
    trifles, of
    unaccountable, vague
    undertaking anything
    vexation, after
Finance, aptitude for
    inaptitude for

Foolish behavior
Forgetful
Forsaken, beloved by his parents, wife,
*   friends, feels of not being*
Frightened easily
**   night, waking, 3h., on**
*   waking, on*
Gamble (*see* Play)
Gestures, makes
    convulsive
    grasping or reaching at something,
        at flocks; carphologia
    picks at bed clothes
    hands, motions, involuntary of the
        head, to the, sleep, during •
        lifting up hand •
        throwing overhead
    usual vocation, of his
    wringing the hands
Gossiping
Greed, cupidity
Grief
    trifles, over
Grimaces, strange faces, makes
Hide, desire to
    fear, on account of
Honor: sense of honor, no
Horrible things, sad stories, affect her
        profoundly
Howling
Hurry, haste
    drinking, on
    movements, in
Hydrophobia
Hypochondriasis
    alone, when •
Hysteria
    fainting, hysterical
Ideas abundant, clearness of mind
Idiocy
Imbecility
Impatience
    heat, with
Impetuous, perspiration, with
Impulse, morbid
Impulsive
Inconsolable
Inconstancy

Indifference, apathy
    duties, to
    everything, to
    life, to
    loved ones, to
    periodical
    perspiration, during
    pleasure, to
    recovery, about his
    sleepiness, with
    welfare of others, to
Indignation
    morning •
Indolence, aversion to work
    sleepiness, with
Industrious, mania for work
Injure himself, fears to be left alone, lest
        he should
Insanity, madness
    anxiety, with
    drunkards, in
    escape, desire to
    fright, from
    grief, from
    heat, with
    melancholy
    paralysis, with
    persecution mania
    prayer, raising hands and kneeling
        as in p. •
    pulse, with frequent
    religious
    restlessness, with
    signs, writes unintelligible •
    suicidal disposition, with
Intolerance
Intriguer
Irresolution, indecision
    projects, in
    trifles, about
Irritability
    morning on waking
    alternating with cheerfulness
    children, in
    chill, during
    eating, after
    headache, during

Irritability
  heat, during
  noise, from
  pain, during
  spoken to, when
  taciturn
  waking, on
Jealousy
  children, between
  men, between
  women, between
Jesting
  aversion to
  malicious •
Joy, misfortune of others, at the •
Jumping, bed, out of
Kill, desire to
  barber wants to kill his customer
  beloved ones
  drunkards, in •
  injure with a knife, impulse to
  knife, with a
  poison, impulse to
  sudden impulse to kill
Killed, desires to be
  stabbing heart, by (after midnight) •
Kleptomania
Lamenting, bemoaning, wailing
  anxiety in epigastrium, about •
  convulsions, during •
  loud, piercing •
  menses, during
Laughing
  agg.
  easily
  never
  spasmodic
  trifles, at
Learns poorly ★
Litigious
Loathing, general, pain, from
Loathing, life, at
Looked at, cannot bear to be
  agg. mental symptoms ★
Loquacity
  perspiration, during
Malicious, spiteful, vindictive

Mania
  anguish, during •
  held, wants to be •
  rage, with
  violence, with deeds of
Memory, active
Memory, weakness of
Menses, mental symptoms agg. during
Mildness
Misanthropy
Mischievous
Moaning, groaning, whining
      evening
        sleep, during •
      night
  menses, during
  sleep, during
Mocking
  sarcasm
  satire, desire for
Mood, alternating
  changeable, variable
  repulsive
Moral feeling, want of
  criminal, disposition to become a,
    without remorse
Morose, cross, fretful, ill-humor, peevish
    morning
        bed,
  alternating with cheerfulness
  children, in
  chill, during
  oneself, with
  waking, on
Morphinism
Mutilating his body
Muttering
  sleep, in
  unintelligible
Obstinate, headstrong
  children
Occupation, diversion amel.
**Offended, easily; takes everything
    in bad part**
Passionate
Partial, prejudiced
Pessimist
Play, passion for gambling

Positiveness
Praying
> *kneeling and*
> quietly
Prostration of mind, mental exhaustion,
> brain-fag
Pull one's hair, desires to
Qualmishness ★
Quarrelsome, scolding
> sleep, in
Quiet disposition
Quiet, wants to be
> chill, during
Quieted, carried, only by being
>> rapidly, only by being ●
Rage, fury
>> evening
>> night
> alternating with sleep ●
> chained, had to be
> convulsions, rage with
> *headache, with*
> pulls hair ★
Refuses every treatment, inspite of be-
> ing very sick
Religious affections
> *children, in*
> melancholia
> *puberty, in*
Remorse
Reproaches himself
> **others**
Reserved
Rest, when things are not in proper place,
> *cannot*
Restlessness
> *evening*
> **night**
> **midnight, after**
>> 3h. after ●
> *alternating with sleepiness till stupor*
>> *(during fever)* ●
> **anxious**
>> **compelling rapid walking**
> **bed, driving out of**
>> **go from one bed to an-**

Restlessness,
> **other, wants to**
>> **tossing about in**
> children, in
>> carried about, relieved by being
> **chill, during**
> *driving, about*
> *headache, during*
> **heat, during**
> hypochondriacal
> **internal**
> *menses, during*
>> suppresed, during
> *move, must constantly*
> pain, from
> *periodical* ●
> sitting, work, while at
> sleepiness, with
> *waking, on*
Reveals secrets, sleep, in
Rocking agg.
Rolling on the floor
Runs about
Sadness, despondency, dejection,
> **mental depression, gloom,**
> **melancholy**
>> morning, waking, on
>> *afternoon, twilight, in*
>> evening
>>> bed, in
>> night
>>> bed, in
> **alone, when**
> anger, after
> *children, in*
> **chill, during**
> consoled, cannot be ●
> darkness, in
> *dinner, after*
> *eating, after*
> *exertion, after*
> *girls before puberty, in*
> headache, during
> **heat, during**
> loss, after financial ●
> menses, suppressed
> *mental exertion, after*

Sadness,
periodical
perspiration, during
puberty, in
quiet
sleeplessness with
talk, indisposed to
wringing the hands
Searching, thieves, at night for •
Self-torture
Senses, acute
dull, blunted
vanishing of
Sensitive, oversensitive
light, to
mental impressions, to
noise, to
voices, to
odors, to
pains, to
sensual impressions, to
Sentimental
Serious, earnest
Shrieking, screaming, shouting
brain cry
delusions, from
pains, with the
waking, on
Sighing
heat, during
menses, during
perspiration, during
sleep, in
comatose •
Sit, inclination to
Slander, disposition to
denouncer
sneak
Slowness
Smiling
never
Speech, abrupt
finish sentence, cannot
hasty
incoherent
epileptic attack, after

Speech,
loud
monosyllabic
slow
unintelligible
wandering
wild
Spit, faces of people, in
Spoken to, averse to being
morning
Starting, startled
evening, asleep, on falling
convulsive
electric shocks, during sleep, wak-
ening her
noise, from
paroxysmal
sleep, on falling
during
from
Strangers, presence of agg.
child coughs at sight of strangers
Strength increased, mental
Striking himself
head, his
knocking his head against wall and
things
Stupefaction, as if intoxicated
morning, 11-18h. •
walking, when
air, in open
Suicidal disposition
night
midnight, after
delusions, from
drunkenness, during
fright, after •
gassing, by
hanging, by
heat, during
intermittent fever, during
knife, with
perspiration, during
poison, by
run over, to be
stabbing, by
throwing himself from a height
windows, from

Sulky
Suppressed or receding skin diseases or
    haemorrhoids, mental symp-
    toms agg. after
Suspicious, mistrustful
    plotting against his life, people, are,
    about the house •
*Talk, indisposed to, desire to be silent,
    taciturn*
    heat, during
    perspiration, during
    sadness, in
    others agg., talk of
Talking, sleep, in
    reveals secrets
Tears himself
Theorizing
Thinking, complaints agg., of
Thoughts: control of t. lost, chilliness,
    during •
    disease, of
    intrude and crowd around each other
        *too weak to keep them off or to
        hold on to one thought •*
    persistent
        alone, when
    rush, flow of
        alone, when •
    tormenting
    vanishing, stooping, on rising from •
Throws things away
Timidity
    evening, going to bed, about
Torments himself
Touched, aversion to being
Tranquillity, serenity, calmness
Unconsciousness, coma, stupor
    evening
    alternating with restlessness
        during fever •
    chill, before
        during
    crowded room, in a
    diarrhoea, after •
        and vomiting •
    epilepsy, after

Unconsciousness,
    exertion, after
    eyes, with fixed
    fever, during
    **frequent spells of unconscious-
        ness,**
        absences
    incomplete
    motion, on least
    stool, before
    vertigo, during
    wakes often, but only for a short time
Unfeeling, hard hearted
Ungrateful
Unsympathetic, unscrupulous
Violent, vehement
    deeds of violence, rage leading to
Vivacious
Walks more as is good for her •
Washing, cleanliness, mania for
Wearisome
Weary of life
    drunkards, in •
Weeping, tearful mood
        night
        midnight, before
            after
    anger, with ★
    causeless
    child, like a
    children, in
    chill, during
    coughing, during
    hysterical
    involuntary, weakness, from
    menses, during
    pains, with
    sleep, in
    whimpering
        sleep, during
Well, says he is, when very sick
Will, weakness of
Work, mental, impossible
Writing, inability for

ARSENICUM HYDROGENISATUM

Anger, irascibility
Answers abruptly, shortly, curtly
    slowly
Anxiety
    chill, before
        during
    health, about
    waking, on
Business, averse to
Company desire for; aversion to solitude,
      company amel.
Complaining, pain, of
Death, conviction of
    thoughts of
Despair
    vomiting, during ●
Discouraged
Doubtful, recovery, of
Eccentricity
Excitement, excitable
    heat, during
Exhilaration
Fear, apprehension, dread
    alone, of being, lest he die
    death when alone, of
Impatience
Indiffernce, apathy
    important news, to ●
Indolence, aversion to work
Loathing at his business ●
Loquacity
Memory, weakness of
Moaning, sleep, during
Mood, changeable, variable
Restlessness
Starting, startled
    sleep, on falling
        during
Unconsciousness, coma, stupor
    vomiting, with

ARSENICUM IODATUM

Ailments from :
    work, mental
Anger, irascibility

Answers, aversion to
Anxiety
    bed, heat of, from ●
Cheerful, gay, mirthful
Concentration, difficult
Confusion of mind
    morning
    evening
Delirium
    night
Delusions, imagination, hallucinations,
    illusions
    dead persons, sees
    fancy, illusions of
Despair
Discontented, displeased, dissatisfied
Discouraged
Dullness, sluggishness, difficulty of think-
    ing and comprehending, torpor
Excitement, excitable
Exertion, agg. from mental
Fear, apprehension, dread
    evil, of
    insanity, losing his reason, of
    misfortune, of
    people, of
Hurry, haste
Impatience
Indifference, apathy
    happiness, to
    loved ones, to
    surroundings, to
Indolence, aversion to work
Insanity, madness
Irresolution, indecision
Irritability
Kill, desire to
    suden impulse to kill
Loquacity
Mildness
Mood, alternating
    changeable, variable
Prostration of mind, mental exhaustion,
    brain-fag
Restlessness
    night
    anxious
    bed, driving out of
    warm bed agg.

Sadness, despondency, dejection, mental depression, gloom, melancholy
Senses, dull, blunted
Sensitive, oversensitive
   noise, to
   sensual impressions, to
Sit, inclination to
Spoken to, averse to being
Starting, startled
   sleep, during
Study agg. ★
Stupefaction, as if intoxicated
Thoughts persistent
   wandering
Timidity
Weeping, tearful mood

ARSENICUM METALLICUM

Ailments from :
   work, mental
Company, aversion to; presence of other
      people agg. the symptoms; de-
      sire for solitude
Death, desires
Delusions, imaginations, hallucinations,
      illusions
   people threatening her, screams,
      horrible •
   spectres, ghosts, spirits, sees
Dullness, sluggishness, difficulty of think-
      ing and comprehending, torpor
Escape, attempts to
Fear, poisoned, of being
   night •
Indolence, aversion to work
Memory, weakness of,
   read, for what has
Sadness, despondency, dejection, mental
      depression, gloom, melancholy
   sleep and never to wake, would like
      to •
Unconsciousness, morning

ARSENICUM SULPHURATUM FLAVUM

Absent-minded, unoberving
Ailments from:
   anger, vexation
Anguish
Answer, aversion to
   slowly
Anxiety
      morning
      evening
            bed, in
      night
      conscience, as if guilty of a crime
      fear, with
      fever, during
      salvation, about
      stool, during
      waking, on
Censorious, critical
   dearest friends, with
Confusion of mind,
      morning, waking, on
Conscientious about trifles
Conversation, aversion to
Death, desires
Delirium,
      night
   raging, raving
Delirium tremens, mania-a-potu
Delusions, imaginations, hallucinations,
      illusions
   falling out of bed
Desires more than she needs
Despair
Dipsomania, alcoholism
Discontented, displeased, dissatisfied
Excitement, excitable
      night
Fear, apprehension, dread
      night
      alone, of being
      crowd, in a
      death, of
      evil, of
      fainting, of

Fear,
>ghosts, of
>people, of
>solitude, of
>torturing, of •
Forgetful
Frightened easily
Gestures, grasping or reaching,
>>picks at bed clothes
Hurry, haste
>always in
Hysteria
Ideas abundant, clearness of mind
Impatience
Indifference, apathy
Indolence, aversion to work
Insanity, madness
>>drunkards, in
>rage •
Irritability
>morning on waking
>chill, during
>bemoaing wailing
Lamenting, alternating with laughing •
Laughing, alternating with groaning
Loathing, life, at
Loquacity
>alternating with maliciousness •
Malicious, spiteful, vindictive
Mania
Memory, active
>alternating with weakness of
>>memory
Muttering
Obstinate, headstrong
Offended, easily; takes everything in
>bad part
Prostration of mind, mental exhaustion,
>brain-fag
Quarrelsome, scolding
Rage, fury
Religious affections
Remorse
Restlessness, evening
>*night*
>bed, tossing about in
>heat, during
>menses, during

Sadness, evening
>heat, during
>perspiration, during
Sensitive, oversensitive
Serious, earnest
Speech, incoherent
>wandering
Spoken to, averse to being
Starting, startled
>evening, asleep, on falling
>easily
>sleep, on falling
>>during
Stupefaction, as if intoxicated
Suspicious, mistrustful
Talk, indisposed to, desire to be silent,
>taciturn
Thoughts, rush, flow of
>vanishing of
Timidity
>bashful
Unreasonable
Vivacious
>alternating with muttering •
Weeping, night
>sleep, in
Work, mental, impossible, after eating •

ARSENICUM SULPHURATUM RUBRUM

Ideas abundant, clearness of mind
Morose, cross, fretful, ill-humor, peevish
Sadness, despondency, dejection, mental
>depression, gloom, melancholy
Talk, indisposed to, desire to be silent,
>taciturn

ARTEMISIA VULGARIS

Ailments from :
>bad news
>*fright*
>grief
Delirium, look fixed on one point, staring
Delusions, imaginations, hallucinations,
>illusions

Excitement, excitable
  epilepsy, before
Fear, apprehension, dread
Hysteria
Imbecility
Irritability
  convulsions, before
  epilepsy, before
Kleptomania
Morose, cross, fretful, ill-humor, peevish
Prostration of mind, epilepsy, in •
Restlessness
Sadness, epilepsy, day and night before
      attack of •
Shrieking, brain cry
  convulsions, before
      during epileptic
Somnambulism
Steals money, without necessity ★
Unconsciousness, coma, stupor
  convulsions, after

ARUM DRACONTIUM

Sadness, despondency, dejection, mental depression, gloom, melancholy

ARUM ITALICUM

Absent minded, unobserving
Restlessness

ARUM MACULATUM

Anxiety
Fear, apprehension, dread
Hypochondriasis
Sadness, despondency, dejection, mental
  depression, gloom, melancholy
Talk, indisposed to, desire to be silent,
  taciturn
Weeping, tearful mood

ARUM TRIPHYLLUM

Absent minded, unobserving
Anger, irascibility

Bite
  fingers, bites
  himself, bites
Confusion of mind
  morning
Contrary
Delirium
  busy
  fever, during
  muttering
  picking at nose or lips, with •
Escape, attempts to
Excitement, excitable
Forgetful
Gestures, grasping or reaching at some-
      thing, at flocks; carphologia
      nose, lips, at
      picks at bed clothes
  plays with his fingers ★
Indifference, apathy
Insanity, madness
Irritability
Mania
Memory, weakness of
Morose, cross, fretful, ill-humor, peevish
Muttering
Obstinate, headstrong
  children
Restlessness
  bed, tossing about in
Sadness, despondency, dejection, mental
      depression, gloom, melancholy
Shrieking, screaming, shouting
Starting, sleep, on falling
      during
Stupefaction, as if intoxicated
Unconsciousness, coma, stupor

ARUNDO MAURITANICA

Anxiety
  air amel., in open
  coughing, from
Cheerful, gay, mirthful
  foolish, and
Dullness, sluggishness, difficulty of thinking and comprehending, torpor
Fancies, lascivious

Hysteria
Ideas, deficiency of
Indifference, pain, to
Lascivious, lustful
Laughing
    easily
Talk, indisposed to, desire to be silent,
    taciturn
Thoughts intrude and crowd around
    each other
    sexual
Weeping, children in night,

ASAFOETIDA

Absent-minded, unobserving
Ailments from:
    excitement, emotional
    sexual excesses
Anger, irascibility
Anguish
    eating, after
Anxiety
    eating, after
    excitement, from
    fever, during
    hypochondriacal
    hysterical
Capriciousness
Chaotic, confused behaviour
Cheerful, gay, mirthful
Company, desire for; aversion to soli-
    tude, company amel.
    alone agg., while
Complaining
Concentration, difficult
Confusion of mind
            morning
            afternoon
            sitting, while
Consolation amel. ★
Contradiction, is intolerant of
Delusions, imaginations, hallucinations,
    illusions
    swollen, is
Dipsomania, alcoholism
Discontented, displeased, dissatisfied
    himself, with ★

Dullness, sluggishness, difficulty of think-
    ing and comprehending, torpor
Excitement, excitable
    leucorrhoea, after suppressed ●
    palpitation, with violent
    suppression of excretions, after
Exertion, agg. from mental
Exaggerates her symptoms ★
Fancies, exaltation of
Fear, apprehension, dread
    abdomen, arising from ●
    alone, of being
    brain, of softening of
    crowd, in a
    death, of
            heart symptoms, during
    eating food, after
    evil, of
    paralysis, of
    solitude, of
    stomach, arising from
Grief, fits of ●
Heedless
Hypochondriasis
Hysteria
    fainting, hysterical
    hysterical complaints in deep
            scrofulous constitutions, psora,
            syphilis ●
    suppression of discharges, after
Ideas abundant, clearness of mind
    deficiency of
Inconstancy
Indifference, apathy
    everything, to
Indolence, aversion to work
Irresolution, indecision
    air, amel. in open ●
    changeable
    projects, in
Irritability
    alternating with indifference
    menses, during
Joy, fits of joy with bursts of laughter
Lamenting, bemoaning, wailing

Laughing
    alternating with shrieking
    joy, with excessive
    spasmodic
Memory, active
Memory, weakness of
Mood, alternating
    changeable, variable
Morose, cross, fretful, ill-humor, peevish
        morning
    cough, before fits of
Nymphomania
Persevere, cannot ★
Prostration of mind, mental exhaustion,
        brain-fag
Quarrelsome, scolding
Reading, mental symptoms agg. from
Restlessness
        night
    anxious
    bed, tossing about in
    chill, during
    hypochondriacal
    hysterical •
Sadness, despondency, dejection, mental
        depression, gloom, melancholy
    anxious
    eating, after
    pressure about chest, from
Selfishness, egotism
Senses, acute
    dull, blunted
Sensitive, oversensitive
    pain, to
Starting, sleep, during
Stupefaction, as if intoxicated
Suicidal, disposition
Sympathy, amel. ★
Symptoms, magnifies her ★
Talks: troubles, of her ★
Unconsciousness, coition, after
    reading, from
    sitting, while
    transient
Walks, hither and thither •
Weeping, alternating with laughter
    pains, with the
Will, weakness of

Writing agg. mind symptoms

ASARUM EUROPAEUM

Absent-minded, unobserving
Absorbed, buried in thought
Anger, irascibility
    cough, before
Anguish
    vomiting, with
Anxiety hypochondriacal
Aversion, everything, to
Business, averse to
Chaotic, confused behavior
Cheerful, gay, mirthful
    alternating with sadness
        talk, aversion to •
Concentration, difficult
    on attempting to concentrate, has a
        vacant feeling
    studying, reading etc., while
Confusion of mind
    morning
        rising and after, on
    concentrate the mind, on attempt-
        ing to
    intoxicated, as if
    sitting, while
    walking, while
Contradiction, is intolerant of
Delusions, imaginations, hallucinations,
        illusions
    air, he is hovering in, like a spirit
    body, lighter than air, is
    floating in air
        walking, while •
    flying, sensation of
    light, incorporeal, he is
    scratching on linen or similar sub-
        stance, some one was •
Dipsomania, alcoholism
Discontented, displeased, dissatisfied
Dullness, sluggishness, difficulty of think-
        ing and comprehending, torpor
    vomiting amel.

Dwells on past disagreeable occurrences
Eccentricity
Euphoria
    alternating with, quietness, desire
       for •
    sadness
    feeling of lightness as after an an-
       esthesia by chlorethylene, with •
Excitement, excitable
    nervous
    pregnancy, during
Exertion, agg. from mental
Exhilaration
Fear, noise, from
    touch, of
Gestures,
    wringing the hands ★
Hysteria
Ideas abundant, clearness of mind
    deficiency of
       vomiting amel. •
Imbecility
Inconsolable
Indifference, apathy
Indolence, aversion to work
    eating, after
Irritability
    alternating with sadness
    noise, cracking of news paper, even
       from
    sadness, with
Jumping
Light, desire for
Loathing, general
Memory, active, names, for proper •
Memory, weakness of
    labor, for mental
Mildness
Mood, alternating
    changeable, variable
Morose, cross, fretful, ill-humor, peevish
    air, amel. in open
    fever, during
Mortification, dreams about received
    mortification •
New, can't do anything ★

Prostration of mind, mental exhaustion,
    brain-fag
Quarrelsome, scolding
Quiet disposition
Restlessness
Sadness, despondency, dejection, mental
    depression, gloom, melancholy
    anxious
    mental exertion, after
    periodical
Senses, acute
    dull, blunted
    vanishing of
Sensitive, oversensitive
    noise, to
       cracking of paper, to
       scratching on linen, silk or
         strings, to •
       slightest, to
       striking of clocks, ringing
         of bells, to
Sit, inclination to
Slowness
Startig, startled
    noise, from
Stupefaction, as if intoxicated
Succeeds, never
Thoughts persistent
    unpleasant subjects, haunted by
    vanishing of
       mental exertion, on
       work, at
Touched, aversion to being
Unconsciousness, coma, stupor
Walking, in open air amel. mental symp-
    toms
Wearisome
Weeping, tearful mood
    anxiety, after
Work, aversion to mental
    impossible

ASCLEPIAS CORNUTI

Dullness, sluggishness, difficulty of think-
    ing and comprehending, torpor
Hysteria
Stupefaction, as if intoxicated

ASCLEPIAS TUBEROSA

Anxiety, walking, after
Cheerful, gay, mirthful
Dullness, sluggishness, difficulty of thinking and comprehending, torpor
Eccentricity
    evening
Gestures, makes
Hysteria
Indolence, aversion to work
Irritability
Morose, cross, fretful, ill-humor, peevish
Prostration of mind, mental exhaustion, brain-fag
Restlessness
    night
Sadness, despondency, dejection, mental depression, gloom, melancholy

ASIMINA TRILOBA

Conversation, aversion to
Thoughts persistent, occurrences of the day at night,
    of the

ASPARAGUS OFFICINALIS

Anxiety
Carried, desires to be
Cheerful, gay, mirthful
Confusion of mind
Excitement, afternoon, feverish
Fear, apprehension, dread
Hydrophobia
Irritability
    trifles, from
Morose, cross, fretful, ill-humor, peevish
    trifles, about
Restlessness, anxious

ASTACUS (CANCER) FLUVIATILIS

Delirium
    chill, during
Fear, apprehension, dread

Sadness, despondency, dejection, mental
    depression, gloom, melancholy
Unconsciousness, coma, stupor

ASTERIAS RUBENS

Ailments from:
    excitement, emotional
Anger, irascibility
    afternoon, 12-14h.
Anxiety
    noon, 12-15h •
    night
    house, in
    sleep, during
        menses, after
    waking, on
    weeping amel.
Bite, desire to
Cheerful
    afternoon
    evening
Confusion of mind
Contradiction, is intolerant of
Delusions
    answers to any d.
    home, away from, is
    strangers, control of, under
    voices, hears
Despair
    sexual craving, from •
Dullness, sluggishness, difficulty of thinking and comprehending, torpor
Excitement, excitable
    night
    alternating with sadness
Fear, noon, 12-15h. •
    apoplexy, of
        night, with feeling as if head
        would burst, at •
    bad news, of hearing
    evil, of
    fainting, of
    misfortune, of
    waking, on
    weeping, amel.
Hysteria
Ideas abundant, headache, after •
    deficiency of

Impatience
  house, in •
Indifference, apathy
Indolence, aversion to work
Insanity, climacteric period, during
Irritability
  noon
  convulsions, before
Lascivious, lustful
Memory, weakness of
  done, for what has just
Moral feeling, want of
Morose, cross, fretful, ill-humor, peevish
Nymphomania
Prostration of mind, mental exhaustion,
  brain-fag
Quarrelsome, scolding
  forenoon., 12-14h. •
Restlessness
  night
Sadness, despondency, dejection, mental
  depression, gloom, melancholy
  alternating with euphoria
Talk, indisposed to, desire to be silent,
  taciturn
Thinking, aversion to
Thoughts, sexual
Unconsciousness, coma, stupor, waking,
  on
Weeping, tearful mood
  desire to weep
  easily
  emotion, after slight
  sexual excitement, with ★

ASTRAGALUS EXCAPUS

Confusion of mind
  morning
Ecstasy
Mental symptoms alternating with
  physical
Mood, changeable, variable
Prostration of mind, evening
Sadness, despondency, dejection, mental
  depression, gloom, melancholy
Thoughts, tormenting
Work, mental, impossible

ATHAMANTA OREOSELINUM

Excitement, evening
Irritability, heat, during

ATROPINUM

Absent-minded, unobserving
Abusive, insulting
Anger, irascibility
  trifles, at
Answers, aversion to
  imaginary questions
  imperfect
  indifferent •
  refuses to answer
Anxiety
  conscience, as if guilty of a crime
Cheerful, gay, mirthful
Company, aversion to; presence of other
  people agg. the symptoms; desire for solitude
Concentration, difficult
Confusion of mind
  closing eyes, on •
Conversation, aversion to
Delirium
  night
  bed and escapes, springs up sud-
    denly from
  books, endeavored to grasp •
  crying, with
  frightful
  headache, from
  raging, raving
  rambling
  restless
  violent
  wild
Delirium tremens, mania-a-potu
Delusions, imaginations, hallucinations,
  illusions
  blood does not circulate well •
  business, ordinary, they are
    pursuing
  engaged in some occupation, is
  ordinary occupation, in
  enlarged, distances are
  objects are

Delusions,
    epilepsy, he has ●
    figures, sees
        gigantic ●
    hearing, illusions of
    images, sees frightful
    newspapers, he sees ●
    nursing her child, she is ●
    objects appear, in open air ●
        seize o., tries to
    past, of events long
    people, sees
        beside him, are
    pleasing
    railway, go off by, he was obliged to ●
    rain, from having wet cloth on head
        thought he had been out in ●
    room, sees people at bed side in
    sewing, she is ●
    shopping with her sister ●
    spectres, ghosts, spirits, sees
        night, sees at
        bed, in ●
    strange, familiar things seem
    talking, imaginary persons, loudly
        and incoherently to
    toys, playing with ●
    visions, horrible
Dream, as if in a
Dullness, sluggishness, difficulty of think-
    ing and comprehending, torpor
        afternoon
Excitement, excitable
Fear, apprehension, dread
    misfortune, of
        heat, during
    observed, of her condition being
Gestures, grasping or reaching at some-
    thing, at flocks; carphologia
        night
        picks at bedclothes
    hands, motions, involuntary throw-
        ing about
Hurry, movements, in
Ideas, deficiency of

Indifference, apathy
Indolence, aversion to work
Insanity, madness
Irritability
Jumping, bed, out of
Laughing, idiotic
    stupid expression, with
    wild
Mania
Meddlesome, importunate
Memory, weakness of
    say, for what is about to
Mistakes, localities, in
        time, in
Morose, cross, fretful, ill-humor, peevish
Muttering
        night
            waking, on
Quarrelsome, scolding
Rage, fury
Restlessness
        night
    anxious
    bed, tossing about in
    heat, during
    internal
    rising, on
Sadness, despondency, dejection, mental
        depression, gloom, melancholy
Senses, acute
Sensitive, oversensitive
Shrieking, screaming, shouting
Sighing
Smiling
Speech, confused, morning on waking ●
    embarassed
    hasty
    incoherent
    irrelevant ●
    loud
    nonsensical
    prattling
    slow
    unintelligible, sleep, in
    wandering
    wild

Starting, startled
  fright, from and as from
  sleep, during
Striking
Talk, indisposed to, desire to be silent,
    taciturn
Thoughts, wandering
    afternoon
Time passes too quickly, appears shorter
Unconsciousness, coma, stupor
  alternating with delirium •
  convulsions, after
  delirium, after
  dream, does not know where he is
Well, says he is, when very sick
Work, aversion to mental

AURUM FOLIATUM

Absent-minded, unobserving
Abusive, insulting
Affections, in general ★
Ailments from :
  anger, vexation
    anxiety, with
    fright, with
    indignation, with
    silent grief, with
    suppressed
  anxiety
  contradiction
  disappointment
  excitement, emotional
  fright
  grief
  love, disappointed
  mortification
  pecuniary loss
  scorn, being scorned
  sexual excesses
  violence
Anger, irascibility
  *absent persons, while thinking of
    them, at*
  alternating with cheerfulness
  contradiction, from
  trembling, with

Anger,
  trifles, at
  violent
Anguish
  palpitation, with
Answers, aversion to
  questions, in •
Antagonism with herself
Anxiety
  **conscience, as if guilty of a
  crime**
  driving from place to place
  eating amel.
  fear, with
  future, about
  noise, from
  pressure on the chest, from
  riding, while
  salvation, about
  suicidal disposition, with
  weary of life, with
Aversion to being approached
  members of family, to
  persons, to certain
Begging, entreating, supplicating
Brooding
  corner or moping, brooding in a
Capriciousness,
  evening
Cares worries, full of
  trifles, about
Censorious, critical
Cheerful, gay, mirthful
  daytime
  evening, bed, in
  alternating with anger
  bursts of indignation
      of passion
    moroseness
    sadness
    violence
  death, while thinking of •
*Company, aversion to; presence of other
      people agg. the symptoms; de-
      sire for solitude*
Complaining
Comprehension, easy
Concentration, difficult

Confidence, want of self
   others have none in him, which makes
      her unhappy, and thinks •
Confusion of mind
   morning
      rising and after, on
   identity, as to his
   mental exertion, after
   rising, after
Conscientious about trifles
Consolation, kind words agg.
Contemptuous,
   self, of
Contented
Contradict, disposition to
Contradiction, is intolerant of
   agg.
Contrary
Conversation agg.
Cowardice
Death, desires
     evening
   alternating with laughing •
   convalescence, during
   thoughts of
     joy, give him •
Deception causes grief and mortifi-
     cation ★
Delirium
   night
   exaltation of strength, with
   gay, cheerful
   headache, from
   loquacious
   raging, raving
   religious
   sleeplessness, and ★
   violent
   waking, on
Delirium tremens, mania-a-potu
Delusions, imaginations, hallucinations,
   illusions
     night
   affection of friends, has lost
   animals, of
   confidence in him, his friends have
     lost all

Delusions,
   deserted, forsaken, is
   dogs, sees
   doomed, being
   faces, sees
     larger, grow
     where ever he turns his eyes,
      or looking out from corners
   fail, everything will
   fancy, illusions of
   friends, affection of, has lost the
   head, monstrous, on distant wall of
     room
   heart, turning around, is •
   hollow, whole body is
   lost, she is
   melancholy
   mortification, after
   neglected his duty, he has
   people, converses with absent
   pursued by enemies
     he was
   religious
   reproach, has neglected duty and
     deserves •
   right, does nothing
   small, things appear
   spectres, ghosts, spirits, sees
     hovering in the air
   succeed, he cannot; does everything
     wrong
   thieves, sees
   unfit for the world, he is •
   waking, on
   wrong, he has done
Dementia, senilis
Despair
   chill, during
   heart disease, in ★
   lost, thinks everything is
   others, about •
     oneself, and
   pains, with
   periodical
   religious despair of salvation
Dipsomania, alcoholism

Discomfort
Discontented, displeased, dissatisfied
    himself, with
Discouraged
Disgust
    everything, with
Doubtful, recovery, of
    soul's welfare, of
Dullness, sluggishness, difficulty of think-
    ing and comprehending, torpor
    mental exertion, from
Eating, amel. of mental symptoms while
Egotism, self-esteem
Emptiness, sensation of
    internal ★
    whole body were hollow, as if ★
Ennui, tedium
    entertainment amel.
Excitement, excitable
        evening, bed, in
    absent persons, about ●
    agg.
    amel.
    chill, during
    hope, as in joyous ●
    pain, during ●
    religious
    trembling, with
Exertion, agg. from mental
Fancies, exaltation of
        night
    lascivious
        night ●
Fear, apprehension, dread
    crowed, in a
    death, of
    desire for death, fear with ●
    duty, to neglect his ●
    evil, of
    heart, of disease of
        arising from
        organic, of
    men, dread, fear of
    noise, from
        door, at
    over powering
    people, of

Fear,
    restlessness from fear
    robbers, of
    stomach, arising from
    tremulous
Foolish, behavior, morning on waking ●
Forgetful
    mental exertion, from
Forsaken feeling
Frightened easily
    falling asleep, on
Gestures, convulsive, thinking of mo-
        tion, when ●
    wringing the hands
Grief
    headache from grief
Hatred
    persons who had offended him, of
    revenge, hatred and
Haughty
Hide, children ●
High places agg.
Homesickness
Hopeful
    lung disease, in ★
*Horrible things, sad stories, affect her
        profoundly*
Howling
Hurry, haste
    eating, while
    mental work, in
    movements, fast enough, cannot do
        things
    occupation, in
        desires to do several things at
        once
Hypochondriasis
    suicide, driving to
Hysteria
Ideas abundant, clearness of mind
    deficiency of
Imbecility
Impatience
    perspiration, during
Impulsive
Indifference, joyless
Indignation

Indolence, aversion to work
Industrious, mania for work
Initiative, lack of
Inquisitive
Insanity, madness
    melancholy
    puerperal
    religious
Introspection
Irresolution, indecision
Irritability
    absent persons, with
    alternating with cheerfulness
        weeping
    chill, during
    sadness, with
    spoken to, when
Jumping
    height, from a, impulse to j. ★
Lamenting, bemoaning, wailing
Lascivious, lustful
Laughing
    agg.
    alternating with loathing of life •
    involuntarily
    spasmodic
    speaking, when
Loathing, general, old age, in
Loathing life, at
        evening
Loquacity
      night
    rapid questioning ★
Love, disappointed
    sadness from
    suicidal disposition from
Malicious, spiteful, vindictive
Mania
Meditation
Melancholy, brooding ★
Memory, active
Memory, loss of; insanity, in
Memory, weakness of
Menses, mental symptoms agg. after
Mental symptoms alternating with
    physical ★
Mildness

Misanthropy
Moaning, sleep, during
Monomania
Mood, alternating
    changeable, variable
        evening
        perspiration, during
    repulsive
Morose, cross, fretful, ill-humor,
        peevish
    alternating with cheerfulness
    oneself, with
Morphinism
Music amel.
Obscene, lewd talk
Obstinate, headstrong
    children
    masturbation, boys after •
Occupation, diversion amel.
Offended easily; takes everything in bad
        part
Passionate
Pessimist
Praying
Prostration of mind, mental exhaus-
        tion, brain-fag
    reading, from
Quarrelsome, scolding
Questions, speaks continually in
Quiet disposition
    alternating with gaiety, trilling,
        singing
Rashness
Reckless, rashness ★
Reflect unable to
Religious affections
    melancholia
        remorse, from
Remorse
Reproaches himself
    others
Reserved
Responsibility, unusual, agg. ★
Restlessness
    afternoon
        lying, when •
    night
    anxious

Restlessness,
   busy
   driving about
   lying, while
   tremulous
Rudeness
Sadness, despondency, dejection,
   mental deprpession, gloom,
   melancholy
     morning
     evening
   age, in old
   alone, when
   alternating with physical energy
   amenorrhoea, in
   anger, from
   climaxis, during
   company, aversion to desire for
     solitude
   diverted from thoughts of himself,
     desires to be
   friends, as if having lost affection of •
   grief, after
   headache, during
   impotence, with
   love, from disappointed
   masturbation, from
   menses, before
     during
     suppressed
   mercury, after abuse of
   periodical
   perspiration, during
   pollutions, from
   puberty, in
   puerperal
   sleeplessness from sadness
   suicidal disposition, with
Schizophrenia
Secretive
Self, criticism ★
Senses, dull, blunted
Sensitive, oversensitive
   certain persons, to
   light, to
   mental impressions, to

Sensitive,
   noise, to
     music amel.
     voices, to
     odors, to
     pains, to
     sensual impressions, to
Serious, earnest
Shrieking, screaming, shouting
   menses, after •
   • must shriek, feels as though she
     sleep, during
Sighing, sleep, in
Sit, inclination to
Sits, still
   wrapped in deep, sad thoughts and
     notices nothing, as if
Smiling, involuntarily
   when speaking •
Speech, foolish
   hasty
   loud
   nonsensical
   wandering
     night
Spoken to, averse to being
   alone, wants to be let
Starting, dream, from a
   noise, from
   sleep, during
     from
Stupefaction, as if intoxicated
   alternating with convulsions •
   convulsions, between
   vertigo, during
Succeeds, never
Suicidal, disposition
   evening
   anxiety, from
   drowning, by
   hanging, by
   hypochondriasis, by
   pains, from
   perspiration, during
   pregnancy, during •

Suicidal,
runover, to be
sadness, from
shooting, by
thoughts
throwing himself from a height
window, from
pain, from •
Sulky
Suspicious, mistrustful
Talk, indisposed to, desire to be si-
lent, taciturn
others agg., talk of
Talking, sleep, in
Talks, himself, to
Theorizing
Thinking, complaints agg., of
Thoughts persistent
Timidity
bashful
Tranquillity, serenity, calmness
Travel, desire to
Unconsciousness, alternating with convulsions
standing, while
Violent, vehement
pain, from
Weary of life
evening
old age, in
perspiration, during
Weeping, tearful mood
night
alternating with laughter
chill, during
involuntary
laughing at same time, weeping
and
meeting people, when •
perspiration, during
sleep, in
spasmodic
whimpering
sleep, during
Wildness
Work, aversion to mental
desire for
fatigues
impossible

AURUM ARSENICUM

Absent-minded, unobserving
Activity
Ailments from:
anger, vexation
silent grief, with
contradiction
grief
sexual excesses
Anger, irascibility
Anguish
Anxiety
daytime
night
conscience, as if guilty of a crime
fear, with
salvation, about
Censorious, critical
Confusion of mind
morning
Conscientious about trifles
Contrary
Death, desires
Delirium,
night
Delusions, imaginations, hallucinations,
illusions
animals, of
fancy, illusions of
wrong, he has done
Despair, chill, during
pains, with
periodical
recovery, of
religious despair of salvation
Discontented, displeased, dissatisfied
Excitement, excitable
chill, during
Exertion, agg. from mental
Fancies, exaltation of
Fear, apprehension, dread
evening
night
alone, of being
crowd, in a
death, of
evil, of
people, of

Forgetful
Frightened easily
Grief
Hurry, haste
Hysteria
Ideas abundant, clearness of mind
Imbecility
Impatience
Indifference, children, to her
    duties, domestic, to
Indolence, aversion to work
Industrious, mania for work
Insanity, madness
    drunkards, in
    fanatics, of
    religious
Irressolution, indecision
Irritability
    alternating with cheerfulness
    chill, during
    spoken to, when
Lamenting, bemoaning, wailing
Laughing
Loathing, life, at
Loquacity
Malicious, spiteful, vindictive
Mania
Memory, active
Memory, weakness of
Neglects, children, her •
    household, the
Obstinate, headstrong
Offended, easily; takes everything in
    bad part
Prostration of mind, mental exhaustion,
    brain-fag
Quarrelsome, scolding
Remorse
Reproaches himself
    others, imaginary insult, for •
Reserved
Restlessness
    night
    anxious
    lying, while

Sadness
    evening
    menses, suppressed
    perspiration, during
Sensitive, oversensitive
    noise, to
        voices, to
Shrieking, screaming, shouting
Speech, wandering
Spoken to, averse to being
Suicidal disposition
    perspiration, during
    throwing himself from window
Talk, indisposed to, desire to be silent,
    taciturn
    alternating with violence •
Thinking, complaints agg., of
Timidity
Untidy
Violent, alternating with tranquillity •
Weary of life
Weeping, tearful mood
    chill, during
    hysterical
    sleep, in

AURUM IODATUM

Anxiety
    daytime
    night
Cheerful, gay, mirthful
    causeless •
    paroxysms, in •
Company, aversion to; presence of other
    people agg. the symptoms; desire
    for solitude
Confidence, want of self
Confusion of mind, morning
Conscientious about trifles
Dementia, senilis
    syphilitics, of
Despair, recovery, of
    religious despair of salvation
Excitement, excitable
Exertion, agg. from mental
Fear, crowd, in a
    evil, of
    people, of
    work, dread of

Hurry, haste
Hysteria
Impatience
Indolence, aversion to work
Insanity, madness
    face, with red
Irresolution, indecision
Irritability
Mania
Mood, alternating
    changeable, variable
Prostration of mind, mental exhaustion,
    brain-fag
Restlessness
Sadness, despondency, dejection, men-
    tal depression,
    gloom, melancholy
Sensitive, noise, to
Timidity
Weeping, tearful mood

AURUM MURIATICUM

Absent-minded
    starts when spoken to
Ailments from:
    anger, vexation
    fright
    grief
    mortification
Anger, thinking of his ailments, when ●
Anxiety, excitement, from
    mental exertion, from
Business, averse to
Capriciousness
Cheerful, gay, mirthful
    afternoon
Company, desire for; aversion to soli-
    tude,
    company amel.
Confusion of mind
    air amel., in open
Contradict, disposition to
Death, desires
Delirium
    congestion, with
    headache, from

Delusions, imaginations, hallucinations,
    illusions
    disease, he has every
Discontented, displeased, dissatisfied
Excitement, excitable
Exertion, agg. from mental
Fear, evil, of
    palpitation, with
    suffocation, of, night
Heedless
Horrible things, sad stories, affect her
    profoundly
Hypochondriasis
Indolence, aversion to work
Irritability
Loathing, life, at
Memory, weakness of
Mood, changeable, variable
Morose, thinking of his ailments
    when alone ●
Music amel.
Religious affections, melancholia
Restlessness
    air amel., in open
    angina pectoris, in ●
    walking, air amel., in open
Sadness, despondency, dejection,
    mental depression, gloom,
    melancholy
    climaxis, during
    mercury, after abuse of
Sensitive, noise, to
Shrieking, screaming, shouting
Starting, startled
    sleep, during
    from
    spoken to, when
    waking, on, suffocated, as if
Suicidal disposition
Thinking, complaints agg., of
Weary of life
Weeping, tearful mood
Work, aversion to mental

AURUM MURIATICUM NATRONATUM

Ailments from:
   anger, vexation
Anxiety
Impatience
Indifference, recovery, about his ★

AURUM SULPHURATUM

Absent-minded, unobserving
Activity, mental
Ailments from :
   grief
Anger, irascibility
   violent
Anxiety
   conscience, as if guilty of a crime
   fear, with
   salvation, about
Brooding
   corner or moping, brooding in a
Censorious, critical
   dearest friends, with
Cheerful, gay, mirthful
   morbidly ●
Company, aversion to; presence of other
    people agg. the symptoms; de-
    sire for solitude
Confidence, want of self
Confusion of mind
      morning
      mental exertion, after
Cowardice
Death, desires
Delusions, animals, of
Despair, recovery, of
   religious despair of salvation
Discontented, displeased, dissatisfied
Dullness, sluggishness, difficulty of
    thinking and comprehending,
    torpor
Excitement, excitable
Exertion, agg. from mental
Fancies, exaltation of

Fear, crowd, in a
   death, of
   evil, of
   people, of
   robbers, of
Forgetful
Frightened easily
Hurry, haste
Hysteria
Ideas abundant, clearness of mind
Imbecility
Indolence, aversion to work
   changing to mania for work ●
Insanity, madness
Irresolution, indecision
Irritability
Lamenting, bemoaning, wailing
Loathing, life, at
Loquacity
Mania
Memory, weakness of
Moaning, groaning, whining
Mood, changeable, variable
Morose, cross, fretful, ill-humor, peevish
Obstinate, headstrong
Offended, easily; takes everything in
    bad part
Prostration of mind, mental exhaus-
    tion, brain-fag
Quarrelsome, scolding
Restlessness
    night
Rudeness
Sadness, despondency, dejection, mental
    depression, gloom, melancholy
    morning
    evening
    perspiration, during
Sensitive, oversensitive
Sits, still
Spoken to, averse to being
Suicidal thoughts
Suspicious, mistrustful
Talk, indisposed to, desire to be silent,
    taciturn
Timidity

Weeping, tearful mood
    night
    alternating with laughter

AURANTII CORTEX

Starting, sleep, during

AVENA SATIVA

Ailments, from:
    work, mental
Dipsomania, alcoholism
Exertion, agg. from mental
Hypochondriasis
Morphinism
Prostration of mind, mental exhaustion,
        brain-fag
    sleeplessness, with

AZADIRACHTA INDICA

Dementia, senillis
Forgetful
Hypochondriasis
Memory, weakness of
    facts, for recent
    names, for proper
Mistakes, speaking, in
        spelling, in
        writing, in
Sadness, despondency, dejection, mental
        depression, gloom, melancholy
Weeping, tearful mood

BACILLINUM BURNETT

Idiocy
Imbecility
Insanity, madness

BADIAGA

Activity, mental
Cheerful, gay, mithful
Despair
Dullness, sluggishness, difficulty of think-
        ing and comprehending, torpor
Excitement, excitable
Memory, active
Mistakes, time, in
Restlessness
    night
Shrieking, screaming, shouting
Thinking, complaints agg., of
Weeping, coughing, during
Work, desire for mental

BAPTISIA TINCTORIA

Answers, sleeps at once, then
        slowly
        stupor returns quickly after answer
Anxiety
    waking, on
Aversion, women, to
Bed, aversion to, shuns bed
    get out of, wants to
Concentration, difficult
Confusion of mind
    heat, during
    identity, as to his
        duality, sense of
        intoxicated, as if
Darkness agg.
Death, conviction of
    presentiment of

Delirium
>   **night**
>   *answers correctly when spoken to*
>   *but delirium and unconscious-*
>   *ness return at once*
>   busy
>   closing the eyes, on
>   constant
>   exhaustion, with
>   *face, red*
>   *fierce*
>   loquacious
>   **mild**
>   *muttering*
>   nonsense, with eyes open
>   *sepsis, from*

Delusions, imaginations, halucinations,
*   illusions* •
>   arms, belong to her, do not
>   cut off, are •
>   *bed, hard, too*
>   sinking is
>   *someone is in bed with him*
>   *body, parts of have been taken away*
>   *scattered about bed, tossed about*
>   *to get the pieces together*
>   *divided into two parts*
>   *double, of being*
>   enlarged
>   *head is*
>   identity, errors of personal
>   *legs don't belong to her*
>   conversing, are
>   *toe is conversing with thumb* •
>   cut off, are
>   limbs are separated
>   sinking, to be
>   succeed, he cannot; does every
>   thing wrong
>   swollen, he is
>   talking to another part of body,
>   one part •
>   three persons, he is

Dementia, senilis
Despair, recovery, of

Dullness, suggishness, difficulty of
**   thinking and comprehend-**
**   ing, torpor**
>   night on waking
>   breakfast, after •
>   *heat, during*

Escape, attempts to
Excitement, excitable
Fancies, confused
Fear, apprehension, dread
>   bed, of the
>   dark, of
>   death, of
>   heart, of disease of
>   poisoned, of being
>   sleep, go to, fear to
>   suffocation, of, sleep, during •

Hysteria
Imbecility
Indifference, apathy
>   everything, to
Indolence, aversion to work
Loquacity
Mania
memory, active
Memory, weakness of
Moaning, sleep, during
Muttering
Prostration of mind, mental exhaus-
**   tion, brainfag**
>   *fever, in*
Resetlessness
>   *night*
>   midnight, after
>   bed, tossing about in
>   heat, during
>   *move, but too weak to* •
Sadness, despondency, dejection, mental
>   depression, gloom, melancholy
Senses, dull, blunted
Sensitive, noise, to
Speech, incoherent
Starting, sleep, falling, on
Stupefaction, as if intoxicated
>   *restlessness, with*
>   sleepiness, with
Suspicious, mistrustful

Talk, indisposed to, desire to be silent,
    taciturn
    sickness or injuries, about •
Thinking, aversion to
    complaints agg., of
Thoughts, vanishing of
    wandering
Timidity, evening, going to bed, about
Unconsciousness, coma, stupor
    answers correctly when spoken to,
        but delirium and unconscious
        ness return at once
    fever, during
    frequent spells of unconciousness,
        absences
Weeping, tearful mood
Wild, feeling in head ★
Wildness
    headache, during •
Work, aversion to mental
    impossible

BARYTA ACETICA

Ailments from:
    work, mental
Anger, sudden •
Anxiety
    trifles, about
Confidence, want of self
Dementia, senilis
Discomfort, eating, after
Exertion, agg. from mental
Fear, people, of; anthropophobia
Indolence, aversion to work
Irresolution, indecision
Irritability
Memory, weakness of
    names, for proper
Mood, changeable, variable
Morose, cross, fretful, ill-humor, peevish
Muttering, sleep, in
Obstinate, headstrong
Sadness, despondency, dejection, mental
    depression gloom, melancholy
    trifles, about
Sit, inclination to
Spit, desire to

Starting, noise, from
Suspicious, mistrustful
Will, weakness of

BARYTA CARBONICA

Absent minded, unobserving
    spoken to, when
Absorbed, buried in thought
Activity
Affectionate
Ailments from :
    anger, vexation
    anticipation, foreboding, presenti-
        ment
Amusement, averse to
Anger, irascibility
    violent
Antagonism with herself ★
Anxiety
            morning
            forenoon
            noon
            evening
            bed, in
                uneasiness and anxiety,
                must uncover
            night
            midnight, before
    air, in open
    bed, in
    business, about
    domestic affairs during pregnancy,
        about
    fear, with
    fever, during
    friends at home, about
    future, about
    lying, side, on
        left
    noise, from
    others, for
    pregnancy, in
    paroxysms, in ★
    stool, before
    sudden
    trifles, about
    walking, while
Awkward, drops things ★

Beside oneself, being
Borrows trouble ★
Brooding, corner or moping, in a
Busy
Capriciousness
Carefulness
Cares, worries, full of
    domestic affairs, about
Cautious, anxiously
Censorious, critical
Cheerful, gay, mirthful
Childish behavior
    old age, in ●
Children covering their face with their
    hands, but looking through
    their fingers ●
Communicative, expansive
Company, aversion to; presence of
    other people
        agg. the symptoms; desire
        for solitude
    alone, amel. when
    presence of strangerss, aversion to
Comprehension, easy
Concentration, difficult
    children, in
    studying, reading etc., while
    learns with difficulty.
Confidence, want of self
Confusion of mind
    morning
        waking, on
    evening
    air, in open, amel.
    old age, in
    sitting, while
    waking, on
Conscientious about trifles
Contradict, disposition to
Contrary
Cowardice
    anger, with sudden ebullition of ●
Credulous
Delirium
    fever, during
    frightful
    loquacious
    sleep, during

Delusions, imaginations, halluciation,
    illusions
    criticised, she is
    dead persons, sees
    deserted, forsaken, is
    die, he was about to
    dying, friend is, beloved ●
    fancy, illusions of
    fire, every noise is a cry of, and
        she trembles ●
    images, phantoms, sees
        frightful
    knees, he walks on
    laughed at, mocked, being
    legs, cut off, are
    people looking at him
    rising, then falling ★
    robbed, is going to be
    sick and dying, a beloved friend is
        being ●
    soldiers, sees
    walks, knees, on his,
    watched, she is being
Dementia, senilis
    talking, with foolish
Despair
    recovery, of
Development of children arrested
Dipsomania, alcoholism
Discontented, displeased, dissatisfied
Discouraged
    anxiety, with
    weeping, with
Doubtful
Dullness, sluggishness, defficulty
    of   thinking and compre-
    hend   ing, torpor
    morning
        waking, on
    children, in
    old people, of
    siesta, after
    waking, on
Ennui
Escape, attempts to
    pregnancy, during ●
    run away, to

Fancies, exaltation of
    night
Fear, apprehension, dread
    evening
    approaching him, of others
    children, in
    crossing a bridge or place, of
    crowd, in a
        public places, of; agoraphobia
    death, of
    evil, of
    happen, something will
    men, dread, fear of
    misfortune, of
    noise, from
        night
        street, in
    people, of; anthropophobia
    children, in
    rail, of going by
    starting, with
    strangers, of
    walking, while
Foolish behavior
Forgetfulness
    errands, of ★
    old people, of
    words while speaking, of; word
        hunting
Forsaken feeling
    evening
Frightened, easily
    trifles, at
Frivolous
Grief
    trifles, over
Hatred, men, of
Heedless
Hide: child thinks all visitors laugh at it
    and hides behind furniture ●
    children, strangers, from ●
Hurry, haste
Hypocrisy
Hysteria
Ideas, deficiency of
Idiocy
Imbecility

Impatience
Indifference, apathy
    puberty, in
Indiscretion
Indolence, aversion to work
    children, in
    dinner, after
    eating, after
    physical
Industrious, mania for work
    menses, before
Infantile behavior
Insanity, madness
    puerperal-
Irritability
Intolerance
Irresolution, indecision
    acts, in
    projects, in
    trifles, about
    Irritability
    evening
Jesting
Laughing
    aversion to
    causeless
    childish
    immoderately
Learns poorly ★
Loquacity
    menses, during
    pregnancy, during ●
Magnetized, desires to be, mesmerism
    amel.
Malicious, spiteful, vindictive
    anger, with
Mania
Memory, weakness of
    do, for what was about to
    done, for what has just
    labor, for mental
        child cannot be taught from
        weakness of
    memory for mental ●
    said, for what has
    say, for what is about to
    words, of
Misanthropy
Mischievous

Moaning, groaning, whining
    old age, in •
    perspiration, during
Mood, alternating
    changeable, variable
Morose, cross, fretful, ill-humor, peevish
    evening
Muttering, old age, in •
    sleep, in
Narrow-minded
Neglects everything
Nibble, desire to
Occupation, diversion amel.
Passionate
Pessimist
Play, aversion to play in children
    sit in corner, and
Prostration of mind, mental exhaustion,
    brain-fag
    old age, in •
Quarrelsome, scolding
Rage, fury
    night
    trifles, at
    violent
Reading, aversion to read
Religious affections
Restlessness
    eating, after
    heat, during
Rudeness
Sadness, despondency, dejection, mental
    depression, gloom, melancholy
    morning
      waking, on
    evening
    eating, after
    talk, indisposed to
    trifles, about
Secretive
Self, odd, at with ★
Senses, acute
Sensitive, oversensitive
    mental impressions, to
    noise, to
      slightest, to
      voices, male, to
    perspiration, during
    sensual impressions, to

Serious, earnest
Sit, inclination to
Sits, still
Slowness
Society, shuns ★
Spineless
Spoiled children
Starting, startled
    asleep, on falling
    dream, from a
    easily
    fright, from and as from
    noise, from
    sleep, falling, on
      during
      from
    tremulous
Strangers presence of strangers agg
    child coughs at sight of strangers
Stupefaction, as if intoxicated
    morning
    night
    vertigo, during
Susceptible
Suspicious, mistrustful
    fear of company
    talking about her, people are •
Talk, indisposed to, desire to be silent,
    taciturn
    sadness, in
    slow learring to
Talking, sleep, in
Thinking, complaints agg., of
Thoughts, disagreeable
    thoughtful
Time, passes too slowly, appears longer
Timidity
    bashful
Travel, desire to
Uncouth ★
Unconsciousness, coma, stupor
    apoplexy, in
    crowded room, in a
    old age, in •
Violent
    deeds of violence, rage leading to

Weeping, tearful mood
> night
>> goes off alone and weeps as if she
>>> had no friends •
> sleep, in
> whimpering, sleep, during
Will, loss of
> *weakness of*
Work, aversion to mental
> impossible

BARYTA IODATA

Anger, irascibility
Anxiety
Brooding
Company, aversion to; presence of other
> people agg. the symptoms; desire
> for solitude
Concentration, difficult
Confusion of mind
Cowardice
Delusions, imaginations, hallucinations,
> illusions
>> dead persons, sees
>> fancy, illusions of
Dulllness, sluggishness, difficulty of think-
> ing and comprehending, torpor
Fear, evil, of
> people, of; anthropophobia
Forgetful
Hurry, haste
Hysteria
Impatience
Indifference, apathy
Indolence, aversion to work
Irresolution, indecision
Irritabillity
Loquacity
Memory, weakness of
Mood, alternating
Prostration of mind, mental exhaustion,
> brain-fag
Restlessness
Sadness, despondency, dejection, mental
> depression, gloom, melancholy

Sensitive, noise, to
Sits, still
Timidity
Weeping, tearful mood

BARYTA MURIATICA

Anger, irascibility
Answers, confusedly as though thinking
> of something else
Anxiety
> *evening*
> *future, about*
> stooping amel. •
Childish behavior
Company, aversion to; presence of other
> people agg. the symptoms; de-
> sire for solitude
Concentration, difficult
> studying, reading etc., while
Confusion of mind
Cowardice
Death, presentiment of
Delusion, changed, everthing is
> knees, he walks on
> strange, everything is
>> familiar things seem
> walks, knees, on his, he
**Dullness, sluggishness, difficulty of
> thinking and comprehend-
> ing, torpor**
> *children, in*
Fear, apprehension, dread
> evil, of
> men, dread, fear of
Foolish, behavior
Idiocy
Imbecility
Indifference, apathy
Insanity, madness
> **erotic**
Irresolution, indecision
Irritability
> evening
Mania
Nymphomania
Play, aversion to play in children
> sit in corner, and

Prostration of mind, mental exhaustion,
  brain-fag
Sadness, despondency, dejection, mental
  depression, gloom, melancholy
    morning
Sit, inclination to
Sits, still
Starting, startled
  easily
Strange, everything seems
Suspicious, mistrustful
Talk, indisposed to, desire to be silent,
  taciturn
Talking, sleep, in
Timidity
Unconsciousness, coma, stupor

BARYTA PHOSPHORICA

Impulse, walk, to ★

BARYTA SULPHURICA

Air, mental symptoms amel. in open ●
Anxiety, evening, bed, in
    night
    midnight, before
  fear, with
  fever, during
  future, about
Capriciousness
Censorious, critical
Company, aversion to; presence of other
    people agg. the symptoms; de-
    sire for solitude
Concentration, difficult
Confusion, morning
    evening
    air, amel. in open
Cowardice
Desires more than she needs
Fear, evening
    conversation, of ●
    crowd, in a
    death, of
    evil, of
    people, of; anthropophobia

Forgetful, words while speaking, of; word
    hunting
Frightened easily
    noon, nap, after
Hurry, haste
Hysteria, grief, from
Imbecility
Impatience
Indifference, apathy
Indolence, aversion to work
Irritability
    evening
Lamenting, bemoaning, wailing
Loquacity
Memory, weakness of
Moaning, groaning, whining
Suspicious, mistrustful
Talking, sleep, in
Timidity, bashful
Unconsciousness, coma, stupor
    periodical
Weeping, tearful mood
    night
Will, loss of
Work, aversion to mental

BARTFELDER AQUA

Anxiety, coffee, after
Serious, earnest
Thoughts, thoughtful

BELLADONNA

Absent-minded, unobserving
Absorbed, buried in thought
Abstraction of mind
Abusive, insulting
Activity, mental
Admonition agg.
    kindly agg.
Affections, in general ★
Ailments from :
    ambition, deceived
    anger, vexation
    anxiety, with
    fright, with
    silent grief, with

Ailments from :
   excitement, emotional
     moral ★
   fear
   fright
   grief
   injuries, accidents, mental symp-
     toms from
   love, disappointed
     unhappy
   mortification
   scorn, being scorned
   work, mental
Amorous
Anger, irascibility
   alternating with weeping
   cough, before
     from anger
   easily
   face, red
   himself, with
   mistakes, about his
   trifles, at
   violent
   waking, on
Anguish
     noon •
     evening
   cardiac
   menses, during
   walking in open air
   weeping, with •
Answers
   aversion to
   foolish
   hastily
   incoherently
   incorrectly
   irrelevantly
   monosyllable
   refuses to answer
Antics, plays
   delirium, during
   drunkenness, during

Anxiety
   daytime
   afternoon
   evening
   night
   air, in open
   alternating with rage •
   company, when in
   crowd, in a
   eating, after
   fear, with
   fever, during
   fits, with
   headache, with
   hypochondriacal
   menses, during
     anger and anxiety
   paroxysms, in ★
   pressure in the chest, from •
   shuddering, with
   sleep, during
   stooping, when
   waking, on
   walking, while
     air, in open
   weary of life, with
Audacity
Automatism, motions (automatic) ★
Aversion, men, to
Barking
   bellowing
   delirium, during
   growling like a dog
Battles, talks about
   war, talks of
Begging, entreating, supplicating
Benevolence
Beside oneself, being
Bite, desire to
     night •
   around him, bites those •
   children, in •
   delirium, during
   objects, bites
   people, bites
   spoon etc., bites •
Boaster, braggart

Break things, desire to
Brooding
    corner or moping, brooding in a
Business, talks of
Calculating, inability for
Capriciousness
Carried, desires to be
    fast
Censorious, critical
Chaotic, confused behavior
Cheerful, gay, mirthful
    evening
    night
    alternating with dancing •
    mania
    moaning
    sadness
    weeping
    dancing, laughing, singing, with
    eating, while
    followed by sleepiness
    foolish, and
    prespiration, during
    quarrelsome, and
    sleep, during
Childbed, mental symptoms during
Childish behavior
Company, aversion to; presence of other
    people agg. the symptoms; desire
    for solitude
    friends, of intimate
    loathing at company
    perspiration, during
Company, desire for; aversion to solitude,
    company amel.
    alone agg., while
Complaining
    sleep, in
Comprehension, easy
Concentration, difficult
    studying, reading, etc., while
Confidence, want of self
Confusion of mind
    morning
        rising and after, on
    evening
    air, in open, amel.

Confusion of mind
    beer, from
    dream, as if in
    drinking, after
    eating, after
    intoxicated, as if
        as after being
    motion, from
    rising, after
    sitting, while
    smoking, after
    spirituous liquors, from
    walking, while
    warm room, in
Consolation, kind words agg.
Contradiction, is intolerant of
Contrary
Conversation, aversion to
Coquettish, not enough
    too much
Cowardice
Crawling on floor
Credulous
Croaking, sleep, in •
Cruelty, inhumanity
    loves to make people and ani-
    mals suffer ★
Cursing, swearing
Dancing
    alternating with moaning •
    wild
Death, conviction of
    desires
        alternating with rage •
        anguish, from •
        anxiety, from
        rage, during intervals from •
        walking in open air, while •
    presentiment of
Deceitful, sly
    fraudulent
Defiant
Delirium
    noon
    evening
    night

Delirium,

   anxious
   arms, throws about •
   bed and escapes, springs up sud-
      denly from
   busy
   carotids pulsating, with •
   chill, during
   closing the eyes, on
   congestion, with
   constant
   convulsions, during
      after
   crying, with
   delusions, with
   dogs, talks about •
   eating amel.
   extravagant language, with •
   face, livid •
      red
   fantastic
   fear of men, with
   fever, during
   fierce
   foolish, silly
   frightful
   furious ★
   gather objects off the wall, tries to
   gay, cheerful
   grimaces, with •
   head, with hot
   haemorrhage, after
   home, wants to go
   hysterical, almost
   injuries to head, after
   jumping, with
   laughing
   loquacious
      indistinct
   maniacal
   menses, before
      during
   moaning, with
   mouth, move lips as if talking •
   muttering
      himself, to

Delirium,

   naked in delirium, wants to be
   noisy
   paroxysmal
   periodic
   pupils, with dilated
   rabid
   raging, raving
   rambling
   recognizes no one
   rocking to and fro
   running, with
   sad
   sleep, during
      falling asleep, on
      after, amel.
   sleepiness, with
   sleeplessness, and ★
   sorrowful
   teeth, grinding •
   terror, expressive of
   trembling, with
   urinates out side the pot •
   violent
   vivid
   waking, on
   water, jumping into
   wild
Delirium tremens, mania-a-potu
   delusions, with
   escape, attempts to
   face, with red, bloated
Delusions, imaginations, hallucina-
      tions, illusions
      evening, falling asleep, on
      night
   activity, with
   animals, of
      beetles, worms etc.
      black animals on walls and fur-
         niture •
      dark colored •
      fire, in the •
      frightful
      persons are, rats, mice, insects
         etc.
      unclean animals •
   arrested, is about to be

Delusions,

assembled things, swarms, crowds
etc.
bats, of ●
beautiful
  things look
bed, bouncing her up and down,
  someone
  sinking, is
  take away the bedclothes, some-
    one tries to ●
  under it, someone is
  knocking
birds, sees
black objects and people, sees
blind, he is
body, putrefy, will
  sink down between the thighs,
    body will ●
  spotted brown, is ●
bulls, of ●
butterflies, of
business, is doing
  ordinary, they are pursuing
butterflies, of
calls, someone
  waking, someone calls on
cats, sees
  black
caught, he will be ●
churchyard, visits a
cockroaches swarmed about the
  room ●
conversing, delusions with
criminals, about
cucumbers, sees on the bed ●
cut through, he is, in two
dead, tall yellow corpse, trying to
  share bed with him and
  promptly ejected ●
  persons, sees
devils, sees
  taken by the devil, he will be
die, he was about to
  time has come to
divided into two parts
  cut in two parts, or

Delusions,

dogs, sees
  black
  he is a dog, growls and barks
  swarm about him
doomed, being
dreaming when awake, imagines
  himself ●
drinking ●
engaged in some occupation, is
● ordinary occupation, in
enlarged
  eyes are
faces, sees
  closing eyes, on
  hideous
falling asleep, on
fancy, illusions of
fiery ●
figures, sees
fire, visions of
  home, on distant ●
  house, on
fishes, flies, etc, sees
floating in air
      evening ●
  bed, swimming in
flying, sensation of
foolish
fright, after
gallows with fear of, vision of ●
gathering objects from pictures and
  walls, making efforts at ●
giants, sees ●
great person, is a
grief and anger, from
groans, with
gun, uses a stick for a ●
head, friend's h. stick out of a bottle,
  sees ●
  shaking the
  transparent and speckled
  brown ●
hearing, illusions of
herbs, gathering
home, away from, is

horses, sees
images, phantons, sees
 night
 black
 closing eyes, on
 dark, in the
 frightful
 pleasant
inanimate objects are persons
injury, is about to receive
insects, sees
 shining •
insulted, he is
journey, he is on a
juggler, he is a •
lascivious
loquacity, with
ludicrous, antics
magician, is a •
masks, sees
 laughing, sees (at night in bed) •
mice, sees
money, he is counting
mortification, after
murdered, he will be
noise, hears
 bed, under •
nose, has a transparent •
objects, brilliantly colored
 glittering •
 seize objects, tries to
officer, he is an
people, sees
 behind him, someone is
 beside him, are
 closing eyes, sees people on
 converses with absent
persecuted, he is
pleasing, morning after sleep •
police man, physician is a •
poor, he is
possessed, being
pursued by enemies
 he was
 police, by
 soldiers, by
rats, sees

Delusions,
 religious
 riding, ox, on an •
 room walls, horrible things on the,
  sees
 sensations, misrepresents his •
 serpent fastening on his neck., a
  crimson •
 shoot with a cane, tries to
 sick, being
 sight and hearing, of
 snakes in and around her
 soldiers, sees
 spectres, ghosts, spirits, sees
  closing eyes, on
  fire, in •
 stabbed a person who passed on
  the street, he had •
 strange, familiar things seem
 strangers, room is full of strange
  men, who snatch at her •
 surrounded by friends, is
 talking, dead people, with
   sister, with his
    church yard, in •
  imaginary persons, loudly and
   incoherently to
  spirits, with
 thieves, sees
 tongue, pulling out his, someone is •
 touching everything •
 transparent, head and nose are
 travelling, of
 trees seem to be people in fantastic
  costume (afternoon, while
 riding) •
 turtles in room, sees large •
 unpleasant
  distinct from surrounding objects
 vexation, after
 violent
 visions, has
  daytime
  beautiful
  closing the eyes, on

Delusions,
  horrible
     dark, in the
     monsters, of
  vivid
  voices, hears
     dead people, of
     distant
     strangers, of
  war, being at
  washing, of
  wealth, of
  well, he is
  whistling, with
  wolves, of
  work, hard at, is
Dementia
  epileptics, of
  senilis
Desires, exercise, for
Despair
  chill, during
  heat, during
Destructiveness
  clothes, of
  drunkeness, during
Dipsomania, alcoholism
Discontented displeased, dissatisfied
  everything, with
  himself, with
Discouraged
Doubtful, soul's welfare, of
Dream, as if in a
Drinking, mental symptoms after
Dullness, sluggishness, difficulty of
  thinking and compreheding,
  torpor
  alternating with dim vision ●
  chill, during
  dreams, after
  drunken , as if
  heat, during ★
  waking, on
Eat, refuses to
  spoon, cannot eat with a ●
Eccentricity
Ecstasy

Escape, attempts to
  run away, to
  springs up suddenly from bed
  street, into, gesticulating and
     dancing in their shirts ●
  window, from
Estranged, ignores his relatives
Excitement, excitable
  eating amel. ●
  perspiration, during
Exertion, agg. from mental
Exhilaration
Extravagance
Extremes, goes to ★
Exuberance
Fancies, exaltation of
  business, of ●
  closing the eyes in bed
     sleeplessness, with
  lascivious
  sleep, falling asleep, on
  vivid, lively
Fear, apprehension, dread
     night
  alone, of being
     lest he die
  alternating with mania ●
     rage ●
  animals, of
     apoplexy, of
  approaching him, of others
  crowd, in a
  dark, of
  death, of
     alone, when
     impending death, of
  dogs, of
  escape, with desire to
  everything, constant of
  evil, of
  gallows, of the ●
  ghosts, of
  imaginary things, of
     animals, of ●
  jumps out of bed from fear
     touch, on ●
  lightning, of

Fear,
- men, dread, fear of
- near, of those standing ●
- *noise, from*
- overpowering
- paralysis, of
- people, of; anthropophobia
- *poisoned, of being*
- putrefy, body will ●
- robbers, of
- solitude, of
- starting, with
- *touch, of*
- *tremulous*
- *waking, on*
  - under the bed, of something ●
- *water, of*

Feigning sick

Fight, wants to

Fire, wants to set things on

Foolish, behavior

Forgetful
- chill, during
- headache, during
- purchases, of; goes off and leaves them

Fright, menses during ●

Frightened easily
- *waking, on*

Frivolous

Gamble (*see* Play)

Gestures, makes
- **breaks pins**
  - *sticks*
  - *clapping of the hands*
  - convulsive
    - drink, at sight of ●
  - drinking, as if ●
  - *grasping or reaching at something, at flocks; carphologia*
  - bystanders, at
  - *picks at bed clothes*
  - hands, motions, involuntary of the
    - *hasty* ●
    - throwing about overhead

Gestures,
- plays with his fingers
- pouring from hand to hand, as if ●
- pulls hair of bystanders ●
- *ridiculous or foolish*
- usual vocation, of his
- *violent*

Grimaces

Grunting

Haughty, stupid and

Heedless

Hide, desire to
- *fear, on account of*

Hides things ●

Home, desires to go
- talks of home

Homesickness

Howling

Hurry, haste
- *drinking, on*
- eating, while
- *movements, in*

Hydrophobia
- *contact renews paroxysms* ●
- *prophylactic* ★

Hypochondriasis

Hysteria

Ideas abundant, clearness of mind
- deficiency of

Idiocy
- **bite, desire to**

Imbecility
- *sexual excitement, with*

Imitation, mimicry

Impatience
- heat, with

Impulse
- **fire, to set on** ★
- rash
- run, to; dromomania

Independent ★

Indifference, apathy
- alternating with sensitiveness ●
- everthing, to
- joyless
- perspiration, during

Indolence, aversion to work

Industrious, mania for work
> menses, before

Insanity, madness
> anger, from
> anxiety, with
> break pins, she will sit and
> busy
> cheerful, gay
> dancing, with
>> *and stripping himself* •
> *drunkards, in*
> eat, refuses to
> erotic
> *escape, desire to*
> *foolish, ridiculous*
> fortune, after gaining
> **fright, from**
> **grief, from**
> heat, with
> lamenting, moaning, only
> loquacious
> melancholy
> *menses, during*
> mortification, from
> *paroxysmal*
> *pregnancy, in*
> *puerperal*
> pulling his tongue out, clicking,
> distortion of face, with •
> religious
> restlessness, with
> *sleeplessness, with*
> *staring of eyes*
> *strength increased, with*
> suppressed eruptions, after
> travel, with desire to
> wantonness, with

Insolence
Intolerance, noise, of
Intriguer
Introspection
Irritability
> *morning, waking, on*
> alternating with indifference
>> weeping
> chill, during

Irritability,
> *consolation agg.*
> headache, during
> menses, during
> noise, from
> sleeplessness, with
> *trifles, from*
> *waking, on*

Jealousy, saying and doing what he
> wouldn't say and do

Jesting
> erotic
> ridiculous or foolish

Jumping
> **bed, out of**
>> *returning to bed continually,*
>> *and* •
>> *children, on chairs, table and stove* •

Kicks
> **sleep, in**

Kill, desire to
> drunkeness, during

Killed, desires to be
Kleptomania
Lamenting, bemoaning, wailing
> alternating with delirium •

Lascivious, lustful
Laughing
> *agg.*
> *alternating with groaning*
> annoying •
> *convulsions, before, during or after*
> grinning •
> immoderately
> involuntarily
> **loudly**
> paroxysmal
> **Sardonic**
> silly
> sleep, during
> *spasmodic*
> speaking, when

Libertinism
Light, desire for
Loathing, general

Loathing, life, at
Loquacity
    alternating with laughing
        silence
    insane
    perspiration, during
Love, disappointed, sadness from
Magnetized, desire to be, mesmerism
    amel.
Malicious, spiteful, vindictive
Mania
    demoniac
    jumps over chairs and tables ●
    rage, with
    scratching themselves ●
    shrieking, in
    singing, with
    spit and bite those around him,
        would ●
    tear, hair, own
    violence, with deeds of
Marriage, obsessed by idea of, excited
    sexual girls are
Mathematics, inapt for
Memory, active
    past events, for
Memory, weakness of
      pains, from, suddenly ★
    do, for what was about to
    expressing oneself, for
    facts, for
        past, for
        recent, for
    headache, during ●
    names, for proper
    persons, for
    read, for what has
    thought, for what has just
Menses, mental symptoms agg. during
Mental symptoms, physical, alternating
    with ★
Mildness
Misanthropy
Mistakes, localities, in
    speaking, in
    work, in

Moaning, groaning, whining
    alternating with dancing ●
    laughing
    songs, gambols ●
    breath, with every ★
    cough, during
    heat, during
    sleep, during
Mood, alternating
    changeable, variable
    opinions, in
    repulsive
Moonlight, mental symptoms from
Moral feeling, want of
    criminal, disposition to become a;
        without remorse
Morose, cross, fretful, ill-humor, peevish
    morning, bed, in
        waking, on
    alternating with weeping ●
    trifles, at
    waking, on
Morphinism
Mutilating his body
Muttering
    evening
Naive
Naked, wants to be
    delirium, in
Noise, inclined to make a
Nymphomania
    puerperal
Objective, reasonable
Obscene, lewd
    talk
Obstinate, headstrong
    children
Offended, easily; takes everything in bad
    part
Passionate
Play
    desire to, hide and seek, at ●
    passion for gambling
    to make money
Pleasure lascivious ideas, only in ●
Pompous, important

Praying
Pregnancy, mental affections in
Prostration of mind, mental exhaustion, brain-fag
Pull one's hair, desires to
    teeth, one's ●
Quarrelsome, scolding
    anger, without
    pugnacious
    sleep, in
Quiet disposition
        alternating with gaiety, trilling, singing
Quiet, wants to be
    repose and tranquillity, desires
Rage, fury
    evening
    night
    alternating with anxiety ●
    cheerfulness
    desire for death ●
    fear ●
    biting, with
    convulsions, rage with
    drinking, while
    epilepsy, rage with
    headache, with
    know his relatives, does not
    malicious
    medicine, from forcible administration of ●
    menses, during
    parturition, during ●
    pulls hair of bystanders ●
    relatives, does not know his ★
    shining objects, from
    shrieking, with
    spitting, with
    staring looks, with ●
    strength increased
    touch, renewed by
    violent
    water, at sight of
Recognize, relatives, does not recognize his
Refuses, treatment, every

Religious affections
Remorse
Reserved
Rest, desire for
Restlessness
    morning
    noon
    night
    anxious
    bed, driving out of
        go from one bed to another, wants to
        tossing about in
    busy
    children roving, wandering
    chill, during
    drink, at the sight of ●
    driving about
    headache, during
    heat, during
    menses, during
    move, must constantly
    pain, from
    stool, during ●
    waking, on
Roving, senseless, insane
Rudeness
Runs about
    against things ●
    shirt, in ●
Sadness, despondency, dejection, mental depression, gloom, melancholy
    night
    anger, after
    continence, from
    heat, during
    love, from disappointed
    menses, before
    perspiration, during
    puerperal
    sexual excitement, with
    waking, on
Scratches with hands
Selfishness, egoism
Self-torture

Senses, acute
  confused
  dull, blunted
  vanishing of
Sensitive, oversensitive
  children
  heat, during
  light, to
  noise, to
    chill, during
    labor, during
    slightest, to
  odors, to
  pain, to
  perspiration, during
  puberty, in
  want of sensitiveness
Serious, earnest
Shamelessness
Shining objects agg.
Shrieking, screaming, shouting
  brain cry
  children, in
    consolation agg. •
    sleep, duiring
  convulsions, before
    between
  cough agg.
  hoarse
  pain, with the
  sleep, during
Sighing
  alternating with dancing and
    jumping •
  heat, during
  sleep, in
Singing
  night
  alternating with groaning •
    weeping
  fever, during
  sleep, in
  trilling
Sit, inclination to
Sits and breaks pins
Slander, disposition to

Slowness
Smiling
  foolish
  involuntarily
  sardonic •
Somnambulism
Speech, affected
  confused
  delirious
    sleep, in •
  foolish
  hasty
  incoherent
    evening •
    night ★
  loud
    sleep, in
  low
  nonsensical
  prattling
  slow
  unintelligible
  violent
  wandering
    night
Spit, desire to
  faces of people, in
Squanders
Staring ★
Starting, startled
  asleep, on falling
  falling, as if
  fright, from and as from
  sleep, falling, on
    during
    from
  touched, when
  waking, on
Strange, crank
Striking
  about him at imaginary objects
  bystanders, at
  desire to strike
Striking himself
  abdomen, his •
  face, his •
  knocking his head against wall
  and things

Stupefaction, as if intoxicated
  air, in open, amel.
  head, from congestion of the ●
  sleepiness, with
  vertigo, during
Suicidal disposition
  drowning, by
  drunkenness, during
  hanging, by
  heat, during
  knife, with
  love, disappointed, from ★
  pains, from
  poison, by
  stabbing, by
  throwing himself from a height
  window, from
  walking in open air, while ●
Superstitious
Suppressed or receding skin diseases or
  haemorrhoids, mental symp-
  toms agg. after
Suspicious, mistrustful
Sympathy, compassion
Talk, indisposed to, desire to be silent,
  taciturn
  alternating with loquacity
  slow learning to
Talking, sleep, in
  confess themselves loud, they
  loud
Talks, dead people, with
  fast ★
  himself, to
Tastes everything ●
Tears things
  hair, her
  himself
  night-dress and bed colthes
Thoughts, business at evening in bed, of
  persistent
  profound
  rapid, quick
  rush, flow of
  sexual
  thoughtful

Thoughts,
  vanishing of
    chill, during
    headache, during ●
  wandering
    night ●
Throws things, persons, at
Timidity
  bashful
Torments, himself
Touch everything, impelled to
Touched, aversion to being
Tranquillity, serenity, calmness
Travel, desire to
Unconsciousness, coma, stupor
  morning
  night
  chill, during
  convulsions, after
  fever, during
  interrupted by screaming ●
  screaming, interrupted by
  sitting, while
  sunstroke, in
  twitching of limbs, with
  vertigo, during
Unreliable, promises, in his
Vanity
Violent, vehement
  deeds of violence, rage leading to
  sick, when ●
Walks, circle, in a
Wanders, restlessly, about
Wearisome
Weary of life
  air, in open
  heat, during
  walking in open air ●
Weeping, tearful mood
  morning
  afternoon
  night
  admonition, from
  agg.
  alternating with cheerfulness
  dancing ●

Weeping, alternating with
- ill-humor
- laughter
- singing
- vexation •
- anger, after
- anxiety, after
- causeless
- *children, in*
- babies, in
- **chill, during**
- consolation agg.
- convulsions, from •
- *convulsions, during*
- **coughing, before**
- *during*
- after
- *easily*
- eating, while, children, in
- **heat, during**
- *involuntary*
- pains, with the
- **perspiration, during**
- refused, when anything is
- remonstrated, when
- sleep, in
- spasmodic
- trifles, at ★
- waking, on
- walking in open air, when
- whimpering

Well, says he is, when very sick
Whistling
Wildness
Work, aversion to mental

BELLIS PERENNIS

Confusion of mind
  surroundings, of
Dullness, sluggishness, difficulty of thinking and comprehending, torpor
Excitement, excitable
Idiocy
Irritability
Restlessness
Slowness

BENZINUM

Censorious, critical
Delusions, hand, vision of white, outspread hand coming towards face in the darkness •
Despair
Weeping, tearful mood

BENZINUM NITRICUM

Dwells on past disagreeable occurrences, night
Excitement, excitable
Irritability
Loquacity
Restlessness, bed, tossing about in
Sighing
Speech, confused
Thoughts, disagreeable, night •
Unconsciousness, coma, stupor

BENZOICUM ACIDUM

Activity, work, at •
Anxiety
  mental exertion, from
  sitting, while
Carried, desires to be
  laid down, will not be (children) ★
Confusion of mind
Delusions, voices, hears
  confused (swallowing or walking in open air agg.)
Dwells on past disagreeable occurrences
Excitement, excitable
Fear, hurry followed by fear •
Forgetful, words while speaking, of; word hunting
Frightened easily
Grief
Hurry, haste
  agg.
Hypochondriasis
Hysteria
Irritability, children, in
Loathing, general

Mistakes, writing, in
    words
Morose, children, desire to be carried
Sadness, despondency, dejection, men-
    tal depression, gloom, melan-
    choly
Shrieking, children, in
Starting, startled
    sleep, during
      from
Thoughts, disagreeable
    persistent ★
Unconsciousness, coma, stupor

BENZOLUM

Delusions, sinking, to be

BERBERIS VULGARIS

Absent minded, unobserving
Abstraction of mind
Ailments from :
    quarrels
Anger, irascibility
Anxiety
      evening, bed, in
    bed, in
    fear, with
    fever, during
    motion, from
    rising from a seat, on
    sleep, before
      evening ●
    standing, while
    stool, before
Concentration, difficult
    interrupted, if
Confusion of mind
    interruption, from
    waking, on
Courageous
Darkness agg.
Death, desires
    menses, during ●

Delusions, imaginations, hallucinations,
    illusions
    enlarged
      head is
    fancy, illusions of
    images, phantoms, sees
      night
    longer, things seem
    spectres, ghosts, spirits, sees, in
    twilight ●
    tall; things grow taller
      pulse is throbbing, as the
      and diminish ●
Discontented, displeased, dissatisfied
Dullness, sluggishness, difficulty of think-
    ing and comprehending, torpor
    morning
      waking, on
    sleep, after sound
      waking, on
Ecstasy
Ennui, menses, during ●
Excitement, night
      waking, on
Exertion, agg. from mental
Fear, apprehension, dread
    afternoon
    evening
      twilight
Forgetful, morning
Frightened easily
Hurry, eating, while
Indifference, apathy
    external things, to
Indolence, aversion to work
    sadness, from
Insanity, madness
Irritability
    menses, before
      during
      after
    waking, on
    walking, when
Loathing, life, at
Malicious, spiteful, vindictive
Meditation
Memory, weakness of

Menses, mental symptoms agg. during
Morose, cross, fretful, ill-humor, peevish
Prostration of mind, mental exhaustion,
    brain-fag
      morning
Reflecting
Sadness, despondency, dejection, mental
    derpression gloom, melancholy
  menses, before
    during
  work shy, in
Sits, supporting body, hands, with ★
Starting, startled
Talk, indisposed to, desire to be silent,
  taciturn
Thinking, aversion to
Thoughts, disconnected
  vanishing of
    interrupted, when
Torpor
Twilight agg. mental symptoms
Unconsciousness, riding, while
Weary of life
  menses, before ●
    during ●
Weeping, tearful mood
Work, aversion to mental
  impossible
    interruption, by least ●

BISMUTHUM SUBNITRICUM

Anguish
  **driving from place to place,
  restlessness, with**
Anxiety
  waking, on
Aversion, everything, to
Cheerful, evening
Clinging to persons or furniture etc.
  take the hands of mother, will always ●
**Company, desire for; aversion to
  solitude, company amel.**
    alone, agg. while

Complaining
Confusion of mind, morning
  intoxicated, as if
Delirium
Delirium tremens, mania-a-potu
Delusions, imaginations, hallucinations,
  illusions
  fancy, illusions of
Dipsomania, alcoholism
Discontented, displeased, dissatisfied
  everything, with
Dullness, sluggishness, difficulty of think-
  ing and comprehending, torpor
  forenoon
  reading, while
Fear, apprehension, dread
  alone, of being
  solitude, of
  waking, on
Frightened easily
  waking, on
Hypochondriasis
Inconstancy
indifference, apathy
  everything, to
Indolence, evening amel.
Introspection
Irresolution, indecision
  changeable
Irritability
  daytime
  evening, amel.
Lamenting, bemoaning, wailing
Mood, alternating
  changeable, variable
Moral feeling, want of
Morose, cross, fretful, ill humor, peevish
Quiet disposition
Reserved
Restlessness
  night
  anxious
  bed, driving out of
  driving, about
Sadness, evening amel.

Starting, startled
    midnight in sleep, before
  easily
  falling, as if
  sleep, on falling
    during
    from
Stupefaction, as if intoxicated
Talk, indisposed to, desire to be silent,
    taciturn
      evening amel.
Unconsciousness, coma, stupor
Undertakes many things, perseveres in
    nothing
Unfeeling, hard hearted
Wearisome
Will, weakness of

BLATTA AMERICANA

Indolence, aversion to work

BOLETUS LARICIS

Absent minded, unobserving
Bilious disposition
Change, dislike of •
Dulllness, sluggishness, difficulty of think-
    ing and comprehending, torpor
Irritabillity
Memory, weakness of
Morose, cross, fretful, ill-humor, peevish
Restlessness
    night
Sadness, despondency, dejection, men-
    tal depression, gloom, melan-
    choly
    heat, during

BOLETUS LURIDUS

Delirium

BOLETUS SATANAS

Discomfort
Restlessness

BOLDO

Delusions; hearing, illusions of

BOMBYX PROCESSIONEA

Delirium

BONDONNEAU AQUA

Anger, irascibility
Anxiety
Excitement, nervous
Irritability
Morose, cross, fretful, ill-humor, peevish

BORAX VENETA

Abusive, insulting
Activity, fruitless ★
Affectionate
Anger, irascibility
    violent
Anxiety
    evening
      untill 23h. •
    night
      children, in
    children, in, when being put in the
      cradle ★
      rocking, during •
    dancing, when •
    motion, from
      aeroplane, of •
      cable-railway, of •
      downward
      lift, of •
    riding, while
      down hill
      rocking, during •
    stool, before
      after
    trifles, about
    waking, on
Awkward ★
Busy, fruitlessly
Carried, desires to be
Censorious, critical

Cheerful, gay, mirthful
    morning
    forenoon
    evening, bed, in
    alternating with vexation
    stools, after
Clinging to persons or furniture etc.
    child awakens terrified, knows
        no one, screams, clings to
        those near
    grasps the nurse when carried
Comprehension, easy
Confusion of mind
    evening
    mental exertion, from
    stool amel.
    walking, while
Contented
    afternoon after stool •
Cursing, swearing
Dancing agg.
Delusions, devils, possessed of a devil, is
    robbed, is going to be
Dipsomania, alcoholism
Discontented, displeased, dissatisfied
    afternoon, stool, before •
    stool, before •
Dullness, sluggishness, difficulty of think
    ing and comprehending, torpor
    morning
    walking, air amel., in open
Eat, refuses to
Ennui, tedium
Excitement, excitable
    evening, bed, in
    agg.
Exertion, agg. from mental
Exhilaration, coition, after •
Fancies, exaltation, night
    sleeplessness, with
Fear, apprehension, dread
    children, in, night
    disease, of impending
    downward motion, of
    falling, of
    infection, of

Fear,
    menses, before
    noise, from
        sudden, of
    riding in a carriage, when
    thunderstorm, of
    trifles, of
    waking, on
Forgetful
Frightened easily
    sneezing, at •
    trifles, at
    waking, on
Gestures, grasping or reaching at some-
    thing, at flocks; carphologia
    mother in sleep, at
Hysteria
Ideas abundant, clearness of mind
    night
Idiocy, shrill shrieking, with
Inconstancy
Indifference, apathy
    irritating disagreeable things, to
Indolence, aversion to work
    afternoon
    siesta, after
    sleep, after
    stool, before •
Insanity, madness
Irritability
    afternoon
        16h. •
    night
    air, in open
    alternating with cheerfulness
    business, about
        important, in an •
    children, in
    chill, during
    eating, after
    stool before
    walking, when
Jesting, aversion to
Lascivious, lustful

Laughing
> **agg.**
> *involuntarily*

Loquacity
Malicious, spiteful, vindictive
Memory, weakness of
> done, for what has just

Mildness
Mistakes, space and time, in
> time, in

Moaning, groaning, whining
> *morning* ●
> children, in

Mood, alternating
> *changeable, variable*
> **epistaxis amel.** ●

Morose, cross, fretful, ill-humor, peevish
> afternoon
> night
> air, in open
> alternating with cheerfulness
> laughing
> children, in
> *eating, after*
> fever, during
> *stool, before*
> waking, on

Nosebleed amel. mental symptoms ●
Offended easily; takes everything in bad
> part

Quarrelsome, scolding
Quiet, wants to be
> repose & tranquility, desires; on
> walking in open   air

Rebels against poultice
Reproaches, others
> 16 h ●

Reserved, walking in open air, while
Restlessness
> night
> bed, tossing about in
> children, in
> chill, during
> eating, when
> menses, during
> mental labor, during and after
> stretching backward amel. ●
> talking, after

Rocking agg.
Sadness, despondency, dejection, mental
> depression, gloom, melancholy

Senses, acute
> vanishing of

Sensitive, oversensitive
> children
> **noise, to**
> > labor, during
> > *slightest, to*
> > sudden reports ●

Serious, earnest
Shrieking, screaming, shouting
> **. children, in**
> > nursed, when being
> > sleep, during
> > waking, on ●
> **sleep, during**
> > stool, before ●
> **urinating, before**

Sit, inclination to
Slander, disposition to
Starting, startled
> *anxious, downward motion, from* ●
> **easily**
> **fright, from and as from**
> **hawking of others, at** ●
> *menses, during*
> **noise, from**
> *sleep, during*
> > **from**
> **sneezing of others, at** ●
> *trifles, at*

Stupefaction, chill, during
> conversation, after animated ●

Suspicious, mistrustful
Talk, indisposed to, desire to be silent,
> taciturn
> heat, during
> slow learning to

Talking agg. all complaints
Thoughts, rush, flow of
> *night*
> sleeplessness, from
> waking, on
> thoughtful
> vanishing of

Thunderstorm, during, mind symptoms
Time, fritters away his
Timidity
Tranquillity
    stool, after •
Unconsciousness, fever, during
    vertigo, during
Undertakes many things, perseveres in
    nothing
Violent
Weary of life, alternating with cheerful-
    ness •
Weeping, tearful mood
    morning
    night
    agg.
    alternating with cheerfulness
        laughter
    child cries when rocked or nursed ★
    children, in
        night
    babies
    coughing, before
    sleep, in
    stool, during
    urination, before
    waking, on
Work, aversion to mental
    impossible

BOTHROPS LANCEOLATUS

Aphasia ★
Confusion of mind
Forgetful, words while speaking, of;
    word hunting
Mistakes, speaking, using wrong words,
    in
Restlessness
Unconsciousness, coma, stupor

BOVISTA LYCOPERDON

Absent-minded, unobserving
Absorbed, buried in thought
Abstraction of mind

Ailments from :
    sexual excesses
Anger, irascibility
    morning
    afternoon
    evening
    alternating with exhilaration
    work, aversion to
Anguish
Anxiety
    afternoon
    evening
    night
    fever, during
    headache, with
    inactivity, with
Audacity
Aversion, everything, to
Capriciousness
    morning
    evening
Chaotic, confused behavior
Cheerful, gay, mirthful
    morning
    company, in •
Company, aversion to; presence of other
    people agg. the symptoms; de
    sire for solitude
    alone, amel. when
Company, desire for; aversion to soli-
    tude, company amel.
    alone, agg. while
Concentration, difficult
    attention, cannot fix ★
Confusion of mind
    morning
    evening
    breakfast, amel. after
    coition, after
    rising, after
    sprituous liquors, from
    standing, while
    stooping, when
    waking, on
    wine, after

Courageous
Cursing, swearing
Delirium, look fixed on one point, staring
    pains, with the
Delusions, enlarged, distances are
        head, is
            objects are
        heart, large, too
        large, parts of body seem too
        spectres, ghosts, spirits, sees
        strange, familiar things seem
        swollen, he is
        vermin, sees, crawl about
        water, of
        worms, creeping of
Despair
    alternating with hope
Dipsomania, alcoholism
Discontented, displeased, dissatisfied
    eating, after
Dullness, sluggishness, difficulty of
    thinking and comprehending,
    torpor
        standing agg.
        waking, on
Exhilaration, morning
Fear, disease, of impending
    insanity, losing his reason, of
    pins, pointed things, of
    waking, dream, from a
Fight, wants to
Frogetful
Grief
Heedless
Hurry, haste
Ideas, deficiency of
Imbecility
Indifference, apathy
    company, society, while in
        amel. •
    everything, to
    external things, to
    life, to
    morose
Indiscretion
Indolence, aversion to work
    eating, after
    sadness, from

Insanity, madness
Introspection
Irritability
    morning
        waking, on
    afternoon
    evening
    coition, after
    headache, during
    sadness, with
    takes everything in bad part
    waking, on
Jesting, aversion to
Lascivious, lustful
Laughing, asthma, with ★
Loathing, life, at
Looking, sky, at, reason, without ★
Loquacity
    openhearted
Memory, active
Memory, weakness of
    done, for what has just
Mildness
Mistakes, localities, in
    space and time, in
    speaking, in
        misplacing words
        words, using wrong
    time, in
    writing, in
        syllables
        wrong words
Mood, alternating
    changeable, variable
Morose, cross, fretful, ill-humor, peevish
    morning
    afternoon
    evening
    alternating with cheerfulness
    eating, after
Naive
Offended, easily; takes everything in bad
    part
Prostration of mind, mental exhaustion,
    brain-fag
Quarrelsome, scolding

Restlessness, evening
      night
      anxious
Sadness, despondency, dejection, mental
      depression, gloom, melancholy
      evening
      alone, when
      company, amel. in •
      work-shy, in
Secretive
Senses, dull, blunted
      vanishing of
Sensitive, oversensitive
Serious, earnest
Society, social functions amel. ★
Speech, jerks, by
Starting, dreams, from a
      sleep, during
         from
Striking
Stupefaction, as if intoxicated
      morning, rising, after
      evening
      vertigo, during
Sulky
Talk, indisposed to, desire to be silent,
      taciturn
Truth, tell the plain
Unconsciousness, coma, stupor
      morning
      dream, does not know where he is
      night •
      eyes, with fixed
      standing, while
      transient
      vertigo, during
Weeping alternating with laughter ★
Wearisome
Weary of life

BRACHYGLOTTIS REPENS

Irritabillity
Restlessness, night
Talking, sleep, in

BROMIUM

Activity, business, in
Answer, stupor returns quickly after
Anxiety
      health, about
Barking
Business, averse to
Capriciousness
Carried, desires to be
      croup, in •
      fast
Censorious, critical
Cheerful, gay, mirthful
Company, aversion to, sits in her room,
      does nothing, •
Company, desires for; aversion to soli-
      tude, company amel.
      evening
      alone agg., while
Comprehension, easy
Concentration, difficult
Confusion of mind
      night, lying down, on
      lying, when
      writing, while
Delirium
      anxious
      congestion, with
Delusions, dead persons, sees
      fasting
      images, phantoms, sees
      journey, he is on a
      jumped upon the ground before
        her, all sorts of things •
      people, sees
        behind him, someone is
      person is in the room, another
      shoulder, people are looking over
        his •
      spectres, ghosts, spirits, sees
        evening, a spectre will appear •
      strangers, looking over shoulder •
      vision, evening
Despair
Disconcerted

Discontented, displeased, dissatisfied
Discouraged
Excitement, excitable
Fear, apprehension, dread
      evening*
    alone, of being
      evening
    apoplexy, of
    behind him, someone is
    dark, of
    ghosts, of
      evening
    imaginary things, of
Forgetful
Howling
Hypochondriasis
Hysteria
    sexual, suppression of s. excitement,
    from ★
Imbecility
Inconsolable
Indifference, apathy
    duties, domestic, to
Indolence, aversion to work
Industrious, mania for work
Insanity, madness
Irritability
    waking, on
Lamenting, bemoaning, wailing
    hoarse ●
Mania
Memory, active
Memory, weakness of
Morose, cross, fretful, ill humor, peevish
    afternoon
    siesta, after
Quarrelsome, scolding
Reading, aversion to read
Rest, desire for
Sadness, despondency, dejection, mental
    depression, gloom, melancholy
    menses, before
      during
Sit, inclination to
Sits, still
Staring, thoughtless

Starting, startled
    sleep, during
Talk, indisposed to, desire to be silent,
    taciturn
Thoughts, thoughtful
Unconsciousness, coma, stupor
Weeping, tearful mood
Work, aversion to Mental
    desire for
    impossible

BRUCEA ANTIDYSENTERICA

Absorbed, buried in thought
Excitement, excitable
    evening
    trembling, with
Morose, morning
Quiet disposition
Sadness, morning
Stupefaction, as if intoxicated

BRYONIA

Activity
Affectionate
Affections, in general ★
Ailments from :
    anger, vexation
      anxiety, with
      silent grief, with
      anticipation, foreboding, presen-
      timent
      excitement, emotional
      fright
      grief
      hurry
      mortification
      scorn, being scorned
      violence
Anger, irascibility
    evening
    contradiction, from
    face, red
    trifles, at
    violent
Answers, hastily

Anxiety
 evening
  bed, in
 night
  midnight, before
 air, in open, amel.
 bed, in
  driving out of
 business, about
 causeless
 conscience, as if guilty of a crime
 do something, compelled to •
 driving from place to place
 fear, with
 fever, during
 future, about
 health, about
 house, in
 hypochondriacal
 thinking about it, from
 waking, on
Asks for nothing
Avarice
Bargaining
Bed, get out of, wants to
Business, talks of
Busy
Capriciousness
Carefulness
Change, desire for
Chaotic, confused behavior
Cheerful, gay, mirthful
Clinging, held, being, amel.
Company, aversion to; presence of other
 people agg. the symptoms; desire
 for solitude
 presence of strangers, aversion to
Company, desires for; aversion to soli-
 tude, company amel.
Complaining
Concentration, difficult
Confidence, want of self
Confusion of mind
 morning
  rising and after, on
  waking, on
 afternoon

Confusion of mind,
 air, in open, amel.
 drinking, after
 eructations amel.
 heat, during
 intoxicated, as after being
 lying, when
 motion, from
 riding, while
 rising, after
 sleeping, after
 standing, while
 waking, on
 walking, while
  air, in open, amel.
 yawning amel.
Conscientious about trifles
Contradiction, is intolerant of
 agg.
Contrary
Cowardice
Cruelty, inhumanity
Death, presentiment of
Delirium
 morning
  day break, at
 noon
 evening
 night
 bed and escapes, springs up suddenly from
 business, talks of
 busy
 closing the eyes, on
 fever, during
 furious ★
 heat agg.
 loquacious
 maniacal
 muttering
  sleep, in
 quiet
 raging, raving
 restless
 sleep, during
  comatose, during
  falling asleep, on

Delirium,
  sleepiness, with
  sleeplessness and ★
  trembling, with
  waking, on
  wild
Delusions, imaginations, hallucination,
    illusions
        morning
        evening
        night
  beaten, he is being
  bed, hard, too
    sinking, is
  business, is doing
  dead persons, sees
  delirious at night, expected to be-
    come ●
  faces, sees; closing eyes, on
  falling asleep, on
  fancy, illusions of
  figures, sees
  head, heavy, his own, seemed too ●
  home, away from, is
    away from, must get there
  injury; injured, is being
  people, sees
    closing eyes, sees people on
  pursued, he was
    soldiers, by
  soldiers, sees
    cutting him down (amel. on get-
      ting cool) ●
  spectres, sees, closing eyes, on
  strange land, as if in a
  strangers, control of, under
    friends appears as
    room, seem to be in the
  unfortunate, he is
  visions, closing the eyes, on
  work, she cannot accomplish the ●
    hard at work, is
Dementia, senilis
Desires, full of
  more than she needs
  present, things not
  unattainable things

Despair
  chill, during
  recovery, of
Dipsomania, alcoholism
Dirtiness, dirting everything
Discomfort
  eating, after
Discontented, displeased, dissatisfied
  himself, with
Discouraged
Dishonest
Disturbed, averse to being
Doubtful, recovery, of
Dream, as if in a
**Dullness, sluggishness, difficulty of
    thinking and comprehend-
    ing, torpor**
  chill, during
  heat, during
  lying, while ●
  motion agg. ●
  spoken to, when
  standing agg.
Ecstasy
Envy ·
Escape, attempts to
    run away, to
    window, from
Excitement, excitable
    noon
Fancies, exaltation of
    evening, bed, in
    night
    sleeplessness, with
Fear, apprehension, dread
  air, in open, amel.
  alone, of being
  death, of
    impending death, of
  disease, of impending
  escape, with desire to
  evil, of
  insanity, losing his reason, of
  misfortune, of
  motion, of
  poisoned, of being

Fear,
>   **poverty, of**
>   riding in a carriage, when
>   *starving, of*
>   stomach, arising from
>   suffering, of
>   *suffocation, of*
>   *thunderstorm, of*
>   *waking, on*

Forgetful
Frightened easily
Gestures hands, motions, involuntary,
>   of the
>   throwing about
>   waving in the air

Home, desires to go
>   *leave home, desire to*
>   *talks of home*

Homesickness
Hurry, haste
>   drinking, on

Hypochondriasis
Hysteria
>   menses, during

Ideas abundant, clearness of mind
>   evening, bed, in
>   deficiency of

Impatience
Impetuous
>   *perspiration, with*

Indifference, apathy
Indignation
Indiscretion
Indolence, aversion to work
Industrious, mania for work
>   menses, before

Insanity, loquacious
>   puerperal
>   restlessness, with
>   travel, with desire to

Insecurity, mental
Irresolution, indecision
Irritability
>   morning, waking, on
>   alone, wishes to be ●

Irritability
>   chill, during
>   alone, wishes to be ●
>   *cough, whooping, in*
>   *eating, after*
>   headache, during
>   *heat, during*
>   *liver trouble, in*
>   menses, during
>   perspiration, during
>   waking, on

Jesting
Jumping, bed, out of
Kleptomania
Lamenting, bemoaning, wailing
>   asleep, while

Malicious, spiteful, vindictive
Mania
Memory, weakness of
Mistakes, localities, in
Moaning, groaning, whining
>   perspiration, during
>   sleep, during

Mocking, sarcasm
Mood, changeable, variable
Morose, cross, fretful, ill humor,
>   **peevish**
>   morning
>   bed, in
>   *cough, whooping, in*
>   eating, after
>   waking, on

Music agg.
Muttering
Obstinate, headstrong
Passionate
Perseverance
Prostration of mind, mental exhaustion,
>   *brain-fag*

Quarrelsome, scolding
Quiet, disposition, heat, during
Quiet, wants to be
>   *amel.* ★
>   **chill, during**

Rage fury
Rebels against poultice

Resignation
Rest, desire for
Restlessness
   night
     midnight, after
     anxious
   bed, driving out of
     tossing about in
   busy
   children roving, wandering
   headache, during
   perspiration, during
Roving, senseless, insane
Sadness, despondency, dejection, mental
     depression, gloom, melancholy
   heat, during
   perspiration, during
Senses, dull, blunted
   vanishing of
Sensitive, oversensitive
   chill, during
   music, to
   noise, to
Shrieking, screaming, shouting
   cough, agg. ★
   pain, with the
   sleep, during
   waking, on
Sighing
   night ●
   heat, during
   perspiration, during
Sit, inclination to
Slowness
Somnambulism
   do day-labor, to
Speech, confused
   delirious, buisness, of ●
     waking, on ●
   foolish
   hasty
   incoherent
   prattling
     morning ●
   wandering
   night

Starting, startled
   asleep, on falling
   bed, in, while lying awake
   fright, from and as from
   sleep, falling, on
     during
     from
   waking, on
Strangers: presence of strangers agg.
Stupefaction, as if intoxicated
Suspicious, mistrustful
Talk, indisposed to, desire to be silent,
    taciturn
     perspiration, during
Talking, sleep, in
Thinking, aversion to
   complaints agg., of
Thoughts, persistent
   desires, of
   unpleasant subjects on waking
   rush, flow of
     evening, in bed
     night
     sleeplessness from
   vanishing of
     chill, during
     reading, on
Throws things away
Thunderstorm, mind symptoms before
   during, mind symptoms
Timidity
Touched, aversion to being
Ugly in behavior ★
Unconsciousness, coma, stupor
   morning
     rising, on ●
   evening
   delirium, after
   fever, during
   rising up, on
Unfortunate, feels
Ungrateful, avarice, from
Violent, vehement
   deeds of violence, rage leading to
Wearisome

Weeping, tearful mood
    daytime
    · night
    midnight, after
    coughing, before
    heat, during
    nervous, all day
    perspiration, during
    sleep, in
    whimpering, sleep, during
Well, before an attack, feels well ★
Will, weakness of

BUFO RANA

Absent-minded, unobserving
Ailments-from :
    fright
    love, disappointed
Anger, irascibility
    convulsions, before •
    misunderstood, when •
Anguish
Anxiety
    music, from
    waking, on
Bilious disposition
Bite, desire to
    objects, bites
Cheerful, gay, mirthful, evening
Childish, behavior
Child-like simplicity remains, while the
    body grows ↔
Company, aversion to; presence of other
    people agg. the symptoms; de-
    sire for solitude
    desire solitude to practise mastur-
    bation
    fear of being alone, yet
    presence of strangers, aversion to
Company, desire for; aversion to solitude,
    compony amel.
    alone agg., while
    yet fear of people
Complaining
    alternating with shrieking •

Concentration, difficult
Confusion of mind
    morning
    eating, after
    intoxicated, as if
Deceitful, sly
Delirium
    fever, during
    head, with hot
Delirium tremens, mania-a-potu
Delusions; fancy, illusions of
Despair
Destructiveness
Dipsomania, alcoholism
Dullness, sluggishness, difficulty of think-
    ing and comprehending, torpor
    evening, amel.
Excitement, excitable.
Fancies, exaltation of
Fear, apprehension, dread
    alone, of being
    animals, of
    crowd, in a
    death, of
    disease, of impending
    happen, something will
    infection, of
    mirrors in room, of
    misfortune, of
    music, from
    waking, on
Foolish behavior
Frightened easily
    trifles, at
Gestures, makes
    grasping, genitals, delirium, dur-
    ing ★
Giggling
Hysteria
Idiocy
    masturbation, with
Imbecility
Impatience
Indifference, apathy

Indolence, aversion to work
    afternoon
Insanity, madness
    erotic
    masturbation, from
Irresolution, indecision
Irritability
      morning, waking, on
      night, retiring, after
    menses, after
    waking, on
Lamenting, bemoaning, wailing
    alternating with crying ●
Lascivious, lustful
Laughing
    causeless
    childish
    serious matters, over
    spasmodic, epilepsy, before, dur-
      ing or after
    trifles, at
Loathing, general
Loquacity
Malicious, spiteful, vindictive
Mania
    erotic↔
Memory, weakness of
    done, for what has just
Mistakes, speaking, in
      misplacing words
      words, using wrong
Moaning, sleep, during
Mood, changeable, variable
Moral feeling, want of
Morose, cross, fretful, ill humor, peevish
    menses, after
Music agg.
    aversion to
Obscene, lewd
    talk
Offended, easily; takes everything in bad
    part.
Prostration of mind, mental exhaustion,
    brain-fag
      evening
Rage, fury
    alone, while ●

Restlessness, convulsions, before
    sleepiness, with
Runs about
Sadness, despondency, dejection, mental
    depression, gloom, melancholy
    waking, on
Senses,   ●
    vanishing of
Sensitive, oversensitive
    music, to
    noise, to
Shamelessness
Shining objects agg.
Shrieking, convulsions, before
    runs, shrieking through house ●
    sleep, during
    unconsciousness, until ●
Sighing, epileptic attacks, before
Speech, foolish
    nonsensical
    unintelligible
      convulsions, before epileptic ●
Starting, startled
    easily
    fright, from and as from
    noise, from
    sleep, during
      from
Strangers, presence of agg.
Strike, desire to
Stupefaction, as if intoxicated
    convulsions, between
    dinner, after
    vertigo, after ●
Suspicious, mistrustful
Symptoms, magnifies her ★
Talk, indisposed to, desire to be silent,
    taciturn
Talking, sleep, in
Ugly (in behavior) ★
Unconsciousness, coma, stupor
    conduct, automatic
    convulsions, after
    epilepsy, after
    transient

Weeping, tearful mood
   sleep, in
   trifles, at
   waking, on

BUFO SAHYTIENSIS

Cheerful, evening
Company, aversion to; presence of other
   people agg. the symptoms; de-
   sire for solitude
Discouraged
Fancies, exaltation of
Fear, people, of; anthropophobia
Forgetful, morning
       evening
Heedless
Imbecility
Indolence, aversion to work
   afternoon
Irresolution, indecision
   projects, in
Memory, weakness of
   happened, for what has
Sadness, despondency, dejection, mental
   depression, gloom, melancholy
Talk, indisposed to, desire to be silent,
   taciturn
Vivacious
   evening
Work, aversion to mental

BUNIAS ORIENTALIS

Anguish
Anxiety
Prostration of mind, mental exhaustion,
   brain-fag
Sadness, despondency, dejection, mental
   depression, gloom, melancholy
Suicidal disposition

BUTYRICUM ACIDUM

Anxiety
Fear, apprehension, dread

Indifference, apathy
Irritability
Sadness, despondency, dejection, mental
   depression, gloom, melancholy

BUTHUS AUSTRALIS

Anger, irascibility
Anguish
   evening, 19h. •
Anxiety
   evening, 19h.
   future, about
   19h. •
Comprehension, easy
Concentration, difficult
Confidence, want of self
Dream, as if in a
Indifference, apathy
   everything, to
   external things, to
Insanity, loquacious
Irresolution, indecision
Irritability
Loquacity
   alternating with silence
Mood, alternating
   changeable, variable
Prostration of mind, mental exhaustion,
   brain-fag
Restlessness
Sadness, climaxis, during
Sensitive, oversensitive
   light, to
   noise, to
Speech, incoherent
Talk, indisposed to, desire to be silent,
   taciturn
   alternating with loquacity
Weary of life
Weeping, tearful mood
Will, weakness of
Work, aversion to mental
   impossible.

CACTUS

Ailments from :
  love, disappointed
Anger, irascibility
  contradiction, from
Answer, aversion to
Anxiety
  afternoon
  evening
  night
  conscience, as if guilty of a crime
  waking, on
Cautious
Cheerful, gay, mirthful
  heart disease, with ★
Company, aversion to; presence of other
  people agg. the symptoms; de-
  sire for solitude
Concentration, difficult
Consolation, kind words agg.
  sympathy agg.
Contradiction, is intolerant of
Death, presentiment of
Delirium
  night
    waking, on ●
  gay, cheerful
  sleep, during
  falling asleep, on
  after, amel.
  waking, on
Delusions, die, he was about to
    heart symptoms, with, rheu-
    matism, in ●
  disease, incurable, has
  injured, is being
  smaller, things grow
  wires, is caught in
Dullness, sluggishness, difficulty of think-
    ing and comprehending, torpor
  sleepiness, with

Excitement, palpitation, with violent
Fear, apprehension, dread
  death, of
    heart symptoms, during
  disease, incurable, of being
  happen, something will
  heart, of disease of
  misfortune, of
  suffocation, of, night
  waking, on
Foolish, grotesque behavior
Forgetful, words while speaking, of; word
    hunting
Frightened easily
  waking, on
Hurry, haste
Hypochondriasis
Hysteria
Impulse to do strange things ★
Insanity, madness
  heat, with
Irresolution, indecision
  projects, in
Irritability
  consolation agg.
Jesting, facetious, desire to do some-
    thing ●
Mania, fear, during ●
Medicine, desire to swallow large doses
  of ●
Memory, weakness of
  words, of
Mildness
Morose, cross, fretful, ill-humor, peevish
Music agg.
  headache from
Remorse
Reserved
Restlessness
  night
  sitting, while
Sadness, despondency, dejection, mental
  depression, gloom, melancholy
  menses, during
  talk, indisposed to
Sensitive, music, to
  noise, to
  talking, of

Shrieking, screaming, shouting
pain, with the
Slowness
behind hand, always •
old people, of
work, in
Speech, incoherent
waking, on
Starting, fright, from and as from
sleep, from
Strange things, impulse to do
Stupefaction, as if intoxicated
Suspicious, mistrustful
Sympathy agg.
Talk, indisposed to, desire to be silent,
taciturn
sadness, in
others agg., talk of
Talking, sleep, in
Unconsciousness, coma, stupor
fever, during
sunstroke, in
Vivacious
Weeping, tearful mood
causeless, without knowing why
consolation agg.
desire to weep
hysterical
menses, before
during
Writing, difficulty in expressing ideas
when

CADMIUM METALLICUM

Anger, reproaches, from
Company, aversion to; presence of other
people agg. the symptoms; de-
sire for solitude
Concentration, difficult
Confusion of mind
Exertion, agg. from mental
Indifference, apathy
Indolence, aversion to work
Irritability
Memory, weakness of
details, for •

Restlessness
Sadness, despondency, dejection, mental
depression, gloom, melancholy
Sensitive, oversensitive
Suspicious, mistrustful
Work, mental, impossible

CADMIUM MURIATICUM

Indifference, everything, to ★
influenza, after
Quietness amel. ★

CADMIUM SULPHURATUM

Ailments from:
anger, vexation
Anxiety
alone, when
company, when in
stool, before
Company, desire for; aversion to solitude,
company amel.
alone agg., while
Dipsomania, alcoholism
Dullness, afternoon
Fear, alone, of being
approaching him, of others
solitude, of
work, dread of
Indolence, aversion to work
Irritability
Moaning, sleep, during
Quiet, wants to be
Restlessness
headache, during
sunlight agg. •
Smiling, sleep, in
Unconsciousness, coma, stupor
cough, between attacks of
Work, aversion to mental

CAELA ZACATECHICHI

Ailments from :
contradiction
grief
Anger, trifles, at

Contradict, disposition to
Grief
Memory, weakness of,
    facts, for recent
Quarrelsome, scolding

CAINCA

Anger, evening
    violent
Anxiety
Ennui, tedium
Forgetful
Irritability, evening
Restlessness, night
    urination, before
Weeping, coughing, during
Work, aversion to mental

CAJUPUTUM

Aversion to being approached
Company, aversion to; walk alone, wants
    to •
Delusions, poisoned, he has been
Dullness, sluggishness, difficulty of think-
    ing and comprehending, torpor
        afternoon
            evening, going to bed, after •
Hysteria
Ideas abundant, clearness of mind
    deficiency of
Indolence, aversion to work
Sadness, despondency, dejection, men-
    tal depression, gloom, melancholy
Speech, slow
Spoken to, averse to being
    alone, wants to be let
Stupefaction, afternoon
Thoughts, rapid, quick
    rush, flow of
Walks, slowly and dignified •

CALADIUM SEGUINUM

Absent-minded, unobserving
Ailments from:
    sexual excesses

Anger, irascibility
    easily
    noise, at, during sleep •
Anguish
Anxiety
    evening
        bed, in
    bed, in
    fear, with
    future, about
    health about
    hypochondriacal
        shaving, while •
Audacity
Borrows trouble ★
Busy
Childish, behavior
Concentration, difficult
Confusion of mind
    waking, on
        breakfast, after
Contrary
Courageous
Delirium
    murmuring
    muttering
    recognizes no one
Discomfort
    pickled fish, after •
Discouraged
Dullness, sluggishness, difficulty of think-
    ing and comprehending, torpor
    sleepiness, with
Emptiness, sensation of ★
Excitement, excitable
Exertion, agg. from mental
Fancies, lascivious
    impotency, with
Fear, apprehension, dread
    evening
    cutting himself when shaving •
    dark, of
    death, of
    disease, of impending
    evil, of
    exertion, of
    infection, of
    injured, of being

Fear,
    misfortune, of
    motion, of
    noise, from
    shadow, of his own
    sleep, before
        go to sleep, fear to
Forgetful
    sexual excesses, after
    sleep, he remembers all he had
        forgotten, during
    tobacco poisoning, from •
Forgotten things come to mind in sleep
Frightened easily
    shadow, his own •
Frivolous
Heedless
Helplessness, feeling of
Howling
Hurry, haste
    eating, while
Hysteria
Indifference, apathy
Indiscretion
Insanity, madness
Irritability
    morning
        7 h.
    coition, after
    sleep, when roused by noise dur-
        ing
    waking, on
Jealousy, impotence, with
Lamenting, bemoaning, wailing
Lascivious, lustful
    impotence, with
    ogling women, on the street ★
Loquacity
    perspiration, during
Mania
Memory, weakness of
    done, for what has just
    occurrences of the day, for
    written, for what he has
Mildness
Moaning, groaning, whining
    anxious ★
    sleep, during

Morose, morning
    eating, after
Muttering
Nymphomania
Prostration of mind, mental exhaus-
    tion, brain-fag
Recognize, relatives, does not his
Restlessness
    forenoon
    headache, during
    smoking, after •
Sadness, despondency, dejection, mental
    depression, gloom, melancholy
    morning
    impotence, with
    masturbation, from
    pollutions, from
Sensitive, noise, to
    sleep, on going to
Shrieking, screaming, shouting
Speech, incoherent
    inconsiderate
    prattling
Starting, startled
    crackling of paper, from •
    door slams, when a
    noise, from
    sleep, during
    from
Stupefaction, as if intoxicated
Thoughts, rush, flow of
Unconsciousness, coma, stupor
    fever, during
    transient
Weeping, night
    child, like a, about illness with
        senseless prattling •
    discontent, self, with ★
    illness, during •
    sleep, in
    vexations, from
Work, mental, impossible

CALCAREA CARBONICA

Abrupt, rough
Absent-minded, unobserving
    menses, during •

Absorbed, buried in thought
Activity, fruitless ★
Affections, in general ★
Admonition agg.
Adulterous
Ailments from:
    anger, vexation
      anxiety, with
      fright, with
    anticipation, foreboding, presentiment
    anxiety
    bad news
    business failure
    cares, worries
    continence ★
    death of a child
      parents or friends, of
    dipsomania
    egotism
    excitement, emotional
    fear
    fright
    grief
    literary, scientific failure
    mortification
    pecuniary loss
    rudeness of others
    sexual excesses
    work, mental
Amativeness
Anger, irascibility
    morning
    evening
    coffee agg.
    coition, after
    cold, after taking ●
    easily
    face, with red
    former vexations, about
    past events, about
    stool, before ●
    trifles, at
    violent
Anguish
    morning
    evening
    heat, during

Anguish,
    horrible things, after hearing ●
    menses, during
    palpitation, with
Anticipation: dentist, physician, before going to
Anxiety
    forenoon
    afternoon
    evening
      twilight, in the
      bed, in
    night
      children, in
    midnight, after
    on waking
   air, amel. in open
   bed, in
   business, about
   children, in
    when lifted from the cradle
   chill, during
   closing eyes, on
   conscience, as if guilty of a crime
   cramp in rectum, during ●
   cruelties, after hearing ●
   dark, in
   dreams, on waking from frightful
   exaggerated ★
   fear, with
   fever, during
   fits, with
   flatus amel, emission of
   flushes of heat, during
   future, about
   headache, with
   health, about
   hypochondriacal
    mania to read medical books
   menses, before
    during
   mental exertion, from
   perspiration amel.
   rain ★
   salvation, about
   shuddering, with
   sleep, on going to

Anxiety,
>   standing, amel. while
>   stool, before
>   *after*
>   *thinking about it, from*
>   thoughts, from •
>   trifles, about
>   waking, on
>   work, anxiety with inclination to •

Automatism ★

Avarice
>   alternating with squandering
>   squandering on oneself, but

Aversion, everything, to
>   *members of family, to*
>   **persons, to certain**
>   to all

Barking

Bed, aversion to; shuns bed

Beside oneself, being

Bite, desire to
>   *spits, barks and bites* •

Blasphemy

Boaster, squander, through ostentation

Borrowing of everyone
>   trouble ★

Brooding

Busy
>   fruitlessly

Calculating, inability for
>   *geometry*

Capriciousness

Carefulness

Cares, worries, full of
>   daily cares, affected by

Cautious ★

Censorious, critical

Charlatan

Cheerful, gay, mirthful
>   afternoon
>   evening
>   *constipated, when*
>   followed by sleepiness
>   foolish, and

Clairvoyance

Company, aversion to; presence of
>   other people agg. the symp
>   toms; desire for solitude

Company,
>   avoids the sight of people
>   country away from people, wants
>   to get into the
Company, desire for; aversion to solitude,
>   *company amel.*
>   alone agg., while

Complaining
>   offences long past, of

Comprehension, easy, drunkenness,
>   during

Concentration, active
>   menses, before •

Concentration, difficult
>   aversion to
>   *menses, after* ★
>   studying, learns with difficulty

Confidence, want of self

Confounding objects and ideas

Confusion of mind
>   *morning*
>   rising and after, on
>   waking, on
>   afternoon
>   evening
>   night
>   bed, while in
>   beer, from
>   breakfast, before
>   coition, after
>   dream, as if in
>   *eating, after*
>   *mental exertion, from*
>   mixes subjective and objective
>   *reading, while*
>   scratching behind the ear in •
>   sitting, while
>   sleeping, after
>   siesta, after a
>   stooping, when
>   waking, on
>   walking, while

Conscientious about trifles

Consolation, kind words agg.

Contrary

Conversation agg.
>   aversion to

Country, desire for ★

Cowardice
Crawling, rolling on the floor
Cruelty, see cruelty in the cinema,
　　children cannot bear to •
Cursing, swearing
Darkness agg.
Death, desires
　　presentiment of
Deceitful, sly
　　fraudulent
Delirium
　　　　night
　　　　anxious
　　　　closing the eyes, on
　　　　fever, during
　　　　fire, talks of •
　　　　frightful
　　　　persecution in d., delusions of
　　　　raging, raving
　　　　sleep, during
　　　　　　falling asleep, on
　　　　sleeplessness, and ★
　　　　throwing from windows
　　　　trembling, with
Delirium tremens, mania-a-potu
　　delusions, with
Delusions, imaginations, hallucina-
　　　　tions, illusions
　　　　　　evening, bed, in
　　　　　　　　falling asleep, on
　　　　animals, of
　　　　annihilation, about to sink into
　　　　anxious
　　　　bed: over it, someone is •
　　　　　　under it, someone is
　　　　　　knocking
　　　　body, dashed to pieces, being •
　　　　cats, sees
　　　　confusion, others will observe her •
　　　　dead persons, sees
　　　　die, he was about to
　　　　disease, incurable, has
　　　　dogs, sees
　　　　　　swarm about him
　　　　faces, sees
　　　　　　closing eyes, on
　　　　　　hideous

Delusions,
　　falling asleep, on
　　fancy, illusions of
　　　　evening in bed
　　　　eyes, on closing
　　fever, during •
　　figures, sees
　　fire, visions of
　　happened, anything, of having
　　hearing, illusions of
　　heart disease, of having
　　home, away from, is
　　images, phantoms, sees
　　　　evening
　　　　night
　　　　closing eyes, on
　　　　frightful
　　inanimate objects are persons
　　insane, she will become
　　　　people think her •
　　lascivious
　　ludicrous
　　mice, sees
　　money, talks of
　　murdered, he will be
　　　　sees someone •
　　noise, hears
　　　　clattering above the bed (when
　　　　　　falling asleep)
　　　　knocking under bed
　　people: behind him, someone is
　　　　beside him, are
　　　　converses with absent
　　persecuted, he is
　　persons; something hanging over
　　　　chair is a person, sitting there •
　　rain, he hears (at night)
　　rats, sees
　　　　running up the leg, a rat
　　room is a house (not: garden) •
　　ruined, he is
　　sick, being
　　　　work, and for this reason will
　　　　　　not
　　smaller, of being
　　snakes in and around her
　　spectres on closing eyes, sees

144

Delusions,
    strange, familiar things seem
    vermin, sees crawl about
    visions, has
      closing the eyes, on
      horrible
        evening
        wonderful
      vivid
      walks beside him, someone
      wat *d. she is being*
      wealth,of
Dementia
Despair
    chill, during
    death, with fear of •
    health, of
    life, of
    pains, with the
    perspiration, during
    recovery, of
    religious despair of salvation
    social position, of
Destructiveness
Development of children arrested
Dipsomania, alcoholism
Discomfort, evening
Discontented, displeased, dissatisfied
    evening
    coition, after
Discouraged
    evening
    impatience, with •
Dishonest
Disobedience
Doubtful, recovery, of
    soul's welfare, of
Dream, as if in a
Dullness, sluggishness, difficulty
    of thinking and compre-
    hending, torpor
    children, in
    damp air, from
    menses, during
    mental exertion, from
    waking, on

Duty, no sense of
    stimulate sense of, to ★
Dwells on past disagreable occurrences
    grief from past offences
    recalls disagreeable memories
Effeminate
Egotism, self-esteem
Ennui, tedium
Envy
    hate, and
    qualities of others, at
Excitement, excitable
    morning
    evening
      bed, in
    night
    agg.
    bad news, after
    chill, during
    coition, after •
    hearing horrible things, after
    menses, return of, excitement
    brings •
    palpitation, with violent
Exclusive, too
Exercise, mental symptoms amel. by
    physical •
Exertion, agg. from mental
    amel.
    physical exertion amel.
Fancies, exaltation of
    evening, bed, in
    night
    closing the eyes in bed
    frightful
    sleeplessness, with
    lascivious
    sleep, falling asleep, on
    waking, on
Fear, apprehension, dread
    evening
      twilight
      bed, in
      night
    alone, of being
    animals, of

Fear,
    bad news, of hearing
    bed, of the
    bugs ★
    children, in
    chill, during
    confusion, that people would observe her ●
    consumption, of
    crowd, in a
      public places, of; agoraphobia
    cruelties, from report of ●
    dark, of
    death, of
      evening
      heat, during
      hunger, from ●
    dentist, of going to ●
    disease, of impending
    disease, of impending, cancer, of ★
      contagious, epidemic diseases, of
      incurable, of being
    dogs, of
    everything, constant of
    evil, of
    falling, of
    fever, of (while chilly)
    ghosts, of
    happen, something will
    heart, of disease of
    infection, of
    insanity, losing his reason, of
      night
    insects, of ★
    lifelong
    menses, before
      suppressed from fear
    misfortune, of
    narrow places, vaults, churches and cellars, of
    observed, of her condition being
    operation, of each ●
    pains, of
    people, of; anthropophobia

Fear,
    position, to lose his lucrative
    poverty, of
    rage, to fly into a
    rags, of ★
    see wounds, to ●
    shadow, of his own
    sleep, before
      go to sleep, fear to
    starving, of
    stomach, arising from
    suffering, of
    thunderstorm, of
    tremulous
    trifles, of
    waking, on
    work, dread of
Fire, thinks and talks of ●
Fishy ★
Fists doubling as if in furious anger ●
Foolish behaviour
Forgetful
    drunkards, forgetfulness in
    headache, during
    mental exertion, from
    words while speaking, of; word hunting
Forgotten something, feels constantly as if he had
Forsaken feeling
    beloved by his parents, wife, friends, feels of not being
Frightened easily
    menses, before ●
    roused, when
    trifles, at
      day before menses ●
    waking, on
Gamble (*see* Play)
Gestures, automatic
    breaks pins
      sticks
    grasping, fingers in the mouth, children put
      everything in the mouth
    plays with his fingers
      counting money, as if

Gluttony
Godless, want of religious feeling
Gossiping
Gourmand
Greed, cupidity
Grief
    headache from grief
    offences, grief from long past
Grumbling, his value is not understood
    by others ★
Hatred
    persons who had offended him, of
    revenge, and
Haughty
    stupid and haughty
Hide, fear, on account of ★
Home, desires to go
Hopeful
Horror ★
**Horrible things, sad stories, affect
    her profoundly**
Hurry, haste
Hydrophobia
Hypochondriasis
    night
    imaginary illness
    suicide, driving to
    weeping, with
Hysteria
    menses, during
Ideas abundant, clearness of mind
    evening in bed
    night
    deficiency of
Idleness
Imbecility
Impatience
Indifference, apathy
    duties, to
    important things, to
    perspiration, during
    recovery, about his
    taciturn
Indiscretion
Indolence, aversion to work
    air amel., in open
    physical
    suddenly ★

Industrious, mania for work
    menses, before
Insanity, madness
    black insanity with despair and
        weary of life from fear of morti-
        fication or of loss of position
    break pins, she will sit and
    chilliness, with
    drunkards, in
    face, with red
    fortune, after losing
    melancholy
    persecution mania
    position, from fear to lose the
Insolence
Irresolution, indecision
    evening
Irritability
    daytime
    morning
        rising, after
        stool, before •
    evening amel.
    air, in open, amel.
    chill, during
    coition, after
    cold, after taking •
    consolation agg.
    dentition, during
    headache, during
    idle, while •
    menses, before
        during
    music, during
    perspiration , during
    sitting, while
    sleeplessness, with
    stool, before
    trifles, from
    warm room, in
Jealousy, brutal, from, gentle husband
    becoming
    sexual excitement, with
    strike his wife, driving to ★
Jesting
    erotic
Jumping, bed, out of

Kill, desire to
Kleptomania
    money, steals •
Lamenting, bemoaning, wailing
Lascivious, lustful
    evening •
Late, always too
Laughing
    chill, during
    convulsions, before, during or after
    spasmodic
    wild
Liar
    charlatan and
    lies, never speaks the truth, does not know what she is saying ★
Libertinism
Light, desire for
Loathing, general
    old age, in
Loathing, life, at
    work, at
Looked at, cannot bear to be
Loquacity
    evening
Love with one of own sex, homosexuality, tribadism
Magnetized, desire to be
Malicious, spiteful, vindictive
    night
Mania
Mathematics, inapt for
    geometry, for
    horror of mathematics
Memory active, short,but
Memory, loss of:
    epileptic fits, after
Memory, weakness of
    facts, for
        past, for
        recent, for
    heard, for what has
    labor, for mental, fatigue, from
    places, for
    said, for what has
    sudden and periodical
    words, of

Menses, mental symptoms agg. before
    during
Mildness
Misanthropy
Mischievous
Mistakes, differentiating of objects, in
    speaking, in
        misplacing words
        reverses words
        words, using wrong
            name of object seen instead of one desired
            names, calls things by wrong
    writing, in
        wrong words
Moaning, groaning, whining
    sleep, during
Mood, alternating
    changeable, variable
    insupportable •
Morose, cross, fretful, ill-humor, peevish
    morning
    evening
    air amel., in open
    children, in
    coition, after
    house, agg. in; amel. on walking in open air
    sleepiness, with
    stool, before
    waking, on
    women, in
Morphinism
Music agg.
    piano playing, from
    violin playing agg.
    cough, m. agg.
        piano, c. when playing
Muttering
Narrating her symptoms agg.
Nibble, desire to ★
Nymphomania
    menses, before
    during
Obscene, lewd
    talk

Obstinate, headstrong
  children, inclined to grow fat •
Occupation, diversion amel.
Offended, easily; takes everything
  in bad part
  offenses, from past
Optimistic
Passionate
Pessimist
Pities herself
Play, passion for gambling
  to make money
Pompous ★
Precocity
Prejudice, traditional
Presumptuous
Prop·· ion, sense of, disturbed ★
Prostration of mind, mental exhaustion, brain-fag
  coition, after
  talking, from
Quarrelsome, scolding
Rage, fury
Reading, mental symptoms agg. from
  passion to read medical books
Rebels against poultice
Religious affections
  bible, wants to read all the day
  children, in
  puberty, in
Remorse
Reproaches others
Reserved
  walking in open air, after
Restlessness
  evening
    20h.
  night
  anxious
  bed, go from one bed to another,
  wants to
    tossing about in
  coition, after
  eructations, from insufficient ★
  faintness, followed by •
  heat, during
  menses, during
Rocking amel.

Rolling on the floor
Runs, about
Sadness, despondency, dejection,
  mental depression, gloom,
  melancholy
  morning
  evening, amel.
    bed, in
    night
  alone, when
  anxious
  children, in
  chill, during
  coition, after
  darkness, in
  exertion, after
  heat, during
  heaviness in legs, with
  idle, while •
  menses, before
    during
    suppressed, from
  misfortune, as if from
  perspiration, during
  puberty, in
  sleepiness, with
  suicidal disposition, with
  walking, while and after, air, in
    open
  warm room, in
Scratches, child, on head on waking •
Selfishness, egoism
Senses, dull, blunted
  vanishing of
Sensitive, oversensitive
  morning
  evening
  certain persons, to
  children
  cruelties, when hearing of •
  mental impressions, to
  music, to
  noise, to
    evening •
    shrill sounds, to
    sleep, on going to
  puberty, in
  rudeness, to
  sensual impressions, to

Sentimental
Serious, earnest
Shamelessness
Shrieking, screaming, shouting
 night
 anxiety, from
 children, in
  day and night •
 convulsions, before
  during epileptic
 must shriek, feels as though she
 sleep, during
Sit, inclination to
Sits and breaks pins
Slowness
 calculation, in •
 motion, in
 old people, of
Somnambulism
Speech, confused
 night in sleep •
 foolish
 wandering
Spineless
Spit, desire to
 anger, from •
 faces of people, in
Squanders
 boasting, from
Starting, startled
  evening, sleep, in
 dreams, from a dream
 easily
 menses, before
 noise, from
 prick of a needle, at the •
 sleep, on falling
  during
  from
 trifles, at
Strange, cranky
 opinions and acts, in
Strength increased, mental, drunkenness,
 more intelligent, during
Stupefaction, as if intoxicated
 afternoon
 night
 stooping, on

Stupefaction,
 vertigo, during
 walking, when
Suicidal disposition
 hypochondriasis, by
 knife, with
 perspiration, during
 sadness, from
 shooting, by
 stabbing, by
Sulky
Susceptible
Suspicious, mistrustful
Talks, indisposed to, desire to be silent,
  taciturn
   perspiration, during
 slow learning to
Talking agg. all complaints
 sleep, in
 unpleasant things agg., of
Talks, himself, to
 murder, fire and rats, of nothing
 but •
Tastlessness in dressing
Testament, refuses to make a
Thinking, complaints agg., of
Thoughts, disagreeable
 frightful
 persistent
  night
 homicide
 murder, fire and rats, of noth-
 ing but •
 rush, flow of
  evening in bed
  night
 sleeplessness from
 sexual
 strange
 thoughtful
 vanishing of
 wandering, menses, during •
Timidity
 awkward, and
 bashful
Torments those about him
  day and night •
Touched, aversion to being

Travel, desire to
Trifles seem important
Twilight agg. mental symptoms
Unconsciousness, coma, stupor
    morning
    evening
    exertion, after
    fever, during
    head, on moving
    stool, after
    stooping, when
    transient
    turning in a circle, during ●
    walking, while
Ungrateful
Unreliable, promises, in his
Violent, vehement
    morning
    deeds of violence, rage leading to
    stool, before ●
Wander, desires to, night
Wearisone
Weary of life
    old age, in
    perspiration, during
Weeping, tearful mood
    evening
    night
    admonition, from
    alternating with laughter
    anxiety, after
    children, in, babies
    chill, during
    consolation agg.
    easily
    heat, during
    irritable
    menses, during
    perspiration, during
    remonstrated, when
    reproaches, from
    sleep, in
    trifles, at
    walking in open air, when
    whimpering
    sleep, during
Whistling
Will, loss of
    weakness of

Work, aversion to mental
    impossible
Writing, difficulty in expressing ideas
    when

CALCAREA ACETICA

Anxiety
    evening, bed, in
    flatus amel., emission of
    future, about
    present, about
Dullness,
    pressing in hypogastrium, from ★
Fear, dark, of
Industrious, mania for work
Loquacity
    evening
Morose, cross, fretful, ill-humor, peevish
    morning
Sadness, despondency, dejection, mental
    depression, gloom, melancholy
Weeping, sleep, in
Will, loss of
    weakness of
Work, mental, impossible

CALCAREA ARSENICOSA

Ailments from:
    anger, vexation
    excitement, emotional
Anger, irascibility
    coition, after
Anguish
Anxiety
    evening
    bed, in
    night
    chill, during
    fear, with
    fever, during
    future, about
    health, about
    salvation, about
    night ●
    waking, on

Censorious, critical
Company, desire for; aversion to solitude, company amel.
Confusion of mind, morning
 evening
 waking, on
Delirium, evening, dark, in the
 dark, in
Delusions, imaginations, hallucinations,
 illusions
 dead persons, sees
 dogs, sees
 fancy, illusions of
 fire, visions of
 floating in air
 images, phantoms, sees
 people, sees disagreeable
 visions, has
Despair, recovery, of
 religious despair of salvation
Dipsomania, alcoholism
Discontented, displeased, dissatisfied
Dullness, sluggisness, difficulty of thinking and comprehending, torpor
Emotion, slightest, causes palpitation ★
Excitement, excitable
 palpitation, with violent
Exertion, agg. from mental
Fear, evening
 night
 alone, of being
 death, of
 night
 disease, of impending
 insanity, losing his reason, of
Indifference, apathy
 pleasure, to
Indolence, aversion to work
Insanity, madness
Irresolution, indecision
Irritability
Lamenting, bemoaning, wailing
Loathing, life, at
Memory, weakness of
Mischievous
Offended, easily; takes everything in
 bad part

Prostration of mind, mental exhaustion, brian-fag
Restlessness
 night
 midnight, after, 3h.
 bed, tossing about in
 heat, during
 menses, during
Sadness, despondency, dejection,
 mental depression, gloom,
 melancholy
 heat, during
 perspiration, during
Sensitive, oversensitive
Starting, startled
 sleep, during
Stupefaction, as if intoxicated
Thoughts, profound
Timidity
Unconsciousness, exertion, after
Weary of life
Weeping, tearful mood
 night
 work, mental, impossible

CALCAREA BROMATA

Anxiety
Irritability
 children, in
Morose, cross, fretful, ill-humor; peevish
Restlessness, children, in

CALCAREA CAUSTICA

Dullness, sluggishness, difficulty of thinking and comprehending, torpor
Restlessness, night

CALCAREA FLUORICA NATURALIS

Anguish
Anxiety
 future, about
 money matters, about
 others, for ★

Avarice
Comprehension, easy
Concentration, active
Concentration, difficult
    eating, amel. from
    studying, reading etc., while
Delusions, poor, he is
    want, he will come to
Eating,. amel. after
Exertion, agg. from mental
Exhilaration
Fear, apprehension, dread
    causeless
    misfortune, of
    poverty, of
    work, daily, of
Hurry, haste
    work, in
Ideas abundant, clearness of mind
Impatience
Indifference, apathy
Indolence, aversion to work
Industrious, mania for work
Irresolution, indecision
Irritability
Jumping, dream, in ★
Prostration of mind, mental exhaus-
    tion, brain-fag.
Restlessness
    back, during tired aching in ●
Sadness, despondency, dejection, mental
    depression, gloom, melancholy
Sensitive, noise, to
    odors, to

CALCAREA HYPOPHOSPHOROSA

Shrieking, screaming, shouting
    brain cry
    sleep, during
Talks, fast ★

CALCAREA IODATA

Anger, trifles, at
Anxiety, paroxysms, in .
    periodical
    trifles, about

Cheerful, gay, mirthful
Company, aversion to; presence of
    other people agg. the symp-
    toms; desire for solitude
Confusion of mind
Delusions, imaginations, hallucinations,
    illusions
    dead persons, sees
Despair
Discontented, displeased, dissatisfied
Discouraged
Dullness, sluggishness, difficulty of
    thinking and comprehending,
    torpor
Exertion, agg. from mental
Fear, insanity, losing his reason, of
    misfortune, of
    people, of; anthropophobia
Impatience
Indifference, apathy
Indolence, aversion to work
Insanity, madness
Irresolution, indecision
Irritability
    headache, during
Mania
Prostration of mind, mental exahustion,
    brain-fag
Restlessness
    anxious
**Sadness, despondency, dejection,
    mental depression, gloom,
    melancholy**
Senses, dull, blunted
Starting, sleep, during
Weeping, tearful mood

CALCAREA MURIATICA

Unconsciousness, coma, stupor

CALCAREA PHOSPHORICA

Absent-minded, unobserving
Ailments from
    anger, vexation
    anxiety
    bad news

Ailments from
 excitement, emotional
 grief
 love, disappointed
 unhappy
 sexual excesses
 work, mental .
Anger, irascibility
 bad news, about •
 contradiction, from
 paralyzed, felt as
 work, cannot •
Anxiety
 children, in
  when lifted from the cradle
 health, about ★
 motion, from ★
 others, for ★
Aversion, school, to ★
Cares, worries, full of
Censorious, critical
Cheerful, gay, mirthful
Clinging, held amel., being
Company, aversion to; presence of other
  people agg. the symptoms; desire
  for solitude
Company, desire for; aversion to solitude, company amel. .
Concentration, difficult,
 studying, learns with difficulty,
 while
Confusion of mind
  morning, waking, on
 coffee, after
 cold bath amel.
 hat agg., putting on
 identity, duality, sense of
 mental exertion, from
 motion, from
 waking, on
 washing the face amel.
Consolation, kind words agg.
Contradiction, is intolerant of
Cretinism
Delirium, sleepiness, with
Delusions, bed, sinking, is
 fancy, illusions of
 fire, visions of

Delusions,
 home, away from, is
  away from, must get there
Dementia .
 senilis
Development of children arrested
Discomfort
Discontented, displeased, dissatis-
 fied
 himself, with
Dullness, sluggishness, difficulty
 of thinking and compre-
 hending, torpor
 bad news, from •
 children, in
 mental exertion, from
 washing, amel. from cold •
Excitement, excitable
 bad news, after
Exertion, agg. from mental
 amel.
 puberty, agg. from mental exertion in
Fear, apprehension, dread
 bad news, of hearing
 dark, of
 disease, of impending, cancer, of ★
 evil, of
 heart, of disease of ★
 starting, with
 thunderstorm, of ★
 work, mental, of
Forgetful
Frightened easily
Fussy ★
Gestures, grasping or reaching at something, at flocks; carphologia
Grief
Home, desires to go
 go out, and when there, to
Homesickness
Ideas abundant, clearness of mind
 deficiency of
Idiocy
Imbecility
Indifference, apathy
Indignation
 dreams, at unpleasant •

Indolence, aversion to work
   evening
Industrious, mania for work
   coition, after •
   menses, before
Insanity, erotic
Irresolution, indecision
Irritability
   children, in
   coffee, after •
   consolation agg.
   dentition, during
   headache, during
   perspiration, during
Jealousy
Lascivious, lustful
Love with one of own sex, homosexuality, tribadism
Memory, active
Memory, weakness of
   do, for what was about to
   done, for what has just
   words, of
Mistakes, speaking, in
      words, using wrong
   writing, in
      repeating words
      wrong words
Mood, changeable, variable
Morose, cross, fretful, ill-humor, peevish
   alternating with cheerfulness
   coffee, after •
Nymphomania
   menses, before
Occupation, diversion amel.
Prostration of mind, mental exhaustion, brain-fag
   talking, from
Quiet, repose and tranquillity, on walk-
      ing in open air, desires
Remorse
Reproaches himself
   others
Restlessness
   anxious
   driving about
   lying on back agg., on side amel. •

Sadness, despondency, dejection, mental
   depression, gloom, melancholy
   anger, from
   bad news, after
   girls before puberty, in
   sleepiness, with
   vexation, after
   waking, on
Sensitive, oversensitive
Sentimental
Shrieking, screaming, shouting
   children, in
      sleep, during
   must shriek, feels as though she
   sleep, during
Sighing
Snappish
Starting, convulsive
   fright, from and as from
   lying on back, while
   sleep, during
Stupefaction, as if intoxicated
Suspicious, mistrustful
Sympathetic ★
Sympathy, compassion ★
Talk, indisposed to, desire to be silent,
      taciturn
   slow learning to
Thinking, complaints agg., of
Travel, desire to
Violent, vehement
   reproached, when hearing an-
      other •
Wander, desires to
Weeping, tearful mood
   consolation agg.
Wildness
   unpleasant news, from •
Work, aversion to mental

CALCAREA SULPHURICA

Absent-minded, unobserving
Absorbed, misfortune, imagines •
Ailments from :
   anger, vexation

Anger, irascibility
Answers; aversion to answer
Anxiety
    morning
    evening
      bed, in
      night
    air, amel. in open
    fear, with
    fever, during
    future, about
    health, about
    lying, while
    salvation, about
    waking, on
Brooding
Capriciousness
    evening
Cheerful, gay, mirthful
    morning
      sad in evening, and
    afternoon
    evening
      18h. λ
    alternating with grief
      sadness
Company, aversion to; presence of
    other people agg. the symp-
    toms; desire for solitide
Confusion of mind
    morning
      waking, on
    evening
    air, amel. in open
    mental exertion, from
Contrary
Cowardice
Delirium tremens, mania-a- potu
Delusions, imaginations, hallucinations,
    illusions
    images, phantoms, sees.
      frightful
        night, while trying to sleep λ
    visions, has
Despair
    heat, during
    recovery, of

Discontented, displeased, dissatisfied
    everything, with
**Dullness, sluggishness, difficulty
    of thinking and compre-
    hending, torpor**
    evening
    eating, after
Excitement, excitable
Fear, apprehension, dread
    night
    birds ↔
    dark, of
    death, of
    evil, of
    insanity, losing his reason, of
    misfortune, of
Forgetful
    eating, after
Hatred persons; agree with him, who
    do not λ
Hurry, haste
Hysteria
Imbecility
Impatience
Indifference, apathy
Insanity, madness
Irresolution, indecision
Irritability
    afternoon
    evening
    coition, after
Jealousy
Lamenting, bemoaing, wailing
    appreciated, because he is not λ
Lascivious, lustful
Loathing, life, at
Malicious, spiteful, vindictive
Memory, weakness of
    do, for what was about to
    sudden and periodical
Mistakes, speaking, in
    misplacing words
Mood, changeable, variable
Morose, cross, fretful, ill-humor, peevish
Obstinate, headstrong

Offended easily; takes everything in
   bad part
Prostration of mind, mental exhaustion, brain-fag
Quarrelsome, scolding
Restlessness
   afternoon
   evening
**Sadness, despondency, dejection,
   mental depression, gloom,
   melancholy**
      morning but cheerful in
        evening
      afternoon
      evening
   bitter •
   perspiration, during
Sensitive, oversensitive
Sits, meditates, and •
Starting, startled
   easily
Stupefaction, as if intoxicated
Suspicious, mistrustful
Talk, indisposed to, desire to be silent,
   taciturn
Thoughts, persistent
   tormenting
   vanishing of
Timidity
   bashful
Unconsciousness, coma, stupor
Vivacious, afternoon
Walk, desire to walk, as soon as she sets
   out desire gone •
Wearisome
Weeping, tearful mood
   perspiration, during
Work, aversion to mental

CALCAREA SILICATA

Absent-minded unobserving
Ailments from :
   fear
   fright
   sexual excesses
   work, mental

Ambition, loss of
Anger, irascibility
   agg.
   mental exertion, after λ
Answers: aversion to answer
   refuses to answer
Anxiety, morning, waking, on
   evening, bed, in
   night
   family, about his
   health, about
   menses, during
   money matters, about
Capriciousness
Cares, worries, full of
Censorious, critical
*Concentration difficult, conversation,
   during*
   studying, reading, etc. while.
Confidence, want of self
Confusion of mind
   morning, waking, on
   evening
   eating, after
   mental exertion, from
   sitting, while
Consolation, kind words agg.
Contrary
Cowardice
Delirium, foolish, silly
   muttering
   quiet
   throwing from window λ
Delusions, dead persons, sees
   dogs, sees
   faces, sees
     hideous
   fancy, illusions of
     night
   images, phantoms, sees, night
   people, sees disagreeable
   starve, family will
   talking, dead people, with
   visions, horrible
   voices, hears
     answers, and λ
     dead people, of
   women, of old and wrinkled

Desires, present, things not
Despair
Discontented, displeased, dissatisfied
    everything, with
Doubtful, recovery, of
Dullness, sluggishness, difficulty of
    thinking and comprehending,
    torpor
Escape, window, from
Excitement, excitable
Exertion, agg. from mental
Fancies, exaltation of
Fear, apprehension, dread
    night
    brain, of softening of
    disease, incurable, of being
    exertion, of
    imaginary things, of
    mental exertion, after •
    poverty, of
    touch, of
    work, dread of
Frightened easily
    noon, nap, after
Hurry, haste
Hysteria
Ideas abundant, night
    deficiency of, daytime •
Imbecility
Impatience
Indolence, aversion to work
Insanity, madness
Irresolution, indecision
Irritability
    morning
    evening
    coition, after
    consolation agg. •
    headache, during
    trifles, from
Lamenting, bemoaning, wailing
Lascivious, lustful
Laughing, weeping or laughing on all
    occasions
Loathing, life, at

Memory, weakness of
    said, for what has just •
Mildness
Mistakes, speaking, in
    misplacing words
Mood, changeable, variable
Morose, cross, fretful, ill-humor, peevish
Muttering
    evening, falling asleep, on •
Occupation, diversion amel.
Prostration of mind, mental exhaus-
    tion, brain-fag
Restlessness, night
    anxious
Sadness, daytime
    morning
    causeless
    heat, during
Senses, dull, blunted
Sensitive, noise, to
    reprimands, to
Shrieking, sleep, during
Sits, still
    weeping
Speech, foolish
    nonsensical
Spoken to, averse to being
Starting, startled
    sleep, during
Stupefaction, as if intoxicated
Suicidal disposition
Talk, indisposed to, desire to be silent,
    taciturn
Talks, dead people, with
Timidity
    bashful
Unconsciousness, coma, stupor
    conduct, automatic
Weary of life
Weeping, night
    sleep, in
Will, loss of
Work, aversion to mental
Yielding disposition

CALENDULA OFFICINALIS

Anxiety
  chill, during
  stool, before
    during
Delirium
  wild
Fear, happen, something will
    terrible ★
Frightened easily
  trifles, at
Irritability
  chill, during
Morose, cross, fretful, ill-humor, peevish
  chill, during
  sleepiness, with
Restlessness
  night
Sensitive, oversensitive
Speech, unintelligible
Starting, fright, from and as from
Unconsciousness, burning, in

CALOTROPIS GIGANTEA

Restlessness
  night

CALTHA PALUSTRIS

Anxiety
Restlessness

CAMPHORA

Abstraction of mind
Abusive, insulting
Ailments from :
  anger, vexation
  anticipation, foreboding, presen-
    timent
  fright
Anger, irascibility
Anguish
Answers; refuses to answer

Anxiety
  night
  apparition while awake, from
    horrible
  bed, in
    tossing about, with
  chill, during
  mental exertion, from
  salvation, about
  sleep, during
  stool, during
Aversion, everything, to
Bed, aversion to, shuns bed
  get out of, wants to
Bite, desire to
Brooding, corner or moping, in a
Cheerful, gay, mirthful
Clinging, grasps at others
Company, aversion to; presence of other
    people agg. the symptoms; desire
    for solitude
Company, desire for; aversion to solitide,
    company amel.
  night
  alone agg., while
Comprehension, easy
Concentration, difficult
Confusion of mind
  heat, during
  identity, as to his
  intoxicated, as after being
  walking, while
Contradict, disposition to
Contrary
Cowardice
Crawling, child crawls into corners,
    howls, cries ●
Dancing, wild
Darkness agg.
Death, sensation of
  thoughts of
Delirium
  night
  anxious
  busy
  convulsions, during
  erotic

Delirium,
 fever, during
 look fixed on one point, staring
 loquacious
 maniacal
 noisy
 quiet
 raging, raving
 repeats the same sentence •
 sleep, during comatose
  falling asleep, on
 sleepiness, with
 thirst, with
 violent
 wild
Delusions, imaginations, hallucina-•
  tions, illusions
   evening, bed, in
    night
 absurd figures are present
 alone, world, she is, in the
 dead, he himself was
 deserted, forsaken, is
 devil, he is a
 enlarged, distances are
 falling asleep, on
 fancy, illusions of
 flying, sensation of
 hell, is in
 images, phantoms, sees
  night
  frightful
 longer, things seem
 objects, brilliantly colored
 sometimes thick, somtimes thin
 (on closing eyes in slumber) •
 people, beside him, are
 smaller, things grow
 spectres, ghosts, spirits, sees
 tall: things grow taller
  pulse is throbbing, as the •
 visions, has
  night
  closing the eyes, on
  horrible
   night
  monsters, of
  wonderful

Despair
 religious despair of salvation
Destructiveness
 clothes, of
Dictatorial, domineering, dogmatical,
  despotic
Dipsomania, alcoholism
Discomfort
Discouraged
Disgust
Dullness, sluggishness, difficulty of thinking and comprehending, torpor
Ecstasy
Ennui, tedium
Escape, attempts to
Excitement, excitable
 wine, as from
Exertion, amel. from mental
Exhilaration
Fancies, confused
 exaltation of
  evening, bed, in
  closing the eyes in bed
 lascivious
 sleep, falling asleep, on
Fear, apprehension, dread
 night
 alone, of being
  night
 bed, of the
 danger, of impending
 dark, of
 death, of
 evil, of
 mirrors in room, of
 people, of; anthropophobia
 sleep, to go to
 thoughts, of his own •
 upward, of being drawn •
 vexation, after
 walking, walks till perspiration
  amel., from fear •
Feces, swallows his own
Foolish, behavior
Forgetful
Forsaken feeling
  isolation, sensation of

Gestures, makes
    convulsive
    involuntary, wild
    strange attitudes and positions
    violent
    wild •
Heedless
Hide, desire to
Howling
Hurry, haste
    movements, in
    occupation, in
Hysteria
Ideas abundant, clearness of mind
    deficiency of
Imbecility
Impulsive
Indifference, apathy
    work, with aversion to
Indiscretion
Indolence, aversion to work
    chill, during •
Insanity, madness
    erotic
    face, with pale
    puerperal
    staring of eyes,
Introspection, night •
Irresolution, indecision
Irritability
    morning, waking, on
    night
    visions, with frightful •
    chill, during
    waking, on
Jealousy
Jumping, bed, out of
Kill, desire to
    somebody, thought he ought to
      kill
    walking in open air and street,
      while
Lamenting, bemoaning, wailing
Laughing, children, winsane •
    convulsions, before, during or after
    sardonic

Learns, easily ★
Lie on bare floor, wants to •
Loquacity
Mania
    abuses everyone
    cold perspiration, with
    rage, with
Memory, active
Memory, loss of :
    catalepsy, after •
Memory, weakness of
    done, for what has just
    facts, for past
Mistakes, time, in
Moaning, groaning whining
    perspiration, during
Mobility ★
Monomania
Mood, repulsive
Morose, cross, fretful, ill-humor, peevish
    night
Muttering, sleep, in
Naked, wants to be
    bares her breast in puerperal
    mania •
Nymphomania
Obscene, lewd
    talk
Obstinate, headstrong
Occupation, diversion amel.
Offended, easily; takes everything in
    bad part
Positiveness
Prophesying
Prostration of mind, mental exhaus-
    tion, brain-fag
    injuries, from
Quarrelsome, scolding
Rage, fury
    biting, with
    foaming mouth, with •
    paroxysms, in
    spitting, with
    tears clothes •
Religious affections
      night, tortured by religious
      ideas

Restlessness
    night
    anxious
    bed, tossing about in
    parturition, during
Sadness, despondency, dejection, mental
    depression, gloom, melancholy
    night
    darkness, in
    diverted from thoughts of him-
    self, desire to be
Satyriasis
Senses, dull, blunted
    vanishing of
Sensitive, oversensitive
    noise, to
Shamelessness
Shining objects agg.
Shrieking, screaming, shouting
    aid, for
    children, in
    convulsions, before
        during epileptic
Sighing
   · sleep, in
Sit, inclination to
Speech, delirious
    foreign tongue, in a
    hasty
    incoherent
    nonsensical
    wandering
    wild
Spoken to, averse to being
Starting, startled
    easily
    noise, from
    sleep, during
Strength increased, mental
Striking
Striking himself
    chest, his
Stupefaction, as if intoxicated
    heat, during
Suicidal disposition, fear of an open
    window or a knife, with
    throwing himself from a height
    window, from

Talk, indisposed to, desire to be silent,
    taciturn
Talking, sleep, in
    gentle voice, all night in a ●
Tears things
Thinking, complaints amel., of
Thoughts, crude ●
    himself, desire to be diverted
    from   thoughts of ●
    intrude and crowd around each
    other
    rush, flow of
    vanishing of
Throws things away
Time passes too slowly, appears longer
Timidity, evening, going to bed, about
Touched, aversion to being
Trance
    plays on piano with closed eyes,
    writes letter in an acquired
    language ●
Unconsciousness, coma, stupor
    chill, during
    conduct, automatic
    cries, with howling ●
    emotion, after
    eyes, with fixed
    fever, during
    sunstroke, in
Violent, vehement
Weeping, tearful mood
    night
    anxiety, after
    causeless
    children, in
    convulsions, during
    desire to weep, all the time
        but eyes are dry ●
    involuntary
    perspiration, during
    sleep, in
Wildness
Will, loss of
Work, mental impossible

CAMPHORA BROMATA

Delusions, dimension of things reversed
•
Excitement, excitable
Hysteria
Irritability
Mistakes, localities, in
Sadness, despondency, dejection, mental
    depression, gloom, melancholy

CANNABIS INDICA

Absent-minded, unobserving
Absorbed, buried in thought
Abstraction of mind
Air, castles (plans), builds, in ★
Amorous
Anguish
    air amel., open
    oppression, with
Answers, incoherently
Antagonism with herself ★
Anxiety
    air, amel. in open
    masturbation, from •
    paroxysms, in ★
    salvation, about
Bite, desire to
Capriciousness
Cares, worries, full of
Caressed: propensity for caresses •
Cheerful, gay, mirthful
    alternating with mania
        sadness
Clairvoyance
    midnight •
Company, aversion to; presence of
    other people agg. the symp-
    toms; desire for sotitude
Comprehension, easy
Concentration, difficult
Confusion of mind
    dream, as if in
Contradiction, is intolerant of
Crawling on floor
Cursing, swearing

Dancing
Death, presentiment of
    sensation of
        chill, during •
    thoughts of
Delirium
    night
    delusions, with
    erotic
    foreign countries, talks of •
    loquacious
    maniacal
    raging, raving
Delirium tremens, mania-a-potu
    delusions, with
Delusions, imaginations, halluci-
    nations, illusions
    night
    absurd, ludircrous •
        figures are present
    angels, seeing
    annihilation, about to sink into
    argument, making an eloquent •
    army passed him in the street, a
        silent (while walking) •
    ball, he is sitting on a
    beautiful
    bells, hears ringing of
        numberless sweet toned •
    bewitched, he is •
    bier, is lying on a
    blood rushed through like roar of
        many waters
    body covers the whole earth •
        divided, is
        greatness of, as to
    brain, has softening of
    butterflies, of
    calls, someone
        him, someone
    changing, suddenly •
    choir, he is in a cathedral on,
        hearing music •
    choked, he is about to be (night on
        waking)
    Christ, himself to be

163

Delusions,

    clothes, fly away and become wandering stars, will (on un-dressing) •

      rags, is clad in •

    clouds, strange, settle upon patients, or dancing about the sun •

    commander, being a

    companions are half men, half plants •

    cowards, persons leaving him are •

    creative power, has •

    cylinder, being a •

    dancing satyres and nodding mandarins •

    dead, corpse on a bier

      he himself was

      person, midnight, on waking, sees •

    delirious, he was •

    deserted, forsaken, is

    devils, sees

      he is a devil

      possessed of a devil, is

      present, are

    die, he was about to

      will die and soon be dissected •

    diminished, all is

    dissected, he will be •

    distances, of

    divided into two parts

    divine, being

    double, of being

      sensations present themselves in a double form •

    dying, he is

    emperor, is an •

    engaged in some occupation, is

    enlarged

      body, parts of

      distances are

      eyelashes are •

      head is

      leg is longer, one •

      objects are

      persons are

    eternity, he was in •

Delusions,

    existence, own, doubted his •

      two existences, to have •

      without form in vast spaces •

    expanding, passers-by are •

    eyelashes prolonged •

    faces, sees

      distinguished people, of •

      hideous

      ridiculous •

      ugly face seem pleasing •

    falling walls

    fancy, illusions of

    finger-nails seem as large as plates (during drowsiness) •

    floating in air

    flowers, of gigantic •

    fluid, surrounded by ethereal, resisting passage •

    flying, sensation of

      abyss, from a rock into dark (on going to bed) •

    giraffe, he is a •

    glow-worms, of •

    gnome, being oneself a •

    great person, is a

    grotesque

    hall, illusions of a gigantic

    head belongs to another

      monstrous head on distant wall of room

      pendulum, head seems an inverted, oscillating •

    hearing, illusions of

    heat, has a furious, radiating from epigastrium •

    heaven, is in

    hell, is in

      shadows of, in (midnight, on waking) •

    hippopotamus, being oneself a •

    home, thinks is at, when not

    horses: horse back, is on •

    house is full of people

      movable, seems •

    hunter, he is a

    ichthyosaurus, seeing an •

Delusions,

identity, errors of personal
    someone else, she is
images, pleasant
injury, is about to receive
ink stand, an, he was •
insane, she will become
journey, he is on a
knowledge, he possesses infinite •
leg is tin case filled with stair rods
    •
legs, long, too •
life, symbols of, all past events
    revolve rapidly in wheels •
    careering from life to •
light, incorporeal, he is
locomotive, he is a •
long, leg is too, one •
ludicrous
maelstrom, carried down a
    psychical •
man, muffled man starts from the
    wall (when walking in the
    streets) •
mandarin, mistook friend for a •
marble statue, felt he is •
mountain, he is on the ridge of a •
murder him, persons are bribed
    to •
music, he hears
    sweetest and sublimest melody
mystery, everything around
    seems a terrifying •
noise, shout of vehicles, hears •
officer, he is an
person is in the room, another
places at a time, of being in
    different
pleasing
pump-log, he was a •
queen, she is a •
rich, as if, he is ★
riding on a horse •
room walls gliding together, seem •
    horrible things on the, sees •
satyrs, visions of dancing
saw, he was a huge, darting up
    and down •

Delusions,

shouting, to be •
singing, to be •
soda water, being a bottle of
soldiers march silently past, sees •
soot, shower of, fell on him •
sorrow, everyone he meets has a
    secret •
soul, body was too small for soul
    or separated from
space, carried into, he was (while
    lying)
        orbit and compelled to de-
            scribe a vast •
        expansion of
sphere, being a •
spinal column is a barometer •
spirit, he is a •
square, surrounded by houses a
    hundred story high, sees a
    colossal •
stars, saw in his plate •
strange, everything is
    familiar things seem
        ludicrous, are
    voice seemed, her own •
strangers, he sees
sun is reeling •
super human, is
surrounded by friends, is
swimming, is
swollen, is
tankard and chased with figures
    of dragons,
    looked an huge •
tartars, of, a band •
thieves, house, in
three persons, he is
time, exaggeration of, passes
    too slowly
transferred, world, to another •
transparent, he is
travelling, of
unearthly, of something •
unreal, everything seems
vegetable existence, leading a •
virgin Mary, being •
visions, has

Delusions,
    beautiful
    grandeur, of magnificient
    monsters, of
    power, of imaginary •
    wonderful
    vitality, vivid consciousness of us-
        ually unnoticed operations of •
    voices, hears
        his own voice sounds strange
        and seems to reverberate like
        thunder •
    walls, is surrounded by high •
    falling
    want, they had come to •
    water, of blue •
        disasters by •
        nectar, water is delicious (when
        drinking)
    wealth, of
    weight, has no
    whimsical •
    wind sighing in chimney sounded
        like the hum of a vast wheel,
        and reverberated like a beat
        of thunder on a grand organ •
    women, of old and wrinkled
    worms, vomitus is a bunch of •
Dementia
Desire, exercise, for
Despair
    recovery, of
Dipsomania, alcoholism
Distances, inaccurate judge of
    exaggerated, are
Dream, as if in a
Dullness, sluggishness, difficulty of
    thinking and comprehending,
    torpor
Eccentricity
    epilepsy, before fit of •
Ecstasy
Excitement, excitable
    afternoon
    sadness, after
Exhilaration
Exultant •

Fancies, exaltation of
    pleasant
    vivid, lively
Fear, apprehension, dread
    approaching him, of others
    brilliant objects, looking-glass or
        cannot endure, of
    coal-scuttle, of •
    control, loss of ★
    dark, of
    death, of
    drowned, of being •
    fit, of having a
    ghosts, of
    injured, of being
    insanity, losing his reason, of
    mirrors in room, of
    things, of real and unreal •
    voice, of using
    water, of
Foolish behavior
Forgetful
    streets, of well known
    words while speaking, of;
        word hunting
Forsaken feeling
    isolation, sensation of
Frightened easily
Gestures, makes
    automatic
    furious
    hands, involuntary motion, of the
        rubbing together •
Giggling
Haughty
Hurry, haste
    everybody must hurry
    movements, in
Hydrophobia
Hysteria
Ideas abundant, clearness of mind
    urination, after •
Impulse, run, to; dromomania
Indifference, apathy
    conscience, to the dictates of
    external things, to
Indolence, eating, after

Insanity, madness
  drunkards, in
  erotic
  puerperal
Introspection
Irresolution, indecision
Irritability
      afternoon
Jesting
      puns, makes ●
Lascivious, lustful
Laughing
  constant
  cyanosis, with
  immoderately
  involuntarily
  sardonic
  serious matters, over
  spasmodic
  trifles, at
  weeping and laughing at same
    time
  word said, at every ●
Loquacity
Mania
  rage, with
Meditation
Memory, active
Memory, loss of
  aphasia, in
Memory, weakness of:
  expressing oneself, for
  heard, for what has
  names, for proper
  read, for what has
  said, for what has
  say, for what is about to
  thought, for what has just
  words, of
  write, for what is about to
  written, for what he has
Mildness
Mischievous
Mistakes, localities, in
  space and time, in
  time, in
  writing, in
      wrong words

Moaning, groaning, whining
Mocking, sarcasm
Morphinism
Music, agreeable, is
    faintness on hearing
Nymphomania
Passionate
Pleasure
Proportion, sense of, disturbed ★
Prostration of mind, mental exhaus-
    tion, brain-fag
    trembling, with
Quiet, wants to be
Rage, fury
    weeping, with
Reading, unable, to read
Recognize, streets, does not, well known
Restlessness
Runs about, against people, in walking ●
Sadness, despondency, dejection, mental
    depression, gloom, melancholy
      morning
Satyriasis
Self, odd at with ★
Senses, acute
Sensitive, noise, to
    want of sensitiveness
Shining objects agg.
Shrieking, screaming, shouting
Singing
Somnambulism
Speech, enthusiastic ●
    extravagant
    finish sentence, cannot
    hasty
    incoherent
    nonsensical
    vivacious
    voice, in a shrill
Spit, faces of people, in
Starting, sleep, during
Strange, everything seems
Strength increased, mental
Stupefaction, as if intoxicated
Suspicious, mistrustful
Talk, indisposed to, desire to be silent,
    taciturn
Talking, sleep, in

Talks, one subject, of nothing but
Theorizing
Thoughts, circles, move in •
  disconnected
  intrude and crowd around each
    other
  past, of the
  persistent
  rapid, quick
  ridiculous
  rush, flow of
  vanishing of
    reading, on
    speaking, while
    writing, while
  wandering
**Time, passes too slowly, appears
  longer**
  ages, a few seconds seem •
Timidity, evening, going to bed, about
Unconsciousness, coma, stupor
  night
  candle light, from •
  conduct, automatic
  dream, as in a
  music, from
  piano, listening of •
  pregnancy, during
  sudden
  transient
Verses, makes
Walking in open air amel. mental
  symptoms
Weeping, tearful mood
  involuntary
Whistling
Witty
Work, aversion to mental
  impossible

CANNABIS SATIVA

Absent-minded, unobserving
Absorbed, buried in thought
Anger, irascibility
  alternating with cheerfulness
    weeping
  trifles, at
  violent

Anxiety
  night
  voice, on raising the •
Bed, aversion to, shuns bed
Capriciousness
  forenoon
  afternoon
Cheerful, gay, mirthful
  afternoon
  alternating with bursts of passion
  mania
  sadness
  seriousness
  chill, during
Comprehension, easy
Concentration, difficult
Confounding objects and ideas
Confusion of mind
  morning, waking, on
  afternoon
  evening
  dream, as if in
  identity, as to his
    duality, sense of
  mixes subjective and objective
Conversation agg.
Dancing amel.
Darkness agg.
Delirium
  delusions, with
  gay, cheerful
  raging, raving
Delirium tremens, mania-a-potu
*Delusions, imaginations, hallucina
  tions, illusions*
  assembled things, swarms,
  crowds, etc.
  distances, of
  double, of being
  enlarged, distances are
  fancy, illusions of
  head belongs to another
  hearing, illusions of
  identity, errors of personal
    someone else, she is
  images, phantoms, sees
  insane, she will become
  journey, he is on a

Delusions,
    music, unearthly
    person, she is some other
    resin, exuding from every pore •
    strange, everything is
       familiar things seem
    talking, some one else is, when he
       speaks
    time, exaggeration of, passes too
       slowly
    unreal, everything seems
    visions, has
    voices, hears
Discontented, displeased, dissatisfied
    everything, with
Distances, inaccurate judge of
Dream, as if in a
Dullness, sluggishness, difficulty of think-
    ing and comprehending, torpor
    afternoon
    evening
    sleepiness, with
    waking, on
    writing, while
Ecstasy
Excitement, excitable
Fancies, exaltation of
    vivid, lively
Fear, apprehension, dread
    bed, of the
    dark, of
    death, of
    noise, from
    stomach, arising from
Foolish behavior
Forgetful
    words while speaking, of; word
       hunting
Forsaken, isolation, sensation of
Frightened easily
Gestures, convulsive
    spinning, around on the feet •
Haughty
Heedless
Hurry, haste
    chill, during •
Hysteria
Ideas abundant, clearness of mind
    deficiency of

Imbecility
Inconstancy
Indifference, apathy
    everything, to
    joyless
Indolence, aversion to work
    evening
Industrious, mania for work
Insanity, madness
    behaves like a crazy person
    cheerful, gay
    malicious, malignant
    puerperal
    weeping, with
Insecurity mental
Irresolution, indecision
    changeable
Irritability
    afternoon
Lascivious, lustful
Laughing
    agg.
    cyanosis, with
    loudly
    spasmodic
Light, desire for
Loquacity
Ludicrous, things seem
Malicious, spiteful, vindictive
Mania
    rage, with
Meditation
Memory, active
Memory, weakness of
    do, for what was about to
    expressing oneself, for
    say, for what is about to
    words, of
Mistakes, differentiating of objects, in
    speaking, in
       misplacing words
       words, using wrong
       wrong answers, gives
    time, in
    writing, in
       omitting words
       repeating words
Mood, alternating
    changeable, variable

Morose, cross, fretful, ill-humor, peevish
    afternoon
Music amel.
Muttering
    unintelligible
Nymphomania
Offended, easily; takes everything in
    bad part
Prostration of mind, mental exhaus-
    tion, brain-fag
Rage, fury
    alternating with cheerfulness
    chill, during
    malicious
    spitting, with
    trifles, at
    weeping, with
Restlessness
    chill, during
Sadness, despondency, dejection, mental
    depression, gloom, melancholy
    forenoon
        evening, amel.
    chill, during
Senses, vanishing of
Sensitive, oversensitive
    eating, after
    noise, to
Serious, earnest
    alternating with cheerfulness
Shamelessness
Singing
Sit, inclination to
Speech, confused
    hasty
    incoherent
Spit, desire to
    faces of people, in
Starting, startled
    electric, as if
    noise, from
    sleep, from
Strange, everything seems
    voices seem •
Stupefaction, as if intoxicated
Suspicious, mistrustful
Talk, indisposed to, desire to be silent;
    taciturn

Thoughts, persistent
    rush, flow of
    stagnation of
    thoughtful
    vanishing of
    wandering
Time, passes too slowly, appears longer
Unconsciousness, coma, stupor
    dream, on waking from a •
Vivacious
    intoxication, as from •
Wearisome
Weeping, tearful mood
    alternating with cheerfulness
        laughter
        rage
    chill, during
Well, says he is, when very sick
Whistling
Will, weakness of
Writing, difficulty in expressing ideas
    when
Yielding disposition

CANTHARIS

Absent-minded, unobserving
Absorbed, buried in thought
Abusive, insulting
Adulterous
Ailments from:
    anticipation, foreboding, presen
    timent
Amativeness
Amorous
Anger, irascibility
    morning, waking, on
    afternoon
    evening
    pains, about
Anguish, walking in open air
Anxiety
    morning
    forenoon
    night
    anticipation, from
    bed, with tossing about in

Anxiety
    conscience, as if guilty of a crime
    dinner, after
    eating, after
    fear, with
    fever, during
    hypochondriacal
    menses, during
    stool, before
        during
Aversion, everything, to ★
Barking
    bellowing
    delirium, during
Bed, aversion to, shuns bed
Bite, desire to
    delirium, during
Blasphemy
    cursing, and
Brooding
Business, talks of
Busy, fruitlessly
Capriciousness
Chaotic, confused behavior
Cheerful, gay, mirthful
    alternating with sadness
Complaining
Concentration, difficult
    morning
Confidence, want of self
Confusion of mind
    morning
    mental exertion, from
    reading, while
Contemptuous
Contradict, disposition to
    afternoon •
Contradiction, is intolerant of
Contrary
    afternoon •
Conversation agg.
Cowardice
Cruelty, inhumanity
Cursing, swearing
Death, conviction of
    presentiment of

Defiant
Delirium
    evening
    night
    anxious
    business, talks of
    crying, with
        help, for
    erotic
    fever, during
    frightful
    look fixed on one point, staring
    maniacal
    nonsense, with eyes open
    rabid
    raging, raving
    violent
    wild
Delusions, imaginations, hallucinations,
    illusions
    night
    bed, bouncing her up and down,
        someone
        raised, is •
        under it, someone is
        knocking
    business, is doing
    choked, icy-cold hands, by •
    dead persons, sees
    elevated in air, bed is raised •
    fancy, illusions of
    floating in air
    footsteps, hears
    hand, midnight vision of somthing
    taking her •
    hearing, illusions of
    images, phantoms, sees
        night
    injured, is being
    move, hears invisible things
    noise, knocking under bed
    possessed, being
    scream, with obliging to
    seized, as if
    shining objects, of •
    tactile hallucinations

Delusions,
>talking, dead people, with
>throat, some one with icy-cold
>hands took her by the •
>visions, has
>>night
>work, is hard at

Despair
Destructiveness
Discontended, displeased, dissatisfied
>everything, with
Discouraged
>anxiety, with
Disobedience
Dullness, shuggishness, difficulty of
>thinking and comprehending,
>torpor
>>morning
Ecstasy
Excitement, excitable
>morning
>chill, during
>convulsive
Exhilaration
Fancies, exaltation of
>morning
>night
>*lascivious*
Fear, apprehension, dread
>bed, of the
>death, of
>eating food, after
>*mirrors in room, of*
>stomach, arising from
>water, of
Foolish behavior
Forgetful
Frightened easily
Gestures, convulsive
>motion of hands, involuntary
>>throwing about
Heedless
Hurry, haste
>walking, while
Hydrophobia
Hypochondriasis
Hysteria

Ideas abundant, clearness of mind
>deficiency of
Impertinence
Inconstancy
Indifference, everything, to
Indolence, aversion to work
>morning
Insanity, madness
>*erotic*
>puerperal
>restlessness, with
>strength increased, with
Insolence
>*afternoon*
Introspection
Irresolution, indecision
Irritability
>morning
>>rising, after
>evening
>insults, from •
>pain, during
Lamenting, bemoaning, wailing
Lascivious, lustful
Laughing, alternating with sadness
Libertinism
Loathing, general
Loquacity
Malicious, spiteful, vindictive
>anger, with
Mania
>erotic ★
>*rage, with*
>tears, hair, own
>>himself to pieces with nails
Meditation
Mistakes, speaking, in
>words, using wrong
Moaning, groaning, whining
Mood, changeable, variable
Morose, cross, fretful, ill-humor, peevish
>morning
>afternoon
Nymphomania
>menses, after suppressed
Obscene, lewd
>songs
Obstinate, headstrong

Passionate
Prostration of mind, mental exhaustion, brain-fag
      morning
Quarrelsome, scolding
Rage, fury
    biting, with
    convulsions, r. with
    drink or touching larynx, when
      trying to •
    paroxysms, in
    shining objects, from
    shrieking, with
    violent
    water, at sight of
Restlessness
    day and night
    night
    anxious
    bed, tossing about in
    driving about
    headache, during
    move, must, constantly
    rage, ending in a •
    waking, on
Roving, senseless, insane
Rudeness
Runs about
Sadness, despondency, dejection, mental
    depression, gloom, melancholy
      morning
      noon
    dinner, after
    eating, after
Satyriasis
Scratches with hand, lime off the walls, the
Senses, dull, blunted
    vanishing of
Sensitive, oversensitive
Sentimental
Shamelessness
Shining objects agg.
Shrieking, screaming, shouting
    convulsions, before
    delusions with
Sit, inclination to

Speech, delirious
    hesitating
    nonsensical
    wandering
Starting, sleep, during
    from
Striking
    about him at imaginary objects
    wall, the •
Succeeds, never
Sulky
Suspicious, mistrustful
Talk, indisposed to, desire to be silent, taciturn
Talks, dead people, with
Tears things
Thoughts, intrude and crowd around each other
    persistent
    rush, flow of
      morning
    strange
    thoughtful
    vanishing of
      mental exertion, on
Timidity
Unconsciousness, coma, stupor
    night on waking
    cold surface, with •
    convulsions, after
    eyes, with fixed
    face, with red
    lying with out-stretched arms,
      screaming and tossing •
    sudden
    transient
    twitching of limbs, with
    uraemic coma
    vertigo, during
    walking in open air, while
Violent, vehement
Wanders restlessly about
Weeping, tearful mood
    morning
    agg.
    anxiety, after
    convulsions, during

Weeping, tearful mood
    pains, with the
        whimpering
Wildness
Work, mental, impossible

CAPSICUM ANNUUM

Absent-minded, unobserving
Absorbed, buried in thought
Abstraction of mind
Ailments from:
    excitement, emotional
    grief
    homesickness
Anger, irascibility
    alternating with cheerfulness
        contentment
        exhilaration
        jesting
    chill, during •
    cough from anger
    easily
Anxiety
    anger, during
    breath, must, he, deeply •
    chill, during
    noise, from
    stool, before
Aversion, everything, to
Awkward ★
Brooding
Busy
Capriciousness
Censorious, critical
Cheerful, gay, mirthful
    alternating with anger
        bursts of indignation
        of passion
Company, aversion to; presence of
        other people agg. the symp-
        toms; desire for solitude
Concentration, difficult
Confusion of mind
    morning
    chill, during
    waking, on
Contented

Contradiction, is intolerant of
Contradictory to speech, intentions are
Contrary
Death, desires
Delirium
    chill, during
Delirium tremens, mania-a-potu
Dipsomania, alcoholism
Dirtiness
Discontented, displeased, dissatisfied
    inanimate objects •
Disgust
Disobedience
Dullness, sluggishness, difficulty of think-
        ing and comprehending, torpor
    morning
        waking, on
    chill, during
    dreams, after
    heat, during
    perspiration, during
    waking, on
Elegance, want of
Ennui, homesickness, with
Excitement, chill, during
    heat from e. •
Extremes, goes to ★
Fear, apprehension, dread
    air, of fresh
    censured, of being •
    death, of
    evil, of
    guilt, of ★
    reproaches, of
    waking, on
Forgetful
    headache, during
Frightened easily
    waking, on
Gestures, awkward in
Grief
Homesickness
    heat in throat, with •
    red cheeks, with •
Howling
Hurry, haste
Hypochondriasis
Idiocy

Imbecility
Indifference, apathy
    everything, to
Indignation
Indiscretion
Indolence, aversion to work
Industrious, mania for work
Insecurity, mental ↔
Introspection
Irritability
    chill, during
    waking on, amel. λ
Jesting
    alternating with anger
    aversion to
    joke, cannot take a
Kisses everyone
Lamenting, bemoaning, wailing
Laughing
Malicious, spiteful, vindictive
    anger, with
Memory, active
Memory, weakness of
    words, of
Mildness
Moaning, groaning, whining
    objects, about λ
Mood, alternating
    changeable, variable
    repulsive
Morose, cross, fretful, ill-humor, peevish
    chill, during
    sleep, amel. in
Obstinate, headstrong
    children, chilly, refractory and
    clumsy λ
Offended, easily; takes everything in
    bad part
Perseverance
Pertinacity
Prostration of mind, mental exhaus-
    tion, brain-fag
Quarrelsome, scolding
Quiet disposition
Rashness
Reproaches others
Reserved

Restlessness
    anxious
    busy
    chill, during
    heat, during
Sadness, despondency, dejection, mental
    depression, gloom, melancholy
    haemorrhoids, suppressed, after λ
Security, desires ↔
Senses, acute
    dull, blunted
Sensitive, chill, during
    external impressions, to all
    noise, to
    chill, during
Shrieking, sleep, during
    waking, on
Singing
Sit, indination to ↔
Sociability, hide insecurity, to ↔
Starting, startled
    dream, from a
    heat, during
    sleep, during
    from
Stupefaction, as if intoxicated
Suicidal disposition
    homesickness, from λ
    thoughts
Suspicious, mistrustful
Talk, indisposed to, desire to be silent,
    taciturn
Thinking, aversion to
Thoughts, disconnected
Tranquillity, serenity, calmness
Unconsciousness, coma, stupor
    chill, during
    fever, during
Uncouth ↔
Wearisome
Weeping, tearful mood
    night
    alternating with laughter
    coughing, after
    heat, during
    sleep, in

Whistling
    fever, during •
Will, contradiction of
Witty
Work, mental, impossible

CARBOLICUM ACIDUM

Absent-minded, unobserving
    starts when spoken to
Abstraction of mind
Activity, mental
Anxiety, cold, becoming, from
Cheerful, gay, mirthful
      evening
      eating, while
Concentration, difficult
    studying, reading etc., while
Confusion of mind
Delirium
Dipsomania, alcoholism
Discontented, displeased, dissatisfied
Dream, as if in a
Dullness, sluggishness, difficulty of think-
    ing and comprehending, torpor
Excitement, excitable
    hydrocephalus, in
Exertion, agg. from mental
Exhilaration
Fear, disease, of impending
    night in bed •
Forgetful
Ideas abundant, clearness of mind
Impatience
Indolence, aversion to work
    physical
Irritability
Memory, weakness of
    do, for what was about to
    facts, for recent
    happened, for what has
    read, for what has
Moaning, groaning, whining
Mood, repulsive
Morose, cross, fretful, ill-humor, peevish
Pleasure

Prostration of mind, mental ex-
    haustion, brain-fag
Reading, mental symptoms agg. from
    aversion to read
Restlessness, night
Sadness, despondency, dejection, mental
    depression, gloom, melancholy
Sensitive, odors, to
Shrieking, screaming, shouting
    brain cry
    sleep, during
Sighing
Starting, startled
    sleep, during
    from
    spoken to, when
Talk, indisposed to, desire to be silent,
    taciturn
Thoughts, rapid, quick
Unconsciousness, coma, stupor
    convulsions, after
    incomplete
Work, aversion to mental
    desire for
    impossible

CARBO ANIMALIS

Affectionate
Ailments from:
    sexual excesses
Anger, irascibility
    morning
      waking, on
    former vexations, about
    past events, about
    waking, on
Anxiety
    morning
      rising on and after
      amel.
      waking, on
    afternoon
    evening
      bed, in
      night
    midnight, 0-2h. after •

Anxiety
    bed, in
    chill,. during
    closing eyes, on
    conscience, as if guilty of a crime
    dark, in
    eating, after
    fever, during
    menses, before
    pollutions, after
    rising, after
      amel.
    shuddering, with
    sitting, while
    waking, on
Avarice
Beside oneself, being
Brooding
Capriciousness
Cheerful, gay, mirthful
    evening, bed, in
    alternating with sadness
      weeping
    foolish, and
Childish behavior
Clinging, held amel., being
Company, aversion to; presence of other people agg. the symptoms; desire for solitude
    alone, amel. when
Concentration, difficult
Confidence, want of self
Confusion of mind
    morning
      waking, on
    evening
    dream, as if in
    epistaxis amel.
    motion of the head, from
    sitting, while
    walking, while
Contrary
Conversation agg.
Cowardice
Darkness agg.
Death, thoughts of
Delirium, intoxicated, as if

Delusions, imaginations, hallucinations, illusions
    evening, bed, in
    changed, everything is
    changing suddenly •
    deserted, forsaken, is
    faces, sees
      diabolical, crowd upon him
      hideous
    fancy, illusions of
    images, phantoms, sees
      evening
      night
      frightful
      sleep, before
        going to, on
    strange, everything is
      familiar things seem
    town, he is in deserted •
    visions, has
      evening
      horrible
Despair
Dipsomania, alcoholism
Discontented, displeased, dissatisfied
    everything, with
Discouraged
    daytime and night •
Dream, as if in a
Dullness, sluggishness, difficulty of thinking and comprehending, torpor
    morning
      waking, on
    forenoon
    dinner, after
    sleepiness, with
Excitement, evening in bed
    night
Fancies, exaltation of
    evening, bed, in
    night
    vivid, lively
Fear, apprehension, dread
    morning
    afternoon
    evening
    night

Fear,
    chill, during
    closing eyes, on
    crowd, in a
    dark, of
    death, of
    disease, of impending
    evil, of
    fainting, of
    fit, of having a
    insanity, losing his reason, of
    narrow places, vaults, churches
        and cellars, of •
    people, of; anthropophobia
    pollutions, after
    suffocation, of
        closing eyes, on •
        lying, while
        mucous in throat, from •
    waking, on
Foolish behavior
Forgetful
    words while speaking, of; word
        hunting
Forsaken feeling
    morning
Frightened easily
    evening
Gestures, hands, involuntary, throw-
        ing, about
Grief
Homesickness
    morning •
Hurry, haste
    walking, while
Imbecility
Indifference, apathy
    sleepiness, with
Indolence, aversion to work
    morning
    sleepiness, with
Insanity, madness
Introspection
Irritability
    morning
        waking, on
    forenoon
    alternating with indifference
    waking, on

Jesting, aversion to
Laughing, spasmodic
Light, desire for
Loathing, life, at
Malicious, spiteful, vindictive
    anger, with
Meditation
Memory, weakness of
    do, for what was about to
    expressing oneself, for
    said, for what has
    say, for what is about to
Mildness
Mistakes, writing, in
Moaning, groaning, whining
    sleep, during
Mood, alternating
    changeable, variable
Morose, cross, fretful, ill-humor, peevish
    morning, waking, on
    sleepiness, with
Music agg.
Obstinate, headstrong
Offended, easily; takes everything in
    bad part
Prostration of mind, mental exhaus-
    tion, brain-fag
    pollutions, after
Reflecting
Remorse
Reserved
Restlessness
    night
    anxious
    bed, driving out of
        tossing about in
    internal
    waking, on
Rocking amel.
Sadness, despondency, dejection,
    mental depression, gloom,
    melancholy
        morning
        amel.
        waking, on
    afternoon
    evening
    night

Sadness,
   anxious
   sleeplessness, with
     waking, on
Senses, vanishing of
Sensitive, oversensitive
   music, to
   noise, to
Shrieking, screaming, shouting
   sleep, during
Speech, intoxicated, as if
   low
   slow
Starting, startled
   sleeep, on falling
     during
Stupefaction, as if intoxicated
   sitting at table, while •
   walking, when
Sulky
Talk, indisposed to, desire to be
   silent, taciturn
   others agg., talk of
Talking, sleep, in
Thoughts, thoughtful
   vanishing of
Timidity
   daytime
   afternoon
   bashful
Unconsciousness, coma, stupor
   morning
   dream, as in a
   head, on moving
   sitting, while
   transient
   vertigo, during
   walking, while
Violent, morning
Wearisome
Weeping, tearful mood
   morning
   evening
   night
     sleep, in
   aloud, wobbing
   alternating with cheerfulness
     queer antics

   eating, while λ
   sleep, in
   waking on
Whistling
   involuntary
   jolly λ
Work, aversion to mental
Writing, difficulty in expressing ideas
   when

CARBO VEGETABILIS

Affectation
Affectionate
Ailments from:
   anticipation, foreboding, presen-
     timent
   debauchery
   sexual excesses
Anger, irascibility
   forenoon
   face, with pale, livid
   violent
   worm affections, in
Anguish
   evening
   cardiac
Answers:
   incorrectly
   irrelevantly
   slowly
Anxiety
   morning
     waking, on
   afternoon
     16-18h. λ
   evening
     twilight, in the
     bed, in
   night
     waking on
   midnight, before
   anticipating, from, an engage-
     ment ↔
   bed, in
   driving out of
   sit up, must λ
   chill, during
   closing eyes, on

Anxiety,
    conscience, as if guilty of a crime
    dark, in
    eating, while
      after
    fear, with
    fever, during
      as from ●
    head, with congestion to
      heat of, with
      perspiration on forehead, with
    headache, with
    lying, while
    menses, before
    pains, from the
    paroxysms, in
    pressure on the chest, from
    shuddering, with
    sleep, before
      on going to
    stool, after
    strangers, in the presence of
    waking, on
Avarice
    generosity towards strangers, ava-
      rice as regards his family
Beside oneself, being
Bite, desire to
    worm affections, bites in ●
Carried, desires to be
Cheerful, gay, mirthful
    evening
      bed, in
    alternating with moroseness
    eating, after
    foolish, and
Childish behavior
Clinging, restlessness, with ●
Company, aversion to; presence of other
    people agg. the symptoms; desire
    for solitude
    presence of strangers, aversion to
Company, desire for; aversion to soli-
    tude, company amel.
Concentration, difficult
Confidence, want of self

Confusion of mind
    morning
      rising and after, on
      waking, on
    afternoon
    evening
    arouse himself, compelled to
    dinner, after
    dream, as if in
    eating, after
    intoxicated, as if
      as after being
    lying, when
    mental exertion, from
      amel. ●
    sleeping, after
    siesta, after a
    waking, on
    walking, while
      air, in open
Cowardice
Darkness agg.
Death, desires
Delirium
    night
    dark, in
    quiet
    waking, on
Delirium tremens, mania-a-potu
Delusions, imaginations, hallucinations,
    illusions
      evening, bed, in
      night
    anxious
    bed, someone is in bed with him
    crime, committed a, he had
    criminals, about
    dark, in the ●
    deserted, foresaken, is
    enlarged, body, parts of
    faces, sees
      closing eyes, on
    fall inwards, walls of room seem
      (before epileptic fit) ●
    fancy, illusions of
    heat, during

Delusions,
  figures, sees
  footsteps, hears
  hand passes over body •
  hearing, illusions of
  images, phantoms, sees
    night
    dark, in the
    frightful
  move, hears invisible things
  noise, hears
  people, beside him, are
  smaller, of being
    epileptic fit, before •
    things grow smaller
  spectres, ghosts, spirits, sees
  visions, has
    evening
    horrible
      evening
      dark, in the
  waking, on
Despair
  heat, during
  pains, with the
  perspiration, during
Dipsomania, alcoholism
Discouraged
  irritability, with
  weeping, with
Doubtful
Dream, as if in a
Dullness, sluggishness, difficulty of think-
    ing and comprehending, torpor
      morning, waking, on
      evening
      damp air, from
      heat, during
      reading, while
      sleepiness, with
Ecstasy, perspiration, during
Excitement, excitable
      evening
        bed, in
      chill, during
      hurried, as if
Exertion, agg. from mental

Extravagance
Fancies, exaltation of
    evening, bed, in
    night
  lascivious
  perspiration, during
Fear, apprehension, dread
    morning
    afternoon
    evening
    night
      waking, after
    accidents, of
    apoplexy, of
      waking, on
    dark, of
    death, of
    eating food, after
    evil, of
    ghosts, of
      night
    happen, something will
    over powering
    people, of; anthropophobia
    sleep, before
    strangers, of
    suffocation, of
    tremulous
Flatterer
Foolish behavior
Forgetful
    periodical
    words while speaking, of; word
      hunting
Forsaken feeling
    morning
Frightened easily
Generous, strangers, for
Gestures: cross fingers ★
Hurry, haste
    occupation, in
Ideas abundant, clearness of mind
    deficiency of
Imbecility
Impatience
Impetuous
    perspiration, with

Indifference, apathy
   duties, to
   everything, to
   family, to his
   joy and suffering, to
   music, which he loves, to
   sleepiness, with
Indolence, aversion to work
     morning
   evening
   sleepiness, with
   drunkards, in
   insanity, haemorrhage, after
Irresolution, marry, to
Irritability
   daytime
   morning
   forenoon
   chill, during
   eating, after
   heat, during
   trifles, from
Jesting
Kicks
   worm-affections, in •
Kleptomania
Lascivious, lustful
Laughing
   agg.
   immoderately
Liar
Libertinism
Loathing, life, at
Mannish habits of girls
Memory, active
Memory, weakness of
   facts, recent, for
   heard, for what has
   periodical
   said, for what has
   sudden and periodical
Moaning, groaning, whining
   sleep, during
Monomania
Mood, changeable, variable
     night •
   supper, after

Morose, cross, fretful, ill-humor, peevish
   eating, after
   trifles, about
   worm affection, in
Music, palpitation when listening to
Nymphomania
Obscene, lewd
Obstinate, headstrong
Offended, easily; takes everything in bad part
Passionate
Prejudice, traditional
Prostration of mind, mental exhaustion, brain-fag
   • morning
   noon
Rage, worm affections, in •
Reading, aloud, agg. ★
Rebels against poultice
Religious affections
Remorse
   afternoon
Restlessness
   afternoon
     16-18 h.
   evening
   night
   anxious
   bed, driving out of
   chill, during
   company, in •
   driving about
   heat, during
Rocking agg.
Sadness, despondency, dejection, mental depression, gloom, melancholy
   evening
     amel.
   anxious
   pain, from slightest •
Senses, dull, blunted
Sensitive, oversensitive
   daytime •
   heat, during
   noise, to

Shrieking, screaming, shouting
    sleep before menses, during
    stool, during •
Sighing, heat, during
Sit, inclination to
Slowness
Smaller, things appear
Spying everything
Starting, startled
    night
    dreams, from a dream
    easily
    fright, from and as from
    noise, from
    sleep, on falling
        during
        from
Striking
    worm affections, in •
Stupefaction, as if intoxicated
Suicidal disposition
    anger driving to suicide •
    despair, from
    hanging, by
    shooting, by
Suspicious, mistrustful
Talk, inapt to talk in public
    indisposed to, desire to be silent,
      taciturn
Talking, sleep, in
Thinking, aversion to
Thoughts, persistent
Timidity
    appearing in public, about
    awkward, and
    bashful
    company, in
Unconsciousness, coma, stupor
    morning
    lies as if dead
    lying, while
    rising up, on
    semi-consciousness
Unfortunate, feels
Verses, makes
Violent, vehement
    morning
    forenoon •

Weary of life
Weeping, tearful mood
    afternoon
    air, in open
    anxiety, after
    chill, during
    sad thoughts, at
    sleep, in
Work, aversion to mental
    impossible

CARBONEUM

Restlessness, night
    bed, tossing about in

CARBONEUM HYDROGENISATUM

Answer, aversion to
    monosyllable
    slowly
Confusion of mind
Contented
Delusions, imaginations, hallucinations,
    illusions
    annihilation, about to sink into
Ecstasy
Excitement
    night
Stupefaction, as if intoxicated
Unconsciousness, coma, stupor
    sudden

CARBONEUM OXYGENISATUM

Activity, mental
Anguish
Answers, difficult
Anxiety
    morning, waking, on
    night. waking, on
Cheerful, gay, mirthful
Concentration, difficult
Confusion of mind
    intoxicated, as if

Delusions, hearing, illusions of
    images, ever changing •
Dullness, sluggishness, difficulty of think-
    ing and comprehending, torpor
Idiocy
Imbecility
Indifference, apathy
Loathing, general
Memory, weakness of
Mistakes, writing, in
Moaning, groaning, whining
Mocking, sarcasm
Mood, changeable, variable
Restlessness
    bed, tossing about in
Sadness, despondency, dejection, mental
    depression, gloom, melancholy
Senses, vanishing of
Sensitive, oversensitive
Shrieking, screaming, shouting
Stupefaction, as if intoxicated
Thoughts, disconnected
Unconsciousness, coma, stupor
    sudden
Weeping, spasmodic

CARBONEUM SULPHURATUM

Absent-minded, unobserving
Activity, mental
Ailments from:
    fright
Anger, irascibility
    alternating with indifference
    violent
Answers, monosyllable
    signs with hands, by •
Anxiety
    morning
    evening
      bed, in
    night
      midnight, before
    conscience, as if guilty of a crime
    fear, with

Anxiety,
    future, about
    menses, before
    salvation, about
    waking, on
Bite, desire to
    father, bites his •
Break things, desire to
Capriciousness
Cheerful, gay, mirthful
    morning
      flatus, after emission of •
Childish behavior
Company, aversion to; presence of
    other ·people agg. the symp-
    toms; desire for solitude
Concentration, difficult
    studying, reading, etc., while
Confusion of mind
    morning
      waking, on
    intoxicated, as if
    mental exertion, from
Conscientious about trifles.
Contradiction, is intolerant of
Delirium
    night
    fantastic
    maniacal
    raging, raving
Delusions, emperor, talked of •
    enemies, surrounded by
    fancy, illusions of
    hearing, illusions of
    injury, is about to recieve
    money, talks of
    strange, objects seem
    swollen, he is
    unpleasant
    visions, has
      grandeur, of magnificient
    voices, hears
Dementia
Despair
    itching of skin, from ★
Destructiveness

Dipsomania, alcoholism
Discontented, displeased, dissatisfied
Discouraged
*Dullness, sluggishness, difficulty of think
    ing and comprehending, torpor*
      morning
    children, in
Excitement, excitable
    night
Exhilaration
Exuberance
Fancies, absurd
    exaltation of
Fear, apprehension, dread
    morning
    night
    death, of
    insanity, losing his reason, of
    misfortune, of
    people, of; anthropophobia
    walking, dark, in the λ
Forgetful
    words while speaking, of; word
      hunting
Frightened easily
Hurry, haste
Hysteria
    attacks, in
Ideas abundant, clearness of mind
Idiocy
Imbecility
Indifference, apathy
    alternating with anger
Indolence, aversion to work
    morning
    amused when not λ
Insanity
Irresolution, indecision
Irritability
    morning
    evening
    spoken to, when
    involuntary
Laughing
Loquacity
    alternating with laughing
Mania

Memory, weakness of
    do, for what was about to
    expressing oneself, for
    facts, for recent
    words, of
Mistakes, speaking, in
    misplacing words
    writing, in
Moaning, groaning, whining
Mood, changeable, variable
Morose, cross, fretful, ill-humor, peevish
Obstinate, headstrong
Occupied with the objects immediately
    around him λ
Offended, easily; takes everything in
    bad part
Passionate
*Prostration of mind, mental exahaustion,
    brain-fag*
Rage, fury
Religious affections
Restlessness
    night
    midnight, before
**Sadness, despondency, dejection,
    mental depression, gloom,
    melancholy**
    evening
    cheerfulness, after λ
    chill, during
    heat, during
    perspiration, during
Sensitive, oversensitive
    noise, to
Shrieking, screaming, shouting
Singing
Sit, inclination to
    still
Speech, embarrassed
    hesitating
    incoherent
Spit, desire to
Spoken to, averse to being
Staring, thoughtless
Starting, startled
    fright, from and as from
    sleep, during
    from

Striking, bystanders, at
    desires to strike
Stupefaction, as if intoxicated
Suicidal, throwing himself, window,
    from
Sulky
Suspicious, mistrustful
Talk, indisposed to; desire to be silent;
    taciturn
Talking, sleep, in
Thoughts, persistent
    tormenting
Timidity
Unconsciousness, coma, stupor
Violent, vehement
Vivacious
Weeping, tearful mood
    irritable
    sleep, in
Whistling
Work, aversion to mental

CARCINOSINUM BURNETT

Ailments from:
    anticipation, foreboding, pre-
        sentiment
    fright
    reproaches
Anxiety
    others, for ★
Cheerful, gay, mirthful
    thunders and at lightenings, when
      it
Concentration, difficult
Confusion of mind
Consolation, kind words agg.
Contradiction, is intorlerant of
Dancing
Discontented, displeased, dissatisfied
    children ★
Dullness, sluggishness, difficulty of think-
    ing and comprehending, torpor
Fastidious
Fear, apprehension, dread
    busy streets ★

Indifference, apathy
Irritability
    forgetful, because ●
Loves animals ★
Memory, weakness of
    everyday things, for
Music agg.
    aversion ⁺o
Obstinate, headstrong
Offended, easily; takes everything
    in bad part
Sensitive, oversensitive
    a very strong sense of rhythm ★
    music, to
    reprimands, to
Shrieking, night
Suicidal disposition
Sympathy, compassion
Talk, indisposed to, desire to be silent,
    taciturn
Thunderstorm, loves ●
Timidity
Travel, desire to

CARDUUS BENEDICTUS

Morose, cross, fretful, ill-humor, peevish
    fever, after
Starting, noise, from

CARDUUS MARIANUS

Anger, irascibility
Dipsomania, alcoholism
Forgetful
Grief
Irritability
Memory, weakness of
    do, for what was about to
    say, for what is about to
Restlessness, night
Sadness, despondency, dejection, mental
    depression, gloom, melancholy
Sensitive, noise, to
Starting, startled
Weeping, tearful mood

CARLSBAD

Absent-minded, unobserving
Absorbed, buried in thought
Anger, irascibility
Anxiety
    air, amel. in open
    house, in
Censorious, critical
Cheerful, gay, mirthful
Confusion of mind
    walking, air amel., in open
Contented
Delirium
Delusions, imaginations, hallucinations,
    illusions
        night
Discouraged
    menses, before •
Dullness, sluggishness, difficulty of
    thinking and comprehending,
    torpor
Excitement, excitable
    trifles, over
Foolish, behavior
Heedless
    talking and writing, in •
Homesickness
Indolence, aversion to work
Introspection
Irritability
    morning, rising, after
Lascivious, lustful
Loquacity
Memory, weakness of
    names, for proper
    say, for what is about to
Mood, changeable, variable
Morose, cross, fretful, ill-humor, peevish
Prostration of mind, mental exhaus-
    tion, brain-fag
Read, aversion to
Restlessness
    bed, tossing about in
    internal

Sadness, despondency, dejection, men-
    tal depression, gloom, melan-
    choly
    afternoon
    air, amel. in open
    menses, before
Speech, confused
Starting, sleep, during
Sulky
Sympathy, compassion
Talk, indisposed to, desire to be silent,
    taciturn
Timidity
    daytime, 9h. •
Weeping, tearful mood
    sympathy with others, from
Work, aversion to mental

CASCARILLA

Anxiety
    fever, during
Delusions, people , behind him, some-
    one is
Frightened, waking from a dream, on
Restlessness
Thinking, aversion to

CASSADA

Moral feeling, want of
Morose, waking, on
Sadness, despondency, dejection, men-
    tal depression, gloom, melan-
    choly
Weeping, tearful mood

CASTOREUM CANADENSE

Anger, irascibility
    morning, waking, on
    menses, during
    waking, on
Anxiety
    morning
        rising, on and after
        amel.

Anxiety,
> night
>> midnight, after
> sleep, during
> waking, on

Capriciousness, daytime
> evening

Cheerful, gay, mirthful
> evening
> alternating with anxiety

Desires, anxious, full of •

Discontented, menses, during

Ecstasy

Excitement, excitable

Exuberance

Fear, apprehension, dread
> afternoon
> evil, of
> misfortune, of
>> afternoon

Frightened, night

Hysteria

Irritability
> morning
> afternoon
> evening
> chill, during
> menses, during
> waking, on

Mildness

Morose, cross, fretful, ill-humor, peevish
> morning
>> bed, in
> evening
> menses, during

Prostration of mind, mental exhaustion, brain-fag
> sleepiness, with

Restlessness
> night
> *anxious*
> *bed, tossing about in*
> women, in

Sadness, despondency, dejection, mental depression, gloom, melancholy
> morning
> afternoon
> evening

Senses, acute

Sensitive, oversensitive
> sensual impressions, to

Sentimental

Shrieking, screaming, shouting
> anger, in
> *sleep, during*

Speech, in sleep, angry •
> unintelligible, in sleep

Starting, midnight, after
> *sleep, during*
> from

Talk, indisposed to, desire to be silent, taciturn
> menses, during

Talking, sleep, in
> angry exclamations, with •
> excited

Unconsciousness, dinner, after

Weeping, tearful mood
> afternoon
> evening, amel.
> *night*
> anxiety, after
> *sleep, in*

CASTOR EQUI

Laughing, serious matters, over

CASTANEA VESCA

Restlessness, night

CASTELLA TEXANA

Anxiety, night, children, in

Capriciousness

Concentration, difficult, studying, learns with difficulty, while

Fear, children, in, night

Irritability

Quarrelsome, scolding

Shrieking, children, in
> sleep, during

Somnambulism

Talking, sleep, in

Violent, vehement

Weeping, children, in

CAULOPHYLLUM

Anger, menses, during
Anxiety, menses, during
Delirium
Delusions, pregnant, she is
Eat, refuses to
Excitement, excitable
    menses, during
Fear, apprehension, dread
    pregnancy, during
Hysteria
    menses, during
        copious
Irritability
    abortion, in •
Morose, cross, fretful, ill-humor, peevish
Prostration of mind, abortion, after •
Restlessness
    afternoon
        15h.
    evening
    night

CAUSTICUM HAHNEMANNI

Abrupt, harsh
Absent-minded, unobserving
Absorbed, buried in thought
Abstraction of mind
Abusive, insulting
Adulterous
Affectation
Affectionate
Ailments from :
    anger, vexation
    anticipation, foreboding, presen-
        timent
    cares, worries
    death of a child
        parents or friends, of
    excitement, emotional
    fear
    fright
    grief
    joy, excessive
    love, disappointed
        unhappy
    mortification

Amativeness
    want of amativeness in women
Ambition, loss of ★
Amorous
Anarchist •
Anger, irascibility
    alternating with cheerfulness
    trifles, at
    violent
    waking, on
Anguish
Answers
    aversion to answer
    refuses to answer
    repeats the question first
Anxiety
    daytime
    morning
        waking, on
    evening
        twilight, in the
        bed, in
    night
    midnight, before
        on waking •
    alone, when
    bed,in
    driving out of
    conscience, as if guilty of a crime
    crowd, in ★
    eating, after
    fear, with
    fits, with
    future, about
    headache, with
    hypochondriacal
    night watching, from
    noise, from
    others, for
    pains, from the
    sitting, while
    sleep, on going to
    stool, before
        during
        after
        ineffectual desire for, from
        straining at, while •
    suicidal disposition, with
    supper, after

Anxiety,
>   thinking about it, from
>   thunderstorm, during
>   trifles, about
>   waking, on
>   weary of life, with

Ardent

Avarice

Aversion, men, to
>   persons, to certain

Bed, aversion to, shuns bed

Beside oneself, being

Brooding

Business, incapacity for

Calculating, inability for
>   geometry

Capriciousness

Cares, worries, full of
>   day and night •
>   *others, about*
>   *relatives, about*

Cautious
>   anxiously

Censorious, critical

Character, lack of ★

Cheerful, gay, mirthful
>   daytime
>   morning
>   forenoon
>   night
>   alternating with irritability
>   *sadness*
>   vexation
>   sleep, during

Childish behavior, epilepsy, before ★

Company, desire for; aversion to soli-
>   tude, company amel.

Complaining

Comprehension, easy

Concentration, active

Concentration, difficult
>   studying, reading, etc., while
>   learns with difficulty

Confidence, want of self

Confusion of mind
>   morning
>   air, in open
>   coition, after
>   eating, after
>   amel.
>   *mental exertion, from*
>   sitting, while
>   stooping, when
>   walking, air, in open
>   after, amel. •

Content, himself, with

Contradict, disposition to

Contrary

Cowardice

Cursing, swearing

Dancing amel.

Darkness agg.

Death, desires
>   anxiety, from
>   thoughts of

Defiant

Delirium, crying, with
>   sleep, falling asleep, on

Delusions, imaginations, hallucinations,
>   illusions
>   absurd figures are present
>   criminals, about
>   dead persons, sees
>   enlarged, persons are
>   faces, sees
>   closing eyes, on
>   diabolical, crowd upon him
>   hideous
>   fancy, illusions of
>   grimaces, sees
>   images, phantoms, sees
>   black
>   *closing eyes, on*
>   *frightful*
>   insects, sees
>   large, people seem too (during
>   vertigo)
>   robbed, is going to be
>   sick, being
>   work, and for this reason
>   will not

Delusions,
    space between brain and skull,
        there is empty λ
    unfortunate he is
    visions, has
        closing the eyes, on
        horrible
Despair
    love, from disappointed
    recovery, of
Dictatorial, domineering, dogmatical,
        despotic
Dipsomania, alcoholism
Discomfort, walking, after
Discontented, displeased, dissatisfied
    himself, with
Discouraged
    disgust, with λ
Disgust
    everything, with
Disobedience
•*Dullness, sluggishness, difficulty of
        thinking and comprehending,
        torpor*
    epilepsy, before λ
    gassing, by
    pollutions, after
    sleepiness, with
    *understands questions only after
        repetition*
Dwells on past disagreeable occur-
        rences, night
Eat, refuses to
Eating, amel. after
Eccentricity, political
Escape, attempts to
    exaltation, politics ↔
Excitement, excitable
    agg.
    chill, during
    debate, during
    joy, from
    talking, while
    walking, after
        after walking in open air λ
    weakness, with
Exertion, agg. from mental

Extravagance
Exuberance
Fanaticism
Fancies, exaltation of
    day and night
    evening
        twilight, in λ
        bed, in
    night
    frightful
    sleeplessness, with
Fear, apprehension, dread
    morning
    evening
        twilight
        night
    alone, of being, night
    animals, of
    approaching him, of others
    bed, of the
    children, in
    closing eyes, on
    crowd, in a
    danger, of impending
    dark, of
    death, of
        alone, when evening in bed
    dogs, of
    eating, of
        after eating, food
    evil, of
    ghosts, of
    happen, something will
        warmth of bed amel.
    misfortune, of
    narrow places, vaults, churches
        and cellars, of
    noise, from
        night
        street, in
    overpowering
    people, of; anthropophobia
    stool, after ↔
    strangers, of
    supper, after λ
    tremulous

Foolish behavior, epilepsy, before ●
Forgetful
    epilepsy, before ●
    purchases, of; goes off and leaves
      them
Forgotten something, feels constantly
    . as if he had
Frightened easily
    trifles, at
Gamble (*see* Play)
Gestures, hands, involuntary motions,
    of the
    strange attitudes and positions
Gluttony
Gossiping
Grief
    day and night ●
    complaining, with ●
Haughty
Heedless
Homesickness
Horrible things, sad stories, affect her
    profoundly
Hurry, haste
    breath, with short ●
    eating, while
Hypochondriasis
    suicide, driving to
Hypocrisy
Hysteria
    menses, during
Ideas abundant, clearness of mind
    evening in bed
    deficiency of
Idiocy, idiotic actions, epilepsy, before ●
Imbecility
    epilepsy, before ●
Impetuous
    afternoon ●
Improvident
Impulse, morbid
Inconsolable
Indifference, apathy
    conscience, to the dictates of
    music, which he loves, to
    weeping, with
    welfare of others, to

Indiscretion
Indolence, aversion to work
    walking, while
    after ●
Industrious, mania for work
Insanity, madness
    fortune, after gaining
    melancholy
    persecution, mania
    suppressed eruptions, after
Intolerance
Introspection
Irresolution, indecision
Irritability
    daytime
    · forenoon
    alternating with cheerfulness
    chill, during
    heat, during
    menses, before
    during
    music, during
    noise, from
    takes everything in bad part
    trifles, from
    waking, on
Jealousy, animal or an inanimate ob-
    ject, for
    sexual excitement, with
    weeping, with
Kleptomania
Lamenting, bemoaning, wailing
Lascivious, lustful
Laughing
    night
    alternating with sadness
    convulsions, before during or af-
    ter
    dream, during
    sardonic
    sleep, during
    spasmodic
    epilepsy, before, during or af-
    ter
    weeping or laughing on all occa-
    sions
Liar
Libertinism

Litigious
Loathing, life, at
Loquacity
     forenoon λ
     drunkenness, during
Love with one of the own sex,
     homosexuality tribadism anal
     coition with a woman
Magnetized, easy to magnetize
Malicious, spiteful, vindictive
Mania
     suppresed eruptions, after
Marriage, obsessed by idea of marriage,
     excited sexual girls are
Mathematics, inapt for algebra
     geometry, for
Memory, weakness of
     names, for proper
Menses, mental symptoms agg. before
           during
Mildness
Mistakes,
     space and time, in
     speaking, in
        misplacing words
        mispronounces words λ
        reverses words
        transposes sounds λ
        wrong syllables, gives
        words, using wrong
     writing, transposing letters in
Moaning, groaning, whining
     sleep, during
     trifles, about every λ
Mocking, sarcasm
Mood, alternating
     changeable, variable
     repulsive
Morose, cross, fretful, ill-humor, peevish
     forenoon
     chill, during
     drunkenness, during
     menses, during
     waking, on
Music agg.
     aversion to
Muttering
Neglects everything
Obscene, lewd
     man searching for little girls

Obstinate, headstrong
Offended, easily; takes everything
     in bad part
Passionate
Pessimist
Play, passion for gambling
Positiveness
Prostration of mind, mental exhaus-
     tion, brain-fag
     sleeplessness, with
Qualmishness ↔
Quarrelsome, scolding
     anger, without
     sleep, in
Quiet disposition
Refuses, treatment, every
     sick, inspite of being very
Religious affections
Remorse
Reserved
Rest, cannot, sleep, during ↔
Restlessness
     afternoon on twilight λ
     evening
     night
        waking λ
     anxious
     bed, driving out of
     tossing about in
     convulsions, before
     menses, before
     move, must constantly
     pain, from
     rising from a seat, on λ
     sitting, while
     walking, while
Sadness, despondency, dejection,
     mental depression, gloom,
     melancholy
     day and night with weeping λ
     morning
     noon
     evening
     night
     alternating with vivacity
     amenorrhoea, in
     anxious
     children, in

Sadness,
    eating, after
    headahe, during
    menses, before
        during
    puberty, in
    suicidal disposition, with
Secretive
Self-control, loss of
Senses, acute
    dull, blunted
Sensitive, oversensitive
    crying of children, to
    music, to
    noise, to
    odors, to
    oppressive influences ★
    touch, to
Sentimental
    drunkenness, weeping or being
    sentimental during
Serious, earnest
Shrieking, screaming, shouting
    convulsions, during epileptic ★
    drunkenness, during
    sleep, during
Sit, inclination to
Slander, disposition to
Slowness
Speech, affected
    confused
    foolish
    hasty
    slow
Squanders
Starting, startled
    fright, from and as from
    noise, from
    perspiration, during
    sleep, on falling
        during
        from
Strangers, presence of strangers agg.
Stupefaction, as if intoxicated
    pollutions, after ●
Suicidal disposition
    hypochondriasis, by
    love, disappointed, from ★
    sadness, from

Sulky
Suppressed or receding skin diseases
    or haemorrhoids, mental symp-
    toms agg. after
Suspicious, mistrustful
Sympathy, compassion
Talk, desire to talk to someone
    forenoon ●
    indisposed to, desire to be silent,
    taciturn
    slow learning to
Talking, sleep, in
Tastelessness in dressing
Teasing
Thinking, complaints agg., of
Thoughts, frightful
    evening ●
    persistent
        evening
        lying, while
    unpleasant subjects, haunted
        by
    rapid, quick
    rush, flow of
        day and night
        evening in bed
        sleeplessness from
    tormenting
        evening
    vanishing of, mental exertion, on
    wandering
        evening ●
Thunderstorm, during, mind symp-
    toms
Timidity
    evening, going to bed, about
    night
Tranquillity, serenity, calmness
Travel, desire to
Trifles, seem important
Twilight, agg. mental symptoms
Unconsciousness coma, stupor
    morning
    evening
    conduct, automatic
    eating, after
    emotion, after
    exertion, after

Unconsciousness
  eyes, with fixed
  sitting, while
  walking in open air, while
Ungrateful
Violent, vehement
  evening, siesta, after •
  trifles, at
Wearisome
Weary of life
Weeping, tearful mood
  night
    sleep, in
  anger, after
  anxious
  children, in
  convulsions, during
Whooping cough, in
  drinking, after
  *drunkenness, weeping or being
    sentimental during*
  easily
  involuntary
  menses, during
  nervous, all day
  offences, about former
  old people for nothing •
  paralysis, in ★
  sleep, in
  spasmodic
  spasms, after •
  sympathy with others, from
  trifles, at
    children at the least worry
    *laughing or weeping on every
      occasion*
    vexation, from old
    whimpering
      sleep, during
Will, weakness of
Work, aversion to mental
  impossible
Writing, inability for
    learning to write in children
    mind symptoms, agg. ★

CEANOTHUS AMERICANUS

Anxiety, work, to become unfit for •
Excitement, chill, during

CECROPIA MEXICANA

Doubtful, recovery, of
Fear, disease, incurable, of being
Pessimist
Sadness, despondency, dejection, men-
  tal depression, gloom, melan-
    choly
  disease, about

CEDRON

Anguish
Anxiety
Aversion, friends, to
Bed, aversion to, shuns bed
Company, aversion to; presence of
  other people agg. the symp-
    toms; desire for solitude
Company, desires; alone agg., while
Confusion of mind, evening
  night
Delirium tremens, trembling, with
Dullness, sluggishness, difficulty of think-
  ing and comprehending, torpor
Excitement, excitable
  chill, before •
  women, in
Fear, bed, of the
  friends, of •
Hydrophobia
Hysteria
Irritability
Lascivious, lustful
Memory, weakness of, persons, for
Mildness
Nymphomania
Restlessness
  night
  driving about
  walᵏing, on
  women, in

Sadness, despondency, dejection, mental
    depression, gloom, melancholy
    coition, after
    heaviness of body, with
Shrieking, screaming, shouting
    convulsions, before
        during epileptic
Sighing
Unconsciousness, coma, stupor
Weeping, tearful mood

CENCHRIS CONTORTRIX

Absent-minded, unobserving
    dreamy
Ailments from:
    anticipation, foreboding, presen-
        timent
Anger, irascibility
    afternoon
    evening, 18h. •
        20 h. •
    alternating with kindness
    interruption, from
Anxiety
    evening, bed, in
    midnight, after
    bed, in
    lying, while
    sleep, on going to
Bed, aversion to, shuns bed
Censorious, critical
Cheerful, alternating with sadness
    sadness, after •
Company, aversion to; presence of
    other people agg. the symp-
    toms; desire for solitude
Company, desire for; averison to soli-
    tude, company amel.
Concentration, difficult
Death, presentiment of
    sudden death, of a •
    sensation of
Delusions, imaginations, hallucinations,
    illusions
    asylum, she will be sent to •

Delusions,
    people, behind him, someone is
        beside him, are
    places, two at the same time, of
        being in
    visions, has
    voices, hears
Discouraged
Dream, as if in a
Dullness, sluggishness, difficulty of
    thinking and comprehending,
    torpor
Duty, aversion to domestic
Envy
Fear, apoplexy, of
    · bed, of the
        death, from dream, of
        heart symptoms, during
        sudden death, of
Forgetful
    going, forgets where she is
Indifference, duties, to
Insanity, madness
Irresolution, indecision
Irritability
Jealousy
Memory, weakness of
Mistakes, writing, in
    wrong words
Mood, alternating
Offended, easily; takes everything in
    bad part
Quarrelsome, scolding
    jealousy, from
Restlessness
    bed, driving out of
    driving about
    move, must constantly
    walking, amel. while
Sadness, depondency, dejection, mental
    depression, gloom, melancholy
    daytime
    causeless
Selfishness, egoism
Shrieking, screaming, shouting
Sighing
Sits, wrapped in deep sad thoughts and
    notices nothing, as if

Staring, thoughtless
Stupefaction, as if intoxicated
Suspicious, mistrustful
    afternoon, 15-20 h. •
    evening
Time passes too slowly, appears longer
Timidity, evening, going to bed, about
Unconsciousness, coma, stupor
Unfeeling, hardhearted
Wander, desire to
Weeping, tearful mood

CENTAUREA TAGANA

Absent-minded, unobserving
Anxiety
Aversion, everthing, to
Cheerful, gay, mirthful
Concentration, difficult
Dullness, sluggishness, difficulty of think-
    ing and comprehending, torpor
Homesickness
Idiocy

CEPHALANTHUS OCCIDENTALIS

Cheerful, gay, mirthful
Excitement, excitable
Restlessness
    bed, tossing about in

CEREUS BONPLANDII

Business, desire for
Busy
Deeds, useful, desire to do •
Delusions, incubus, being weighed down
    by •
    influence, is under a powerful
Dullness, morning
Impulsive
Indolence, aversion to work
Industrious, mania for work
Insanity, madness
    alternating mental with physical
      symptoms

Irritability
Loathing, life, before menses, at •
Mistakes, time, in
Praying
Restlessness
Sighing
Time passes too slowly, appears longer
Tranquillity, serenity, calmness
Useful, desire to be ★

CEREUS SERPENTINUS

Anger, trifles, at
    violent
Cursing, swearing
Ennui, tedium
Irritability
Lascivious, lustful
Mistakes, speaking, in
    writing, in
Moral feeling, want of
Praying, night
Sensitive, oversensitive
Work, mental, impossible

CERVUS BRASILICUS

Restlessness
Sadness, daytime

CHAMOMILLA

Absent-minded, unobserving
    inadvertence
Absorbed, buried in thought
Abstraction of mind
Abusive, insulting
    menses, before ★
Affections, in general ★
Ailments from:
    anger, vexation
      anxiety, with
        silent grief, with
        suppressed
      contradiction
      fright
      honor, wounded
      mortification
    scorn, being scorned

Anger, irascibility
    agg.
    children, in
    consoled, when
    cough from anger
    easily
    face, with red
    interruption, from
    pains, about
    spoken to, when
    suffocative attack, with ●
    trembling, with
    trifles, at
    violent
    wakes in ★
    waking, on
Anguish
    tossing about, with
Answers: aversion to answer
    civil, cannot be
    incorrectly
    snappishly
Anxiety
    evening, bed, in
        night
    bed, in
        driving out of
    children, in infants
    coffee, after
    conscience, as if guilty of a crime
    eating, after
    fever, during
    future, about
    hypochondriacal
    mental exertion, from
    morphine, habits of ★
    nursing, after
    paroxysms, in
    periodical
    sleep, during
    stool, before
        during
            as for s⁺ool
    urination, during
        with urging to
Beside oneself, being

Bite, spoon etc., bites
Brooding
Capriciousness
Carried, desires to be
Censorious, critical
Change, desire for
Cheerful, gay, mirthful
**Company, aversion to; presence of
    other people agg. the symp-
    toms; desire for solitude**
    friends, of intimate
Complaining
Concentration, difficult
    afternoon
    studying, reading etc., while
Confusion of mind
    morning
    rising and after, on
    afternoon
    evening
    chill, during
    dream, as if in
    epistaxis amel.
    heat, during
    lying, when
    mental exertion, from
    paroxysms of pain, during
    waking, on
Conscientious about trifles
Consolation, kind words agg.
Contemptuous
Contradiction, is intolerant of
Contrary
Cowardice
Cross, crossness, (anger) ★
Death, thoughts of
Delirium
    night
    chill, during
    delusions, with
    fantastic
    fever, during
    nonsense, with eyes open
    pains, with the
    raging, raving
    sleep, during

Delusions, imaginations, hallucinations,
  illusions
    night
  animals, of
    bed, under •
    frightful
  council, holding a
  faces, sees
  fancy, illusions of
  groans, with
  head, shaking the
  hearing, illusions of
  images, phantoms, sees
    night
  insulted, he is
  large, people seem too (during
    vertigo)
  noise, hears
  people, converses with absent
  vexations and offences, of
  visions, has
    night
  vivid
  voices, hears
    night •
    distant
    strangers, of
Despair
  chill, during
  heat, during
  pains, with the
  perspiration, during
  recovery, of
Dictatorial, domineering, dogmatical,
  despotic
Dipsomania, alcoholism
Discontented, displeased, dissatisfied
  everything, with
  himself, with
  surroundings, with
  wrong, everything another does is •
Discouraged
  anxiety, with
  moaning, with
Dream, as if in a

*Dullness, sluggishness, difficulty of think-
  ing and comprehending, torpor*
    morning, rising, on
  chill, during
  heat,during
  think long, unable to
*Dwells on past disagreeable occur-
  rences*
Ecstasy
Escape, attempts to
Exaggerates her symptoms ★
Excitement, excitable
  agg.
  chill, during
  heat, during
    puerperal, during
  perspiration, during
Exertion, agg. from mental
Eyes, walks with downcast
Fancies, exaltation of
  evening
    night
    sleeplessness, with
  vivid, lively
Fear, apprehension, dread
    night
  evil, of
  heat, during
  noise, from
  overpowering
  recurrent
  touch, of
  tremulous
  vexation, after
  waking, on
  wind, of
  work, dread of
Forgetful
  words while speaking, of; word
    hunting
Frightened easily
  night, waking, 3h., on
  waking, on
Frown, disposed to ★
*Gestures, grasping or reaching at some
    thing, at flocks; carphologia
  fingers in the mouth, children put*
  picks at bed clothes

Grief, offences, from long past
Heedless
Howling
Hurry, haste
Hypochondriasis
Hysteria
    fainting hysterical
    menses, during
Ideas abundant, clearness of mind
    night
    deficiency of
Idiocy
Imbecility
Impatience
    heat, with
    pain, from
    slowly, everything goes too •
Impetuous
Inconsolable
Indifference, apathy
    alternating with vexation
    everything, to
    external things, to
    life, to
    pleasure, to
Indignation
Indolence, aversion to work
    physical
Insanity, immobile as a statue
Insecurity, mental
Intolerance, interruption, of
    spoken to, of being •
Introspection
Irresolution, indecision
    projects, in
Irritability
    morning
        rising, after
        waking, on
        night
    abortion, in threatened •
    children, in
    chill, during
    dentition, during
    dinner, after
    eating, after
    heat, during
    liver trouble, in

Irritability
    menses, before
        during
    pain, during
    parturition, during
    perspiration, during
    pregnancy, during •
    questioned, when
    sends the doctor home, says
        he is not sick
            out of the room •
    spoken to, when
    suspicious
    talking, while
    waking, on
Kicks
    stiff and kicks when carried, be-
        comes
Lamenting, bemoaning, wailing
    asleep, while
    pains, about
Loathing, general
Looked at, cannot bear to be
    agg. mental symptoms ★
Loquacity, speeches, makes
Malicious, spiteful, vindictive
Mania
Memory, weakness of
    persons, for
    words, of
Menses, mental symptoms agg. at be-
    ginning of
    mental symptoms agg. during
Mistakes, localities, in
    persons, in
    reading, in
    speaking, in
        intend, what he does not
        misplacing words
        omitting words
        words, using wrong
    writing, in
    omitting syllables
        words
Moaning, groaning, whining
    children, in
        wanted, piteous because
        they cannot have what
        they •

Moaning,
    dentition, in
    heat, during
    ill-humor, from •
    involuntary
    offences happened long ago, for
        trifling •
    pain, from
    restlessness, with
    sleep, during
    sleepiness, with •
Mood, changeable, variable
Moral feeling, want of
Morose, cross, fretful, ill-humor,
    peevish
        daytime
        night
    children, in
    carried, desire to be
    dentition, in •
    eating, after
    interruption, from •
    menses, before
        during
    pain, after
    trifles, about
    waking, on
Morphinism
Music agg.
    piano playing, from
    aversion to
    cough, m. agg.
        piano, cough when playing
    earache from m.
Muttering
Naked, wants to be
Obstinate, headstrong
    children
    menses, upon appearance of •
Offended, easily; takes everything in
    bad part
    offences, from past
Prostration of mind, mental exhaus-
    tion, brain-fag
        evening

Quarrelsome, scolding
    menses, at begining of •
    parturition, during •
Quiet disposition
Quieted, carried, only by being
Rage, fury
    pain, from
Rebels against poultice
Religious affections
Remorse
Reproaches others
Reserved
Restlessness
    evening in bed
    night
    anger, restlessness from
    anxious
    bed, driving out of
        go from one bed to another,
        wants to
        tossing about in
    children, in
        carried about, relieved by
        being
    chill, during
    headache, during
    heat, during
    menses, during
    metrorrhagia, during
Rocking amel.
    desire for being rocked
Rudeness
    naughty children, of
    women, in •
Sadness, despondency, dejection,
    mental depression, gloom,
    melancholy
    chill, during
    eating, after
    music, from
Senses, acute
    dull, blunted
    vanishing of
Sensitive, oversensitive
    children
    coffee, after •
    external impression, to all
    music, to

Sensitive,

  noise, to
  odors, to
  pain , to
  puberty, in
Serious, earnest
Shrieking, screaming, shouting
  anger, in
  brain cry
  children, in
    night
    colic, with
      weeping and
    obstinate •
    pain, with the
    sleep, during
    waking, on
Sighing
  heat, during
  perspiration, during
Sit, inclination to
Sits, erect
  stiff
  still
Snappish
Somnambulism
Speech, abrupt
  confused, night •
  delirious, chill, during •
  incoherent
  loud
  sharp
  strange
  unintelligible, in sleep
  vexations, about old •
  wandering
Spoken to, averse to being
  agg. (or addressed) ★
Starting, startled
  dentition, during •
  heat, during
  perspiration, during
  sleep, during
    from
  sleepiness, with
  tremulous
  trifles, at

Striking, children, in
Stupefaction, as if intoxicated
  morning on waking
Suspicious, mistrustful
Symptoms, magnifies her ★
Talk, indisposed to, desire to be silent,
  taciturn
  heat, during
  obstinacy, from •
Talking, sleep, in
  obstacles removed •
Thinking, complaints agg., of
Thoughts, persistent
  rapid, fever, during •
  thoughtful
  vanishing of
    mental exertion, on
Throws things away
Touched, aversion to being
Touchy ★
Tranquillity, serenity, calmness
  reconciled to fate
Ugly (in behavior) ★
Unbearable, pains ★
Unconsciousness, coma, stupor
  emotion, after
  menses, suppression of
Unsympathetic, unscrupulous
Violent, vehement
  pain, from
Wearisome
Weeping, tearful mood
    night
      sleep, in
  agg.
  aloud, sobbing
  anger, after
  carried, child is quieted only
    when
  children, in ·
    babies
  chill, during
  convulsions, during
  coughing, during
  heat, during
  obstinate •
  offence, imaginary, at least •

Weeping, tearful mood
  pains, with the
  perspiration, during
  piteous
  refused, when anything
  sleep, in
  sleepiness, with •
  stool, during
  vexation, from
  whimpering
    sleep, during
Work, aversion to mental

CHELIDONIUM MAJUS

Absent-minded, unobserving
Absorbed, buried in thought
Anger, irascibility
  causeless
  trembling, with
  trifles, at
  violent
Anxiety
  morning, waking, on
  afternoon
  evening
    18 h.
    amel.
  night, waking, on
  chill, after
  conscience, as if guilty of a
  crime
  exaggerated ★
  exercise amel.
  fear, with
  future, about
  house, in
  noise, from
  rising, after
  salvation, about
  sudden
  waking, on
Brooding
Cares, worries, full of
Carried, desires to be
Cheerful, evening
Children, desires to beat •

Concentration, difficult
Confusion of mind
  morning
    rising and after, on
  afternoon
  night
    waking, on
  sleeping: siesta, after a
  waking, on
Conversation agg.
  aversion to
Death, desires
  presentiment of
  thoughts of
Delirium
  night
  fever, during
  muttering
  quiet
  raging, raving
  waking, on
Delusions, imaginations, hallucinations,
    illusions
  crime, committed a
  criminals, about
  die, he was about to
  disease, incurable, has
  health, he has ruined his •
  insane, she will become
  soldier, being a (at night)
  think, she cannot •
Despair
  heat, during
  religious despair of salavation
Dipsomania, alcoholism
Discontended, displeased, dissatisfied
  surroundings, with
Doubtful, soul's welfare, of
Dullness, sluggishness, difficulty of think-
    ing and comprehending, torpor
  morning, bed, in
  condition, could not think of her •
  eating, after
  waking, on
Escape, attempts to
  run away, to
Excitement, excitable
  evening
  night

Exhilaration
Fancies, exaltation of
    evening
Fear, apprehension, dread
    death, of
       night
    happen, something will
    health, ruined, that she has •
    insanity, losing his reason, of
    noise, from
    observed, of her condition being
    pneumonia, of •
Forgetful
    shaving or dressing, of •
Imbecility
Indifference, apathy
    sleepiness, with
Indolence, aversion to work
    morning
    afternoon
        14 h. •
    dinner, after
    eating, after
    physical
    sleepiness, with
Insanity, madness
Irresolution, indecision
Irritability
    afternoon
    waking, on
Loathing, general
Loquacity
Mania
Memory, weakness of
    business, for
    do, for what was about to
    done, for what has just
Mildness
Morose, cross, fretful, ill-humor, peevish
    afternoon
    causeless
    trifles, about
    waking, on
Muttering
Obstinate, headstrong
Offended, easily; takes everything in
    bad part

Quarrelsome scolding
Rage, fury
Religious affections
Remorse
Restlessness
    day and night
    anxious
    conscience, of
    internal
Sadness, despondency, dejection, mental
    depression, gloom, melancholy
Senses, dull, blunted
    vanishing of
Sensitive, noise, to
Shrieking, sleep, during
Sit, inclination to
Slowness
Speech, incoherent
Starting, startled
    noon
    noise, from
    sleep, during
    from
    sleepiness, with
Striking, children, in
Stupefaction, as if intoxicated
    morning on waking
    night
Suicidal disposition
Sulky
Talk, indisposed to, desire to be silent,
    taciturn
Thoughts, disease, of
    persistent
    vanishing of
Tranquillity, serenity, calmness
    morning on waking
Unconsciousness, coma, stupor
    morning
        waking, on
    night
    delirium, after
    jaundice, in •
    pneumonia, in
    rubbing soles of feet amel. •
    transient
    vertigo, during
    waking, on

Unfortunate, feels
Weeping, tearful mood
   night
   carried. when •
   despair, from
Work, aversion to mental
   impossible

CHENOPODIUM ANTHELMINTICUM

Aphasia ★
Conversation, desire for
Fear, heat, from •
Forgetful, words while speaking, of;
   word, hunting
Hysteria •
Mistakes, speaking, using wrong words
   in
Repeated, same action ★
Restlessness, bed, tossing about in
Striking, bystanders, at
Unconsciousness, coma, stupor
Weeping, tearful mood
   menses, suppression of, in

CHIMAPHILA UMBELLATA

Delusions, ball, he is sitting on a
Dipsomania, alcoholism
Dullness, sluggishness, difficulty of think-
   ing and comprehending, torpor
Hysteria
Restlessness
Sadness, despondency, dejection, mental
   depression, gloom, melancholy

CHIMAPHILA MACULATA

Irritability, heat, during
Mildness
Unconsciousness, transient

CHINA OFFICINALIS

Absent-minded, unobserving
Absorbed, buried in thought
Admonition, kindly agg.
Affections, in general ★

Ailments from:
   anger, vexation
      silent grief, with
   anticipation, foreboding, presen-
      timent
   bad news
   sexual excesses
   work, mental
Air, castles (plans), plans, in ★
Anger, irascibility
   alternating with indifference
   caressing, from •
   stabbed any one, so that he could
      have
   trifles, at
   vex others, inclined to •
Anguish
Anorexia mentalis
Answers: aversion to answer
   refuses to answer
   unintelligibly
Anxiety
      morning
         waking, on
      evening
      night
      midnight, after
      2 h.
   bed, driving out of
   chill, before
      during
   conscience, as if guilty of a crime
   dreams, on waking from frightful
   eating, after
   fear, with
   fever, during
      prodrome of, during
   future, about
   trifles, about
   waking, on
   weary of life, with
Aversion, persons, to all
Bed, jumps out of; wants to destroy
   himself but lacks courage •
   . slides, down in ★
Beside oneself, being
Capriciousness

Cares, worries, full of
    trifles, about
Censorious, critical
Chaotic, confused behavior
Cheerful, gay, mirthful
        morning, waking, on
        evening
        night
            until 2 h. •
        alternating with sadness
            seriousness ★
        desires to be cheerful •
Company, aversion to; presence of other
    people agg. the symptoms; de-
    sire for solitude
Complaining
Concentration, difficult
Confidence, want of self
Confusion of mind
        morning
        afternoon
        night, waking, on
        beer, from
        dream, as if in
        excitement amel.
        heat, during
        intoxicated, as after being
        perspiration, during
        waking, on
Conscientious about trifles
Consolation, kind words agg.
Contemptuous
        everything, to
Contradiction, is intolerant of
Contradictory to speech, intentions are
Contrary
Conversation agg.
Corrupt, venal
Cowardice
Cruelty, inhumanity
Death, desires
Delirium
        bed and escapes, springs up sud-
            denly from
        depletion, after •
        fever, during
        haemorrhage, after

Delirium
        loss of fluids, from
        quiet
        raging, raving
        sleeplessness, and ★
        sleep: falling asleep, on
        trembling, with
Delirium tremens, mania-a-potu
Delusions, imaginations, hallucinations,
    illusions
        evening, bed, in
        deserted, forsaken, is
        faces on closing eyes, sees
            dark, in the
        falling asleep, on
        fancy, illusions of
        images, phantoms, sees
            night
        frightful
        sleep, going to, on
        obstructed, being •
        people, sees
            closing eyes, on
            persecuted, he is
            pursued by enemies
        rain, he hears (at night)
        spectres on closing eyes, sees
        tormented, he is
        unfortunate, he is
        vexations and offences, of
        visions, evening
            closing the eyes, on
        work, is hindered at •
Desires, indefinite
Despair
        pains, with the
Dictatorial, domineering, dogmatical,
    despotic
Dipsomania, alcoholism
Discontented, displeased, dissatisfied
Discouraged
Disobedience
        children, in •
Dream, as if in a
Dullness, sluggishness, difficulty of think-
    ing and comprehending, torpor
        morning
        waking, on

Dullness,
>> dreams, after
>> *loss of fluids, after*
>> periodical •
>> perspiration, during
>> sleepiness, with
>> waking, on

Dwells on past disagreeable occurrences
>> night

Ecstasy, heat, during
Ennui, tedium
Envy, avidity, and
Escape, attempts to
>> springs up suddenly from bed

Excitement, excitable
>> morning
>> evening
>> agg.
>> bad news, after
>> coffee, as after
>> *haemorrhage, after* •
>> **hearing horrible things, after**

Exertion, agg. from mental
Exhilaration, evening
Extravagance
Fancies, exaltation of
>> morning, bed, in •
>> evening
>> *bed, in*
>> *night*
>> going to bed, after
>> heat, during
>> *sleeplessness, with*
>> *lascivious*
>> *impotency, with*
>> sleep, falling asleep, on

Fear, apprehension, dread
>> morning
>> *night*
>> **animals, of**
>> death, of
>> **dogs, of**
>> *evil, of*
>> falling, of
>> ghosts, of
>> night

Fear,
>> hurt, of being
>> *killing, of*
>> knaves, of
>> knives, of
>> noise, from
>> overpowering
>> people, of; anthropophobia
>> pitied, of being •
>> rage, to fly in to
>> rags, of ★
>> suffocation, of, night
>> touch, of
>> waking, dream, from a
>> work, dread of

Foolish behavior
Foppish
Forgetful
>> night
>> *loss of fluids, from*
>> periodical
>> waking, on

Forsaken, feeling
Frightened, waking from a dream, on
Gamble (*see* Play)
Gestures, grasping or reaching at something, at   flocks; carphologia
>> picks at bed clothes
>> light

Gluttony
Gourmand
Greed, cupidity
Grief
Haughty
Hurt, feeling of others, disposition to ★
Hypochondriasis
>> eating, after
>> suicide, driving to

Hysteria
>> *loss of fluids, after*
>> menses, during
>> after

Ideas abundant, clearness of mind
>> **evening**
>> bed, in
>> *night*
>> *deficiency of*
>> fixed ★

Imbecility
Impatience
Inconsolable
   suicide, even to •
Indifference, apathy
   alternating with vexation
   eating, to
   everything, to
   fever, during
   money-making, to
   periodical
   typhoid, in
Indignation
Indolence, aversion to work
   dinner, after
   eating, after
   physical
   sleepiness,with
Industrious, mania for work
   menses, before
Insanity, drunkards, in
   gluttony, with
   haemorrhage, after
   heat, with
   restlessness, with
   travel, with desire to
Intolerance, noise, of
Introspection
Irresolution, indecision
   acts, in
Irritability
      morning
         children, in •
      night
      alternating with cheerfulness
      children, in
      chill, during
      coition, after
      consolation agg.
      excited , when
      headache, during
      waking, on
      weakness, with
Jealousy, sexual excitement, with
Jumping, bed, out of

Kill, desire to
   beloved ones
   injure with a knife, impulse to
   knife, with a
Lamenting, bemoaning, wailing
Lascivious, lustful
   impotence, with
Laughing agg.
Libertinism
Loathing, life, at
   work, at
Looked at, cannot bear to be
Magnetized, desires to be, mesmerism
   amel.
Malicious, spiteful, vindictive
   anger, with
Mania
Meditation
Memory, active
Memory, weakness of
   periodical
   sudden and periodical
   words, of
Mistakes:
   speaking, in
      misplacing words
      reverses words
      words, using wrong
   writing, in
      transposing letters
Moaning, groaning, whining
   perpiration, during
   sleep, during
Mocking
Mood, alternating
   changeable, variable
Moral feeling, want of
Morose, cross, fretful, ill-humor, peevish
   morning
      evening, bed, in
      night
   alternating with cheerfulness
   caressing agg.
   talk, indisposed to
Naive, intelligent, but very

Nymphomania
   menses, after suppressed
     puerperal
Obscene, lewd
Obstinate, headstrong
   children
Occupation, diversion amel.
Offended, easily; takes everything in
     bad part
Plans, making many
   evening
   night •
Play, passion for gambling
Pregnancy, mental affections in
Prostration of mind, mental exhaustion, brain-fag
Quarrelsome, scolding
Rage, fury
Reading, desires to be read to
Reproaches others
Reserved
Restlessness
   night
   anxious
   bed, driving out of
     tossing about in
   eating, after
   headache, during
   heat, during
   waking, on
Roving, senseless, insane
Rudeness, naughty children, of
Runs about
Sadness, despondency, dejection, mental depression, gloom, melancholy
   chill, during
   eating, after
   heat, during
   menses, after
   perspiration, during
   pregnancy, in
   suicidal disposition, with
Senses, acute
   dull, blunted

Sensitive, oversensitive
   chill, during
   moral impressions, to
   noise, to
     labor, during
     slightest, to ★
   perspiration, during
   sensual impressions, to
   touch, to
   want of sensitiveness
Sentimental
Serious, earnest
Shrieking, screaming, shouting
   cheerful mood, causeless during •
   mirth, during •
   pain, with the lumbar region
   sleep, during
Sighing
   evening
   perspiration, during
Singing
Sit, inclination to
Slowness
Speech, foolish
   wandering
Starting, startled
   fright, from and as from
   sleep, on falling
     during
     from
Strange, crank
Stupefaction, as if intoxicated
   morning
Suicidal disposition
   evening
   night
   courage, but lacks
   fear of death, with
   fear of an open window or a knife, with
   hypochondriasis, by
   intermittent fever, during
   sadness, from
   shooting, by
   throwing, window, from
Suspicious, mistrustful

Talk, indisposed to, desire to be silent,
 taciturn
  perspiration, during
  others agg., talk of
Theorizing
 evening •
 night
Thinking, aversion to
Thoughts, disagreeable
 disconnected
 foolish thoughts in the night •
 persistent
 rapid, quick
 rush, flow of
  morning in bed •
  evening
  in bed
  night
  sleeplessness from
  waking, on
 sexual, day and night
 stagnation of
 thoughful
 vanishing of
  periodically •
Timidity
 bashful
 company, in
Touched, aversion to being
Tranquillity, serenity, calmness
Unattractive, things seem •
Unconsciousness, coma, stupor
 erect, if he remained •
 menses, after
  suppression of
 standing, while
 waking, on
Unfortunate, feels
Unsympathetic, unscrupulous
Unworthy, objects seem •
Verses, makes
Violent, vehement
 deeds of violence, rage leading to
Vivacious
Wearisome
Weary of life
 heat, during

Weeping, tearful mood ·
 night
 admonition, from
 caressing, from
 children, in
 consolation agg.
 coughing, during
 easily
 need, about a fancied •
 perspiration, during
 sleep, in
 whimpering
  sleep, during
Will, weakness of
Work, aversion to mental
 desire, for
 impossible
Writing, desire for

CHININUM ARSENICOSUM

Ailments from:
 sexual excesses
Anger, irascibility
Answers
 refuses to answer
Anxiety
 daytime
 evening
 night
 chill, during
 fear, with
 fever, during
 health, about
 sitting, must sit bent •
 waking, on
Capriciousness
Censorious, critical
 dearest friends, with
Complaining
Confusion of mind
 morning
  waking, on
Conscientious about trifles
Delirium
 night
 haemorrhage, after

Delusions, imaginations, hallucinations,
    illusions
        night
    fancy, illusions of
    haemorrhage, after •
    images, phantoms, sees
        frightful
    prostration, cannot endure such
        utter •
Despair
    chill, during
    heat, during
    pains, with the
Discontented, displeased, dissatisfied
    everything, with
Discouraged
Disturbed, averse to being
Dullness, sluggishness, difficulty of think-
    ing and comprehending, torpor
Excitement, excitable
    trifles, over
Exhilaration
Fancies, exaltation of
Fear, apprehension, dread
    night
    disease, of impending, cancer, of ★
    evil, of
        night •
    ghosts, of •
        night
Forgetful
    words while speaking, of; word
        hunting
Ideas abundant, clearness of mind
    night
Impatience
    intermittent fever, in •
Indifference, apathy
    pleasure, to
Indolence, aversion to work
Irritability
    chill, during
    headache, during
    waking, on

Jumping, bed, out of
    fever, during
Loathing, life, at
Memory, loss of:
    injuries, after
Memory, weakness of
Moaning, groaning, whining
    chill, during
    heat, during
Offended easily; takes everything in
    bad part
Prostration of mind, mental exhaus-
    tion, brain-fag
Restlessness
    afternoon
    night
    anxious
    bed, driving out of
    exhaustion, with •
    heat, during
Sadness, despondency, dejection, mental
    depression, gloom, melancholy
    chill, during
    heat, during
    perspiration, during
Sensitiveness, oversensitive
    noise, to
Sentimental
Sit, inclination to
Sits, still
Speech, wandering
Starting, startled
    sleep, on falling
    waking, on
Stupefaction, as if intoxicated
    heat, during
Suicidal disposition
Suspicious, mistrustful
Talk, indisposed to, desire to be silent,
    taciturn
Thinking, complaints agg., of
Thoughts, persistent
    rush, night
Timidity
Weary of life
Weeping, tearful mood
Work, aversion to mental

CHINA (CINCHONA) BOLIVIANA

Absent-minded
    conversing, when
Blasphemy, cursing, and
Cheerful, evening
Cowardice
Cursing, swearing
Forsaken feeling
Morose, alternating with cheerfulness
Rage, paroxysms, in
Remorse
Resignation
Sadness, despondency, dejection, mental
       depression, gloom, melancholy
    alternating with tranquillity •
Sensitive, noise, to
Thoughts, future, of the
Weeping, desire to weep

CHININUM MURIATICUM

Dipsomania, alcoholism

CHININUM SULPHURICUM

Activity, 21 h. after walking in open air •
Anger, waking, on
Anguish, perspiration, during
Answer, aversion to
    unintelligibly
Anxiety
        noon
        night
        midnight, after
        bed, in
           driving out of
        fear, with
        fever, during
        future, about
Business, averse to
    incapacity for
Cheerful, gay, mirthful
    evening
Concentration, difficult

Confusion of mind
    morning
    evening
    intoxicated, as if
Delirium
    night
    bed and escapes, springs up sud-
        denly from
    crying, with
    fever, during
    intoxicated, as if
    maniacal
    raging, raving
Delirium tremens, mania-a-potu
Delusions, bed, sinking, is
    fancy, illusions of
    will power, loss of •
Despair
Discouraged
    weeping, with
Dullness, sluggishness, difficulty of think-
    ing and comprehending, torpor
    heat, during
    writing, while
Excitement, excitable
    morning
    forenoon
    coffee, as after
    heat, during
    wine, as from
Exhilaration
Exuberance
Fear, evil, of
    afternoon •
    dark, of ★
    misfortune, of
Gestures, makes
    slow
Hysteria
Ideas abundant, clearness of mind
    night
Indifference, apathy
    fever, during
    pleasure, to
    typhoid, in

Indolence, aversion to work
      morning on waking •
      noon
    sleep, after
    walking, while
Insanity, madness
Irresolution, indecision
Irritability
    headache, during
    waking, on
Jumping, bed, out of
Mania
Memory, confused
Memory, weakness of,
    names, for proper
Mistakes, adding, in •
    calculating, in
    speaking, in
      words, using wrong, putting
      right for left or vice versa
    work, in
    writing, in
    wrong words
Morose, cross, fretful, ill-humor, pee-
    vish
Obstinate, headstrong
    forenoon •
Plans, making many
    evening
Rage, fury
Restlessness
    afternoon, 17 h.
    evening
    anxious
    bed, driving out of
    tossing about in
    heat, during
Sadness, despondency, dejection, mental
    depression, gloom, melancholy
    afternoon
    misfortune, as if from
Senses, dull, blunted
Sensitive, oversensitive
Shrieking, anxiety, from
Sighing
Speech, slow

Starting, morning, after waking
    sleep, from
Stupefaction, as if intoxicated
Tranquillity, serenity, calmness
Unconsciousness, coma, stupor
    morning
    parturition, during
    semi-consciousness
    vertigo, during
Weeping, tearful mood
    night
      waking, on
    sleep, in
    waking, on
Will, loss of
    walking, while •
Work, aversion to mental
    impossible

CHIONANTHUS VIRGINICA

Ailments from:
    quarrels
Irritability

CHLOROFORMIUM

Confusion of mind
Delirium
    quiet
    violent
Delirium tremens, mania-a-potu
    excitement, with
Delusions, floating in air
    motion of chair and table in differ-
    ent directions (while sitting) •
Dullness, sluggishness, difficulty of
    thinking and comprehending,
    torpor
Familiarity •
Hysteria
Indifference, apathy
Memory, weakness of
Moaning, groaning, whining
Obscene, lewd, talk
Restlessness
    bed, tossing about in
    parturition, during

Singing
Speech, nonsensical
      slow
Unconsciousness, coma, stupor
      excitement, after
      shock from injury, in
Weeping, tearful mood

CHLORALUM HYDRATUM

Answers, aversion to answer
      difficult
      incoherently
Anxiety
         night, children, in
Childish, behavior
Concentration, difficult
Confusion of mind
Dancing
Deceitful, sly
Delirium
      rambling
      wild
Delirium tremens, mania-a-potu
Delusions, imaginations, hallucinations,
      illusions
      bed, stands at the foot menacing,
         someone
      figures, hurled bottle at, sees
      visions, has
         fantastic
      voices, hears
Despair, recovery, of
Excitement, night
Fear, apprehension, dread
Frightened, waking, on
Hide, desire to
Home, desires to go
Hydrophobia
Hysteria
         pregnancy and labor, during
Idiocy
Imbecility
Insanity, madness
         puerperal

Irresolution, indecision
Irritability
      morning
Jumping, bed, out of
Mania
Memory, weakness of
Morose, cross, fretful, ill-humor, peevish
Restlessness
*Sadness, despondency, dejection, men-
      tal depression, gloom, melan-
      choly*
Sensitive, noise, to
Shrieking, children, in, night
      chorea, in
      sleep, during
Speech, hasty
      incoherent
      nonsensical
Stupefaction, as if intoxicated
Talk, indisposed to, desire to be silent,
      taciturn
Talks, himself, to
Terror: night-terror, of children ↔
Thoughts, monotony, of
      vacancy of
      wandering
Unconsciousness, coma, stupor
Witty

CHLORUM

Activity, mental
Anger, irascibility
      drinking coffee and wine, while λ
Answers, incoherently
Anxiety
         night, children, in
Cheerful, gay, mirthful
Confidence, want of self
Confusion of mind
Deceitful, sly
Delirium, alternating with restlessness λ
      rambling
      quiet ↔
         alternating with restlessness λ
Delirium tremens, mania-a-potu

Delusions, imaginations, hallucinations,
    illusions
    figures, hurld bottle at, sees
    insane, she will become
Escape, attempts to
    fever, during
Excitement, excitable
    champagne, after
    feverish
Fear, apprehension, dread
    disease, of impending
    insanity, losing his reason, of
    poverty, of
Forgetful, names of persons ★
Frightened easily
Hide, desire to
Homesickness
Hydrophobia
Hysteria
Ideas abundant, clearness of mind
Imbecility
Insanity, noisy
Irritability
    drinking wine and coffee, while •
    eating, during
    after
Memory, weakness of
    names, for proper
    persons, for
    read, for what has
Morose, cross, fretful, ill-humor, peevish
    morning
Music, desire to play piano
Muttering
Nymphomania
Rage, eating, during and after •
Restlessness
Sadness, despondency, dejection, mental
    depression, gloom, melancholy
Shrieking, screaming, shouting
Stupefaction, as if intoxicated
Tranquillity, serenity, calmness
Unconsciousness, coma, stupor
    fever, during
    incomplete
Wildness

CHLORAMPHENICOLUM

Confusion of mind
Delirium
Delusions, imaginations, hallucinations,
    illusions
Despair, rising, amel. on
Euphoria
Indifference, apathy
Restlessness, evening in bed
Sadness, despondency, dejection, mental
    depression, gloom, melancholy

CHLORPROMAZINUM

Ailments from:
    anticipation, foreboding, presen-
      timent
Anguish
    forenoon, 10 h. •
Concentration, difficult
Confusion of mind
Delusions, imaginations, hallucinations,
    illusions
    visions, has
Indifference, apathy
Irritability
Memory, weakness of
Sadness, despondency, dejection, mental
    depression, gloom, melancholy
Schizophrenia, catatonic
    hebephrenia
Thoughts, automatic •

CHROMICUM ACIDUM

Confusion of mind
Delirium
    meningitis, cerebrospinalis
    scolding
Dullness, sluggishness, difficulty of think-
    ing and comprehending, torpor
Memory, weakness of
    letters, how to make several •
    write, for what is about to
Mistakes, writing, in

Restlessness
    night
    pain, during
    waking, on
Sadness, despondency, dejection, mental
    depression, gloom, melancholy
Stupefaction, as if intoxicated

CICUTA VIROSA

Absent-minded, unobserving
Absorbed, buried in thought
Abstraction of mind
Abusive, insulting
Activity
Admiration, excessive
Ailments from:
    anticipation, foreboding, presen
        timent
    injuries, accidents; mental symp-
        toms from
    quarrels
Anger, irascibility
Answers abruptly, shortly, curtly
    spoken to, answers when; yet
        knows no one •
Antics, plays
Anxiety
    noon
    convulsions, before •
    faintness, with
    fear, with
    fits, before •
    future, about
Aversion, men, contempt for •
        loss of confidence in •
        shuns the foolishness of •
Bite, desire to
Catatonia
Censorious, critical
Cheerful, gay, mirthful
    bed, jumps out of •
    clapping one's hand
Childish behavior
Clinging, convulsions, before •
**Company, aversion to; presence of
    other people agg. the symp-
    toms; desire for solitude**

Company,
    avoids the sight of people
    menses, desires to be let alone
        during
    **presence of strangers, aver-
        sion to**
Concentration, difficult
Confusion of mind
    morning
        rising and after, on
    bed, jump out of, makes him
    chill, during
    sitting, while
    standing, while
    walking, while
Contemptuous
Contented
    himself, with
Dancing
    grotesque
Death, sensation of
Delirium
    bed and escapes, springs up sud-
        denly from
    foolish, silly
    frightful
    maniacal
    muttering
    raging, raving
    singing
Delusions, imaginations, hallucinations,
    illusions
    absurd figures are present
    child, he is again a •
        acts like a, and •
    church yard, dancing in, he is
    fancy, illusions of
    figures, sees
    home, away from, is
    identity, erorrs of personal
    images, phantoms, sees
    living under ordinary relations, is
        not •
    ludicrous, antics
    pursued by enemies
    smell, of
    strange, everything is
        familiar things seem

Delusions, strange,
 places seemed
  surroundings ★
 toys, objects seemed as attractive
  as
 unreal, everything seem
 visions, has
  monsters, of
Dipsomania, alcoholism
Discontented, displeased, dissatisfied
Doubtful
Dullness, sluggishness, difficulty of think-
 ing and comprehending, torpor
 evening amel.
 chill, during
 injuries of head, after
Ecstasy
 periodical
  twice a day, seems to be dying •
Escape, attempts to
Excitement, excitable
 convulsions, with
 hearing horrible things, after
Exertion, amel. from mental
Fancies, exaltation of
Fear, apprehension, dread
 company, of •
 convulsions, before ★
 crowd, in a
 danger, of impending
 disease, of impending
 door, in opening
 men, dread, fear of
  confidence in, loss of •
  contempt for •
  shuns the foolishness of •
 misfortune, of
 noise, from
  door, at
 people, of
Foolish behavior
 night •
Forgetful
Frightened easily
Gestures, makes
 clapping of the hands
 involuntary motions, of the
 ridiculous or foolish

Grief
Hatred
 revenge, and
Haughty
Heedless
Home, desires to go
Horrible things, sad stories, affect
 her profoundly
Horror ★
Howling
Hysteria
Ideas, deficiency of
Idiocy
Imbecility
Indifference, apathy
 concussion of brain, after
 everything, to
 external things, to
Indolence, aversion to work
Insanity, madness
 dancing, with
 foolish, ridiculous
 melancholy
 paroxysmal
 puerperal
Introspection
Irritability
Jesting
 ridiculous or foolish
Jumping
 bed, out of
Lamenting, bemoaning, wailing
Laughing
 night
 silly
 spasmodic
Loathing, life, at
 eating, amel. on •
Malicious, spiteful, vindictive
Mania
 night
  dancing, laughing, striking,
  with •
 shrieking in
 singing, with
Meditation

Memory, loss of :
    epileptic fits, after
    injuries of head, after
Memory, weakness of
Mildness
Misanthropy
Mistakes, localities, in
    space and time, in
    time, in
        confouds, future with the past
        present with past
Moaning, groaning, whining
    sleep, during
Monomania
Mood, changeable, variable, night agg. λ
Morose, cross, fretful, ill-humor, peevish
    fever, during
Morphinism
Muttering
Naive
Narrating her symptoms agg.
Occupation, diversion amel.
Offended, easily; takes everything in
    bad part
Play, desire to, toys with childish λ
Prostration of mind, mental exhaus-
    tion, brain-fag
Quiet disposition
Rage, fury
Reckless, rashness ↔
Recognize: relatives, does not recognize
    his
Reproaches others
Restlessness
    night
    bed, tossing about in
Sadness, despondency, dejection, men-
    tal depression, gloom, melancholy
    anxious
    injuries of the head, from
    stories, from sad
Schizophrenia, catatonic
Self, over-estimation of ↔
Senses, dull, blunted
    vanishing of
Sensitive, oversensitive
    noise, to
    sad stories, to λ

Shrieking, screaming, shouting
    brain cry
    convulsions, before
        epileptic
        during epileptic
    must shriek, feels as though she
    pain, with the
    sleep, during
Sighing, epileptic attacks, before
Singing
Somnambulism
Speech, delirious
    wandering
Staring, thoughtless
Starting, startled
    bed, in
    easily
    fright, from and as from
    noise, from
    sleep, during
Strange, everything seems
Stupefaction, as if intoxicated
    convulsions, between
    injury to head, after
Suicidal disposition
Suspicious, mistrustful
    solitude, desire for
Sympathy, compassion
Talk, indisposed to, desire to be silent,
    taciturn
Talking, unpleasant things agg., of
Thinking, complaints amel., of
Thoughts, thoughtful
    errors of others, about the λ
    vanishing of
    wandering
Torpor
Tranquillity, serenity, calmness
Unconsciousness, coma, stupor
    chill, during
    conduct, automatic
    convulsions, after
    dream, as in a, does not know
        where he is
    eyes, with open
    fever, during

Unconsciousness,
    knows no one but answers cor-
       rectly when touched or spoken
      to
    periodical
      prolonged ★
Violent, vehement
    deeds of violence, rage leading to
Weeping, tearful mood
    aloud, sobbing
    convulsions, during
    waking, on
    whimpering
Work, desire for mental, evening

CICUTA MACULATA

Anxiety
Delirium
Gestures, violent
Unconsciousness, coma, stupor

CIMICIFUGA RACEMOSA

Ailments from:
    anger, vexation
    anxiety
    business failure
    excitement, emotional
    fright
    love, disappointed
Anger, irascibility
    menses, during
Answers: aversion to answer
       loquacious at other time ●
    hastily
    evasively ●
    irrelevantly
    refuses to answer
Anxiety
    climacteric period, during
    menses, during
Business, averse to
    talks of
Busy
Capriciousness
Cares, worries, full of

Cheerful, gay, mirthful
    alternating with sadness
Climacteric period agg.
Company, aversion to; presence of
    other people agg. the symp-
    toms; desire for solitude
Concentration, difficult
Confusion of mind; morning, waking,
    on
    menses, before
      during
Death, presentiment of
Delirium
    answers abruptly
    fever, during
    headache, during
    loquacious
    pupils, with dilated
    raging, raving
Delirium tremens, mania-a-potu
    sleeplessness, with
Delusions, imaginations, hallucinations,
    illusions
    animals, of
      persons are rats, mice, insects
      etc.
    arms are bound to her body ●
    bed, strange objects, rats, sheep,
      in ●
    clouds, heavy black, enveloped
      her
    dark objects and figures, sees ●
    encaged in wires ●
    figures, sees
    home, away from, is
      away from, must get there
    images, phantoms, sees
    insane, she will become
    mice, sees
      mouse running from under a
    chair
    poisoned, he has been
    rats, sees
      running across the room
    sheep, sees ●
    visions, has
      monsters, rats and strange
      objects ●
    wires, is caught in

Dementia, epileptics, of
Despair, life, of
   recovery, of
Dipsomania, alcoholism
Dullness, sluggishness, difficulty of thinking and comprehending, torpor
   afternoon
Excitement, excitable
   climacteric period, during
   menses, during
   pregnancy, during
Exertion, agg. from mental
Fear, apprehension, dread
   abortion from fear, threatening
   danger, of impending
   death, of
   disease, of impending
      incurable, of being
   insanity, losing his reason, of
      climacteric period, during •
   murdered, of being
   poisoned, of being
   pregnancy, during
   rats, of ★
Forgetful
Frightened, night
Grief
Homesickness
Hurry, haste
   occupation, in
   work, in
Hypochondriasis
Hysteria   .
   climacteric period, at
   fainting, hysterical
   menses, during
      copious
Ideas abundant, clearness of mind
Impatience
Inconstancy
Indifference, apathy
   duties, to domestic
      everything, to
Industrious, mania for work

Injure himself, fears to be let alone, lest he should
Insanity, madness
   business, from failure in
   climacteric period, during
   neuralgia, with disappearance of pregnancy, in
   puerperal
Irresolution, indecision
Irritability
   menses, during
   trifles, from
Loquacity
   alternating with silence
   changing quickly from one subject to another
   rambling ★
Mania
   lochia, from suppressed
Memory, active
Memory, weakness of
   expressing oneself, for
   words, of
Menses, mental symptoms agg. during
Mental symptoms alternating with physical
Moaning, groaning, whining
Mood, changeable, variable
Morphinism
Playful
Rage, fury
   headache, with
Refuses to take the medicine
Restlessness
   forenoon
   afternoon
   night
   midnight, after, 3h.
   anxious
   driving about
   exertion, after •
   feverish
   menses, during suppressed
   move, must constantly
Sadness, despondency, dejection, mental depression, gloom, melancholy

Sadness,
    afternoon
    climaxis, after
    cold, from becoming
    drunkards, in
    headache, during
    labor, during
    menses, during
        suppressed, from
    pregnancy, in
    puerperal
    sleeplessness, with
    suicidal disposition, with
Sensitive, oversensitive
    noise, to
        labor, during
Sighing
    menses, during
Sits, still
Speech, finish sentence, does not •
    hasty
    incoherent
Starting, startled
    sleep, from
Suicidal disposition
    sadness, from
Suspicious, mistrustful
    climacteric period, during •
    medicine, will not take •
Talk, indisposed to, desire to be silent,
    taciturn
    alternating with loquacity
Thoughts, rapid, quick
    rush, flow of
Touchy ★
Travel, desire to
Unconsciousness, coma, stupor
    parturition, during
Wander, desires to
Weeping, tearful mood
    spoken to, when
Will, weakness of
Writing, difficulty in expressing ideas
    when

CIMEX LECTULARIUS

Anxiety
    chill, during
    drinking, after ★
Confusion of mind
Destructiveness
Disgust
Dullness, sluggishness, difficulty of
    thinking and comprehending,
    torpor
    chill, during
Irritability
    chill, during
Rage, chill, during
Tears things

CINA MARITIMA

Ailments from:
    anger, vexation
    fright
Anger, irascibility
    cough, before
    trifles, at
    worm affections, in
Anguish
    walking in open air
Anxiety
        evening
        night
            children, in
            waking, on
    air, in open
    children, in
    conscience, as if guilty of a crime
    cough, after whooping •
    fear, with
    menses, during
    standing, while
    touched, anxiety to being
    waking, on
    walking, while
        air, in open
Avarice
Bite, spoon etc.
    desire to, ★
Capriciousness
Carressed, aversion to being

221

Carried, desires to be
 shoulder, over
Complaining
 waking, on
Confusion of mind
 morning, rising and after, on
 cough, before paroxysm of •
Contemptuous
 everything, to
Contradiction, is intolerant of
Contrary
Croaking
Cross, crossness (anger) ★
Defiant
Delirium
 crying, with
 raging, raving
 sleep, during
 waking, on
Delusions, imaginations, hallucinations,
 illusions •
 animals, of
 crime, committed a, he had
 criminals, about
 dogs, sees
 fancy, illusions of
 figures, sees
 images, sees frightful
 smell, of
 taste, of
 visions, has
 evening
 wrong, he has done ★
Desires, full of
 numerous, various thing
Discomfort
Discontented, displeased, dissatisfied
 everything, with
Excitement, excitable
Exertion, agg. from mental
Fear, apprehension, dread
 approaching him, of others,
 children cannot bear to have
 anyone come near them
 evil, of
 evening, walking in open air,
 while •
 touch, of

Fear,
 tremulous
 waking, on
 dream, from a
 walking, while
 air, in open
Frightened, waking, on
Gestures, grasping or reaching at something, at flocks; carphologia
 nose, lips, at
 pick at bed clothes
 strange attitudes and positions
Gluttony
Grimaces
Grunting
Haughty
Howling
Hurry, drinking, on
Impatience
Indifference, apathy
 agreeable things, to
 caresses, to •
 everything, to
 irritating, disaggreeable things,
 to
 joy and suffering, to
Irresolution, indecision
Irritability
 children, in
 cough, from •
 dentition, during
 heat, after
 during ★
 menses, during
 rocking fast amel.
 waking, on
 worm affections, in
Jesting, aversion to
Jumping, children in evening •
 sudden pain, as from
Kicks, sleep, in
 stiff and kicks when carried, becomes
 worm affections, in
Lamenting, bemoaning, wailing
 morning on waking •
 asleep, while
 waking, on

Looked at, cannot bear to be
agg. mental symptoms ★
Malicious, spiteful, vindictive
Mildness
Moaning, groaning, whining
afternoon •
children, in
cough, during
waking, on
Mood, changeable, variable
Morose, cross, fretful, ill-humor, peevish
daytime
children, in
puberty, in
waking, on
worm affections, in
Obstinate, headstrong
children
Offended, easily; takes everything in
bad part
Play: aversion to play in children
Quieted, cannot be •
Rage, fury
Refuses to take help •
Religious, affections
Remorse
Restlessness
morning on waking
night
bed, go from one bed to another,
wants to
tossing about in
children, in, relieved by being
carried about
heat, during
nausea, from
waking, on
Rocking amel.
Rudeness, naughty children, of
Sadness, despondency, dejection, mental
depression, gloom, melancholy
Senses, acute
Sensitive, oversensitive
touch, to
Serious, earnest
Shrieking, screaming, shouting
children, in
evening

Shrieking,
convulsions, before
during epileptic
cough agg.
hydrocephalus, in
must shriek, feels as though she
sleep, during
waking, on
Speech, hasty
wandering
Starting, startled
sleep, on falling
during
from
Stranger, presence of strangers agg.
Striking
children, in
Stupefaction, as if intoxicated
air, in open
walking in open air, when
Sulky ★
Talk, indisposed to, desire to be silent,
taciturn
Talking, sleep, in
Throws things away
Touch everything, children, in, im-
pelled to •
Touched, aversion to being
caressed, aversion to being
Ugly (in behavior) ★
Unconsciousness, coma, stupor
Walk, walking in open air agg. mental
symptoms
Weeping, tearful mood
night
carried, child cries piteously if
taken hold or
child is quiet only when c.
causeless
children, in
will is not done •
convulsions, during
after
coughing, during
after
involuntary
pains, with the
sad thoughts, at
sleep, in

Weeping,
  spasmodic
  stool, during
  touched, when
  trifles at
  waking, on

CINCHONINUM SULPHURICUM

Cheerful, gay, mirthful

CINNABARIS

Ailments from:
  bad news
Anger, irascibility
Cheerful, gay, mirthful
  morning
  walking in open air and after, on
Company, aversion to; presence of
  other people agg. the symp-
  toms; desire for solitude
Concentration, difficult
Confusion of mind
Delusions, well, he is
Discontented, displeased, dissatisfied
  himself, with
Dullness, daytime
  air, amel. in open
  think long, unable to
Ecstasy, walking in open air, when λ
Elevation, mental
  morning on walking in the open
  air λ
Excitement, bad news, after
  nervous
  trifles, over
Exhilaration
  morning
  walking in open air, while λ
Forgetful
Ideas abundant, clearness of mind
Indifference, sleepiness, with
Indolence, aversion to work
  sleepiness, with

Irritability
  forenoon
  noon
  night after retiring
  noise, from
Memory, weakness of, do, for what was
  about to
Mocking, sarcasm
Morose, cross, fretful, ill-humor, peevish
  afternoon
Offended, easily; takes everything in
  bad part
Prostration of mind, mental exhaustion, brain-fag
  menses, before λ
Restlessness
  night
  bed, tossing about in
  eating, after
Sadness despondency, dejection, mental
  depression, gloom, melancholy
Sensitive, noise, to
  slightest, to
Shrieking, children, in, evening
  sleep, from
Sulky, afternoon λ
Talking, sleep, in
Thoughts, intrude and crowd around
  each other
Well, says he is, when very sick
Work, aversion to mental

CINNAMOMUM CEYLANICUM

Anxiety
Delusions, diminished, all is
  left side of body is smaller λ
Discontented, displeased, dissatisfied
  himself, with
Forgetful
Hysteria
  loss of fluids, after
Shrieking, screaming, shouting chil-
  dren, in, evening
Weeping, tearful mood

CISTUS CANADENSIS

Ailments from:
    anger, vexation
        excitement, emotional
Anger, paralysed, felt as
Cheerful, evening
    eating, while
    supper, after λ
Excitement, excitable
    agg.
Exertion, agg. from mental
Fear, apprehension, dread
Restlessness
    night
    bed, tossing about in

CITRICUM ACIDUM

Frightened easily
Indolence, housework, aversion to her
    usual λ

CITRUS LIMONUM

Duty, aversion to domestic
Indifference, duties, to domestic
Unconsciousness, coma, stupor

CITRUS VULGARIS

Delusions, disabled, she is λ
Excitement, excitable
    motions, quick, brusque, per
        formed, with uncontrollable
        zeal λ
Industrious, mania for work
Restlessness
    night
    bed, tossing about in
    lying, while
    working, while
Starting, sleep, from
Stupefaction, as if intoxicated
Weeping, tearful mood

CLEMATIS ERECTA

Absent-minded, unobserving
Absorbed, buried in thought

Activity
    mental
Ailments from:
    grief
    homesickness
Anger, irascibility
    trifles, at
Anxiety
    forenoon
    night
    fear, with
    sleep, on starting from
    walking, while
Brooding
Cheerful, gay, mirthful
    morning, waking, on
    forenoon
    evening
    alternating with sadness
    followed by irritability
    followed by prostration
    perspiration, during
Company, aversion to; presence of
    other people agg. the symp-
    toms; desire for solitude
    fear of being alone, yet
Company, desire, for; aversion to soli-
    tude, company amel.
    alone agg., while
    yet fear of people
Concentration, difficult
Confusion of mind
    morning
        rising and after, on
        waking, on
    afternoon
    air amel., in open
    intoxicated, as after being
    waking, on
Death, desires
    thoughts of
Delirium
    raging, raving
Delusions, fire, visions of
    motion of bed and ground, (on
        waking) λ
Despair

Discomfort
  eating, after
Discontented, displeased, dissatisfied
    cause, without ★
*Dullness, sluggishness, difficulty of think-
    ing and comprehending, torpor*
  sleepiness, with
  toothache, from
  waking, on
Ennui, homesickness, with
Excitement, excitable
Exhilaration
Fear, apprehension, dread
  alone, of being
  misfortune, of
  people, of, yet agg. if alone ★
  solitude, of
Forgetful
Frightened easily
Gestures, light
Going out, aversion to
Heedless
Homesickness
Hurry, eating, while
Ideas, deficiency of
Indifference, apathy
Indolence, aversion to work
    morning
      evening amel.
  sleepiness, with
Industrious, mania for work
Introspection
Irresolution, indecision
Irritability
  perspiration, during
  waking, on
  walking, when
Malicious, spiteful, vindictive
Meditation
Memory, weakness of
Mildness
Misanthropy
Moaning, sleep, during
Moral feeling, want of
Morose, cross, fretful, ill-humor, peevish
Prostration of mind, mental exhaus-
    tion, brain-fag

Quiet disposition
Read, aversion to
  desires to be read to
Remorse
Reserved
Rest, desire for
Restlessness
    evening
    night
    midnight, after, 4h.
  anxious
  bed, tossing about in
  heat, during
Runs, about, lightness and rapidity,
    with great ●
*Sadness, despondency, dejection, mental
    depression, gloom, melancholy*
  eating, amel., after
  supper amel.
Senses, acute
Sensitive, oversensitive
  external impressions, to all
  mental impressions, to
Sighing, head, during heat of ●
Slowness
Starting, morning, after waking
  sleep, from
Strength increased, mental
Stupefaction, as if intoxicated
Suicidal disposition
Talk, indisposed to, desire to be silent,
    taciturn
      evening amel.
Thoughts, thoughtful
Tranquillity, serenity, calmness
Unconsciousness, coma, stupor
    morning
    fever, during
    hydrocephalus, in
Wearisome
Weeping, tearful mood
    evening
Will, loss of
Work, aversion to mental
  desire for

COBALTUM METALLICUM

Ailments from:
  excitement, emotional
Cheerful, gay, mirthful
Confidence, want of self
Confusion of mind, morning
  motion, from
Delusions, criminal, he is a
          and others know it λ
Discontented, displeased, dissatisfied
  himself, with
Excitement, excitable
  agg.
Exhilaration
Frightened easily
Hysteria
Ideas abundant, clearness of mind
Indolence, aversion to work
  physical
Memory, active
Reproaches himself
Restlessness
Sadness, despondency, dejection, mental
          depression, gloom, melancholy
Sighing
Stupefaction, as if intoxicated
  morning
Thoughts, rapid, quick
Vivacious
Work, aversion to mental
  desire for

COBALTUM NITRICUM

Activity
Anguish
  night
        paralysing, impossble to call
        and move, with
        heat in head λ
Anxiety
  night
        paralyzed, as if
Concentration, difficult
  headache, with

Delusions enlarged, distances are
Dwells on past disagreeable occur-
  rences
Euphoria
Excitement, excitable
Fear, apprehension, dread
  failure, of
  high places, of
  sleep, before
Forgetful,.waking, on
Indolence, aversion to work
Industrious, mania for work
Irritability
  morning
Memory, weakness of
Mood, alternating
Morose, cross, fretful, ill-humor, peevish
Prostration of mind, mental exhaus-
          tion, brain-fag
Restlessness
  heat, during
Sadness, despondency, dejection, mental
          depression, gloom, melancholy
  waking, on

COCCUS CACTI

Anxiety
  midnight, after
        2-4 h. λ
  eating, after
Cheerful, gay, mirthful
  evening
  alternating with sadness
Confusion of mind
  morning, rising and after, on
  waking, on
  evening
  air amel., in open
  breakfast, after
  eating, after
  heat, during
  waking, on
  walking, while
Delusions, body, adherent to woollen
        sack (night while half awake) λ
  enlarged

Dipsomania, alcoholism
Dullness, sluggishness, difficulty of think-
 ing and comprehending, torpor
Excitement, night on waking
 beer, after •
 waking, on
Fear, apprehension, dread
 evening
Ideas abundant, clearness of mind
Indifference, irritating, disagreeable
 things, to
Indolence, aversion to work
Irritability
 dinner, after
Lascivious, lustful
 morning •
Loquacity
Memory, active
Moaning, sleep, during
Morose, cross, fretful, ill-humor, peevish
Restlessness
 night
 midnight, after, 3h.
Sadness, despondency, dejection, mental
 depression, gloom, melancholy
 afternoon
 waking, on
Sensitive, oversensitive
Shining objects agg.
Spit, desire to
Stupefaction, as if intoxicated

COCA

Activity
Ailments from:
 shock, mental
 work, mental
Anguish
Anxiety
 evening
 pressure on the chest, from
Bilious disposition
Business man, worn out

Cheerful, gay, mirthful
Company, aversion to; presence of
 other people agg. the symptoms; desire for solitude
Concentration, difficult
Confusion of mind
 coffee amel.
 drowsiness, confusion while re-
 sisting •
 washing the face amel.
Contented
Deceitful, sly
Delusions, imaginations, hallucinations,
 illusions
 beautiful
 figures, sees
 images, phantoms, sees
 frightful
 neglected, appearance, his own ★
 space, carried into, he was (while
 lying)
 visions, has beautiful
 voices, hears
Dementia
Desire, exercise, for
 physical •
Dream, as if in a
Dullness, sluggishness, difficulty of
 thinking and comprehending,
 torpor
 evening
Ecstasy
Elated
Exhilaration
Fancies, exaltation of
 pleasant
Fear, apprehension, dread
 downward motion, of
 falling, letting things fall, of •
 walking, when
Forgetful, words while speaking, of;
 word hunting
Forsaken, isolation, sensation of

Gestures, impatient •
    hands, involuntary motions, of
      the
Hurry, movements, in
    writing, in
Hysteria
Ideas abundant, clearness of mind
    night
Indifference, apathy
    external things, to
Indolence, aversion to work
    evening
    nervous exhaustion, in •
Industrious, 7-9 h. •
    night •
Irresolution, indecision
Irritability
    morning on waking
    headache, during
    waking, on
Laughing: ludicrous, everything seems
Liar
Malicious, spiteful, vindictive
Mania
Memory, active
Memory, weakness of
    expressing oneself, for
    words, of
Mistakes, speaking, in
Moaning, groaning, whining
    evening
Mood, changeable, variable
Moral feeling, want of
Morose, morning on waking
Obstinate, headstrong
Prostration of mind, mental exhaus-
    tion, brain-fag
Quiet, wants to be
Reading, aversion to
    difficult, is
Rest, desire for
Restlessness
    night
    bed, tossing about in

Sadness, despondency, dejection, mental
    depression, gloom, melancholy
    afternoon, 18h.
    evening amel.
    exertion, after
    heat, during
Society
    social functions agg. ★
    ill at ease, in ★
Speech, incoherent
Suspicious, mistrustful
Thinking, aversion to
Thoughts, persistent
    rush, flow of
    night
Time passes too quickly, appears longer
Timidity
    bàshful
Tranquillity, serenity, calmness
Unconsciousness, semi-consciousness
Washing her hands always
Weeping, evening
Will, loss of
Work, desire for mental

COCAINUM
HYDROCHLORICUM

Ambition
Audacity
Delusions, imaginations, hallucinations,
    illusions
    criticised, she is
    hearing, illusions of
    pursued by enemies
    worms, covered with, he is •
Industrious, mania for work
Jealousy
    irrational ★
Loquacity
Moral feeling, want of

COCCULUS INDICUS

Absent-minded, unobserving
Absorbed, buried in thought
Ailments from:
  anger, vexation
    anxiety, with
    fright, with
    silent grief, with
  anticipation, foreboding, presen-
    timent
  excitement, emotional
  fear
  fright
  grief
  noise •
  rudeness of others
  sexual excesses
  work, mental
Anger, irascibility
  alternating with cheerfulness
    jesting
    vivacity
  contradiction, from
  easily
  interruption, from
  trifles, at
Answer, aversion to
  difficult
  hastily
  reflects long
  slowly
Anxiety
    morning
      waking, on
    evening
      bed, in
    night
      midnight, before
  bed, in
  chill, during
  conscience, as if guilty of a crime
  excitement, from
  fear, with
  fever, during
    intermittent, during
  fits, with
  future, about

Anxiety
  health, about
    relatives, of
  menses, before
    during
  motion, from
  night watching, from
  nursing, after
  others, for
  paroxysms, in ★
  periodical
  sleep, during
    loss of
      menses, after
  sudden
  trifles, about
  waking, on
Asks for nothing
Aversion, everything, to
Brooding
  corner or moping, brooding in a
Busy
Capriciousness
Cares, worries, others, about
Censorious, critical
Cheerful, gay, mirthful
  alternating with irritability
Complaining
Concentration, difficult
Confusion of mind
    morning
  drinking, after
  eating, after
  identity: duality, sense of
  head separated from body, as if
  intoxicated, as after being
  menses, during
  mental exertion, from
  reading, while
  vertigo, with
  waking, on
Conscientious about trifles
  trifles, occupied with
Contented
Contradiction, is intolerant of
Contrary
Conversation agg.

Cowardice
Dancing
Death, agony before
Delirium
    alternating with sopor
    angry •
    encephalitis
    menses, during
**Delusions, imaginations, halluci-
nations, illusions**
    criminals, about
    dead persons, sees
    fancy, illusions of
    figures, sees
    grimaces, sees
    hollow in organs, being
    spectres, ghosts, spirits, sees
    strange, familiar things seem
    *time, seems earlier, passes too
quickly*
    unreal, everything seems
    visions, closing the eyes, on
Despair
    menorrhagia, in •
Dipsomania, alcoholism
Discontented, displeased, dissatisfied
    everything, with
    himself, with
Discouraged
Disturbed, averse to being
Drinking, mental symptoms after
*Dullness, sluggishness, difficulty of think-
ing and comprehending, torpor*
    morning, bed, in
    dreams, after
    mental exertion, from
    understands questions only after
        repetition
    waking, on
Dwells on past disagreeable occur-
    rences
Eat, refuses to
Ecstasy
Emptiness, sensation of ★
Escape, attempts to

Excitement excitable
    agg.
    hearing horrible things, after
    palpitation, with violent
    perspiration, during
    trembling, with
Exertion, agg. from mental
Exhilaration
Fancies, exaltation of
    evening, bed, in
    sleeplessness, with
Fear, apprehension, dread
    night
    danger, of impending
    death, of
        heat, during
    events, of sudden •
    evil, of
    ghosts, of
        night ★
        waking, on
    happen, something will
    health of others, about ★
    narrow places, in; claustrophobia
    noise, from
        sudden, of
    overpowering
    people, of; anthropophobia
    recurrent
    waking, on
Foolish, behaviour
Forgetful
    heat, during
    words while speaking, of; word
        hunting
Frightened easily
    waking, on
Gestures, makes
    grasping or reaching at some
        thing, at flocks; carphologia
        picks at bed clothes
        strange attitudes and positions
Grief
Homesickness
Horrible things, sad stories affect her
    profoundly
Hurry, haste
Hypochondriasis
    afternoon

Hysteria
    fainting, hysterical
      menses, before
        during
Ideas abundant, clearness of mind
      evening, bed, in
    deficiency of
Imbecility
Indifference, apathy
    lies with eyes closed
    pleasure, to
Indignation
Indolence, aversion to work
     morning
    difficulties, in face of •
Industrious, mania for work
    menses, before
Insanity, madness
    amenorrhoea, from •
    grief, from
    masturbation, from
    sleeplessness, with
Intolerance, interruption, of
Introspection
Irresolution, indecision
Irritability
     morning
    alternating with cheerfulness
      jesting •
    chill, during
    noise, from
    trifles, from
Jesting
    alternating with vexation •
    aversion to
Lamenting, bemoaning, wailing
    menses, during
Laughing, spasmodic
Loquacity
    perspiration, during
Malicious, spiteful, vindictive
Mania
    singing, with
Mathematics, apt for
Meditation
Memory, active

Memory, weakness of
    expressing oneself, for
    happened, for what has
    read, for what has
    thought, for what has just
    words, of
Menses, mental symptoms agg. before
Mildness
Mistakes, speaking, in
     misplacing words
     words, using wrong
    time, in
Moaning, groaning, whining
    menses, during
    sleep, during
Mood, changeable, variable
Moral feeling, want of
Morose, cross, fretful, ill-humor, peevish
Muttering
    apoplexy, in
Nymphomania
    menses, suppressed, after
Offended, easily; takes everything in
    bad part
Playful
Prostration of mind, mental exhaus-
    tion, brain-fag
Quiet, disposition
Rage, fury
    malicious
    violent
Reading, mental symptoms agg. from
Recognizes everything, but cannot move
    (catalepsy)
Reflecting, sadness, in
Remorse
Reserved, morning
    bed, in •
Restlessness
    bed, tossing about in
    menses, during
Reverence for those around him
Rocking agg.
Romantic ★

Sadness, despondency, dejection, mental depression, gloom, melancholy
   afternoon
   chill, during
   diarrhoea, during
   heat, during
   insult, as if from •
   masturbation, from
   trifles, about
Sensitive, oversensitive
   external impressions, to all
   noise, to
    slightest, to
    talking, of
    voices, to
   rudeness, to
Sentimental
Serious, earnest
Shrieking, screaming, shouting
   anxiety, from
   menses, during
   sleep, during
Sighing
   heat, during
   menses, during
   perspiration, during
Singing
   trilling
Sit, inclination to
Sits, desire to
   still
   wrapped in deep sad thoughts and notices nothing, as if
Slowness
   motion, in ★
Speech, hasty
   slow
Starting, startled
   easily
   noise, from
   sleep, during
    from
   touched, when
   trifles, at
Stupefaction, as if intoxicated
   eating, agg. after
   sleepiness, with
Suspicious, mistrustful

Sympathy, compassion
Talk, indisposed to, desire to be silent, taciturn
   morning
   waking, on
   waking, on
   others agg., talk of
Talking agg. all complaints
Thinking, complaints amel., of
Thoughts
   business, at evening in bed, of
   disagreeable
   persistent
    unpleasant subjects, haunted by
   profound
   rush, flow of
    evening in bed
   sleeplessness from
   thoughtful
Time, fritters away his
   passes too quickly, appears shorter
Timidity
   bashful ★
Touched, aversion to being
Tranquillity, serenity, calmness
Unconsciousness, coma, stupor
   morning
   exertion, after
   menses, during
   muttering
   semi-consciousness
   stool, after
   sudden
   vertigo, during
Violent, vehement
   deeds of violence, rage stet leading to
Vivacious
Wearisome
Weeping, tearful mood
   night
   aloud, sobbing
   anger, after
   convulsions, during
   menses, during
   sleep, in

Weeping, tearful mood
  trifles, at
  whimpering
Wicked following amenorrhoea ★
Witty
Work, mental
  fatigues
  impossible
Yielding disposition

COCCINELLA SEPTEMPUNCTATA

Hydrophobia

COCHLEARIA OFFICINALIS

Ailments from:
  anger, vexation
  excitement, emotional
Anxiety
Despair, pains, stomach, in the, with
Dullness, sluggishness, difficulty of think-
  ing and comprehending, torpor
Excitement, excitable
Irresolution, indecision
Sadness, despondency, dejection, mental
  depression, gloom, melancholy
Stupefaction, as if intoxicated

CODEINUM PURUM AUT PHOSPHORICUM AUT ACETICUM

Ailments from:
  excitement, emotional
Anxiety
Concentration, active
Concentration, difficult
Confusion of mind
Delirium
Dullness, sluggishness, difficulty of think-
  ing and comprehending, torpor
    afternoon
    evening
Exhilaration
Fancies, lascivious
    pleasant

Foolish behavior
Indifference, apathy
Lascivious, lustful
Pleasure
Restlessness
Sadness, headache, during
Sit, inclination to
Strength increased, mental
Unconsciousness
  waking, on
Vivacious

COFFEA CRUDA

Absent-minded, unobserving
Activity, creative ●
  mental
  midnight, until
Affectionate
Ailments from:
  anger, vexation
  anxiety, with
  fright, with
  anticipation, foreboding, presen-
    timent
  excitement, emotional
  fear
  fright
  joy, excessive
  laughing, excessive ●
  love, disappointed
  scorn, being scorned
  surprises, pleasant
  violence
Air, castles (plans); builds, in ★
Anger, irascibility
  alternating with sadness
  throws things away
  violent
Anguish
  menses, during
  tossing about, with
Animation agg. ★
Answers abruptly, shortly, curtly
  aversion to answer
  disconnected

Anxiety
    evening
    night
    conscience, as if guilty of a crime
    fear, with
    fever, during
    flatus, from
    inactivity, with
    menses, during
Benevolence
Beside oneself, being
Blissful feeling
Capriciousness
Cares, worries, full of
Carried, aversion to being •
Cheerful, gay, mirthful
    alternating with moaning
        sadness
    drunkenness, during
Climacteric period agg.
Clinging to persons or furniture etc.
Complaining
Comprehension, easy
Concentration, active
Concentration, difficult
    studying, reading etc., while
Confusion of mind
    chill, during
    paroxyms of pain, during
    walking, while
        air, in open
Consolation
    sympathy agg.
Conversation agg.
Death, conviction of
    thoughts of
        fear, without
Delirium
    night
    fever, during
    maniacal
    waking, on
Delirium tremens, mania-a-potu
Delusions, imaginations, hallucinations,
    illusions
    beautiful landscape, of
    criminals, about
    excited •

Delusions,
    fancy, illusions of
    hearing, illusions of
    home, away from, is
    light, incorporeal, he is
    noise, hears
    paradise, he saw •
    visions, has
        grandeur, of magnificience
    voices, hears
Desires, this and that
    uncontrollable, itching of / for ★
Despair
    pains, with the
        stomach, in the
    parturition, during •
Dipsomania, alcoholism
Discontented, displeased, dissatisfied
    everything, with
Discouraged
    air, in open, amel.
Dream, as if in a
Dullness, sluggishness, difficulty of think-
    ing and comprehending, torpor
    reading, while
    sleepiness, with
Eccentricity
Ecstasy
    heat, during
Excitement, excitable
    night
    agg.
    chill, during
    climacteric period, during
    heat, during
        puerperal, during
    hurrried, as if
    joy, from
    palpitation, with violent
    perspiration, during
    reading, while
    weakness, with
Exertion, agg. from mental
Exhilaration
Fancies, exaltation of
    night
    heat, during
    sleeplessness, with

Fancies,
   reading, on
   vivid, lively
Fear, apprehension, dread
   air, of fresh
   alternating with exhilaration •
   apoplexy, of
   danger, going to sleep, on •
   death, of
     labor during
     pain, from •
   evil, of
   falling, of
     sleep, on going to •
   labor, during
   menses, during
   noise, from
   overpowering
   surprises, from pleasant •
   touch, of
   tremulous
Forgetfulness
   old people, of
Forsaken feeling
Frightened easily
Gestures, light
Grief
   silent
Heedless
Homesickness
Howling
Hurry, haste
   agg.
   drinking, on
   eating, while
   movements, in
Hypochondriasis
Hysteria
   menses, during
Ideas abundant, clearness of mind
   evening
   night
   deficiency of
Inconsolable
   air, amel. in open
Inconstancy

Indifference
   irritating, disagreeable things, to
Indolence, aversion to work
   walking, while
Industrious, mania for work
Insanity, madness
   drunkards, in
Irresolution, indecision
Irritability
   morning, rising, after
   air, in open, amel.
   chill, during
   pollution, after
   sleeplessness, with
Jealousy
Jesting ★
Joy
   headache from excessive joy
   sleeplessness from excessive •
Lamenting, bemoaning, wailing
   trifles, over •
Laughing
   immodrately
Learns, easily ★
Loquacity
   heat, during
Mania
Meditation
Memory, active
     evening, midnight, until •
Memory, weakness of
   facts, for past, old people, in •
   read, for what has
Menses, mental symptoms agg. during
Moaning, groaning, whining
   heat, during
   pain, from
   sleep, during
Mood, changeable, variable
Morose, cross, fretful, ill-humor, peevish
   morning
   air, in open, amel.
Morphinism
Music, agg.
   headache, from
Nymphomania
Passionate

Plans, making many
Prostration of mind, mental exhaus-
   tion, brain-fag
   sleeplessness, with
Quarrelsome, scolding
Quick to act
Religious affections
Remorse
Restlessness
   night
   anxious
   menses, during
Roving, senseless, insane
Runs, room, in
   unsteady ●
Sadness, depondency, dejection, mental
   depression, gloom, melancholy
   air, in open, amel.
   walking, air, in open
Senses, acute
   vanishing of
Sensitive, oversensitive
   music, to
   noise, to
      agg. pains ●
      labor, during
      painful sensitiveness to
      slightest, to
      stepping, of
      striking of clocks, ringing
         of bells, to
      talking, of
      odors, to
      pains, to
      touch, to
Sentimental
Serious, earnest
Shrieking, screaming, shouting
   children, in
   pain, with the
Sighing, heat, during
Speech, delirious, fever, during
   incoherent
Starting, fright, from and as from
   sleep, falling, on
      during
      from
   touched, when

Stupefaction, as if intoxicated
Surprises, pleasant, agg. ★
Sympathy, agg.
   resents ★
Talk, indisposed to, desire to be silent,
   taciturn
Talking, sleep, in
Theorizing
   night
Thoughts, rapid, quick
   rush, flow of
   night
   air amel., open ●
   reading, while
   vanishing of
Throws things away
Timidity
   bashful
Touched, aversion to being
Tranquillity, serenity, calmness
Unbearable, pains ★
Unconsciousness, coma, stupor
   emotion, after
   parturition, during
Veneration ●
Verses, makes
Violent, vehement
Vivacious
Walk
   walking in open air agg. mental
      symptoms
Weeping, tearful mood
   air, in open, amel.
   aloud, wobbing
   alternating with laughter
   anger, after
   children, in
      babies
      easily
   headache, with
   heat, during
   hysterical
   involuntary
   joy, from
   lamenting, and ★
   menses, during
   mortification, after
   pains, with the

Weeping, tearful mood
   parturition, during •
   trifles, at
   walking in open air, when
Well, says he is, when very sick
Will, weakness of
Witty
Work, Mental
   fatigues
   impossible

COFFEA TOSTA

Ailments from:
   excitement, emotional
Answers, incoherently
   unintelligibly
Anxiety
   motion, from downward
Benevolence
Concentration, active
Confusion of mind
   knows not where she is not when-
     ever came to objects around
     her
Deeds, good, desire to perform •
Delusions, enchantment, of •
Eccentricity
Excitement, excitable
   heat, during
Fancies, exaltation of
Fear, apprehension, dread •
Hysteria
Ideas abundant, clearness of mind
Killed, desire to be,
   labor, in •
Memory, active
Prostration of mind, mental exhaus-
   tion, brain-fag
Reason increased, power of •
Restlessness
Speech, repeats same thing
Starting, fright, from and as from
Striking, desires to push things •
Talk, indisposed to, headache, during.
Thoughts, rush, flow of
Unconsciousness, coma, stupor

COFFEINUM

Confusion of mind
Excitement, nervous
Restlessness

COLCHICUM AUTUMNALE

Absent-minded, unobserving
Abstraction of mind
Ailments from :
   grief
   rudeness of others
Anger, irascibility
Answers: questioned when, nothing,
   says ★
Anxiety
   evening
   midnight, after
Beside oneself, being
Cheerful, gay, mirthful
Concentration, difficult
Confounding objects and ideas
Confusion of mind
   morning
   air, in open
   sitting, while
Contradiction, is intolerant of
Delirium
   night
   collapse, with
   fever, during
   frightful
   headache, during
   laughing
   maniacal
   muttering
   raging, raving
   waking, on
   wild
Delusions, imaginations, hallucinations,
   illusions
   animals, of
   bed, on
   bed: under it, someone is
   knocking
   fancy, illusions of

Delusions,
   hearing, illusions of
   insane, she will become
   mice, sees
   noise, hears
   rats, sees
   waking, on
Despair
   pains, with the
Discomfort
Discontented, displeased, dissatisfied
   everything, with
Discouraged
   pain, from
   rage, with
Dullness, sluggishness, difficulty of thinking and comprehending, torpor
   alternating with clearness of mind •
   interrupted, when •
   sleepiness, with
Excitement, excitable
   agg.
   alternating with sadness
   feverish
Exertion, agg. from mental
Exhilaration
Fear, apprehension, dread
   night
   evil, of
   insanity, losing his reason, of
   mice, on waking, of •
   misfortune, of
   touch, of
Forgetful
   words while speaking, of; word hunting
Gestures, grasping or reaching at something, at flocks; carphologia
   picks at bed clothes
Hurt, little pains, terribly ★
Ideas abundant, clearness of mind
   night
   deficiency of, interruption, from any •
Impatience

Indifference, complain, does not, unless questioned, then says nothing of his condition •
   typhoid, in
Indolence, aversion to work
   sleepiness, with
   stool, after •
Insanity, madness
   pain, from intolerable
Interruption agg. mental symptoms
Irritability
   afternoon
   alternating with indifference
   pain, during
   sardonic
   spasmodic
Laughing sardonic spasmodic
Mania
Memory, weakness of
   expressing oneself, for
   labor, for mental, fatigue, from
   read, for what has
   say, for what is about to
   thought, for what has just
   write, for what is about to
Mistakes, writing, in
   omitting letters
   syllables
Moaning, groaning, whining
Morose, cross, fretful, ill-humor, peevish
   forenoon
   afternoon
Muttering
Prostration of mind, mental exhaustion, brain-fag
Quarrelsome, scolding
Quietness, amel. ★
Rage, fury
Reading, mental symptoms agg. from
   understand, does not
Rest, desire for
Restlessness
   night
   pregnancy, during
Sadness, despondency, dejection, mental depression, gloom, melancholy

Senses, acute
Sensitive, oversensitive
　　chill, during
　　external impressions, to all
　　light, to
　　noise, to
　　odors, to
　　pain, to
　　rudeness, to
Sighing
Sit, inclination to
Starting, startled
　　dream, from a
　　sleep, during
　　　from
Stupefaction, as if intoxicated
Talk, indisposed to, desire to be silent,
　　taciturn
　　others agg., talk of
Thinking, complaints agg., of
Thoughts, disconnected
　　rapid, quick
　　rush, night
　　wandering
Touched, aversion to being
Unconsciousness, coma, stupor
　　fever, during
　　lying, while
　　sitting upright, while
Wearisome
Weeping, tearful mood
　　amel.
　　whimpering
Wildness, bright light, strong odors,
　　touch, from •
　　misdeeds of others, from •
Work, aversion to mental
Writing, inability for, connectedly

COLLINSONIA CANADENSIS

Ailments from:
　　excitement, emotional
Delirium, nonsense, with eyes open
Excitement, excitable
　　agg.

Exhilaration
Irresolution, indecision
Restlessness

COLOCYNTHIS

Absent-minded, unobserving
Ailments from:
　　anger, vexation
　　　indignation, with
　　　silent grief, with
　　business failure
　　grief
　　embarrassment
　　indignation
　　misfortune of others ★
　　mortification
　　　anger, with •
　　reproaches
　　scorn, being scorned
Anger, irascibility
　　answer, when obliged to
　　delusions during climaxis,
　　　with
　　pains, about
　　throws things away
Anguish
Answer, aversion to
Anxiety
　　pains, from the
　　salvation; faith, about loss of his
　　stool, after
Avarice
Aversion, everything, to
　　friends, to ★
Beside oneself, being
Capriciousness
Carried, desires to be
Cheerful, gay, mirthful
Company, aversion to; presence of
　　other people agg. the symp-
　　toms, desire for solitude
　　friends, of intimate
Company, desires for; aversion to soli-
　　tude, company amel.
Complaining
　　day and night •
Concentration, difficult

Confusion of mind
 morning
 afternoon
 evening
 beer, from
 eating, after
 heat, during
 intoxicated, as after being
 stooping, when
 walking, while
 wine, after
Contradiction, is intolerant of
Cowardice
Delirium
 night
 alternating with sopor
 *bed and escapes, springs up sud-
  denly from*
 escapes in abortion •
 frightful
 nonsense, with eyes open
 raging, raving
 sleep, comatoes during
 sleepiness, with
 sleeplessness, and ★
Delusions, imaginations, hallucinations,
  illusions
 night
 fancy, illusions of
 transferred to another room •
Despair, recoverry, of ★
Discomfort, evening
Discontented, displeased, dissatisfied
 everything, with
Discouraged
Disgust
Dullness, sluggishness, difficulty of thinking and comprehending, torpor
 morning
 beer, after •
Duty, no sense of
Escape, attempts to
 fever, during
Excitement, excitable
 agg.
Fancies, exaltation, sleeplessness, with

Fear, apprehension, dread
 escape, with desire to
 faith, to lose his religious ★
 happen, something will ★
 thunderstorm, of ★
 work, dread of
Forgetful
*Gestures, strange attitudes and posi-
  tions*
Godless, want of religious feeling
Grief
 silent, indignation, with •
Ideas, abundant, clearness of mind
 deficiency of
Impatience
Indifference, apathy
 religion, to his
Indignation
Indolence, sleepiness, with
Insanity, madness
Irritability
 night
 pain, during
 questioned, when
 taciturn
Jealousy
Lamenting, bemoaning, wailing
 pain, about
Malicious, spiteful, vindictive
Memory, weakness of
Moaning, groaning, whining
 pain, from
Moral feeling, want of
Morose, cross, fretful, ill-humor, peevish
Obstinate, headstrong
*Offended, easily; takes everything in
  bad part*
Prostration of mind, mental exhaus-
  tion, brain-fag
Rage, fury
Religious feeling, want of
Reserved
Restlessness
 afternoon
 night
 anger, restlessness from
 anxious

Restlessness
> bed, tossing about in
> headache, during
> itching, after •
> menses, before
> pain, during
> sleepiness, with

Reverence, lack of

Sadness, despondency, dejection, mental depression, gloom, melancholy

Sensitive, oversensitive
> reprimands, to

Shrieking, menses, during
> *pain, with the*

Speech, wandering
> night

Stupefaction, as if intoxicated
> dinner, after

Talk, indisposed to, desire to be silent, taciturn

Thoughts, rush, flow of
> sleeplessness from
> wandering

Throws things away

Unconsciousness, coma, stupor
> evening
> *alternating with, escape, desire to* •

Violent, vehement

Wearisome

Weeping, tearful mood
> headache, with
> mortification, after

Will, weakness of

Work, aversion to mental

Wrong, everything seems

COLOCYNTHINUM

Restlessness
> night
> heat, during

COMOCLADIA DENTATA

Ailments from:
> love, disappointed

Cheerful, forenoon

Clairvoyance, sleep, during •

Confusion of mind

Contemptuous
> opponents, for

Contented

Dullness night on waking

Indifference, ordinary matters, to •
> sleepiness, with

Industrious
> menses, before •

Malicious, spiteful, vindictive

Restlessness
> night
> midnight, after, 2h.

Talking, sleep, in
> business, of

CONIUM MACULATUM

Absent-minded, unobserving
> *old age, in*

Absorbed, buried in thought

Abstraction of mind

Abusive, insulting
> somebody, on the road, to ★

Affectation

Ailments from:
> *celibacy, continence* ★
> cares, worries
> *excitement, emotional*
> grief
> *love, disappointed*
> mortification
> **reverses of fortune**
> *sexual excesses*
> work, mental

Amativeness
> want of amativeness in men

Ambition

Anger, irascibility
> easily
> *face, with pale, livid*
> *trifles, at*
> voices of people

Answers; aversion to answer
> *slowly*

Anxiety
> morning
> afternoon
> 15-18 h. •
> until evening

Anxiety,
    night
      waking, on
    midnight, on half waking,
      after •
    breakfast, after
    conscience, as if guilty of a crime
    continence prolonged, from •
    eating, after
    fear, with
    fever, during
    future, about
    hypochondriacal
    hysterical
    menses, before
      during
    present, about
    sexual excitement, from suppressed ★
    sleep, during
    thinking about it, from
    trifles, about
    waking, on
Approach of persons agg.
Attention amel. •
Avarice
Aversion
    friends
      during pregnancy, to •
    members of family, to
    men, to
    women, to
Bed, remain in, desire to
Beside oneself, being
Brooding
    corner or moping, brooding in a
Business, averse to
    desire for
Busy
Calculating inability for, (geometry, to)
Cares, worries, full of
    company, with aversion to
Cheerful, gay, mirthful
    morning

Company, aversion to; presence of other
    people agg the symptoms; desire
    for solitude
    alone, amel. when
    fear of being alone, yet
    heat, during
    menses, during
    presence of strangers, aversion to
Company, desire for; aversion to solitude, company amel.
    alone agg., while
    yet fear of people
Complaining, sleep, in
Concentration, difficult
    studying, learns with difficulty
Confusion of mind
    morning
    air, in open
    beer, from
    chill, during
    drinking, after
    headache, with
    old age, in
    sleeping, after
      siesta, after a
    spirituous liquors, from ★
    waking, on
    walking, while
    wine, after
Contradiction, is intolerant of
Contrary
Cowardice
Dancing
Death, thoughts of
    morning
Delirium
    morning
      daybreak, at
    night
    constant
    fantastic
    gay, cheerful
    intermittent
    laughing
    maniacal
    paroxysmal
    running, with
    violent

Delusions, imaginations, hallucinations,
    illusions
        morning
        night
    animals, of
    bed, dancing on the •
    assembled things, swarms,
    crowds, etc.
    dead, corpse, brother and child,
    corpse of multilated corpse
        persons, sees
    door, someone was coming in at the
        (at night) •
    entering, someone is (at night) •
    fancy, illusions of
    geese, threw themselves into wa-
        ter, thinking themselves to be
    goose, he is a •
    hearing, illusions of
    house is full of people
    images, sees, frightful
    injury, is about to receive
    mutilated bodies, sees
    noise, hears
    people, sees
        entering the house at night
        front of him, in •
    persecuted, he is
    person is in the room , another
    pursued by enemies
        he was
    room, sees people at bedside in
    thieves, house, in
    time, exaggeration of, passes too
        slowly
    visions, has
Dementia
    senilis
        talking, with foolish
Despair
    heat, during
Destructiveness
Dictatorial, domineering, dogmatical,
    despotic
Dipsomania, alcoholism

Discontented, displeased, dissatisfied
    himself, with ★
Discouraged
    afternoon •
Discrimination, lack of
Disgust
    everything, with
Dream, as if in a
Dress, averse to (in melancholia) •
Drinking, mental symptoms after
Dullness, sluggishness, difficulty of think-
    ing and comprehending, torpor
        noon
        afternoon
    old people, of
    reading, while
    thinking long, unable to
    waking, on
Dwells on past disagreeable occur-
    rences
Ennui, tedium
Estranged, from her family
Excitement, excitable
    morning
    agg.
    alternating with sadness
    perspiration, during
    weakness, with   .
    weeping, till
    women, in
Exertion, agg. from mental
Extravagance
Extremes, goes to ★
Fancies, confused
    exaltation of
        morning
        night
    lascivious
    wild •
Fastidious
Fear, apprehension, dread
    night
        waking, after
        midnight
    alone, of being
        desire of being alone, but •
    approaching him, of others
    crowd, in a

Fear,
> death, of
>> morning
>> waking, on
> door, in opening
> men, dread, fear of
> menses, before
>> during
> people, of; anthropophobia
>> yet agg. if alone ★
> pregnancy, during
> robbers, of
> thunderstorm, of ★
> waking, on
> work, dread of
>> mental, of
>>> *persuaded to, cannot be* ●

Foolish behavior
Forgetful
> chill, during
> (-ness) old people, of
> words, while speaking, of; word
>> hunting

Frightened easily
> night, 3h., on waking
> waking, dream, from

Frivolous
Gestures, grasping or reaching at some-
> thing, at flocks; carphologia
>> picks at bed clothes
> plays with his fingers

Grief
Gritty, feeling ● ★
Ground gives way ★
Haughty
> *clothes, likes to wear his best* ●

Heedless
Horrible things, sad stories, affect her
> profoundly

Hurry, haste
> movements, in

Hypochondriasis
> *air, in open*
> *menses, suppression of* ●
> morose
> **sexual abstinence, from**
>> **excess, from**
> suicide, driving to

Hysteria
> coition amel.
> menses, before
> sexual excesses, after
>> **suppression of sexual excite-**
>>> **ment, from** ●

Ideas, deficinecy of
Imbecility
Impressionable
> *unpleasanlty by everything* ●

Indifference, apathy
> afternoon
> air, in open
> chill, during
> conscience, to the dictates of
> ennui, with
> everything, to
> external impressions, to
> **fever, during**
> morose
> *walking in open air, while* ●

Indiscretion
Indolence, aversion to work
> intelligent, although very

Insanity, madness
> alternating with other mental
>> symptoms
> *dresses in his best clothes* ●
> *periodical*
> *purchases, makes useless* ●

Intolerance
Irresolution, indecision
Irritability
> morning
>> waking, on
> afternoon
>> 17-18 h. ●
> *evening*
> air, in open
> breakfast, after ●
> **chill, during**
> eating, after
> headache, during
> menses, during
> *walking, when*

Jealousy, sexual excitement, with
Jesting, trifles with everything

Lascivious, lustful
Laughing
   agg.
   convulsions, before, during or after
   exhausted condition, during •
   involuntarily
   irritation in stomach and hypo-
     chondria, from •
   sardonic
   spasmodic
   weakness, during •
Liar
Libertinism
Light, shuns
Loathing, work, at
Loquacity
Magnetized, desire to be, mesmerism
   amel.
Malicious, spiteful, vindictive
Mania
   alternating with depression
Mathematics, inapt, geometry, for
Meddlesome, importunate
Meditation
Memory, weakness of
   dates, for
   labor, for mental
   orthography, for
   words, of
Menses, mental symptoms agg. before
Mental symptoms alternating with
   physical •
Misanthropy
Mistakes, calculating, in
   speaking, in
     misplacing words
     words, using wrong
   time, in
   writing, in
   sleep, during
Mood
   alternating
   changeable, variable
   repulsive
Moral feeling, want of

Morose, cross, fretful, ill-humor, peevish
   morning
   forenoon
   afternoon
     17-18 h. •
   evening
   air, in open
   trifles, about
Muttering, evening
   sleep, in
Narrow minded
Neglects important things
Obscene, lewd
Occupation, diversion amel.
Passionate
Play, desire to
Pregnancy, mental affections in
Prophesying
Prostration of mind, mental ex-
   haustion, brain-fag
   trembling, with
Quarrelsome, scolding
   alternating with silent sadness •
Quiet disposition
   light is intolerable, bright •
   noise, intolerable to •
   repose and tranquillity, desires ★
Rage, night
Reading: aversion to read
Religious, affections
   melancholia
   remorse, from
Remorse
Reproaches himself
Restlessness
   anxious
   bed, driving out of
     tossing about in
   heat, during
   menses, before
   sleepiness, with
Runs about
Sadness, despondency, dejection, mental
   depression, gloom, melancholy
   morning
   afternoon
   evening

Sadness,
   air, in open
   alone, when
   alternating with quarrelsomeness
   aversion to see her children from
      sadness •
   breakfast, after •
   chill, during
   climaxis, during
   coition, after
   company, aversion to; desire for
      solitude
   continence, from
   eating, after
   headache, during
   heat, during
   injuries, from, head, of the
   masturbation, from
   menses, before
      suppressed
   periodical
      fourteen days, every •
   perspiration, during
   pollutions, from
   sexual excitement, suppressed,
      from ★
   sexual excesses, from
   suicidal disposition, with
   walking, while and after
      air, in open
Satyariasis
Senses, acute
   dull, blunted
Sensitive, oversensitive
   light, to
   noise, to
   painful, sensitiveness to
   talking, of
   voices, to
   want of sensitiveness
Sentimental
Serious, earnest
Shrieking, waking, on
Sit, inclination to
Sits on place for 3 or 4 days during
   headache •

Slowness
   motion, in
   old people, of
Speech, babbling
Spoken to, averse to being
Squanders
Starting, startled
   fright, from and as from
   noise, from
   sleep, from
   twitching •
Strangers, presence of strangers agg.
Striking
Striking himself, knocking his head
      against wall and things
Stupefaction, as if intoxicated
   chill, during
   injury to head, after
   sleepiness, with
Suicidal, hypochondriasis, by
   sadness, from
Sulky
Superstitious
Suspicious, mistrustful
Talk, indisposed to, desire to be silent,
   taciturn
   alternating with quarrelsomeness •
   headache, during
   others agg., talk of
Talking, sleep, in
Thinking, complaints agg., of
Thoughts, intrude, sexual
   rush, flow of
   morning
   night
   sexual
   tormenting
   sexual
Time passes too slowly, appears longer
Timidity
   afternoon
   bashful
Touched, aversion to being

Unconsciousness, coma, stupor
  morning
    night, waking, on
    chill, during
    conduct, automatic
    crowded room, in a
    dream, as in a
    menses, suppression of
    mental insensibility
    vertigo, during
    waking, after
Unfeeling, hard hearted
Unreliable, promises, in his
Violent, vehement
    deeds of violence, rage leading to
    talks of others, from
Walk, walking in open air agg. mental
    symptoms
Wearisome
Weary of life
Weeping, tearful mood
    night
      sleep, in
    alone, when
    aloud, sobbing
    alternating with laughter
    chill, during
    menses, before
      during
      after
    periodical every four weeks •
    sleep, in
    trifles, at
Will, loss of
    weakness of
Work, aversion to mental
    fatigues
    impossible

CONIINUM

Concentration, difficult
Delusions, hearing, of
Dullness, sluggishness, difficulty of think-
    ing and comprehending, torpor
Gestures, labored •
    slow
Muttering
    sleep, in

CONIINUM BROMATUM

Inactivity •
Indifference, apathy

CONVOLVULUS DUARTINUS

Discouraged
Fancies, exaltation of
Moral feeling, want of
Prostration of mind, mental exhaus-
    tion, brain-fag
Sadness, despondency, dejection, mental
    depression, gloom, melancholy
Starting, sleep, from

CONVOLVULUS STANS

Ailments from:
    excitement, emotional
Anxiety
    night, children, in
Company, aversion to; presence of
    other people agg. the symp-
    toms; desire for solitude
    alone, amel. when
Confusion of mind
Delirium
    muttering
Delusions, imaginations, hallucinations,
    illusions
    visions, has
Excitement, excitable
Hysteria
Memory, weakness of
Prostration of mind, mental exhaus-
    tion, brain-fag
Restlessness
Sadness, despondency, dejection, mental
    depression, gloom, melancholy
Schizophrenia, catatonic
Sensitive, oversensitive
    noise, to
Weeping, tearful mood

COPAIVA

Anger, irascibility
  trembling, with
Anxiety, health, about
Business, averse to
Company, aversion to; presence of
  other people agg. the symp-
  toms; desire for solitude
Confusion of mind
Contemptuous, self, of
Delirium
Delusions, tall, he is
Dullness, sluggishness, difficulty of think-
  ing and comprehending, torpor
Dwells on past disagreeable occur-
  rences
Excitement, morning
    night
    menses, during
Fancies, lascivious
Fear, death, of
Hysteria
Irritability
Lascivious, lustful
  emotions, with violent •
Loathing, general, eruption, before •
  fear of death, during •
Loathing, life, at
Memory, weakness of
Misanthropy
Moaning, hemicrania, with •
Morose, cross, fretful, ill-humor, peevish
Quarrelsome, recrimination about
  trifles •
Restlessness
  night
  coition, after
Sadness, despondency, dejection, mental
  depression, gloom, melancholy
    morning
      waking, on
        after
    afternoon
    evening
    menses, during
    periodical
    walking amel., while and after

Sensitive, music, to
  noise, to
Weeping, tearful mood
    afternoon
    bells, sound of
    music of bells, from
    piano, of
Work, mental, impossible

CORALLIUM RUBRUM

Abusive, insulting
  pains, with the •
Anger, irascibility
Blank ★
Complaining
Confusion of mind
  beer, from
  intoxicated, as after being
  spirituous liquors, from
Cursing, swearing
  amel. •
  pains, at
Delirium
    night
Fear, suffering, of
Gestures, covers mouth with hands ★
Hysteria
Irritability
Lamenting, bemoaning, wailing
Laughing
Morose, cross, fretful, ill-humor, peevish
Quarrelsome, scolding
  pains, from •
Restlessness
    night
    bed, tossing about in
Slander, disposition to
Starting, dream, from a
  sleep, on falling
    during
    from
Stupefaction, wine, after •
Unconsciousness, coma, stupor

CORIARIA MYRTIFOLIA

Gestures, convulsive

CORIARIA RUSCIFOLIA

Astonished
Complaining
Delirium, intoxicated, as if
    maniacal
    raging, raving
Delirium tremens, mania-a-potu •
Delusions, born, feels as if newly, into
    the world and was overwhelmed
    with wonder at the novelty of his
    surroundings •
Excitement, excitable
Fear, pain, of
    suffering, of
Foolish, grotesque behavior
Insanity, strength increased, with
Irritability
Laughing
Mania
Memory, loss of
    coma, after •
Memory, weakness of
Rage, fury
Stupefaction, as if intoxicated
Unconsciousness, coma, stupor
    convulsions, after

CORNUS CIRCINATA

Anxiety
Concentration, difficult
    studying, reading, etc., while
Confusion of mind
    morning
        rising and after, on
    evening
    night
    stooping, when
Dullness, sluggishness, difficulty of think-
    ing and comprehending, torpor
Forgetful
Ideas, deficiency of

Indifference, apathy
    morning
    agreeable things, to
Indolence, aversion to work
Irritability
Memory, weakness of
    read, for what has
Morose, cross, fretful, ill-humor, peevish
Prostration of mind, mental exhaus-
    tion, brain-fag
Reading, aversion to
Restlessness
    night
Sadness, despondency, dejection, mental
    depression, gloom, melancholy
Sighing
Stupefaction, as if intoxicated
Thinking, aversion to
Thoughts, wandering
Violent, vehement
Work, aversion to mental

CORNUS FLORIDA

Prostration of mind, sleepiness, with
Reading, understand, does not

CORTICOTROPINUM

Abstraction of mind
Activity, mental
    night, from 4h. •
Anxiety
    alone, when
Catatonia
Company, aversion to; presence of
    other people agg. the symp-
    toms; desire for solitude
    alone, amel. when
Concentration, difficult
Confusion of mind
Death, desires
    thoughts of
Delusions, imaginations, hallucinations,
    illusions
    mice, sees
    visions, has ·

Dullness, sluggishness, difficulty of think-
    ing and comprehending, torpor
Exhilaration
Fear, apprehension, dread
    age, of own, of people •
Foolish behavior •
Forgetful
Forsaken feeling
    isolation, sensation of
Heedless
Irresolution, indecision
Irritability
    alone, when
Mania
Memory, weakness of
    do, for what was about to
    names, for proper names
Mistakes, speaking, in
    spelling, in
    words, using wrong
Mood, alternating
    changeable, variable
Prostratoion of mind, mental exhaus-
    tion, brain-fag
Restlessness, working, while
Sadness, despondency, dejection, mental
    depression, gloom, melancholy
Schizophrenia, catatonia
Speech, babbling
    hesitating
Talk, indisposed to, desire to be silent,
    taciturn
Talking, sleep, in
Timidity
    company, in
Unconsciousness, coma, stupor
    dream, does not know where he is
    head, bending forward, on •
    stooping, when
Undertakes many things, perseveres in
    nothing
Will, loss of

CORTISONUM

Concentration, difficult
Confusion of mind
Death, thoughts of

Dullness, sluggishness, difficulty of think-
    ing and comprehending, torpor
Euphoria
    alternating with sadness
Excitement, alternating with indeci
    sion •
    sadness
Exertion, agg. from mental
Exhilaration
Forgetful
Insanity, madness
Irritability
    travel is too slow, when the •
Memory, weakness of
Mood, alternating
Sadness, despondency, dejection, mental
    depression, gloom, melancholy
Slowness
    bus, sensation of slowness of •
Talk, indisposed to, desire to be silent,
    taciturn
Weeping, tearful mood
    causeless

COTYLEDON UMBILICUS

Absent-minded, unobserving
Anxiety
Cheerful, gay, mirthful
Company, desire for; aversion to soli-
    tude, company amel.
Confusion of mind
Dullness, sluggishness, difficulty of
    thinking and comprehending,
    torpor
Excitement, desire for •
Foolish behavior
Heedless, morning on waking •
Hysteria
Memory, weakness of
    expressing oneself, for
    say, for what is about to
Restlessness, midnight, before
Sadness, despondency, dejection, mental
    depression, gloom, melancholy
Singing
Unconsciousness, night, on waking
Wildness, night, on waking •

CRATAEGUS OXYACANTHA

Despair
Irritability

CROCUS SATIVUS

Absent-minded, unobserving
Abstraction of mind
Abusive, insulting
Affectionate
Ailments from:
    anger, vexation
    excitement, emotional ★
    joy, excessive
Anger, irascibility
    evening
    alternating with cheerfulness
      laughing
      repentence, quick
      singing •
      tenderness •
      tranquillity
    laughing, with burst of •
    reproaches, from
    trifles, at
    violent
Antics, plays
Anxiety
Bite, desire to
    evening •
    convulsions, with
Capriciousness
    evening
Cheerful, gay, mirthful
    alternating with anger
      bursts of indignation
        of passion
      irritability
      mania
      quarrel
      sadness
      vexation
      violence
    music, from •
    sleep, during
Childish behavior
Concentration, difficult

Confusion of mind
    air amel., in open
    drinking, after
    eating, after
    intoxicated, as after being
    writing,while
Contrary
Cruelty, inhumanity
Dancing
Delirium
    evening
    quiet
Delusions, imaginations, hallucinations,
    illusions
    business, unfit for, he is •
    die, he was about to die
    fancy, illusions of
    fire, visions of
    images, sees frightful
    light, incorporeal, he is
    music, he hears
    pregnant, she is
    religious
    strange, familiar things seem
Dementia
Dipsomania, alcoholism
Disgust
Doubtful, soul's welfare, of
Dullness, sluggishness, difficulty of think-
    ing and comprehending, torpor
    sleepiness, with
Eat, refuses to
Ecstasy
Excitement, excitable
    menses, during
    pregnancy, during
Exertion, amel. from mental
Exhilaration
    alternating with sadness
Extravagance
Exuberance
Fancies, exaltation of
    vivid, lively
Fear, apprehension, dread
    death, of
    evil, of
    tremulous

Foolish behavior
Forgetful
Gestures, ridiculous or foolish
Godless, want of religious feeling
Grief
Groping, as if in the dark
Heedless
Hypochondriasis
Hysteria
    man, in a
    sleeplessness, with
Ideas, deficiency of
Imbecility
Impetuous
Impressionable
Impulsive
Indifference, apathy
    everything, to
    pleasure, to
    sleepiness, with
Indignation
Indiscretion
Indolence, aversion to work
    sleepiness, with
Insanity, madness
    alternating mental with physical
    symptoms
    behaves like a crazy person
    cheerful, gay
    face, with pale
    mild
    religious
Irritability
    alternating with cheerfulness
    takes everything in bad part
Jesting
    ridiculous or foolish
Jumping
Kisses everyone
Lascivious, lustful
Laughing
    alternating with quarrelsomeness ●
        shrieking
        sleep during
        tenderness ●
        vexation, ill-humor
        violence
        childish
        immoderately

Laughing,
    involuntarily
    loudly
    sardonic
    shrieking
    silly
        children, on all occasions, in ●
    sleep, during
    spasmodic
    unbecoming ●
Loathing, work, at
Loquacity
    cheerful, exuberant
    jesting, with
    witty ●
Malicious, spiteful, vindictive
Mania
    rage, with
Memory, active
    music, for ●
Memory, weakness of
    names, for proper
    persons, for
    said, for what has
    write, for what is about
Mental symptoms alternating with
    physical
Mildness
    evening ●
    alternating with hardness
Mistakes, speaking, in
    time, in
        confounds future with the past
        present with the past
    writing, in
Mobility ★
Mood, aggreeable
    alternating
    changeable, variable
        evening
        perspiration, during
    repulsive
Moral feeling, want of
Morose, cross, fretful, ill-humor, peevish
    alternating with cheerfulness
        laughing
        singing ●

Music agg
    amel.
Nymphomania
Obstinate, headstrong
Occupation, diversion amel.
Offended, easily; takes everything in
    bad part
Passionate
Playful
Prostration of mind, mental exhaus-
    tion, brain-fag
Quarrelsome, scolding
    alternating with gaiety and laugh-
    ter
        singing •
Rage, fury
    evening
    alternating with affectionate dis-
        position •
        cheerfulness
    biting, with
    headache, with
    paroxysms, in
    repentence, followed by
    violent
Reading agg. ★
Religious, affections
    feeling, want of
    melancholia
Remorse
    quickly, repents
Restlessness
    anxious
    menses, during
Sadness, despondency, dejection, mental
    depression, gloom, melancholy
    anxious
    menses, from suppressed
Sensess, vanishing of
Sensitive, oversensitive
    mental impressions, to
    music, to
Shrieking, screaming, shouting
    sleep, during
Sighing

Singing
    night
    alternating with anger •
        quarrelsomeness •
        vexation
    involuntarily
        on hearing a single note sung •
    sleep, in
Sit, inclination to
Smiling, sleep, in
Somnambulism
Starting, dreams, from a dream
    sleep, during
Stupefaction, as if intoxicated
    vertigo, during
Sympathy, compassion
Thoughts, rush, flow of
    vanishing of
Timidity
Tranquillity, serenity, calmness
Unconsciousness, coma, stupor
    morning
    conduct, automatic ★
Unfeeling, hardhearted
Violent, vehement
    alternating with mildness •
    deeds of violence, rage leading to
Weeping, tearful mood
    night
    agg.
    alternating with laughter
    sleep, in
Whistling
Wildness
    evening •
Will, loss of
    weakness of
Witty
Yielding, disposition

CROTALUS CASCAVELLA

Anguish
Answers, monosyllable
    "no" to all questions
Anxiety
Childish behavior
Clairvoyance

Company, desire for; aversion to soli-
    tude, company amel.
Confusion of mind
Death, thoughts of
    alone, when •
Delirium
Delusions, imaginations, hallucina-
    tions, illusions
    eyes, falling out •
    falling out of bed
    fancy, illusions of
    footsteps, hears
      behind him •
    groans, he hears •
    hearing, illusions of
    people, behind him, someone is
      converses with absent
    skeletons, sees
    spectres, death appears as a gi-
      gantic black skeleton •
    visions, has
    voices, hears
      hears, that he must follow
    walks behind him, someone
Desires, exercise, for
Fancies, exaltation of
Fear, night
    alone, of being
    behind him, someone is
    death, of
Frightened, night
Gestures, plays with his fingers
Hurry, haste
Indifference, apathy
Insanity, madness
    alternating with metrorrhagia •
Laughing alternating with groaning •
    metorhagic •
    silly
Loquacity
Mania
    evening •
    alternating with metrorrhagia •
Memory, weakness of
    orthography, for
Moaning, groaning, whining
    sleep, during
    sleeplessness, with •

Restlessness
    drinking agg. •
**Sadness, despondency, dejection,
    mental depression, gloom,
    melancholy**
    weep, cannot
Shrieking, screaming, shouting
    convulsions, before
Speech, confused
Starting, sleep, during
Suicidal, throwing, window, from
Talk, indisposed to, desire to be silent,
    taciturn
Unconsciousness, coma, stupor
Weeping, tearful mood
    aloud, wobbing

CROTALUS HORRIDUS

Absent-minded, unobserving
Ailments from:
    anticipation, foreboding, presen-
      timent
    fright
Anger, irascibility
    easily
Anguish
Answers
    disconnected
Anxiety
    faintness, with
    fever, during
    perspiration, with cold
Aversion, members of family, to
    his own mind, to ★
    persons, to certain
Calculating, inability for
Cheerful, gay, mirthful
Company, desire for; aversion to soli-
    tude, company amel.
Confusion of mind
    morning
Death, thoughts of
Delirium
    night
    bed and escapes, springs up sud-
      denly from

Delirium,
   convulsions, during
   crying, with
   fever, during
   headache, during
   loquacious
   maniacal
   moaning, with
   muttering
   nonsense, with eyes open
   sepsis, from
   sleepiness, with
Delirium tremens, mania-a-potu
   face, with red, bloated
Delusions, imaginations, hallucinations,
   illusions
   animals, of
      frightful
   body, only half alive •
   enemy, surrounded by enemies
   falling, forward, she is, out of
      bed ★
   images, phantoms, sees
      night
   journey, he is on a
   pursued by enemies
   voices, hears
Dementia
   senilis
Dipsomania, alcoholism
Dirtiness
Dullness, sluggishness, difficulty of
   thinking and comprehending,
   torpor
   alternating with vivacity •
   sleepiness, with
Ecstasy
      morning on waking •
      sublime •
Escape, attempts to
   springs up suddenly from bed
Excitement, agg. from mental
Fear, apprehension, dread
   crowd, public places, of; agora
      phobia
   evil, of
   medicine, of not being able to
      bear any kind of,
      selecting remedies, when •

Fear,
   people, of
   sadness, with
   serious thoughts, of
Forgetfulness
   old people, of
   streets, of well known
   words while speaking, of; word
      hunting
Hydrophobia
Hysteria
Imbecility
Indifference, apathy
   epilepsy, in
Indolence, aversion to work
Insanity, madness
   chilliness and coldness of skin •
   drunkards, in
   puerperal
   pulse, with frequent
Irresolution, indecision
Irritability
Laughing
Loquacity
Mania
Memory, weakness of
   dates, for
   expressing one self, for
   names, for proper
   persons, for
   places, for
   words, of
Misanthropy
Mistakes, calculating, in
   speaking, in
      misplacing words
      spelling, in
      words, using wrong
   writing, in
      old age, in
Moaning, groaning, whining
Morose, cross, fretful, ill-humor, peevish
Muttering
Obstinate, headstrong
Plaintive ★
Quarrelsome, scolding
Rage, fury

Restlessness
    anxious
    driving about
    sleeplessness, with
Sadness, despondency, dejection, mental
    depression, gloom, melancholy
    diarrhoea, during
    headache, during
Senses, vanishing of
Sensitive, oversensitive
    certain persons, to
    noise, to
    reading, to
Sentimental
Shrieking, convulsions, during epileptic
Slowness, motion, in
Somnambulism
Speech, affected
    bombast, worthless
    confused
    incoherent
Starting, sleep, during
Stupefaction, as if intoxicated
Suicidal disposition
    throwing himself from a height
Suspicious, mistrustful
Talks, himself, to
Thoughts, wandering
Timidity
Torpor
Unconsciousness, coma, stupor
    apoplexy, in
    fever, during
    incomplete
    vertigo, during
Vivacious
Weeping, tearful mood
    questioned, when ★
    reading, while
Work, mental, impossible

CROTON TIGLIUM

Anger, irascibility
Answers, incoherently
Anxiety
    afternoon
    air, amel. in open

Anxiety,
    stool, before
    after
Confusion of mind
    afternoon
    night
    air, in open
    beer, from
    bread agg.
Dancing
Despair
Discomfort, eating, dinner, after
Discontented, displeased, dissatisfied
Dullness, sluggishness, difficulty of think-
    ing and comprehending, torpor
Fear, diarrhoea with
    happen, something will
    misfortune, of
    people, of
Hysteria
Indolence, aversion to work
    sadness, from
Insanity
    staring of eyes
Irritability
Memory, weakness of
Morose cross, fretful, ill-humor, peevish
    pain, after
Restlessness
    night
    bed, tossing about in
Sadness, despondency, dejection, mental
    depression, gloom, melancholy
    anxious
    work shy, in
Selfishness, egoism
Stupefaction, as if intoxicated
    solitude, desire for
Suspicious, mistrustful solitude desire
    for
Talk, indisposed to, desire to be silent,
    taciturn
Thoughts: himself, cannot think of
    anyone beside •
Time, fritters away his

CRYPTOPINUM

Excitement, excitable

CUBEBA OFFICINALIS

Anxiety
  waking, on
Bite, desire to
Delusions, unfortunate, he is
Eccentricity
Envy
Excitement, excitable
  feverish
Impatience
Irritability
Memory, active
Memory, weakness of
Obscene, lewd
  talk
Prostration of mind, mental exhaustion, brain-fag.
Restlessness
  heat, during
Shamelessness
Speech, incoherent
  sleep, during
Starting, noise, from
Striking
Unfortunate, feels

CULEX MUSCA

Anxiety
Delusions, poisoned, he has been
Fear, death, of
Impatience
Indolence, aversion to work
Interruption agg. mental symptoms
Memory, weakness of
Quarrelsome, scolding
Restlessness
  walking, amel. while

CUNDURANGO

Confusion of mind
Delusions, snakes in and around her
  snakes, black ★
Sadness, despondency, dejection, mental
  depression, gloom, melancholy

CUPRUM ACETICUM

Abusive, insulting
Ailments from:
  work, mental
Anguish
Answers, slowly
Anxiety
  night
  bed, in
    tossing about, with
    mental exertion, from
    paroxysms, in
Beside oneself, being
Bite, desire to
Croaking, frogs, as of
Death, conviction of
Delirium
  crying, with
  home, wants to go
  quiet
  raging, raving
  sleep, during
Delusions, imaginations, hallucinations,
  illusions
  chairs, he is repairing old
  objects, immaterial o. in room
  officer, he is an
  spectres, ghosts, spirits, sees
  thieves, sees
    house, in
  vegetables, he is selling green
  voices, hears
Dementia, epileptics, of
Despair
Dipsomania, alcoholism
Eccentricity
  chorea, with
Escape, attempts to, waking, on ●
Excitement, agg.
Exertion, agg. from mental
Fear, apprehension, dread
  approaching him, of others
  falling, of, child holds on to
    mother
  fire, things will catch
  injured, of being
Frightened easily

Home, desire to go
· *go out, and when there to*
Insanity, puerperal
    pulse, with frequent
Irritability
    cough, in whooping
Jumping, bed, out of
    mania, in
Lamenting, bemoaning, wailing
Mania
Memory, weakness of
Moaning, groaning, whining
    cough, during whooping •
Morose, cross, fretful, ill-humor, peevish
    cough, in whooping
Prostration of mind, mental exhaus-
    tion, brain-fag
Restlessness
Sadness, despondency, dejection, mental
    depression, gloom, melancholy
Sensitive: want of sensitiveness
Shrieking, screaming, shouting
    brain cry
    chorea, in
    sleep, during
Speech, delirious
    distorted •
    fluent
    incoherent, perspiration, ending
        with
Spit, faces of people, in
Stupefaction, as if intoxicated
Thoughts, disconnected
Unconsciousness, coma, stupor
    apoplexy, in
    scarlatina, in
Weeping, tearful mood
    child, like a
    despair, from

CUPRUM METALLICUM

Absent-minded, unobserving
Absorbed, buried in thought
Ailments from:
    anger, vexation
        anxiety, with
        fright, with

Ailments from:
    bad news
    excitement, emotional
    fear
    fright
    work, mental
Anguish
    afternoon
Answers
    aversion to answer
    incoherently
    reflects long
    slowly
Antics, plays
    delirium, during
Anxiety
    afternoon
    conscience, as if guilty of a crime
    cough, before
        whooping cough, before •
    epilepsy, during intervals of
    fear, with
    fits, with
    fright, after
    future, about
    head, with congestion to
        heat of, with
    hypochondriacal
    laughing and crying, ending in
    profuse perspiration, from anxi-
        ety •
    mental exertion, from
    night watching, from
    pains, from the abdomen
    paroxysms, in
    parturition, during •
Aversion, everything, to
Barking, bellowing
Bed, aversion to, shuns bed
Beside oneself, being
Bite, desire to
    convulsions, with
    delirium, during
    spoon etc., bites
Brooding, corner or moping, in a
Cautious

Cheerful, gay, mirthful
    evening
    night
    alternating with sadness
Company, aversion to; presence of other
    people agg. the symptoms; de-
    sire for solitude
    avoids the sight of people
Concentration, difficult
Confusion of mind
    dream, as if in
    intoxicated, as if
Contradict, disposition to
Cowardice
Croaking
    frog, as of
Darkness agg.
Death, agony before
    presentiment of
    thoughts of
Deceitful, sly
Delirium
    evening
        dark, in the
    anxious
    bed and escapes, springs up sud-
        denly from
    bellows like a calf •
    collapse, with
    convulsions, during
    crying, with
    dark, in
    laughing
    looks fixed on one point, staring
    loquacious
    maniacal
    quiet
    raging, raving
    sleep, during
    violent
    wild
Delusions, imaginations, hallucina-
    tions, illusions
    arrested, is about to be
    business, is doing
    chairs, he is repairing old
    commander, being a
    devils, sees

Delusions,
    die, he was about to
    engaged in some occupation, is
    faces, sees
        distorted, on lying down, day-
        time
    fancy, illusions of
    figures, sees
    general, he is a •
    great person, is a
    herbs, gathering
    images, phantoms, sees
        night
        closing eyes in bed, on
    officer, he is an
    police officer called on him ★
    pursued by enemies
        police, by
    rank, he is a person of
    spectres, ghosts, spirits, sees
    thieves, sees
    vegetables, he is selling green
    visions, has, evening
        closing the eyes, on
Dementia, epileptics, of
Despair
    chill, during
Destructiveness
Development of children arrested
Dictatorial, domineering, dogmatical,
    despotic
    command, talking with air of
Discontented, displeased, dissatisfied
    everything, with
Discouraged
Dream, as if in a
Dullness, sluggishness, difficulty of
    thinking and comprehending,
    torpor
    sleepiness, with
Eccentricity
    chorea, with
Ecstasy
Ennui, tedium
Escape, attempts to
    run away, to
Excitement, excitable
    bad news, after
Exertion, agg. from mental

Exhilaration
Fancies, absorbed in
    exaltation of
Fear, apprehension, dread
        evening
    accidents, of
    approaching him, of others
        children cannot bear to have
    any one come   near them
        delirium, in
    bed, of the
    dark, of
    death, of
        impending death, of
    downward motion, of
    escape, with desire to
    evil, of
    falling, of
    fire, things will catch
    insanity, losing his reason, of
    misfortune, of
    people, of
        fever, in •
    strangers, of
    tread lightly or will injure him-
        self, must •
    tremulous
    waking, on
    water, of
Feces passed on the floor
Foolish behavior
Forgetful
        fright, after •
Frightened, easily
Gestures, ridiculous or foolish
    covers mouth with hands ★
Grimaces
Hatred
Haughty
Heedless
Hide, desire to
    fear, on account of
Home, desire to go
Howling
Hurry, eating, while
Hydrophobia
Hypochondriasis

Hysteria
    fainting, hysterical
    menses, before
        during
        after
Ideas, deficiency of
Imbecility
Imitation, mimicry
Impulsive
Indifference, apathy
Indolence, aversion to work
Insanity, madness
    anxiety, with
    cheerful, gay
    convulsions, with
    escape, desire to
    haemorrhage, after
    malicious, malignant
    perspiration, fits of insanity, with,
        following •
    puerperal
    pulse, with frequent
    wantonness, with
Irresolution, indecision
Irritability
            morning, waking, on
    children, in
    waking, on
Jesting
Jumping, bed, out of
Kill, desire to
Lamenting, bemoaning, wailing
Laughing
        evening
    agg.
    anxiety, after
    immoderately
    overwork, after •
    perspiration, ending in profuse •
    spasmodic
Loquacity
    excited
    perspiration with ★
    sleep, during
**Magnetized, desire to be, mesmer-
    ism amel.**
Malicious, spiteful, vindictive
    laughing •

Mania
    rage, with
Melancholy, death, with fear of ★
Memory active
Memory, confused
Memory, weakness of
    words, of
Menses, mental symptoms agg. before
Mildness
    alternating with obstinacy •
Misanthropy
Mischievous
Mistakes
    speaking, in
        words, using wrong
Moaning, groaning, whining
    night
    chill, during
    perspiration, during
    sleep, during
Mood, alternating
    changeable, variable
Morose, cross, fretful, ill-humor, peevish
Occupation, diversion amel.
Play, desire to, night
Pompous, important
Prostration of mind, mental exhaustion, brain-fag
    sleepiness, with
Pull one's hair, desire to
Quarrelsome, scolding
    sleep, in
Rage, fury
    biting, with
    epilepsy, rage with
    malicious
    paroxysms, in
    pulls hair ★
    shrieking, with
    striking, with
    violent
    water, at sight of
Recognize, relatives, does not, his
Remorse
Restlessness
    night
    anxious
    bed, tossing about in
    driving about

Runs about
Sadness, despondency, dejection, mental depression, gloom, melancholy
    air, in open
    anxious
    chill, during
    company, aversion to, desire for solitude
    walking, air, in open
        stand still, or sit down, must •
Senses, acute
    vanishing of
Sensitive, oversensitive
    music, to
    pain, to
    want of sensitiveness
Sentimental
Shamelessness
Shrieking, screaming, shouting
    brain cry
    children, in
    convulsion, before
    epileptic
    during epileptic
    cramps, during •
    in abdomen
    menses, during
Sighing
    perspiration, during
Singing
Sit, inclination to
Slowness
Speech, incoherent
    nonsensical
    prattling
    slow
    voice, in a shrill
    wandering
Spit, desire to
    faces of people, in
Starting, startled
    anxious
    sleep, during
Striking
    about him at imaginary objects
    convulsions, after •

Stupefaction, as if intoxicated
**suppressed exanthemata,
  from** •
Suppressed or receding skin diseases
  or haemorrhoids, mental symptoms agg. after
Suspicious, mistrustful
Talk, indisposed to, desire to be silent,
  taciturn
Talking, sleep, in
Tears things
Thoughts, persistent
  vanishing of
  wandering
Timidity
  appearing, talk in public, to
  bashful
Torpor
Touched, aversion to being
Tricky ★
Unconsciousness, coma, stupor
  apoplexy, in
  eyes, with fixed
  incomplete
  menses, after
  twitching of limbs, with
Violent, vehement
  deeds of violence, rage leading to
Vivacious
Wearisome
Weeping, tearful mood
  agg.
  aloud, wobbing ★
  alternating with queer antics
  **convulsions, during
    epileptic
    emotion, after slight**
  heat, during
  **involuntary
  perspiration, during**
  spasmodic
  speeches, when making •
  whimpering
Wildness

CUPRUM AMMONIAE SULPHURICUM

Ecstasy

CUPRUM ARSENICOSUM

Anxiety
  night
Confusion of mind
  vertigo, with
Delirium
Dipsomania, alcoholism
Dullness, sluggishness, difficulty of think-
  ing and comprehending, torpor
Eccentricity
Excitement, excitable
  night
Fear, apprehension, dread
Irritability
Restlessness
Runs about
Sadness, despondency, dejection, mental
  depression, gloom, melancholy
Shrieking, screaming, shouting
Stupefaction, as if intoxicated
Unconsciousness, incomplete

CUPRUM SULPHURICUM

Anxiety
Indifference, apathy
Irritability
Mania, wild look, with •
Quiet, wants to be
Restlessness
  night
Unconsciousness, coma, stupor

CURARE

Anger, irascibility
Anxiety
Bite, desire to
Chases persons •
Company, aversion to; presence of
  other people agg. the symp-
  toms; desire for solitude
  avoids the sight of people
  shuts herself up •
Confusion of mind
Cruelty, inhumanity

Delirium, waking, on
    watching, vigil, from
Delusions, dirty, everything is •
    foul, everything appears •
    images, sees, night
Desires, grandeur, for •
Despair
Destructiveness
Dullness, waking, on
Ecstasy
    night •
Enuui, tedium
Envy
Fear, death, of
    falling, of
Hurry, haste
Hydrophobia
Hypochondriasis, menses, during •
Insanity, madness
Irresolution, indecision
    debility, in nervous •
Kill, desire to
Kleptomania
Moral feeling, want of
Restlessness
    bed, tossing about in
Sadness, despondency, dejection, mental
    depression, gloom, melancholy
    menses, during
Sighing
Somnambulism
Spoken to, averse to being
Starting, startled
    sleep, during
Steals money without necessity ★
Striking himself
Stupefaction, as if intoxicated
Suicidal disposition
Tears himself
Travel, desire to
Unconsciousness, conduct, automatic
Weeping, tearful mood
    sleep, in
Wicked, disposition

CYCLAMEN EUROPAEUM

Absent-minded, unobserving
Absorbed, buried in thought
Abstraction of mind
Activity amel.
Ailments from:
    grief
    joy, excessive
Anger, irascibility
Answers, incoherently
Anxiety
    night
    chill, during
    conscience, as if guilty of a crime
    fever, during
    future, about
    head, with congestion to
    sleep, during
Brooding
    disease, imaginary, over ★
Censorious, critical
Cheerful, gay, mirthful
    evening
    alternating with moroseness
Company, aversion to; presence of other
    people agg.   the
    symptoms; desire for soli-
    tude
    alone, amel. when
    weeping, agg. •
Concentration, difficult
Confusion of mind
    evening
    eating, after
    excitement amel.
    identity, duality, sense of
    washing the face amel.
Conscientious about trifles
Contemptuous
Contented
Delusions, alone, world, she is alone in
    the
    animals creeping in her
    bed, two person in bed with her •
    crime, committed a, he had
    criminal, he is a
    deserted, forsaken, is
    doomed, being

Delusions,
> double, of being
> images, sees pleasant
> money, he is counting
> neglected his duty, he has
> persecuted, he is
> pregnant, she is
> pursued by enemies ★
> wrong, he has done

Despair: religious despair of salvation

Doubtful, soul's welfare, of

Dullness, sluggishness, difficutly of think-
> ing and comprehending, torpor
> morning
> alternating with desire for work •
> stool, after •
> working amel. •

Eccentricity

Excitement, excitable

Exhilaration, evening

Fancies, exaltation of
> evening
> pleasant
> vivid, lively
> evening

Fear, apprehension, dread
> death, of
> evil, of
> lightning, of
> misfortune, of
> chilliness, during •
> heat, during

Forgetful

Forsaken feeling

Going out, aversion to

Grief
> undemonstrative

Hypochondriasis

Ideas, deficiency of

Imbecility

Indifference, apathy
> *climacteric period, in* •

Indolence, aversion to work
> amenorrhoea, in •
> physical

Industrious, mania for work

Insanity, madness
> climacteric period, during

Introspection

Irritability
> daytime
> morning
> > *waking, on*
> afternoon
> evening
> alternating with cheerfulness
> chill, during
> headache, during
> *waking, on*

Jesting, aversion to

Joy alternating with irritability •
> headache from excessive joy

Lamenting, bemoaning, wailing

Malicious, spiteful, vindictive

Mania

Meditation

Memory, active
> alternating with weaknesss of
> memory

Memory, weakness of
> labor, for mental

Menses, copious flow amel. mental
> symptoms, during

Mistakes, speaking, in
> misplacing words
> reverses words

Mood, alternating
> changeable, variable

Morose, cross, fretful, ill-humor, peevish
> afternoon, siesta, after
> evening
> alternating with cheerfulness
> causeless
> menses, in suppressed •
> *trifles, about*
> waking, on

Obstinate, headstrong

Occupation, diversion amel.

Offended, easily; takes everything in
> *bad part*

Reading, aversion to read
    unable, to read
Religious affections
Remorse
Reproaches himself
Reserved
Restlessness
    night
    headache, forehead, at night from
    pain in •
    menses, during
Sadness, despondency, dejection, mental
    depression, gloom, melancholy
    evening
    amenorrhoea, in
    chill, during
    menses, before
    during, agg.
    amel.
    suppressed, from
    misfortune, as if from
Senses, dull, blunted
Sensitive: want of sensitiveness
Serious, earnest
    alternating with cheerfulness
Sit, inclination to
Somnambulism
Speech, incoherent
Starting, sleep, during
    from
Stupefaction, as if intoxicated
Talk, indisposed to, desire to be silent,
    taciturn
Thinking, bad act has committed, as if ★
    duty, has not done her ★
Thoughts, future, of the
    profound
      future, about his
    rush, flow of
    thoughtful
Tranquillity, serenity, calmness
Unconsciousness, coma, stupor
    mental insensibility
    reading, from
Vivacious
Wearisome

Weeping, tearful mood
    agg.
    amel.
    menses, during
      which does her no good •
    suppression of, in
    silently ★
Work, aversion to mental
    impossible
Writing agg. mind symptoms

CYNODON DACTYLON

Anger, causeless
Indolence, aversion to work
Irritability
Quarrelsome, scolding
Rage, fury
Sensitive, noise, to
Spoken to, averse to being

CYNARA SCOLYMOS

Anger, irascibility
Company, desire for; aversion to soli-
    tude, company amel.
Irritability
Malicious, spiteful, vindictive
Nymphomania
Satyriasis
Speech, prattling
Thoughts, sexual
Violent, vehement

CYPRIPEDIUM PUBESCENS

Ailments from:
    excitement, emotional
    grief
Anger, irascibility
    violent
Anxiety
Capriciousness
Cheerful, gay, mirthful
Delirium tremens, mania-a-potu
    mild attacks •

Ecstasy
  night on waking •
Hysteria
Indifference, apathy
  everything, to
Laughing
  children, in
  convulsions, before, during or after
  shrieking
  sleep, during
Prostration of mind, pollutions, after
Restlessness
Sadness, despondency,dejection, mental
  depression, gloom, melancholy
  amenorrhoea, in
  pollutions, from
Shrieking, screaming, shouting
  night
  sleep, during
Starting, startled
Weeping, speeches, when making •

CYSTISUS LABURNUM

Anger, irascibility
Anguish
Anxiety
Delirium
Delusions, imaginations, hallucinations,
  illusions
Excitement, excitable
Fear, apprehension, dread
Indifference, apathy
Irritability
Mania, alternating with depression
Restlessness
Sadness, despondency, dejection, men-
  tal depression, gloom, melan-
  choly
Stupefaction, as if intoxicated
Unconsciousness, coma, stupor

D

DAPHNE INDICA

Absent-minded, unobserving
Anger, irascibility
  trembling, with
Confusion, identity: head separated
  from body, as if
Delusions, body
  parts of body have been taken
    away
  scattered about bed, tossed
  about to get the pieces to-
    gether
  cats, sees
  fire, visions of
Excitement, excitable
  evening
Fear, apprehension, dread
  heart, of disease of
  pain about heart, from •
Frightened easily
Heedless
Irresolution, indecision
Irritability
Morose, cross, fretful, ill-humor, peevish
Restlessness, headache, during
Sadness, despondency, dejection, mental
  depression, gloom, melancholy
Sensitive, oversensitive
  pain, to
  want of sensitiveness
Starting, sleep, on falling
Timidity

DATURA ARBOREA

Clairvoyance
Confusion of mind
Delusions, imaginations, hallucinations,
  illusions
  beautiful atmosphere, in
  feet touching scarcely the ground •
  floating in air
  ideas floating outside of brain •

DATURA FEROX

Delirium, aroused, on being
     raging, raving
Mania

DATURA METEL

Delirium, crying, with
     loquacious
Mania
Timidity
     delirium, during
Unconsciousness, coma, stupor

DATURA SANGUINEA

Unconsciousness, coma, stupor

DERRIS PINNATA

Anguish
Anxiety
Censorious, critical
     dearest friends, with
Company, desire for; aversion to soli-
     tude, company amel.
Death, desires
Delusions, sea sick, he is •
Despair
Discouraged
Fear, falling, on turning head, of •
     killing, of
          knife, with a
          pains, of
          suffering, of
Foolish behavior
Ideas abundant, clearness of mind
Irritability
Mania
Memory, weakness of
Sadness, despondency, dejection, men-
     tal depression, gloom, melan-
     choly
Sighing
Singing
     alternating with weeping

Spit, desire to, morning •
     eating, after •
Striking
     desires to strike
Suicidal disposition
Thoughts, rush, flow of
Unconsciousness, coma, stupor
Weeping, tearful mood

DESOXYRIBONUCLEINICUM ACIDUM

Anger, irascibility
Anguish
     motion, amel. from •
     waking, on
Concentration, difficult
Confusion, identity, duality, sense of
Development of children arrested
Discouraged
Dullness, sluggishness, difficulty of
     thinking and comprehending,
     torpor
Irritability
Lascivious, lustful
Morose, cross, fretful, ill-humor, peevish
     forenoon
Restlessness
Sensitive, oversensitive
Somnambulism
Will, loss of

DICHAPETALUM

Eating, amel. after
Frightened, waking, dream, from a
Indolence, aversion to work
Industrious, mania for work
     weariness, although •
Morose, cross, fretful, ill-humor, peevish

DICTAMNUS ALBUS

Somnambulism

DIGITALIS PURPUREA

Absorbed, buried in thought
Activity, mental, night •
    restless
    sleeplessness, with
Ailments from:
    anticipation, foreboding, presen-
        timent
    debauchery
    grief
    reverses of fortune
    sexual excesses
Anger, irascibility
Anguish
    cardiac
    nausea, with
    waking, on
Answers, vaguely •
Anxiety
    evening
        twilight, in the
        18h.
    night
    conscience, as if guilty of a
    crime
    faintness, with
    fear, with
    future, about
    motion, from
    music, from
    pressure on the chest, from
    sitting, while
    sleep, during
    urination, before
        after •
    waking, on
    walking, after
    weeping amel.
Capriciousness
Cares, worries, full of
    evening
Company, aversion to; presence of other
    people agg. the symptoms; de-
    sire for solitude
Complaining
Confusion of mind
    evening
    intoxicated, as if
        as after being

Conscientious about trifles
Cowardice
Death, presentiment of
    thoughts of
Delirium
    night
    bed and escapes, springs up sud-
        denly from
    convulsions, during
    delusions, with
    frightful
    maniacal
    raging, raving
    sleeplessness, and •
    violent
Delirium tremens, mania-a-potu
Delusions, imaginations, hallucinations,
    illusions
    night
    criminal, he is a
    criminals, about
    fancy, illusions of
    insects, sees
    light, incorporeal, he is
    people, converses with absent
    water, of
    wrong, he has done
Despair
Dipsomania, alcoholism
Discouraged
    irritability, with
Disobedience
Doubtful, soul's welfare, of
Dullness, sluggishness, difficulty of
    thinking and comprehending,
    torpor
    evening
    painful
    sleepiness, with
    waking, on
Escape, attempts to
    run away, to
Excitement, excitable
    night
    stammers when talking to strang-
        ers •
Exertion, agg. from mental

Fancies, exaltation of
  lascivious
  vivid, lively
Fear, apprehension, dread
  afternoon
  evening
  death, of
    heart symptoms, during
  escape, with desire to
  evil, of
  insanity, losing his reason, of
  lightning, of
  misfortune, of
  music, from
  over powering
  people, of; anthropophobia
  reproaches, of
  stomach, arising from
  suffocation, of
    night
    heart disease, in
  walking, while
  weeping amel.
Forgetful
  immediately, of everything ●
  masturbations, after
Frightened easily
  waking, on
Grief
Hurry, haste
Hypochondriasis
Hysteria, fainting, hysterical
Ideas, deficiency of
Imbecility
Inconsolable
Indifference, apathy
  daytime
  evening
  everything, to
  sleepiness, with
Indolence, aversion to work
  morning, rising, on
  eating, after
  masturbation, after
  sleepiness, with
Industrious, mania for work

Insanity, madness
  drunkards, in
  escape, desire to
  obstinate in
  paroxysmal
  secretive ●
Introspection
Irresolution, indecision
Irritability
  coition, after
  sadness, with
Lamenting, bemoaning, wailing
Lascivious, lustful
  prostate enlarged, with ★
Mania
Memory, active
Memory, weakness of
Moaning, groaning, whining
Mood, changeable, variable
Morose, cross, fretful, ill-humor, peevish
  pollutions, after
Music agg.
Nymphomania
Obstinate, headstrong
  night ●
Perseverance
Prostration of mind, mental exhaustion, brain-fag
Quarrelsome, scolding
Rage, fury
Religious affections
Remorse
Reproaches himself
Reserved
Restlessness
  night
  bed, tossing about in
  busy
  coition, after
Sadness, despondency, dejection, mental depression, gloom, melancholy
  afternoon
    18h.
  evening
  anxious

Sadness,
disappointment, from •
heat, during
music, from
pollutions, from
sighing, amel.
trifles, about
weeping amel.
Secretive
Senses, dull, blunted
Sensitive, oversensitive
mental impressions, to
moral impressions, to
music, to
sensual impressions, to
Shrieking, screaming, shouting
hydrocephalus, in
sleep, in
Sighing
Speech, delirious, night
wandering, night
Starting, dream, from a
falling, as if
fright, from and as from
palpitation, from •
sleep, during
from
Strength increased, mental
Stupefaction, as if intoxicated
Suspicious, mistrustful
Talk, indisposed to, desire to be silent,
taciturn
can not ★
sleep, in
Talks, absent persons, with, night •
Thoughts, disconnected
sexual, day and night
wandering
Unconsciousness, coma, stupor
morning
coition, after
stool, before
Unsympathetic, unscrupulous
Vivacious
Wander, desires to, night
Wearisome

Weeping, tearful mood
afternoon
amel.
anxiety, after
disappointments, about •
music, from
Work, mental, impossible

DIGITALINUM

Anger, trifles, at
Anxiety, evening
sitting, while
Delusions, imaginations, hallucinations,
illusions
wrong, he has done
Discomfort
Excitement, excitable
Fear, misfortune, of
Impatience
Irritability
Morose, cross, fretful, ill-humor, peevish
Prostration of mind, mental exhaus-
tion, brain-fag
Restlessness, night
Sensitive, oversensitive
Stupefaction, as if intoxicated
Unconsciousness, night, waking, on

DIGITOXINUM

Restlessness, night
pulse, from intermittent •

DIOSCOREA VILLOSA

Ambition, loss of
Anxiety, waking, on
Aversion, women, to
Cheerful, alternating, looking down on
the street
Company, aversion to; presence of
other people agg. the symp-
toms; desire for solitude
Confusion of mind
evening

Conversation agg.
Delusions, head, standing, on ★
Dullness, sluggishness, difficulty of think-
　　ing and comprehending, torpor
　　　afternoon
　　　evening
Fear, crowd, in a
　　men, dread, fear of
　　people, of; anthropophobia
Imbecility
Indolence, aversion to work
　　evening
　　pollutions, after
Irritability
　　evening
Loathing, speaking, at
Memory, weakness of
　　words, of
Mistakes, names, in
　　speaking, in
　　　words, using wrong
　　　　names, calls things by wrong
　　　　putting right for left or vice
　　　　versa
　　　　say plums, when he means
　　　　pears
　　writing, in
Morose, cross, fretful, ill-humor, peevish
　　evening
Quiet, wants to be
Restlessness
　　afternoon
　　　16h. ●
　　evening
　　night
　　midnight, after
　　bed, in
　　pain, during
　　walking, amel. while
Sadness, despondency, dejection, mental
　　depression, gloom, melancholy
　　pollutions, from
Talk, indisposed to, desire to be silent,
　　taciturn

DIPHTHERINUM

Clinging, held amel., being
Delirium
　　answers correctly when spoken
　　　to, but delirium and uncon-
　　　sciousness return at once
Unconsciousness, answers correctly
　　when spoken to, but delirium
　　and unconsciousness return at
　　once

DIRCA PALUSTRIS

Absent-minded, unobserving
Anger, irascibility
Anxiety, future, about
Confusion of mind
Fear, bad news, of hearing
Indolence, aversion to work
Memory, weak, write, for what is about
　　to
Mistakes, speaking, in
　　words, using wrong
　　time, in
　　writing, in
　　　wrong words
Morose, cross, fretful, ill-humor, peevish
Restlessness
　　night
Talk, indisposed to, desire to be silent,
　　taciturn
Time passes too slowly, appears longer
Unconsciousness, coma, stupor
Work, mental, impossible

DORYPHORA
DECEMLINEATA

Anxiety, sleep, during
Business, talks of
Delirium
　　business, talks of
　　exhaustion, with
　　face, with red
　　fever, during
　　look fixed on one point, staring

Delirium,
    loquacious
    muttering
    sepsis, from
Delirium tremens, mania-a-potu
Irritability
Restlessness
    night
Shrieking, children, in
    sleep, in
Unconsciousness, coma, stupor
    fever, during
    muttering
    vomiting, with

DROSERA ROTUNDIFOLIA

Ailments from :
    bad news
    grief
Anger, irascibility
    trifles, at
    violent
Anxiety
    evening
        19 h.
        19-20h.
        20h.
    night
        waking, on
    alone, when
    fear, with
    fever, during
    flushes of heat, during
    future, about
    hypochondriacal
    suicidal disposition, with
    waking, on
    weary of life, with
Barking
Beside oneself, being
Capriciousness
Cares, worries, full of
Cheerful, gay, mirthful
Clinging, held amel., being

Company, desire for; aversion to soli-
    tude, company amel.
    evening
    alone agg., while
Concentration, difficult
    studying, reading etc., while
Confidence, want of self
Confusion of mind
    evening
    chill, during
    heat, during
    walking, while
Courageous
Cowardice
Deceitful, sly
Delusions, calls, someone
    deceived, being ★
    fancy, illusions of
    hearing, illusions of
    images, phantoms, sees
    longer, things seem
    persecuted, he is
    pursued by enemies
    tall: things grow taller
    vexations and offences, of
    visions, has
Discouraged
    future, about
Dullness, sluggishness, difficulty of think-
    ing and comprehending, torpor
    chill, during
    reading, while
Fear, apprehension, dread
    evening
    night
    alone, of being
        evening
    bad news, of hearing
    death, of
    evil, of
    ghosts, of
    misfortune, of
Forsaken feeling
Grief
Homesickness
Impatience
Inconstancy
Indifference, apathy

Indolence, aversion to work
    sadness, from
Introspection
Irresolution, indecision
Irritability
Laughing agg.
Loathing, life, at
    evening
Loquacity, cough, after ★
Mania
Mood, alternating
    changeable, variable
Morose, cross, fretful, ill-humor, peevish
Obstinate, headstrong
    execution of plans, in ●
Offended, easily; takes everything in
    bad part
Perseverance
Pertinacity
Plans, carrying out, insists on ●
Rage, fury
Reading
    subject, must change the ●
Reserved
Restlessness
    anxious
    driving about
    internal
    reading, while
Sadness, despondency, dejection, mental
    depression, gloom, melancholy
    daytime
    alone, when
    anxious
    work-shy, in
Senses, dull, blunted
Sensitive, oversensitive
    noise, striking of clocks, ringing
    of bells, to
    odors, to
Starting, sleep, on falling
    during
    from
Suicidal disposition
    evening
    drowning, by
    thoughts

Suspicious, mistrustful
Talk, indisposed to, desire to be silent,
    taciturn
Thinking, complaints agg., of
Tranquillity, serenity, calmness
Violent, vehement
Weary of life
    evening
Weeping, tearful mood
Work, aversion to mental

DUBOISINUM

Delirium

DUBOISIA MYOPOROIDES

Delirium
Delusions, imaginations, hallucinations,
    illusions
Excitement, excitable
Grasp reaching
Jumping, bed, out of
Restlessness
Unconsciousness, coma, stupor

DULCAMARA

Absent-minded, unobserving
Abusive, insulting
    angry, without being ●
Anger, irascibility
    easily
Anxiety
    night
    midnight, after
    fear, with
    future, about
    others, for ★
    sleep, during
    vomiting, on
Cares, worries, full of, midnight ●
Capriciousness
Censorious, critical
    afternoon ●
Complaining
Concentration, difficult
    headache, with

Confusion of mind
    evening
    air amel., in open
    intoxicated, as after being
    paroxysms of pain, during
Delirium
    morning
      waking, on
      night
    easy ★
    fantastic
    fever, during
    pains, with the
    raging, raving
    sleeplessness, and ★
    sorrowful
    waking, on
Delusions, imaginations, hallucinations,
    illusions
      morning, bed, in
      night
    bed, sinking, is
    calls, waking, someone calls on
    devils, sees
    fancy, illusions of
    images, phantoms, sees
    spectres, ghost, spirits, sees
      morning on waking, a spectre
      continues to enlarge until it
      disappears ●
    waking, on
    weeping, with
Desires, full of
Dictatorial ★
Discontented, displeased, dissatisfied
Dullness, sluggishness, difficulty of think-
    ing and comprehending, torpor
    evening
    sleeplessness with
Fear, apprehension, dread
    night
    evil, of
Foolish behavior
Forgetful, words while speaking, of;
    word hunting
Gestures, grasping or reaching at some-
    thing, at flocks; carphologia
      picks at bed clothes
    stamps the feet
Haughty

Hurry, haste
    always in
Ideas wander ★
Imbecility
Impatience
    morning
Indifference, apathy
    sleepiness, with
Indolence, aversion to work
    sleepiness, with
Insanity, madness
Irresolution, indecision
Irritability
    daytime
    children, in
    headache, during
**Jumping, bed, out of, frightful dream,
    from a** ●
Lamenting, bemoaning, wailing
Loquacity
Mania
Memory, weakness of
    expressing oneself, for
    words, of
Mistakes, speaking, in
    words, using wrong
    writing, in
Moaning, groaning, whining
    night, tossing about, with ●
Morose, cross, fretful, ill-humor, peevish
Muttering
Nymphomania
Prostration of mind, mental exhaus-
    tion, brain-fag
Quarrelsome, scolding
    afternoon
    anger, without
Rage, fury
Restlessness
    morning
    night
    bed, tossing about in
    headache, during
    waking, on
Rudeness, naughty children, of
*Sadness, despondency, dejection, mental
    depression, gloom, melancholy*
    morning
      bed, in ●

Sadness,
> night
> *headache, during*
Senses, dull, blunted
Shrieking, screaming, shouting
> brain, cry
> children, in
> sleep, in
Sit, inclination to
Slowness
Speech, babbling
> incoherent
> wandering
Starting, evening
> > asleep, on falling
> *sleep, on falling to*
> during
> from
Stupefaction, as if intoxicated
> evening
> vertigo, during
Sulky
Thoughts, wandering
Throws things away
> morning
Unconsciousness, coma, stupor
> fever, during
Violent, vehement
Weeping, tearful mood
> morning
> delusions, after •
> impatience, from •
Will, weakness of
Work, aversion to mental
> impossible

(BACILLUS) DYSENTERIAE

Confidence, want of self
Cowardice
Fear
> *crowd, in a public place* ★
> thunderstorm, of
Timidity, appearing in public, about
Weeping, causeless
> *telling of her sickness, when*

EAUX BONNES AQUA

Activity, mental
Restlessness
Strength increased, mental

ECHINACEA

Confusion of mind
> sleepiness, with
Contradiction, is intolerant of
Dullness, sluggishness, difficulty of think-
> ing and comprehending, torpor
Exertion, agg. from mental
Fear, apprehension, dread
Sadness, despondency, dejection, mental
> depression, gloom, melancholy
> afternoon
Stupefaction, as if intoxicated
Thinking, aversion to
Work, aversion to mental

ELAEIS GUINEENSIS

Abusive, insulting
Anger, irascibility
Cheerful, gay, mirthful
Disobedience
Laughing
Morose, cross, fretful, ill-humor peevish
Sadness, despondency, dejection, mental
> depression, gloom, melancholy
Sighing

ELAPS CORALLINUS

Absent-minded, unobserving
Absorbed, buried in thought
> daytime •
Abstraction of mind
Ailment from anticipation, foreboding,
> *presentiment*

Anger, irascibility
  spoken to, when
Anxiety
  rain ★
Bite himself
Company, aversion to; presence of
  other people agg. the symptoms; desire for solitude
  country away from people, wants
    to get into the
  fear of being alone, yet
*Company, desire for; aversion to soli-
  tude, company amel.*
  alone agg., while
  *happen, as if something horrible
    might* •
Concentration, difficult
Country, desire for •
Delusions, imaginations, hallucinations,
  illusions
  beaten, he is being
  falling forward, she is
  head standing, on ★
  hearing, illusions of
  injured, is being
  talking, he hears •
  voices, hears
Desires, cavern, to be in •
Dream, as if in a, daytime
Ennui, tedium
Excitement, excitable
  forenoon
  evening
Fancies, exaltation of
  daytime •
Fear, apprehension, dread
  alone, of being
  apoplexy, of
  disease, of impending
  happen, something will
  rain, of
  robbers, of
  solitude, of
Forgetful
Homesickness
Hysteria
  menses, before
Indifference, apathy

Indolence, aversion to work
Irritability
  afternoon
  spoken to, when
Memory, weakness of
  time, in
Morose, cross, fretful, ill-humor, peevish
  afternoon
Play in the grass, desire to •
Playful
Prostration of mind, mental exhaus-
  tion, brain-fag
Quarrelsome, scolding
Restlessness
Sadness, despondency, dejection, mental
  depression, gloom, melancholy
  wet weather, during
Shrieking, screaming, shouting
  must shriek, feels as though she
Sits, still
  wrapped in deep, sad thoughts
    and notices nothing, as if
Spoken to, averse to being
Striking
  desires to strike
Talk, indisposed to, menses, during
  others agg., talk of
Time passes too quickly, appears shorter
Travel, desire to
Unconsciousness, coma, stupor
  conduct, automatic

ELATERIUM OFFICINARUM

Fear, of disaster, of
Home: leave home, desire to
Homesickness
Sadness, heat, during
Starting, sleep, during
Wander, desire to, night

EPIGAEA REPENS

Ailments from:
  work, mental
Exertion, agg. from, mental

EPILOBIUM PALUSTRE

Dullness, sluggishness, difficulty of thinking and comprehending, torpor

EPIPHEGUS VIRGINIANA

Ailments from :
    excitement, emotional
    work, mental

EQUISETUM HYEMALE

Frown, disposed to
Irritability
Prostration of mind, mental exhaustion, brain-fag
Restlessness, evening

EQUISETUM ARVENSE

Shrieking, screaming, shouting
Work, mental, impossible

ERECHTHITES HIERACIFOLIA

Desire, exercise, for

ERGOTINUM

Anxiety
Sadness, despondency, dejection, mental depression, gloom, melancholy
Slowness

ERIGERON CANADENSIS

Ambition, loss of
Cheerful, urination, after
Concentration, difficult
Frightened, waking, dream, from a
Indolence, aversion to work
    afternoon
    evening
Irritability, morning
Mistakes, omitting letters
    words
Restlessness
    night

Sadness, despondency, dejection, mental depression, gloom, melancholy
Weeping, urination, during

ERIODYCTION CALIFORNICUM

Exhilaration
Memory, weakness of
Moaning, sleep, during

ERYNGIUM AQUATICUM

Concentration, difficult
    afternoon
Confusion of mind
    afternoon
Dullness, sluggishness, difficulty of thinking and comprehending, torpor
    night on waking
    think long, unable to
Ecstasy
Restlessness
Sadness, despondency, dejection, mental depression, gloom, melancholy
    pollutions, from
Soberness
Thoughts, wandering

ERYNGINUM MARITINUM

Cheerful, gay, mirthful
    morning, waking, on
Singing, morning on waking

ERYTHROPHLAEUM JUDICIALE

Quiet, wants to be

ESPELETIA GRANDIFLORA

Concentration, difficult
Dullness, noon
Dullness, noon
Hurry, haste
Hypochondriasis
Indifference, apathy

Mistakes, speaking, in
      words, using wrong
Sadness, despondency, dejection, mental
    depression,, gloom, melancholy
    age, in old

EUCALYPTUS GLOBULUS

Activity, mental
Buoyancy
Cheerful, gay, mirthful
Desire, exercise, for
Dullness, sluggishness, difficulty of think-
    ing and comprehending, torpor
Excitement, excitable
Exhilaration
Industrious, mania for work
Prostration of mind, mental exhaus-
    tion, brain-fag

EUGENIA JAMBOSA

Cheerful, gay, mirthful
    urination, after
Company, aversion to; presence of other
    people agg. the symptoms; de-
    sire for solitude
Confusion of mind
Delusions, beautiful, urination, all things
    seem beautiful after •
Discontented, displeased, dissatisfied
    everything, with
Exhilaration
Hide, desire to
Indolence, aversion to work
Loquacity
Meditation
Morose, alternating with cheerfulness
Reflecting
Restlessness
Rudeness
Sadness, despondency, dejection, men-
    tal depression, gloom, melan-
    choly
    urination, amel.
Work, desire for mental
Wrong, everything seems

EUONYMUS EUROPAEA

Anxiety
Confusion of mind, mental exertion,
    from
Delusions, floating in air
    flying, sensation of
Heedless
Indolence, aversion to work
Irritability
Morose, cross, fretful, ill-humor, peevish
Sadness, despondency, dejection, men-
    tal depression, gloom, melan-
    choly

EUONYMUS ATROPURPUREA

Memory,weakness of, names, for proper
Wearisome

EUPATORIUM AROMATICUM

Hysteria

EUPATORIUM PERFOLIATUM

Anxiety
Clinging, held amel., being
Conversation amel. •
Despair
Dipsomania, alcoholism
Excitement, excitable
Fear, night
    insanity, losing his reason, of
    suffering, of
Homesickness
Irritability
Moaning, groaning, whining
    chill, during
    heat, during
    pain, from
    sleep, during
Mood, changeable, variable

Restlessness
    chill, during
    heat, during
Sadness, despondency, dejection, mental
    depression, gloom, melancholy
    heat, during
    sleepiness, with
Sensitive, odors, to
Shrieking, screaming, shouting
Sighing
Unconsciousness, fever, during
Weeping, tearful mood

EUPATORIUM PURPUREUM

Ailments from:
    homesickness
Confusion of mind
Delusions, imaginations, hallucinations,
    illusions
    hearing, illusions of
    sight and hearing, of
Dullness, sluggishness, difficulty of think-
    ing and comprehending, torpor
Fear, disease, of impending
Homesickness
Hysteria
Loquacity
Moaning, groaning, whining
Sadness, despondency, dejection, mental
    depression, gloom, melancholy
Shrieking, screaming, shouting
Sighing
Weeping, tearful mood

EUPHORBINUM OFFICINARUM

Anxiety
    future, about
Company, aversion to; presence of other
    people agg. the symptoms; de-
    sire for solitude
Delirium
Delusions, enlarged
    man, the same, is walking before
    and after him •

Delusions,
    walking, the same one is, after him
    that is walking before him •
Fear, apprehension, dread
    evil, of
    poisoned, has been
    stomach, arising from
Industrious, mania for work
Insanity, madness
    prayer at the tail of his horse,
    insists upon saying his •
Introspection
Meditation
Mildness
Praying
Quiet disposition
Quiet, wants to be
Reflecting
Reserved
Restlessness, midnight, before
    tremulous
Sadness, despondency, dejection, men-
    tal depression, gloom, melan-
    choly
    company, agg. in
Serious, earnest
Shrieking, sleep, in
Speech, unintelligible
Starting, night
    bed, while lying awake in
    electric, as if
    shocks through the body while
    wide awake
Stupefaction, as if intoxicated
    sleepiness, with
Talk, indisposed to, desire to be silent,
    taciturn
Thoughts, thoughtful
Tranquillity, serenity, calmness
Unconsciousness, coma, stupor
    daytime
    noon and afternoon •
Weeping, night
    sleep, in

EUPHORBIA AMYGDALOIDES

Delusions, imaginations, hallucinations,
   illusions
   smell, of
Morose, cross, fretful, ill-humor, peevish
   evening amel.
Restlessness, night

EUPHORBIA CORROLATA

Anxiety
   perspiration, with cold
Death, desires
Weary of life

EUPHORBIA HYPERICIFOLIA

Concentration, difficult

EUPHORBIA LATHYRIS

Restlessness

EUPHRASIA OFFICINALIS

Absorbed, buried in thought
Answers, aversion to
Anxiety, future, about
Brooding
Chaotic, confused behaviour
Concentration, difficult
Confusion of mind
   morning
      waking, on
   evening
   cold bath amel.
   dinner, after
   eating, after
   waking, on
   washing the face amel.
Delusion, faces, on closing eyes, sees
   fancy, illusions of
   fasting
   head seems too large, heads
      make grimaces (evening on
      closing eyes) ●

Dullness, sluggishness, difficulty of think-
   ing and comprehending, torpor
Fancies, exaltation of
Fear, apprehension, dread
Frightened, night, waking, on
   waking, on
Hypochondriasis
   interest in his surrounding, takes
   no ●
Indifference, apathy
   external things, to
Indolence, aversion to work
Industrious, mania for work
Introspection
Irritability
Memory, weakness of
Mildness
Morose, cross, fretful, ill-humor, peevish
Quiet disposition
Reserved
Restlessness
   night
Sadness, despondency, dejection, men-
   tal depression, gloom, melan-
   choly
Sensitive, want of sensitiveness
Serious, earnest
Sit, inclination to
Speech, hesitating
Starting, fright, from and as from
   sleep, during
   from
Stupefaction, as if intoxicated
Talk, indisposed to, desire to be silent,
   taciturn
Thoughts, persistent
   thoughtful
Unconsciousness, coma, stupor
   morning
Weeping, lying, while ●

EUPIONUM

Anguish, afternoon
Anger, irascibility
Cheerful, gay, mirthful
Confusion of mind

Delusions, imaginations, hallucinations,
    illusions
      glass, wood etc., being made of
      jelly, the body is made of ●
Frightened, waking, on
Ideas abundant, clearness of mind
Irritability
    menses, intermision of, during
    an ●
Memory, weakness of
Rage, fury
Restlessness
    night
    internal
    evening, in bed ●
Thoughts, rush, flow of

EYSENHARDTIA POLYSTACHIA

Concentration, difficult

FAGOPYRUM ESCULENTUM

Activity, mental, 5h.
Cheerful, gay, mirthful
Concentration, difficult
    studying, reading etc., while
Confusion of mind
    eating amel., after
Dullness, sluggishness, difficulty of think-
    ing and comprehending, torpor
    eating amel., after
Fear, death, of
Irritability
    evening
Morose, evening
Restlessness, morning
    forenoon
    afternoon
    evening
    night
    midnight, 3-4 h. after ●
    mental labor, during and after
    rising, on
    study, when attempting to
Sadness, despondency, dejection, men-
    tal depression, gloom, melan-
    choly
Spoken to, averse to being
Talk, indisposed to, desire to be silent,
    taciturn
    afternoon
Work, aversion to mental
    forenoon, 11 h. ●
    impossible, afternoon

FAGUS SILVATICA

Delirium
Fear, water, of
Hydrophobia

Sadness, despondency, dejection, mental
  depression, gloom, melancholy
    night
Wildness

FEL TAURI

Business, desire for
Busy
Irritability
Morose, cross, fretful, ill-humor, peevish

FERRUM METALLICUM

Abusive, insulting
Ailments from:
  anger, vexation
  excitement, emotional
  scorn, being scorned
Anger, irascibility
  contradiction, from
  easily
  sympathy, agg. ★
  violent
Anxiety
    night
    midnight, before
  bed, in
    tossing about, with
  beer, after ●
  conscience, as if guilty of a crime
  eating, after
  fear, with
  fever, during
  fits, with
  paroxysms, in ★
  perspiration, with cold
  sleep, during
  trifles, about
Aversion, friends, to
Capriciousness
Chaotic, confused behavior
Cheerful, gay, mirthful
  evening
  alternating with sadness
Company, aversion to; presence of other
  people agg. the symptoms;
  desire for solitude

Company, aversion to
  alone, amel. when
  avoids the sight of people
  friends, of intimate
Concentration, difficult
Confusion of mind
  morning, waking , on
  afternoon
  evening
  eating, after
  motion, amel. from
  walking, while
Conscientious about trifles
Contradict, disposition to
Contradiction, is intolerant of
  agg.
Conversation agg.
  aversion to
Death, thoughts of
Delusions, people, behind him when
  walking in the dark, someone is
  criminal, about
  large, surroundings seem too ●
  surroundings are capacious ●
  war, being at
  water, of
Dictatorial, domineering, dogmatical,
  despotic
Dipsomania, alcoholism
Discomfort
Discontented, displeased, dissatisfied
Dullness, sluggishness, difficulty of think-
  ing and comprehending, torpor
  afternoon
  sleepiness, with
Ennui, tedium
Excitement, excitable
  evening
  night
  agg.
  contradiction, from sightest ●
  heat, during
  menses, during
  after ●
  trifles, over
Exertion, amel. from mental

Fear, apprehension, dread
  apoplexy, of
  crossing a bridge or place, of
  crowd, in a
    public places, of; agoraphobia
  death, of
  evil, of
  misfortune, of
    evening
  noise, from
  palpitation, with
  people, of; anthropophobia
  rail, of going by
Foolish behavior
Forgetful
  eating, after
Haughty
  look, self-contented
Horrible things, sad stories, affect her
    profoundly
Hypochondriasis
Hysteria
Impetuous, perspiration, with
Indifference, apathy
Indolence, aversion to work
Irresolution, indecision
Irritability
  heat, during
  menses, during
  noise, from
    crackling of news papers, even
    from
Laughing
  immoderately
  menopause, during ★
Memory, weakness of
Mental symptoms alternating with
    physical ★
Menses, mental symptoms agg. at be-
    ginning of
    after suppressed
Mood, alternating
  changeable, variable
Morose, cross, fretful, ill-humor, peevish
  fever, during
  menses, during
    after

Obstinate, headstrong
Occupation, diversion amel.
Positiveness
Prostration of mind, mental exhaus-
    tion, brain-fag
Quarrelsome, scolding
Religious affections
Remorse
Restlessness
  evening
  night
  midnight, before
    after, 2h.
  anxious
  bed, driving out of
    go from one bed to another,
    wants to
    tossing about in
  heat, during
  sitting, while
  warm bed agg.
Rudeness
**Sadness, despondency, dejection,
    mental depression, gloom,
    melancholy**
  evening
  alone, when
  alternating with exuberance
  diarrhoea, during
  exertion, amel. after •
  menses, before
    during
    after
Senses, acute
sensitive, oversensitive
  noise, to
    aversion to
    crackling of paper, to
    slightest, to
Serious, earnest
Sit, inclination to
Soberness
Strength increased, mental
Stupefaction, as if intoxicated
Talk, indisposed to, desire to be silent,
    taciturn
    others agg., talk of

Talking agg. all complaints
Thinking, aversion to
Thoughts, wandering
Tranquillity, serenity, calmness
Trifles seem important
Unconsciousness, coma, stupor
night amel. •
    vertigo, during
Vivacious, evening
Weeping, tearful mood
    desire to weep, all the time
    immoderately ★
    laughing at climacteric period •
Work, aversion to mental
    impossible

FERRUM ACETICUM

Morose, eating, after
Restlessness, heat, during
Sadness, alone, when

FERRUM ARSENICOSUM

Absent-minded, unobserving
Anger, irascibility
    contradiction, from
Anxiety
    night
    conscience, as if guilty of a crime
    fear, with
    fever, during
Cheerful, gay, mirthful
Concentration, difficult
Confusion of mind
    morning
    waking, on
    evening
Conscientious about trifles
Death, thoughts of
Discontented, displeased, dissatisfied
Excitement, excitable
Fear, apprehension, dread
    crowd, in a
    death, of
    evil, of
    misfortune, of
    people, of; anthropophobia
Forgetful

Hysteria
Indifference, apathy
Irresolution, indecision
Irritability
Laughing
Mood, alternating
    changeable, variable
Obstinate, headstrong
Quarrelsome, scolding
Religious, affections
Remorse
Restlessness
    night
    bed, driving out of
    tossing about in
    heat, during
Sadness, despondency, dejection, mental depression, gloom, melancholy
    evening
    alone, when
Sensitive, oversensitive
    noise, to
    voices, to
Serious, earnest
Stupefaction, as if intoxicated
Talk, indisposed to, desire to be silent,
    taciturn
    others agg., talk of
Tranquillity, serenity, calmness
Unconsciousness, coma, stupor
Weeping, tearful mood

FERRUM BROMATUM

Sadness, pollutions, from

FERRUM CARBONICUM

Anxiety, future, about

FERRUM IODATUM

Anger, irascibility
Anxiety
Cheerful, gay, mirthful
Company, aversion to; presence of
    other people agg. the symptoms; desire for solitude

Concentration, difficult
    studying, reading, etc., while
Confusion of mind, evening
    hat agg., putting on
    reading, while
    smoking, after
    writing, while
Conscientious about trifles
Dementia, epileptics, of
Dullness, sluggishness, difficulty of think-
    ing and comprehending, torpor
    reading, while
Excitement, excitable
Hysteria
Indifference, apathy
Indolence, evening
Irresolution, indecision
Irritability
Mood, alternating
    changeable, variable
Restlessness
    night
Sadness, despondency, dejection,
    mental depression, gloom,
    melancholy
Starting, startled
    sleep, during
        from
Stupefaction, as if intoxicated
Weeping, tearful mood

FERRUM MAGNETICUM

Anger, irascibility
Cheerful, gay, mirthful
Dullness, sluggishness, difficulty of
    thinking and comprehending,
    torpor
Haughty
    look, self-contented
Hopeful
Introspection, eating, after
Irresolution, indecision
Morose, cross, fretful, ill-humor, peevish
Slowness
Starting, dream, from a
    sleep, on falling
        during

Talk, indisposed to, eating, after
Walk self-sufficient air of importance,
    along with a •

FERRUM MURIATICUM

Anger, irascibility
Anxiety
    eating, after
    perspiration, with cold
Bed
    remain in, desire to, morning
Irresolution, indecision
Loquacity
Optimistic
Restlessness
    bed, tossing about in
Sadness, despondency, dejection, mental
    depression, gloom, melancholy
Sighing, involuntary
Unconsciousness, coma, stupor

FERRUM PHOSPHORICUM

Ailments from:
    anger, vexation
Anger, irascibility
    trembling, with
    violent
Anxiety
    night
    conscience, as if guilty of a crime
    eating, after
    fear, with
    fever, during
    future, about
    hypochondriacal
Busy
Cheerful, gay, mirthful
Company, aversion to; presence of
    other people agg. the symp-
    toms; desire for solitude
    alone, amel. when
Concentration, difficult
Confusion of mind
    morning
    evening

Confusion of mind
  eating, after
  motion, amel. from
  walking, amel. while
  washing the face amel.
Courageous
Delirium
  crying, with
Delirium tremens, mania-a-potu
Discontented, displeased, dissatisfied
Discouraged, evening
Dullness, sluggishness, difficulty of
    thinking and comprehending,
    torpor
Excitement, excitable
    evening
    alternating with sadness
Fear, apprehension, dread
  apoplexy, of
  crowd, in a
  death, of
  evil, of
  misfortune, of
  people, of; anthropophobia
Firmness, morning •
Forgetgful
Hurry, afternoon •
Hypochondriasis
Hysteria
Ideas abundant, clearness of mind
Impetuous
  evening •
Indifference, apathy
  exciting events, to •
  pleasure, to
Indolence, aversion to work
Insanity, puerperal
Intolerance, afternoon •
  hinderance, of •
  vexation, of •
Irresolution, evening
Irritability
Loquacity
Mania
Memory, weakness of
Mood, alternating

Morose, cross, fretful, ill-humor, peevish
Obstinate, headstrong
Precision of mind increased ★
Pushed, forward ★
Restlessness
  night
  bed, driving out of
    tossing about in
  heat, during
Sadness, despondency, dejection, mental
    depression, gloom, melancholy
  evening
  menses, before
Sensitive, oversensitive
  noise, to
  pain, to
Shrieking, screaming, shouting
Singing
Starting, heat, during
  sleep, during
    from
Stupefaction, as if intoxicated
Talk, indisposed to, desire to be silent,
    taciturn
Thinking, aversion to
Timidity, afternoon
Unconsciousness, coma, stupor
Weeping, tearful mood
Work, aversion to mental

FERRUM PICRICUM

Exertion, agg. from mental
**Prostration of mind, mental ex-
    haustion, brain-fag**

FERRUM SULPHURICUM

Moaning, groaning, whining

FERRUM TARTARICUM

Fear, apoplexy, of
Firmness, morning •

FERULA GLAUCA

Anger, irascibility
Impatience
Indolence, aversion to work
        erotic
Nymphomania
Restlessness, night
Sadness, despondency, dejection, mental
        depression, gloom, melancholy
Starting, sleep, from
Weeping, tearful mood

FICUS RELIGIOSA

Restlessness
Sadness, despondency, dejection, mental
        depression, gloom, melancholy

FILIX-MAS

Anxiety
Irritability, worm affections, in
Morose, worm affections, in
Unconsciousness, coma, stupor

FLUORICUM ACIDUM

Absent-minded
        periodical attacks of, short lasting
Ailments from:
        anticipation, foreboding, presen-
            timent
        debauchery
        work, mental
Anger, irascibility
Anxiety
            morning, rising, amel. on and
            after
                evening
            fever, during
            future, about
            headache, with
            walking rapidly, which makes him
            walk faster
Aversion
        his own mind, to ★
            others ★
        friends, to

Aversion
        members of family, to
            talks pleasantly to others ★
        parents, to ●
        wife, to his ●
Buoyancy
Business, averse to
Capriciousness
        evening
Cheerful, gay, mirthful
        morning
        alternating with sadness
        menses, before
        during
        walking in open air and after, on
Company, aversion to; presence of
        other people agg. the symp-
        toms; desire for solitude
Company, desire for; aversion to soli-
        tude, company amel.
        alone agg., while
Concentration, difficult
Confusion of mind
        night
        breakfast, before
Contented
Conversation agg.
Deceitful, sly
Destructiveness ★
Delusions, imaginations, hallucinations,
        illusions
        betrothal must be broken ●
        children out of the house, he must
            drive ●
        danger, impression of
        dead persons, sees
        fancy, illusions of
        images, phantoms when alone,
            sees
        marriage, must dissolve ●
        repulsive fantastic ●
        servants, he must get rid of ●
Dipsomania, alcoholism
Discontented, displeased, dissatisfied
        evening
        eating, after
Ecstasy
Excitement, excitable
        evening
        walking, after

Exertion, agg. from mental
Exhilaration
Fancies, anxious exaltation of
    anxious •
    repulsive, when alone
Fear, apprehension, dread
    apoplexy, of
    death, of
    happen, something will
    misfortune, of
    people, of; anthropophobia
    suffering, of ★
Forgetful
    morning amel. •
    evening
    wind his watch, to •
Gestures, decided •
    hands, motions, involuntary, of
    the
Hatred, absent person, of; better on
    seeing them •
    revenge, h. and
Home, leave home, desire to
Hurry, walking, while
Imbecility
Impulse, walk, to ★
Indifference, apathy
    business affairs, to
    important things, to
    loved ones, to
        strangers, but animated to •
    relations, to
Industrious, mania for work
Insanity, madness
    immobile as a statue
Irritability
    absent persons, with
    sends nurse home •
Lascivious, lustful
    ogling women, on the street ★
Libertinism
Malicious, spiteful, vindictive
Mannish habits of women •
Memory, active
    morning •
Memory, weakness of
    business, for
    dates, for
    do, for what was about to

Memory, weakness of
    done, for what has just
    names, for proper
    thought, for what has just
Mistakes, localities, in
    speaking, misplacing words in
        spelling, in
    words, wrong
        putting right for left or vice
    versa
    time, in
    writing, in
    wrong words
Morose, cross, fretful, ill-humor, peevish
Nymphomania
Optimistic
Prostration of mind, mental exhaus-
    tion, brain-fag
Quarrelsome, scolding
Rage, fury
Reading, mental symptoms agg. from
Reserved
Responsibility, inability to realize ★
Restlessness
    night
Sadness, despondency, dejection, mental
    depression, gloom, melancholy
    evening
Satyriasis
Sensitive, oversensitive
    noise, to
        morning •
Shrieking, sleep, in
Sits still
Stunning ★
Suppressed or receding skin diseases
    or haemorrhoids, mental symp-
    toms agg. after
Talk, indisposed to, desire to be silent,
    taciturn
Thoughts, intrude and crowd around
    each other
    rush, flow of
Tranquillity, serenity, calmness
Unconsciousness, coma, stupor
    periodical

Vivacious, morning
Weeping, sleep, in
Women, mannish ●

FLAVUS

Sadness, despondency, dejection, mental depression, gloom, melancholy

FOLLICULINUM

Anguish
    evening
Excitement, alternating with sadness
Sensitive, noise, to
    touch, to

FLOR DE PIEDRA

Activity, mental
Ideas abundant, clearness of mind
Sadness, despondency, dejection, mental depression, gloom, melancholy
Slowness

FORMICA RUFA

Activity, mental
Agility, mental ●
Ailments from :
    bad news
    mortification
Anger, irascibility
Cheerful, gay, mirthful
    alternating with moroseness
    pain, after ★
Confusion of mind
Delusions, imaginations, hallucinations, illusions
Discomfort
Dullness, sluggishness, difficulty of thinking and comprehending, torpor
    morning
Dwells on past disagreeable occurrences

Eccentricity
Excitement, excitable
    bad news, after
Exhilaration
Fear, apprehension, dread
    evening
Forgetful
    evening
Hysteria, menses, during
Indolence, aversion to work
    evening
Irritability
Memory, weakness of
Mood, changeable, variable
Morose, cross, fretful, ill-humor, peevish
    evening
Restlessness
    night
Sadness, despondency, dejection, mental depression, gloom, melancholy
Work, aversion to mental
    impossible, night ●

FRANZENSBAD AQUA

Anxiety, afternoon
Indolence, physical
Morose, cross, fretful, ill-humor, peevish
Restlessness, night

FRAXINUS AMERICANA

Fear, waking from a dream
Restlessness
    anxious
Sadness, despondency, dejection, mental depression, gloom, melancholy
Talk, must ★

FUCUS VESICULOSUS

Activity

FULIGO LIGNI

Suicidal disposition

GADUS MORRHUA

Death, desires
Despair
Dullness, sluggishness, difficulty of think-
    ing and comprehending, torpor
Memory, weakness of, expressing one-
    self, for
Sadness, despondency, dejection, mental
    depression, gloom, melancholy

GALLICUM ACIDUM

Abusive, insulting
Cursing, swearing
Delirium
    bed and escapes, springs up sud-
        denly from
    wild, night
Desires, watched, to be •
Fear, solitude, of
Irritability
Jealousy
Jumping, bed, out of
Restlessness, night
Rudeness
Speech, strange

GALINSOGA PARVIFLORA

Confusion of mind
Mistakes, calculating, in
    writing, in
        wrong letters, figures
Optimistic, in spite of the weakness

GAMBOGIA

Anger, irascibility
Anxiety
        afternoon
        warmth, from

Cheerful, gay, mirthful
Despair
Gestures: strange attitudes and posi-
        tions
Indolence, aversion to work
Industrious, mania for work
Irritability
        morning, waking, on
        waking, on
Loquacity
Morose, cross, fretful. ill-humor, peevish
Restlessness, morning
Sadness, despondency, dejection. men-
        tal depression, gloom, melan-
        choly
        diarrhoea, during
Violent, morning

GASTEIN AQUA

Delusions, vivid
Excitement, bath, during •
Loquacity
Restlessness
Sighing

GAULTHERIA PROCUMBENS

Unconsciousness, coma, stupor

GELSEMIUM SEMPERVIRENS

Activity, mental
Ailments from:
    anger, vexation
    anxiety, with
    fright, with
    silent, grief, with
    anticipation, foreboding, pre-
        sentiment
    bad news
    death of a child
    embarrassment
    excitement, emotional
    fear
    fright
    grief

Ailments from:
  mortification
  reproaches
  shock, mental
  work, mental
Anger, irascibility
  easily
Anguish
Answers, abruptly, shortly, curtly
  monosyllable
  slowly
Anticipation, complaints from
  dentist, physician, before going to
  examination, before
  stage-fright
  singers and speakers, in
Anxiety
  midnight, before
  anticipation, an engagement,
  of
  children, in
  when being put in the cradle ★
  chill, during
  fright, after
  future, about
  motion, from downward
  thunderstorm during
  time is set, if a
Attention amel. ★
Brooding
Cheerful, gay, mirthful
  alternating with sadness
  followed by melancholy
Clinging to persons or furniture etc.
  grasps the nurse when carried
  held, wants to be
  amel., being
Company, aversion to; presence
  of others people agg. the
  symptoms; desire for soli-
  tude
  avoids the sight of people
Company, desire for; aversion to soli-
  tude, company amel.
  alone agg., while
Concentration, difficult
  alternating with uterine pains •
  on attempting to concentrate has
  a vacant feeling
Confidence, want of self

Confusion of mind
  concentrate the mind, on attempting to
  identity, duality, sense of
  masturbation, from •
  mental exertion, from
  smoking, after
  waking, on
Conversation, aversion to
Cowardice
Delirium
  muttering
  sleep, in
  paroxysmal
  sleep, during
  falling asleep, on
  wild
Delirium tremens, mania-a-potu
  sleeplessness, with
Delusions, double, of being
  enlarged, distances are
  head is
  objects are
  grave, he is in his
  identity, someone else, she is
  images, sees frightful
  sick, someone else is •
  snakes, white ★
  snakes in and around her
Despair
Dipsomania, alcoholism
Disturbed, averse to being
Dullness, sluggishness, difficulty
  of thinking and compre
  hending, torpor
  masturban after
  sleepiness, with
  think long, unable to
  urine amel., copious flow of
Excitement, excitable
  agg.
  anticipating events, when
  bad news, after
  hearing horrible things, after
  pregnency during
Exertion, agg. from mental
Exhilaration
  recall things long forgotten, can •

Fear, apprehension, dread
   alone, of being
   appearing in public, of
   church or opera, when ready to go
   **crowd, public places, of; ago-
     raphobia**
   dark, of
   death, of
   diarrhoea from
   downward motion, of
   examination, before
   failure, of
   falling, of
     child holds on to mother
   happen, something will
   *heart, cease to beat unless con
     stantly on the move, will* •
   insanity, losing his reason, of
   motion, of
   ordeals, of
   people, of; anthropophobia
   self-control, of losing
   shivering from fear •
   sleep, before
   thunderstorm, of
   water, of
Forgetful
Grief, cry, cannot
   silent
Grimaces
Heedless
High places agg.
Horrible things, sad stories, affect her
   profoundly
Hypochondriasis
Hysteria
   grief, from
   plethoric subjects, in
   pregnancy and labor, during
Ideas abundant, clearness of mind
Impatience
Inattention, agg. ★
Indifference, apathy
Indolence, aversion to work
   afternoon
   masturbation, after

Insanity, madness
   paroxysmal
Irritability
   chill, during
   spoken to, when
Jumping, height, from a, impulse to j. ★
Light, desire for
Loquacity
   heat, during
Mania
Memory, active
Memory, weakness of
   labor, for mental
   fatigue from
Moaning, groaning, whining
   sleep, during
Mood, changeable, variable
Morose, cross, fretful, ill-humor, peevish
*Prostration of mind, mental exhaus-
   tion, brain-fag*
   pollutions, after
Quiet disposition
   heat, during
Quiet, wants to be
Reclining, half ★
Restlessness
   morning
   night
   bed, tossing about in
   heat, during
   menses, during
   storm, before
   during
**Sadness, despondency, dejection,
   mental depression, gloom,
   melancholy**
   heat, during
   impotence, with
   masturbation, from
   sleeplessness with sadness
   weep, cannot
Senses, dull, blunted
Sensitive, oversensitive
   noise, to
   chill during

Shrieking, screaming, shouting
   pains, with the
   thunderstorm, during •
   waking, on
Sighing
Singing
   alternating with talking •
Sits, still
Slowness
Speech, affected
   babbling
   confused
   incoherent
     night
   sleep, during
   intoxicated, as if
Spit, desire to, afternoon
Spoken to, averse to being
Starting, sleep, during
Stupefaction, as if intoxicated
   vertigo, during
Suicidal disposition
   throwing himself from a height
     window, from
Surprise, agg. ★
Talk, indisposed to, desire to be silent,
   taciturn
   heat, during
   sleep, in
Thinking, aversion to
   complaints agg., of
Thoughts, disconnected
   vacancy of
   vanishing
   mental exertion, on
Timidity
Torpor
Touched, aversion to being
Unconsciousness, coma, stupor
   alcoholic
   eyes, cannot open •
   fever, during
   meningitis, in
   parturition, during
   prolonged ★
   scarlatina, in

Vivacious
   rising, after •
Weeping, tearful mood
Will, muscles, obey, feebly
   refuse to obey the will when
   attention is turned away
Work, aversion to mental
   desire for
   impossible

GENTIANA CRUCIATA

Confusion of mind
   eructations amel.
Fear, apprehension, dread
Restlessness, headache, during
Talk, indisposed to, desire to be silent,
   taciturn
Weeping, tearful mood

GENTIANA LUTEA

Confusion of mind
   writing, while
Dullness, sluggishness, difficulty of
   thinking and
   comprehending, torpor
Morose, cross, fretful, ill-humor, peevish
Restlessness, night
Stupefaction

GETTYSBURG AQUA

Dullness, sluggishness, difficulty of thinking and comprehending, torpor
Restlessness, night
   midnight, after, 1h.
Work, aversion to mental, forenoon

GINKGO BILOBA

Anger, irascibility
Delusions, unreal, everything seems
Loquacity
Reproaches himself
Tears things

GINSENG

Anxiety
    dinner, after
    future, about
Confusion of mind
Contented
Courageous
Delirium, sleep, falling asleep, on
Dullness, sluggishnes, difficulty of
    thinking and comprehending,
    torpor
Fear, apprehension, dread
    accidents, of
    misfortune, of
    riding in a carriage (car drive),
      when
Hurry, movements, in
Impatience
Impulsive
Indolence, aversion to work
Insanity, erotic
Memory, weakness of
Restlessness
    internal
Starting, sleep, from
Stupefaction, as if intoxicated
Thinking, aversion to
Tranquillity, serenity, calmness
Weeping, tearful mood
Work, impossible, mental

GLONOINUM

Ailments from :
    anger, vexation, fright, with
    excitement, emotional
    fear
    fright
    injuries, accidents; mental symp-
    toms from
    quarrels
Answers; aversion to answer
Anxiety
    climacteric period, during
    headache, with
    health, about
    waking, on
Aphasia ★

Aversion, children, to her own
    husband and children, to
Cheerful, gay, mirthful
Climacteric period agg.
Clinging, held amel., being
Concentration, difficult
Confusion of mind
    night, waking, on
    air amel., in open
    intoxicated, as if
    as after being
    loses his way in well-known
    streets
    stooping, when
    talking, while
    waking, on
    walking, while
    air, in open
    will amel., strong effort of ●
Contradiction, is intolerant of
Death, desires
Delirium
    bed and escapes, springs up sud-
    denly from
    headache, during
    raging, raving
Delirium tremens, mania-a-potu
Delusions, imaginations, hallucina-
    tions, illusions
    chin is too long ●
    disorder, objects appear in
    divine, being
    double, of being
    enlarged
      chin is
      distances are
      head is
      objects are
    head, standing, on ★
    house, place, not in right (while
      walking in the street after
      headache) ●
    lip is swollen, lower ●
    long, chin seems too ●
    nose, longer, seems
    objects, crooked ●
    strange, familiar things seem
    streets, loses his way in, the
    houses seem

Delusions,

   strange •

      places seemed, after head-
      ache •

   swollen, he is

Dipsomania, alcoholism

Discomfort

Distances, inaccurate judgement of
   exaggerated, are

Dream, as if in a

*Dullness, sluggishness, difficulty of think-
   ing and comprehending, torpor*

   gassing, by

   mental exern, from

   reading, while

   writing, while

Dwells on past disagreeable occurrences

   offences come back to him, long
   forgotten

   recalls old grievances

Eccentricity

   fancies, in

Escape, attempts to

   run away, to

   springs up suddenly from bed

   window, from

Excitement, excitable

   climacteric period, during

Exertion, agg. from mental

Fancies, confused

Fear, apprehension, dread

   apoplexy, of

      waking, on

   crowd, public places, of; agoraphobia

   climacteric period, during •

   death, of

   misfortume, of

   poisoned, of being

      has been

   *throat, fear from sensation of
   swelling of*

Forgetful

   headache, during

   **house was, on which side of
   the street, his**

   street, of well-known

   words while speaking, of; word
   hunting

Frightened easily

Gestures, makes: fingers spread apart ★

Ideas abundant, clearness of mind
   deficiency of

Idleness

Impulse, run, to; dromomania

Indifference, apathy

Insanity, madness

Jesting

Jumping, bed, out of

Loquacity

Malicious, spiteful, vindictive

Mania

Memory, active

Memory, loss of, sunstroke, after

Memory, weakness of

   names, for proper

Mistakes, localities, in

   space and time, in

   time, in

Prostration of mind, mental exhaustion, brain-fag

Rage, fury

Recognize anyone, does not

   relatives, does not recognize his

   **streets, does not recognize
   well known**

Restlessness

   night

Runs, about

*Sadness, despondency, dejection, men-
   tal depression, gloom, melancholy*

Senses, confused

   vanishing of

Sensitive, noise, to

Shining objects agg.

Shrieking, screaming, shouting

   brain cry

   children, in

Sighing

Sits, head on hand and elbows on
   knees, with

Speech, affected

Spit, desire to

Strange, everything seems

   standing agg. •

Striking
  convulsions, after puerperal •
Suicidal, throwing himself from a height
  window from
**Talk, indisposed to, desire to be
  silent, taciturn**
Terror, sudden ★
Thoughts, persistent
  offended him, of persons who
    had •
  rush, flow of
  wandering
**Time passes too slowly, appears
  longer**
Unconsciousness, coma, stupor
  morning
  noon
  alcoholic
  cold water dashed in face amel.
  convulsions, after
  *dream, as in a, does not know
    where he is*
  face, with red
  incomplete
  sighing, with •
  sunstroke, in
Vivacious
Weeping, tearful mood
  pain, with the
    during intermission of •
  sleep, in
Work, impossible, mental

GLYCERINUM

Concentration, difficult
Indifference, apathy
Memory, weakness of
Work, impossible mental

GNAPHALIUM
POLYCEPHALUM

Restlessness, night
Unconsciousness, coma, stupor

GOSSYPIUM HERBACEUM

Ailments from:
  excitement, emotional
Anxiety
Brooding
Capriciousness
Complaining
Concentration, difficult
Discontented, displeased, dissatisfied
Dwells on past disagreeable occur-
  rences
Excitement, nervous
Eating, amel. after
Impatience
Restlessness
  bed, tossing about in
Sadness, despondency, dejection, men-
  tal depression, gloom, melan-
  choly
Travel, desire to
Weeping, tearful mood

GRANATUM

Anger, irascibility
Anxiety
Censorious, critical
Confusion of mind
  carousual, after a
Delusions, imaginations, hallucinations,
  illusions
Discomfort
Discouraged
Dullness, sluggishness, difficulty of think-
  ing and comprehending, torpor
Excitement, excitable
Fear, work, during headache, of •
Haughty
Hypochondriasis
Indolence, aversion to work
Irritability
Memory, weakness of; do, for what was
  about to
Morose, cross, fretful, ill-humor, peevish
Prostration of mind, mental exhaus-
  tion, brain-fag
Quarrelsome, scolding
Reproaches others

Sadness, despondency, dejection, mental
    depression, gloom, melancholy
Sensitive, oversensitive
Shrieking, sleep, during
Sighing
Stupefaction, as if intoxicated
    vertigo, during
Tranquillity, serenity, calmness

GRAPHITES NATURALIS

Absent-minded, unobserving
Abstraction of mind
Activity, mental, evening
    midnight, until
Affectation
Affectionate
Ailments from:
    anger, vexation
    anticipation, foreboding, pre-
    sentiment
    discords between chief
      and sabordinate parents
      and friends ★
    fear
    fright
    grief
    work, mental
Ambition
Amorous
Anger, irascibility
    night
    easily
    interruption, from
    violent
Anguish
    daytime
    amenorrhoea, in
    menses, before
Answers, hesitating
Anxiety
    morning
      waking, on
    evening
      bed, in
    night
      waking, on
    midnight, before

Anxiety
    midnight, after
      2h.
    air amel., in open
    bed, in
      driving out of
    conscience, as if guilty of a crime
    dreams, on waking from frightful
    fear, with
    fever, during
    flushes of heat, during
    future, about
    hypochondriacal
    manual labor, during
    menses, before
    others, for ★
    pains, from the stomach
    salvation, about
    sedentary employment, from
    sitting, while
    sleep, during
    trifles, about
    waking, on
    warmth, amel. from
    weeping amel.
    working, while ●
Avarice
Aversion, men, to
Beside oneself, being
    anxiety, from
Business, averse to
Calculating, inability for
Cares, worries, full of
    evening, bed, in
Cautious
Censorious, critical
Cheerful, gay, mirthful
    morning
      sad in evening, and
    forenoon
    evening
    alternating with grief
    sadness
    weeping
    followed by melancholy
    sad, evening ★

Company, aversion to; presence of
   other people agg. the symptoms; desire for solitude
Concentration, difficult
   children, in
Confusion of mind
   morning
      rising and after, on
      waking, on
   afternoon
   evening
   intoxicated, as if
   menses, during
      after
   sleepiness, after
   waking, on
   walking in open air amel.
Conscientious about trifles
   trifles, occupied with
Consolation, kind words agg.
Conversation agg.
Cowardice
   opinions, without courage of own
Darkness agg.
Death, presentiment of
   sensation of
   thoughts of
Delirium
   night
   closing the eyes, on
   delusions, with
   fantastic
   raging, raving
Delusions, imaginations, hallucinations,
   illusions
      evening, bed, in
   assembled things, swarms, crowds
      etc.
   bed, someone is in, with him
   criminals, about
   dead persons, sees
   fancy, illusions of
   heart disease, of having
   images, phantoms, sees
      night
      closing eyes, on
      frightful
   sick, being

Delusions,
   strange, everything is
      familiar things seem
   unfortunate, he is
   visions, has
      closing the eyes, on
   water, of
Despair
   chill, during
   heat, during
   perspiration, during
   trifles, over ●
Dipsomania, alcoholism
Discontented, displeased, dissatisfied
   everything, with
Discouraged
   night ●
   anxiety, with
   waking, on
Doubtful
Dullness, sluggishness, difficulty
   of thinking and compre
   hending, torpor
   morning
   afternoon
   air amel., in open
   eating, after
   mental exertion, from
   perspiration, during
   siesta, after
   walking, air amel., in open
Dwells on past disagreeable occurrences
Excitement, excitable
   evening
   night
   talking while
Exertion, agg. from mental
Exhilaration
   evening
Fancies, exaltation of
   evening in bed
   night
   closing the eyes in bed
   sleeplessness, with
   lascivious
Fastidious

Fear, apprehension, dread
   morning
   evening in bed
   night
   business, of
   crowd, in a
   death, of
   evil, of
     evening
   happen, something will
   insanity, losing his reason, of
   misfortune, of
   people of; anthropophobia
   suffocation, of, eating amel. ●
   thunderstorm, of ★
   tremulous
   waking from a dream, on
   weeping amel.
   work, dread of
     mental, of
Fishy ★
Forgetful
   afternoon
Frightened easily
   waking, on
     dream, from a
Gestures: cross fingers ★
Grief
   evening ●
   night in bed
   constant and chronic ●
Hesitates ★
   at trifles ★
Hurry, haste
Hypochondriasis, afternoon
   morose
   suicide, driving to
Hysteria
Ideas abundant, clearness of mind
   night
   deficiency of
Impatience
Impertinence
Inconstancy
Indifference, apathy
   conscience, to the dictates of
   pleasure, to
Indiscretion

Indolence, aversion to work
   air amel., in open
   intelligent, although very
Insanity, megalomania
Insolence
Irresolution, indecision
   anxious ●
Irritability
   morning
   afternoon
   children, in
   coition, after
   disturbed, when
   eating, after
   headache, during
   spoken to, when
   stool, after
   trifles, from
Lascivious, lustful
Laughing
   morning
   forenoon
   immoderately
   reprimands, at ●
   reproach, at ●
   trifles, at
Magnetized, mesmerism amel.
Manual work, fine work, mind symptoms from
Mathematics: inapt for algebra
Memory, weakness of
   done, for what has just
   facts, for recent
   happened, for what has
   labor, for mental
Menses, mental symptoms agg. during
Mistakes, speaking, in
   misplacing words
   words, using wrong
   writing, in
Moaning, groaning, whining
   dreaming, while ●
   impulse to ★
   sleep, during
   weakness, from
Mood, alternating
   changeable, variable
   opinions, in

Morose, cross, fretful, ill-humor, peevish
   children, in
   eating, after
Music agg.   ·
Noise amel. ★
Nymphomania
Offended, easily; takes everything in
   bad part
Prostration of mind, mental exhaus-
   tion, brain-fag
Quarrelsome, without waiting for an-
   swer ★
Rage, fury
Religious affections
Remorse
Restlessness
   night
      midnight on waking
         2h. after
      air amel., in open
      anxious
      bed, driving out of   .
         tossing about in
      driving about
      hypochondriacal
      lascivious thoughts, during ●
      mental labor, during and after
      perspiration, during
      sitting, while at work
      waking, on
      walking, air amel., in open
      working, while
Rudeness
Sadness, despondency, dejection,
   mental depression, gloom,
   melancholy
   morning
      amel.
   forenoon
      amel.
   afternoon
   evening
      bed, in
         but cheerful in morning ●
      night
         bed, in
   anxious
   chill, during

Sadness,
   eating, after
   heat, during
   heaviness in feet, with ●
   menses, during
   music, from
   perspiration, during
   pressure about chest, from
   puberty, in
   suicidal disposition, with
   trifles, about
Senses, dull, blunted
   vanishing of
Sensitive, oversensitive
   morning
   mental impressions, to
   music, to
   noise amel. ★
   odors, to
   pain, to
   sensual impressions, to
Shrieking, sleep, during
Sighing
   menses, during
Sit, inclination to
Slowness
   purpose, of ●
Speech, anxious, in sleep
   hesitating
Spoken to, averse to being
Starting, startled
   sleep, during
   from
Strange, everything seems
Stupefaction, as if intoxicated
   morning
   vertigo, during
Suicidal disposition
   hypochondriasis, by
   sadness, from
Suspicious, mistrustful
Sympathy, compassion
Talk, indisposed to, desire to be silent,
   taciturn
   sleep, in
      anxious
      excited
Thinking, complaints agg., of

Thoughts, intrude, sexual
  persistent
    evening
    night
    midnight, before •
    lying, while
    unpleasant subjects, haunted by
    walking in open air amel. •
  rush, flow of
    evening, in bed
    night
    tormenting
    evening
    sexual
  wandering
Timidity
Trifles seem important
Unconsciousness, coma stupor, morning
Undertakes many things, perseveres in nothing
Unfortunate, feels
Violent, vehement
  morning
Walking in open air amel. mental symptoms
Wearisome
Weeping, tearful mood
  evening
  night
  alternating with cheerfulness
  irritability and laughter at trifles •
  laughter
  amel.
  anxiety, after
  anxious
  causeless
  children, in
  heat, during
  menses, during
  music, from
    organ., on hearing •
  perspiration, during
  sleep, in

Will, weakness of
Work, aversion to mental
  fatigues
  impossible
  siesta, after •

GRATIOLA OFFICINALIS

Absent-minded, unobserving
Absorbed, buried in thought
Ailments from :
  pride of others •
Anger, irascibility
  contradiction, from
  violent
Answers, reflects long
Anxiety
  air amel, in open
  fever, during
  future, about
  health, about
  hypochondriacal
Aversion, everything, to
Capriciousness
Cheerful, gay, mirthful
Company, aversion to; presence of other people agg. the symptoms; desire for solitude
Concentration, difficult
Confusion of mind
  air amel., in open
  dream, as if in
  eating, after
  intoxicated, as if
  lying, when
  standing, while
  waking, on
  walking, while
Contradict, disposition to
Contradiction, is intolerant of
Dancing
Delirium tremens, mania-a-potu
Delusions, diminished, all is
  small, he is •
Discomfort
Discontented, displeased, dissatisfied
  afternoon
  everything, with

Dullness, waking, on
Eat, refuses to
Fear, apprehension, dread
    eating, of
    fit, of having a
    hungry, when •
Hurry, haste
Hypochondriasis
    morose
Hysteria
Indifference, sleepiness, with
Indolence, aversion to work
    sleepiness, with
Insanity, erotic
Irresolution, indecision
Irritability
       morning
       forenoon
Jumping
Loathing, life, at
Loquacity
    cheerful, exuberant
Mania
Memory, active
Misanthropy
Morose, cross, fretful, ill-humor, peevish
    forenoon
    hypochondriasis, in
Nymphomania
Persevere, cannot ★
Prostration of mind, mental exhaustion, brain-fag
Quarrelsome, scolding
Reserved
Sadness, despondency, dejection, mental depession, gloom, melancholy
    afternoon
Satyriasis
Serious, earnest
Suicidal disposition
Talk, indisposed to, desire to be silent, taciturn
    afternoon
Thoughts, profound
    rush, sleeplessness from
    thoughtful

Unconsciousness, coma, stupor
    riding, while
    vertigo, during
    walking, while
Violent, vehement
Wearisome
Weary of life
Will, loss of
    weakness of
Work, aversion to mental
    impossible

GRINDELIA ROBUSTA

Anxiety
Confusion of mind, intoxicated, as if ★
Fear, dark, of
    suffocation, of
Light, desire for
Longing, sunshine, light and society, for
Starting, sleep, during

GUACO

Hydrophobia

GUAIACUM OFFICINALE

Absent-minded, unobserving
    morning
Abstraction of mind
    morning •
Anxiety, constriction in stomach, from •
    pressure in epigastrium •
Audacity
Censorious, critical
Confusion, dream, as if in
Contemptuous
Contrary
Defiant
Delirium, sleep, falling asleep, on
Delusions, evening on falling asleep
    falling asleep, on
    narrow, everything seems too
Disobedience
Dullness, sluggishness, difficulty of thinking and comprehending, torpor
    morning
    standing agg.

Fear exertion of
Forgetful
    names, of, persons ★
Frightened easily
Haughty
Heedless
Ideas, deficiency of
Indifference, apathy
Indolence, aversion to work
Irritability
Malicious, spiteful, vindictive
Memory, weakness of
    names, for proper
    read, for what has
Misanthropy
Mocking
Morose, cross, fretful, ill-humor, peevish
Obstinate, headstrong
Restlessness
    morning, bed, in
    night
    bed, tossing about in
    waking, on
Sadness, despondency, dejection, mental
    depression, gloom, melancholy
Shrieking, sleep, during
    waking, on
Sit, inclination to
Staring, thoughtless, morning •
Starting, sleep, during
    from
Talk, indisposed to, desire to be silent,
    taciturn
Thoughts, vanishing of
Unconsciousness, coma, stupor
Wearisome
Weeping, night
    nightmare, after •
    waking, on

GUARANA

Cheerful, gay, mirthful
Delirium
Excitement, excitable
Extravagance

Restlessness
    convulsive •
Sadness, headache, during
Vivacious

GUAREA TRICHILOIDES

Anxiety
    fever, during
Excitement, excitable
Forgetful, heat, during
Indifference, apathy
Industrious, mania for work
Irresolution, indecision
Loquacity
Memory, weakness of
Mood, changeable, variable
Perseverance
Restlessness, evening

GUATTERIA GAUMERI

Irresolution, indecision
Irritability
Memory, weakness of
Sadness, despondency, dejection, mental
    depression, gloom, melancholy
Thoughts, tormenting

GYMNOCLADUS CANADENSIS

Dullness, sluggishness, difficulty of think-
    ing and comprehending, torpor
Forgetful
Indifference, apathy
Memory, weakness of
Work, mental impossible

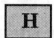

HAEMATOXYLUM CAMPECHIANUM

Anger, irascibility
Anxiety
 night
Dullness, sluggishness, difficulty of
 thinking and comprehending,
 torpor
Malicious, spiteful, vindictive
Memory, weakness of
 expressing oneself, for
Mistakes, speaking, in
Rest, desire for
Restlessness
Sensitive, oversensitive
Stupefaction, as if intoxicated
Weeping, tearful mood
Will, weakness of
Work, mental impossible,

HALL AQUA

Restlessness, night

HALOPERIDOLUM

Anguish
Company, aversion to, alone, amel.
 when
Concentration, difficult
Confusion of mind
 time, of
Delusions, legs are cut off
Dullness, sluggishness, difficulty of think-
 ing and comprehending, torpor
Exertion, agg. from mental
Memory, weakness of
 everyday things, for
 read, for what has

Mistakes, time, in
Pessimist
Restlessness, anxious
 bed, in
Sadness, despondency, dejection, mental depressiontion, gloom, melancholy
  evening, amel.
Schizophrenia
 catatonic
 hebephrenia
Slowness

HAMAMELIS VIRGINIANA

Absent-minded, unobserving
Absorbed, buried in thought
Anger, irascibility
·Company, aversion to; presence of
 other people agg. the symp-
 toms; desire for solitude
Concentration, difficult
Conscientious about trifles
Conversation, desire, sublime, to hear •
Delirium
Delusion insane, she will become
Discontented, displeased, dissatisfied
 everything, with
Desires, respect, due to him, shown ★
Dullness, sluggishness, difficulty of think-
 ing and comprehending, torpor
  morning on rising
  waking, on
  afternoon
  waking, on
  walking, while
Excitement, excitable
Fancies, confused
Fear, insanity, losing his reason, of
Forgetful
 words while speaking, of; word
 hunting
Haughty
Ideas abundant, morning, after restless
 sleep •
Indifference, apathy
 afternoon
 business affairs, to

Indolence, aversion to work
    morning ★
Irritability
Meditation
Memory, weakness of
    read, for what has
    words, of
Mistakes, speaking, in
Morose, cross, fretful, ill-humor, peevish
Opinions, expects others to pay respect
    to her •
Prostration of mind, mental exhaus-
    tion, brain-fag
Reading, unable, to read
Restlessness
Reverence for those around him
Sadness, despondency, dejection, mental
    depression, gloom, melancholy
    evening amel.
    masturbation, from
    pollutions, from
Sensitive, oversensitive
Sit, inclination to muse, and •
Spoken to, averse to being
Stupefaction, as if intoxicated
Talk, indisposed to, desire to be silent,
    taciturn
Thinking, constantly of his ailments •
Thoughts, wandering, studying, while
Tranquillity, serenity, calmness
    haemoptysis, haemorrhages, in •
Unconsciousness, coma, stupor
Work, aversion to mental
    desire for
    impossible

HARPAGOPHYTUM PROCUMBENS

Indifference, apathy

HEDERA HELIX

Anguish
Anxiety
Cares, worries, full of

Fear, apprehension, dread
    extreme •
    heart, of disease of

HELLEBORUS NIGER

Absent-minded, unobserving
Absorbed, buried in thought
Abstraction of mind
Ailments from :
    homesickness
    love, disappointed
Anger, irascibility
    consoled, when
    easily
    interruption, from
    spoken to, when
    trifles, at
Answers, aversion to
    confusedly as though thinking of
        something else
    difficult
    reflects long
    refuses to answer
    repeats the question first
    slowly
Anxiety
    fear, with
Asks for nothing
Asks for nothing
Attention amel. ★
Automatism
Aversion to being approached
Awkward, drops things ★
Barking, growling like a dog
Bilious disposition
Bilious disposition
Blank ★
Brooding
Chaotic, confused behavior
Cheerful, alternating with sadness
Company, aversion to; presence of other
    people agg. the symptoms; de-
    sire for solitude
    alone, amel. when
Complaining
Concentration, active
Concentration, difficult

Confusion of mind
    afternoon
    chill, during
    stooping, when
    thinking of it agg.
    waking, on
Consolation, kind words agg.
    sympathy agg.
Contemptuous
Contradiction, is intolerant of
Darkness agg. ★
Death, presentiment of
    predicts the time
Deeds, feels as if he could do great ●
Delirium
    morning
      waking, on
    answers correctly when spoken to,
    but delirium and unconscious-
    ness return at once
    bed and escapes, springs up sud-
      denly from
    fever, during
    maniacal
    meningitis cerebrospinalis
    muttering
    raging, raving
Delirium tremens, mania-a-potu
Delusions, imaginations, hallucina-
    tions, illusions
      morning, bed, in
      assembled things, swarms,
      crowds, etc.
    devils, sees
    die, he was about to
    doomed, being
    fancy, illusions of
      evening in bed
    figures, sees
    images, phantoms, sees
      dark, in the
    lost, she is (salvation)
    neglected his duty, he has
    new, everything is
    pursued by enemies
    spectres, ghosts, spirits, sees

Delusions,
    talking with dead people, she is
    visions, has, closing the eyes, on
    horrible, dark in the
    walks, cannot, must run or hop
    wrong, he has done
Dementia
Desires, has no more ★
Despair
    recovery, of
    religious despair of salvation
Dipsomania, alcoholism
Discomfort
Discontented, displeased, dissatisfied
Discouraged
Dream, as if in a
Dresses indecently
Dullness, sluggishness, difficulty
    of thinking and compre-
    hending, torpor
    afternoon
    chill, during
    says nothing
    understands questions only after
      repetition
Envy
Escape, attempts to
    fever, during
Excitement, excitable
Exertion, agg. from mental
    amel.
Fancies, exaltation of
    evening in bed
    going to bed, after
    vivid, lively
    evening
Fear, apprehension, dread
    alone, of being, night
    death, of
    evil, of
    imaginary things, of
    misfortune, of
Foolish behavior
Forgetful
Forsaken feeling
Frown, disposed to

Gestures, automatic
    grasping or reaching at some
      thing, at flocks; carphologia
    picks at bed clothes
Grief
Grimaces
Grunting
Haughty
Heedless
Helplessness, feeling of
Hide, desire to
Homesickness
Hurry, drinking, on
Hypochondriasis
Hysteria
Ideas, abundant, clearness of mind
    deficiency of
    fixed ★
Idiocy
Imbecility
    shrieks on being engaged
Impatience
Inattention, agg. ★
Inconstancy, thought, of
Indifference, apathy
    desire, has no, no action of the
      will
    everything, to
    external things, to
    family, to his
    joy and suffering, to
    loved ones, to
    pleasure, to
    relations, to
    suffering, to
    taciturn
Indolence, aversion to work
Insanity, madness
    apoplexy, after ★
    drunkards, in
Introspection
    afternoon ●
Irresolution, indecision
Irritability
    consolation agg.

Lamenting, bemoaning, wailing
Laughing
Looked at, cannot bear to be
Mania
    demoniac
    hands, wringing, runs about day
      and night ●
Meditation
Memory, weakness of
    heard, for what has
    said, for what has
    say, for what is about to
    words, of
Mildness
Moaning, groaning, whining
    sleep, during
    weeping, with ●
Monomania
Mood, changeable, variable
Morose, cross, fretful, ill-humor, peevish
Muttering
    unintelligible
Obstinate, headstrong
Occupation, diversion amel.
Prostration of mind, mental exhaus-
    tion, brain-fag
Puberty, mental affections in
Quiet disposition
Rage, fury
Reproaches himself
Reserved
Restlessness
    night
    anxious
    bed, tossing about in
Rudeness
Runs about
Sadness, despondency, dejection,
    mental depression, gloom,
    melancholy
    girls before puberty, in
    happy, on seeing others
    menses, before
      during the first m. ●
      after

Sadness,
  puberty, in
  quiet
  thinking of his position, on •
  typhus, after
Self, accusation ★
Senses, dull, blunted
Sensitive, oversensitive
  noise, to
Shamelessness
Shrieking, screaming, shouting
  brain cry
  children, in
  must shriek, feels as though she
  ' *sleep, during*
Sighing
  involuntary
Sit, inclination to
Sits still
Slowness
  old people, of
Speech, slow
Spoken to, averse to being
  alone, wants to be let
Staring, thoughtless
Starting, evening, jerking or twitching,
  ceasing on falling asleep
  sleep, during
    from comatose sleep •
Strange, crank
    dressing, in
Striking
Stupefaction, as if intoxicated
  chill, during
  convulsions, between
  injury to head, after
  rouses with difficulty
  vertigo, during
Suicidal, disposition
  drowning, by
  hanging, by
Suspicious, mistrustful
Sympathy, agg.
Talk, indisposed to, desire to be silent,
    taciturn
      forenoon
    others agg., t. of

Talking, sleep, in
Talks, dead people, with
Tastelessness in dressing
Thinking, complaints agg., of
    amel.
Thoughts, persistent
  thoughtful, afternoon
  vanishing of
Touched, aversion to being
Tranquillity, serenity, calmness
Unconsciousness, coma, stupor
  answers correctly when spoken to,
    but delirium and unconscious-
    ness return at once
  conduct, automatic
  hydrocephalus, in
  meningitis, in
  mental insensibility
  stooping, when
Unfortunate, feels
Weeping, tearful mood
  amel.
  consolation agg.
  despair, from
  sleep, in ★
Will, loss of
  muscles obey, feebly ★
  muscles refuse to obey the will
    when attention is turned away
Work, mental, impossible
Wrong, doing something

HELLEBORUS FOETIDUS

Anxiety

HELLEBORUS VIRIDIS

Restlessness, night

HELODERMA SUSPECTUM

Concentration, difficult
Forgetful, words while speaking, of;
    word hunting
Indifference, apathy
Indolence, aversion to work

Industrious, mania for work
Memory, weakness of
Mistakes, speaking, in, omitting words
    spelling, in

HELONIAS DIOICA

Activity, amel.
Ailments from:
    joy, excessive
Anger, contradiction, from
Aversion to being approached
Censorious, critical
Company, aversion to; presence of other
    people agg. the symptoms; desire
    for solitude
Conscious of uterus
Contradiction, is intolerant of
    agg.
Conversation, agg. ★
Despair
Dullness, sluggishness, difficulty of think-
    ing and comprehending, torpor
    diabetes, in
Exertion, amel. from mental
Hypochondriasis
Indolence, aversion to work
    morning ★
Industrious, mania for work
Irritability
    diabetes, in
    headache, during
Memory, weakness of
Morose, cross, fretful, ill-humor, peevish
Occupation, diversion amel.
Restlessness
    women, in
Sadness, despondency, dejection, men-
    tal depression, gloom, melan-
    choly
    company, aversion to, desire for
    solitude
    happy, on seeing others
    puberty, in
Slander, disposition to
Spoken to, averse to being
    alone, wants to be let
Starting, easily
Stupefaction, as if intoxicated

Suggestions, will not receive •
Talk, indisposed to, desire to be silent,
    taciturn
    others agg., t. of
Thinking, complaints agg., of
Unconsciousness, coma, stupor

HEPAR SULPHURIS CALCAREUM

Abrupt rough harsh
Absent minded, unobserving
    vertigo, during •
Abusive, insulting
    drunkenness, during
Ailments from :
    anger, suppressed
    discords, between parents,
      friends
      servants ★
Anger, irascibility
    children, in
    noise at
    stabbed any one, so that he
      could have
    trifles, at
    violent
Anguish
    evening
    suicide, attempts to commit •
Answers, hastily
    sleep at once, a. then
Anxiety
    evening
      bed, in
    night
    midnight, before
      after
      1-3h. •
    air, in open
    alone, when
    bed, in
      driving out of
    dreams, on waking from frightful
    family, about his
    fear, with
    fever, during
    future, about
    health, relatives, of

Anxiety, `
  lying, while
  others, for
  sleep, going to
    during
  suicidal disposition, with
  touched, a. to being
  waking, on
  walking, while
    air, in open
  weary of life, with
Asks for nothing
Audacity
Avarice
Aversion, of family, to members
    persons, to certain ★
    places, to ★
Capriciousness
Cares, alone, when •
  relatives, about
  walking in open air •
Change, desire for
Cheerful, morning
  bed, in •
  never
Company, aversion to; presence of other
    people agg. the symptoms; de-
    sire for solitude
Company, desire for; aversion to soli-
    tude, company amel.
    alone agg., while
Complaining
Confusion of mind
  mental exertion, from
  sleeping, after
  stretching on the couch, on •
  waking, on
Conscientious about trifles
Contradict, disposition to
Contradiction, is intolerant of
Contrary
Cowardice
Cruelty, inhumanity
Death, desires
  presentiment of
Deceitful, perjured
Delirium
    morning
      waking, on

Delirium,
    night
    anxious
    aroused, on being
    fever, during
    frightful
    muttering
    raging, raving
Delusions, imaginations, hallucina-
    tions, illusions
    morning, bed, in
    clouds, sees
    dead persons,
      morning on waking, fright-
      ened by images of •
    fancy, illusions of
    fire, visions of
      house is on
      nighbour's house on (morning
        waking in a fright) •
      world is on
    images, phantoms, sees
      frightful
    murdered, he will be
    poor, he is
    sick, members of the family are •
    spectres, ghosts, spirits, sees
    unpleasant
    visions, has
      horrible
Despair
  chill, during
Destructiveness
Dipsomania
Discontented, displeased, dissatisfied
  always
  everything, with
  himself, with
  others, with ★
Discouraged
  pains, from
Discrimination, lack of
Disgust
Dream, as if in a
Dullness, sluggishness, difficulty of think-
    ing and comprehending, torpor
  cough, during •
  mental exertion, from
Duty: no sense of duty

Dwells on past disagreeable occurrences
recalls disagreeable memories
Estranged from her family
Excitement, excitable
chill, during
Exertion, agg. from mental
Fancies
exaltation of
night
sleeplessness, with
Fear, apprehension, dread
evening
night
air, in open
alone, of being
crowd, in a
death, of
disease, of impending
walking in open air, agg. •
disfigured, of being •
evil, of
health of loved persons, about
ruined, that she has, of
those she loves ★
hurt, of being
menses, before
people, of
recover, he will not
snakes, of ★
thunderstorm, of
touch, of
waking, on
walking, while
Fire, wants to set things on
Forgetful
Frightened, waking, on
Fur, wraps up, in summer
Gestures, frightful
furious
grasping, picks at bedclothes
violent
Hatred, revenge, and
Heedless
Horrible things, sad stories, affect her
profoundly
Hurry, haste
drinking, on
eating, while
occupation, in

Hypochondriasis
suicide, driving to
Ideas, abundant, clearness of mind
night
deficiency of
Imbecility, sexual excitement, with
Impatience
Impetuous
perspiration, with
Impolite
Impulse, morbid
fire, to set on ★
Impulsive
Indifference, apathy
morning on waking
pleasure, to
relations, to
Indolence, aversion to work
morning
Insanity, madness
drunkards, in
suppressed eruptions, after
Irritability
morning, rising, after
chill, during
heat, during
pain, during
perspiration, during
trifles
Kill, desire to
barber wants to kill his customer
beloved ones
drunkenness, during
knife, with a
offence, sudden impulse to kill for
a slight
sudden impulse to kill
threatens to kill
wife and children •
throw child into fire, sudden impulse to
Laughing, never
Loathing, general
evening
Loathing, life, at
evening
Loquacity
drunkenness, during
listen, would not •

Malicious, spiteful, vindictive
    anger, with
Mania
    suppressed eruptions, after
Memory, weakness of
        pains, from, suddenly ★
        names, for proper
        places, for
        said, for what has
        words, for
Mistakes, speaking, in
        misplacing words
        words, using wrong
        writing, in
Moaning, night
Mood, repulsive
Moral feeling, want of
    criminal, disposition to become a,
        without remorse
Morose, cross, fretful, ill-humor, pee-
    vish
        morning
        evening
        children, in
        chill, during
        pain, after
        trifles, about
Music, aversion to
Muttering
Objective, reasonable
Obstinate, headstrong
Passionate
Philosophy, ability for
Play, aversion to play in children
Prostration of mind, mental exhaus-
    tion, brain fag
Quarrelsome, scolding
    sleep, in
Rage, fury
    kill people, tries to
Reserved, morning
Restlessness
        evening
            bed, in
            night
        anxious
        bed, driving out of
        sleepiness, with

Sadness, despondency, dejection, men-
    tal depression, gloom, melan-
    choly
    morning
    evening
air, in open
anxious
chill, during
mercury, after abuse of
suicidal disposition, with
walking, air, in open
Senses, dull, blunted
    vanishing of
Sensitive, oversensitive
    chill, during
    external impressions, to all
    mental impressions, to
    noise, to
    pain, to
    sensual impressions, to
Shrieking, aid, in sleep, for
        springs up from bed
    cough agg. ★
    sleep, during
        jumping out of sleep and shr.
    for aid
Sit, inclination to
Sits, still
Slowness
Speech, delirious, chill, aroused, dur-
    ing, on being ●
        hasty
    incoherent
Squanders
Starting, startled
    noon
    anxious
    eating, after ●
    sleep, falling, on
    during
    from
Striking, drunkenness, during
Stupefaction, as if intoxicated
Suicidal. disposition
    evening
    drowning, by

Suicidal,
    fire, to set oneself on •
    hypochondriasis, by
    perspiration, during
    sadness, from
    shooting, by
    thoughts
Talk indisposed to, desire to be silent,
    taciturn
        morning
    sits, does not move
Testament, refused to make a
Thoughts, disagreeable
    rush, flow of
        night
            sleeplessness, from
    thoughtful
    vanishing of
        mental exertion, on
        work, at
Threatening
    kill, threatens to
Time, passes too slowly, appears longer
Touchy ★
Trifles seem important
Unbearable, pain ★
Unconsciousness, coma stupor
        morning
        night waking, on
    chill, during
    pain, from
    transient
    walking, in open air
Unfeeling, hard hearted
Violent, vehement
        evening, trifles, at
        **deeds of violence, rage lead-
        ing to**
        pain, from
        trifles, at
Vivacious
Walk, walking in open air agg. mental
        symptoms
Wearisome
Weary of life
        evening
        perspiration, during

Weeping, tearful mood
        night
        agg.
    aloud, w., sobbing
        bitterly •
        chill, during
        coughing, before
            during
            after
        sleep, in
Work, aversion to mental
        impossible
        needs wine for mental work •
Wrong, everything seems

HERACLEUM
SPHONDYLIUM

Capriciousness
Fear, eating, of
Hypochondriasis
Indolence, aversion to work
Morose, cross, fretful, ill-humor, peevish
Sadness, despondency, dejection, men
        tal depression, gloom, melan-
        choly
Talk, indisposed to, desire to be silent,
        taciturn

HIPPURICUM ACIDUM

Anxiety
        conscience, as if guilty of a crime
Irritability

HIPPOMANES

Anger, fever, during •
Anxiety, evening
        future, about
Aversion to being approached
Business, averse to
*Company, aversion to; presence of other
        people agg. the symptoms; de-
        sire for solitude*

Concentration, difficult
  attention, cannot fix ★
Confusion of mind
  evening
Coffee, after, amel.
Delirium
Discomfort
  morning
Discontented, displeased, dissatisfied
  morning
  evening
  everything, with
Discouraged
  morning
Dullness, sluggishness, difficulty of thinking and comprehending, torpor
  evening
  reading, while
Excitement, excitable
Fancies, exaltaion of, night
  lascivious
  forenoon •
Fear, evening
  noise, of
Fight, wants to
Forgetful
Homesickness
  evening •
Indolence, morning
  forenoon
Insanity, climacteric period, during
Irritability
  morning
  forenoon
  headache, during
  heat, after
Memory, active
Memory, weakness of
  read, for what has
Moaning, pollutions, after
Morose, cross, fretful, ill-humor, peevish
  morning
  forenoon
  fever, after
*Prostration of mind, mental exhaus-
  tion, brain fag*
Quarrelsome, scolding
Restlessness
  move, must constantly

**Sadness, despondency, dejection,
  mental depression, gloom,
  melancholy**
  morning after waking
  heat, during
  sits in corner and does not want
    to have anything to do with
    the world •
Singing
Sit, inclination to
Sits, still
  *wrapped in deep, sad thoughts
  and notices*
    nothing, as if
Spoken to, averse to being
  alone, wants to be
Starting, noise, from
Stupefaction, as if intoxicated
Suicidal, disposition
Talk, indisposed to, desire to be silent,
  taciturn
  forenoon
Travel, desire to
Vivacious
Weary of life
Weeping, night
  pollutions, after
Work, aversion to mental
  impossible

HIPPOZAENIUM

Delirium
  night

HIRUDO MEDICINALIS

Anger, irascibility
Concentration, difficult
Dullness, sluggishness, difficulty of think-
  ing and comprehending, torpor
Irritability
Quarrelsome, scolding
Sadness, despondency, dejection, mental
  depression, gloom, melancholy
  alternating with physical energy
Weeping, tearful mood

HISTAMINUM MURIATICUM

Abusive, insulting
Ailments from :
    bad news
Anxiety
    rest, during
    waking, amel. while
Concentration, difficult
Death, thoughts of
Dullness, sluggishness, difficulty of think-
    ing and comprehending, torpor
Impatience
Irritability
    trifles, from
Memory, weakness of
    names, for proper
    words, for
Mood, alternating
Quarrelsome, scolding
Restlessness
    anxious
    driving, about
    waiting, during •
Sadness, despondency, dejection, men-
    tal depression, gloom, melan-
    choly
    walking, amel. while and after
Sensitive, oversensitive
Slowness
Spoken to, averse to being
Talk, indisposed to, desire to be silent,
    taciturn
Walk: hard walking amel. mental symp-
    toms •
Wander, amel. mental symptoms •
Weeping, tearful mood

HOITZIA COCCINEA

Anguish
Delusions, imaginations, hallucinations,
    illusions
Eccentricity
Excitement, excitable
Fear, apprehension, dread
Moaning, groaning, whining

HOMERIA COLLINA

Unconsciousness, coma, stupor

HURA BRASILIENSIS

Absent-minded, unobserving
    work, when at •
Activity
Affectionate
Ailments from :
    grief
Anger, irascibility
    contradiction, from
Anxiety
    evening
    chill, during
    salvation, about
Bite, desire to
    hands, bites
    himself, bites
Break things, desire to
Cheerful, gay, mirthful
    morning
        8 h. •
Concentration, difficult
Confusion of mind
Contradiction, is intolerant of
Death, desires
    thoughts of
Delusions, imaginations, hallucinations,
    illusions
    affection of friends, has lost
    alone in the world, she is
    confidence in him, his friends
        have lost all
    dead persons, sees
    deserted, forsaken, is
    despised, is
    floating in air
    friends, she is about to lose a •
        affection of, has lost the •
    hanging, sees persons,
        three feet from the ground (on
        falling asleep) •
    lost, she is (salvation)
    repudiated by relatives, he is
    spectres, ghosts, spirits, sees
    unfortunate, he is

Despair
   recovery, of
   religious despair of salvation
Destructiveness
Discontented, displeased, dissatisfied
   everything, with
Dullness, mental exertion, from
Ennui, tedium
Excitement, excitable
   noon

   night
Fear, falling when walking, of
   fever, on going to bed, of •
   misfortune, of
   afternoon
     14 h. •
   noise, from
Forsaken feeling
   isolation, sensation of
Hysteria
Impatience
   noon •
   pain, from
Indifference, apathy
   pleasure, to
Indolence, aversion to work
Irritability
Laughing
   morning
     7-8 h. •
   chilliness, followed by •
   paroxysm of pain, from every •
Love with one of the own sex homosex-
   uality, tribadism perversity
Mistakes, localities, in
   time, in
Obstinate, headstrong
Passionate
Reading, difficult, is
Religious affections
Reproaches himself
Restlessness, night
   bed, in
Sadness, despondency, dejection, men-
   tal depression, gloom, melan-
   choly
   morning
Sensitive, noise, to

Sighing
Starting, startled .
   morning, after waking
   bed, in
   door is opened, when a
   easily
   noise, from
   sleep, during
   trifles, at
Sulky
Thinking, complaints agg., of
Unfortunate, feels
Weeping, tearful mood
   forenoon
   evening
   air, in open
   causeless
   singing, when •

HYDRASTIS CANADENSIS

Absent-minded, unobserving
Anger, irascibility
   leucorrhoea ceases, as soon as •
Anguish
Cheerful, gay, mirthful
   morning, rising, on •
   waking, on
Company, aversion to; presence of
   other people agg. the symp-
   toms; desire for solitude
Concentration, difficult
Confusion of mind
Cursing, swearing
   mother, throws food or medicine
   across room, curses his
Death, desires
Delirium
   night
Dipsomania, alcoholism
Discouraged
Dullness, sluggishness, difficulty of
   thinking and comprehending,
   torpor
Ennui, tedium
Exhilaration
Fancies, exaltation of, night
   frightful

Fear, crowd, public places, of; agora
    phobia
    death, of
    disease, of impending
Forgetful
    words while speaking, of; word
      hunting
Going out, aversion to
Hatred and revenge
High-spirited
Hopeful
Indifference, everything, to •
Indolence, aversion to work
Irritability
    dinner, after
    eating, after
    leucorrhoea ceases, i. as soon as •
Loathing, life, at
Malicious, spiteful, vindictive
Memory, weakness of
    do, for what was about to
    facts, for recent
    happened, for what has
    orthography, for
    read, for what has
    say, for what is about to
Mildness
Mistakes, writing, in
Moaning, groaning, whinning
    pain, from
Morose, cross, fretful, ill-humor, peevish
    drunkenness, during
Reading, aversion to read
Restlessness, night
Sadness, despondency, dejection, men-
    tal depression, gloom, melan-
    choly
Singing
Snub one who differed from him, desire
    to •
Striking
    desire to strike
      evening amel. •
Stupefaction, as if intoxicated
    vertigo, during
Talk, indisposed to, desire to be silent,
    taciturn

Thinking, complaints agg., of
Weeping, tearful mood
Work, aversion to mental
    impossible
Writing, aversion to

HYDROCYANICUM ACIDUM

Anger, irascibility
Anguish, uraemia, in •
Anxiety
Bite, desire to
    delirium, during
Concentration, difficult
Confusion of mind
    air amel., in open
Cowardice
Delirium, wild
Delusions, imaginations, hallucinations,
    illusions
      friends: surrounded by friends,
        shaking hands and calling
        them by name •
Despair
Discomfort
Discouraged
Dullness, sluggishness, difficulty of
    thinking and comprehending,
    torpor
Excitement, excitable
Fancies, exaltation of, frightful
Fear, apprehension, dread
    approaching vehicles, of
    crowd, in a
      public places, of; agoraphobia
    everything, constant fear of ★
    misfortune, of
    run over, of being (on going out)
    sleep, to go to
    troubles, of imaginary •
Forgetful
Gestures, convulsive
    hands, motion, involuntary, of
    the, throwing over-head
Hydrophobia
Hypochondriasis
Hysteria
    injure herself, desire to •
Indifference, apathy

Indolence, aversion to wok
Insanity, insensibility, painlessness, with general
Irritability
    afternoon
Laughing, loudly
    sardonic
Mania, excitement in gesture or speech •
Menses, mental symptoms agg. during
Moaning, groaning, whining
Morose, cross, fretful, ill-humor, peevish
    afternoon
Restlessness
    bed, tossing about in
Sadness, despondency, dejection, mental
    depression, gloom, melancholy
    afternoon
Senses, acute
    dull, blunted
Sensitive, want of sensitiveness
Sentimental
Shrieking, screaming, shouting
    convulsions, before
        epileptic
        involuntary ★
        waking, on
Sighing, hysteria, in
Speech, incoherent
Staring, thoughtless
Starting, startled
Stupefaction, as if intoxicated
    vertigo, during
Suicidal, disposition
Talk, indisposed to, desire to be silent,
    taciturn
Tranquillity, serenity, calmness
Unconsciousness, coma, stupor
    prolonged ★
    sudden
Weeping, violent
Work, mental, impossible

HYDROCOTYLE ASIATICA

Cheerful, gay, mirthful
Communicative, expansive
Confiding
Ennui, tedium
Fear, people, of; anthropophobia

Indifference, apathy
Loquacity
Misanthropy
Moaning, groaning, whining
Optimistic
Sadness, despondency, dejection, mental
    depression, gloom, melancholy
Vivacious

HYDROPHIS CYANOCINCTUS

Anxiety
Clairvoyance
Concentration, difficult
Dullness, sluggishness, difficulty of think-
    ing and comprehending, torpor
Forgetful
Irritability
Loathing, life, at
Sadness, despondency, dejection, men-
    tal depression, gloom, melan-
    choly
    climaxis, during
Starting, sleep, from
Weeping, tearful mood

HYOSCYAMUS NIGER

Absent-minded, unobserving
Absorbed, buried in thought
Abstraction of mind
Abusive, insulting
    children insulting parents
Activity
    mental
Affectations ★
    gestures and acts, in
Affections, in general ★
Ailments from:
    anger, vexations
        anxiety, with
        silent grief, with
    anticipation, foreboding, presen-
    timent
    anxiety
    excitement, emotional
    fright

Ailments from:
  grief
  injuries, accidents; mental symp-
    toms from
  jealousy
  love, disappointed
  love, unhappy
  scorn, being scorned
Amativeness
Amorous
Anger, irascibility
  red face, with
  menses, during
  violent
Anguish
Animation agg. ★
Answers abruptly, shortly, curtly
  aversion to answer
  imaginary questions
  incoherently
  incorrectly
  irrelevantly
  monosyllable, "no" to all ques-
    tions
  refuses to answer
  slowly
  **stupor returns quickly after
    answer**
  unintelligibly
Antics, plays
  delirium, during
Anxiety
  night
  conscience, as if guilty of a crime
  dinner, after
  eating, after
  fear, with
  fits, with
  hypochondriacal
  menses, during
  motion, from
  paroxysms, in ★
  pursued, as if
Asks for nothing
Automatisms ★
Avarice
  generosity towards strangers,
    avarice as
      regards his family
  squandering on oneself, but

Aversion, everything, to
Battles, talks about
  war, talks of
Bed, get out of, wants to
  chill, during
  remain in, desires to
Bite, desires to
  disturbs him, bites everyone who ●
  objects, bites ●
Break things, desire to
Brooding, corner or moping, b. in a
Business, talks of
Busy
Cautious
Censorious, critical
cheerful, gay, mirthful
  night
  alternating with bursts of passion
  sadness
  dancing, laughing, singing, with
  followed by irritability
  menses, before
  sleep, during
  urination, after
Childish, behaviour
Clairvoyance
Climb, desire to
*Company, aversion to; presence of other
    people agg. the symptoms;
    desire for solitude*
  heat, during
**Company, desires for; aversion to
    solitude, company amel.**
  alone agg., while
Complaining
  supposed injury, of ●
Comprehension, easy
Concentration, active
  difficult
    attention, cannot fix ★
Confidence, want of self
Confounding objects and ideas
Confusion of mind
  morning
  afternoon
  air, in open
  chill, during
  eating, after

Confusion of mind
    heat, during
    intoxicated, as if
    mixes subjective and objective
Conscientious about trifles
Contemptuous
Contradict, disposition to
Contradiction, is intolerant of
Cruelty, inhumanity
Cursing, swearing
Dancing
Deceitful, sly
Delirium
    answers correctly when spoken to,
    but delurium and unconscious-
    ness return at once
    anxious
    attacks people with knife •
    bed and escapes, springs up sud-
    denly from
    business, talks of
    busy
    comical
    delusions, with
    embraces the stove •
    erotic
    exaltation of strength, with
    exhaustion, with
    face, with pale •
        red
    fantastic
    fever, during
    fierce
    foolish, silly
    frightful
    gather objects off the wall, tries to
    gay, cheerful
    hysterical, almost
    injuries to head, after
    jealousy, from •
    laughing
    loquacious
        indistinct
    maniacal
    menses, before
        during

murmuring
    himself, to
muttering
    himself, to
naked in delirium, wants to be
noisy
nonsense, with eyes open
pains, from
persecution in delirium, delusions
    of
quiet
raging, raving
rambling
recognizes no one
reproachful
restless
rocking to and fro
scolding
sleepiness, with
sleeplessness, and ★
trembling, with
vexation, from •
violent
waking, on
watching, vigil, from
wedding, prepares for •
wild
wraps up in fur during summer •
wrong, of fancied •
Delirium tremens, mania-a-potu
    sleeplessness, with
    trembling, with
Delusions, imaginations, halluci-
    nations, illusions
    activity, with
    animals, of
        beetles, worms etc.
        cup, moving in a •
        persons are
    ants, letters are •
    birds, picking feathers from, he
        is •
    bitten, will be
    calls, absent persons, for •
    catches at imaginary appearances

Delusions,
  cats, sees
  changeable •
  climbing up •
  crabs, of •
  criminal, he is a
  criminals, about
  criticised, she is
  dead persons, sees
  debate, of being in •
  demoniacal, thinks he is ★
  deserted, forsaken, is
  devils, sees
    possessed of a devil, is
  devoured by animals, had been •
  doomed, being
  driving peacocks •
  engaged in some occupation, is
  enlarged, body, parts of
    distances are
    objects are
  fall, things will
  fancy, illusions of
    heat, during
  figures, sees
  foolish
  friends affection of, has lost the
  geese, sees •
  grotesque, people appear •
  harlequin, he is a •
  hear, he cannot
  hearing, illusions of
  hens bound with chains •
  home, thinks is at, when not
    away from, is
    away from, must get there
  images, phantoms, sees
    frightful
  injury, is about to receive
  injured, is being, surround-
    ings, by his
  insects, sees
  journey, he is on a
  large, parts of body seem too
  loquacity, with
  ludicrous

HYOSCYAMUS NIGER

Delusions,
  married, is going to be •
  mice, sees
  murder someone, he has to
  murdered, he will be
  neglected his duty, he has
  noises, hears
  nuts, cracking •
  objects: seize o., tries to
  offended people, he has
  past, of events long
  peacocks, chasing •
    frightening away •
  people, sees
    converses with absent
  persecuted, he is
  places, wrong, in •
  poisoned, he has been
    he is about to be
  policeman come into house, he
    sees
  possessed, being
  present, someone is
  pursued by enemies
    he was
    police, by
  rats, sees
  religious
  room wall, horrible things on the,
    sees
  screaming, with
  see, cannot
  seized, as if
  small, things appear
  snakes in and around her
  sold, being •
  sounds, listens to imaginary •
  spectres, ghosts, spirits, sees
    clutches at •
  spinning, is
  stove, mistake stove for a tree •
    climb it, wants to •
  strange, familiar things seem
    ludicrous, are
    places seemed
  study, after

Delusions,
  suicide, driving to
  surroundings, strange ★
  swine, people are
  talking, dead people, with
      sister, with his
  violent
  visions, has
      fantastic
  vivid
  voices, hears
  war, being at
  watched, she is being
  wedding, of a
  well, he is
  wife is faithless
  wrong, he has done
      suffered, has
Dementia
Despair
  love, from disappointed
Destructiveness
  clothes, of
Dipsomania, alcoholism
Discouraged
Distances, inaccurate judge of
Doubtful, soul's welfare, of
Dream, as if in a
Dresses indecently,
Dullness, sluggishness, difficulty
    of thinking and compre-
    hending, torpor
      afternoon
  air, in open
  heat, during
  perspiration, during
  sleepiness, with
Dwells on past disagreeable occur-
    rences
  recalls disagreeable memories
Eat, refuses to
Eccentricity
Ecstasy
Escape, attempts to
  run away, to
  springs up suddenly from bed,
      change bed, to
  street, into ●
  springs up suddenly fumbed
      changes, bed to ●

Estranged: ignores his relatives
Excitement, excitable
  agg.
  menses, during
Exertion, agg. from mental
Faces, made ill-mannered ●
Fancies
  confused
  exaltation of
      night
  vivid, lively
Fear, apprehension, dread
  alone, of being
  betrayed, of being ●
  death, of
  dogs, of
  eating, after e., food
  enemies, of
  everything, constant of
  evil, of
  ghosts, of
  injured, of being
  knaves, of
  knives, of
  long-lasting ★
  men, dread, fear of
  noise, rushing water, of
  people, of
  poisoned, of being
  pursuit, of ●
  sold, of being ●
  starting, with
  syphilis, of
  waking, on
  water, of
  work, dread of
Fight, wants to
Fire, wants to set things on
Foolish behavior
Forgetful
  chill, during
Frightened easily
  waking, on
Frown, disposed to ★
Fur, wraps up, in summer
Generous, strangers, for

Gestures, makes
    actor, like an •
    automatic
    brushing the face or something
      away, as if •
    frightful
    grasping or reaching at some-
      thing, at flocks; carphologia
    genitals, delirium, during ★
      picks at bed clothes
    intoxicated, as if •
    hands, motions, involuntary,
      of the
    spinning and weaving ★
    nuts, as if opening •
    plays with his fingers
    ridiculous or foolish
    spinning, imitates •
    stamps the feet
    strange attitudes and positions
      arms, of
    sublime
    violent
Gossiping
Greed, cupidity
    grasping greedily with both hands
      anything offered him •
Grief
Grimaces
Groping as if in the dark
Haughty
Heedless
Hide, desire to
High-spirited
Home, desires to go
Homesickness
Honor, sense of h., no
Hurry, haste
    movements, in
Hydrophobia
    prophylactic ★
Hypochondriasis
Hysteria
    menses, before
      during

Ideas abundant, clearness of mind
    deficiency of
Idiocy
Imbecility
    laughing for nothing
    sexual excitement, with
Imitation, mimicry
Impatience
Impertinence
Impetuous, perspiration, with
Impulse, rash
    fire, to set on ★
Inciting others •
Indifference, apathy
    complain, does not
    everything, to
    exposure of her person, to
    naked, to remain
Indiscretion
Indolence, aversion to work
    afternoon
Industrious, mania for work
    menses, before
Inquisitive
Insanity, madness
    alternating mental with physical
      symptoms
    behaves like a crazy person
    convulsions, with
    dancing, with
    drunkards, in
    erotic
    foolish, ridiculous
    gluttony alternating with refusal
      to eat
    haughty
    heat, with
    immobile as a statue
    insensibility, painlessness, with
      general
    lamenting, moaning, only
    loquacious
    masturbation, from
    megalomania
    melancholy
    mental labor, from

Insanity,
 pregnancy, in
 puerperal
 quarrelsome ★
 religious
 restlessness, with
 sleeplessness, with
 strength increased, with
 suicidal disposition, with
 travel, with desire to
 wantonness, with
Insolence
Intriguer
Introspection,
Irresolution, indecision
 afternoon ●
 sleepiness, with ●
Irritability
 chill, during
 masturbation, after ●
 parturition, during
 sleeplessness, with
 spoken to, when
Jealousy
 animal or an inanimate object, for
 crime, to a, driving
 drunkenness, during
 kill, driving to ●
 rage, with ●
 vindictive ●
Jesting
 erotic
 ridiculous or foolish
Jumping
 bed, out of
 fever, during
Kill, desire to
 drunkenness, during
 everyone he sees ●
 injure with a knife, impulse to
 knife, with a
 somebody, thought he ought to
  kill
 walking in open air and street,
  while
Kisses everyone
Lamenting, bemoaning, wailing

Lascivious, lustful
 uncovers sexual parts ●
Laughing
 agg.
 alternating with quietness ●
  whining, moaning
 constant
 dream, during
 forced ●
 imbecility
 immoderately
 involuntarily
 love, from disappointed ●
 loudly
 ludicrous, everything seems
 menses, before
 sardonic
 silly
 sleep, during
 spasmodic
 trifles, at
Libertinism
Light, shuns
Loathing, general
Loathing, life, at
 work, at
Loquacity
 hasty
 insane
 perspiration, during
 rambling ★
 vivacious
Love, disappointed
 jealousy, anger and incoherent
 talk, with
 laugh, with inclination to ●
 rage after ●
 sadness from
 suicidal disposition from
Malicious, spiteful, vindictive
 insulting
Mania
 demoniac
 erotic ★
 rage, with
 violence, with deeds of
Meddlesome, importunate

Meditation
Memory, active
  involuntary recollections ★
  past events, for
Memory, weakness of
  business, for
  done, for what has just
  heard, for what has
  persons, for
  read, for what has
  said, for what has
  thought, for what has just
Menses, mental symptoms agg. before
  during
Misanthropy
Mischievous
Mistakes, differentiating of objects, in
  reading, in
  speaking, in
    misplacing words
    words, using wrong
Moaning, groaning, whining
  sleep, during
    why, does not know ●
Mocking
  ridicule, passion to
Mood, alternating
  changeable, variable
Moral feeling, want of
Morose, cross, fretful, ill-humor, peevish
  sleepiness, with
Morphinism
Multilating his body
Muttering
  sleep, in
  sleeplessness, with ●
  unintelligible
Naive, intelligent, but very
Naked, wants to be
  morning in bed
  delirium, in
  drunkenness, during ●
  hyperaesthesia of skin, in ●
  sleep, in
Nymphomania
  menses, during
    suppressed, after

Obscene, lewd
  songs
  talk
Obstinate, headstrong
  children
Offended, easily; takes everything in
  bad part
Overactive
Passionate
Pessimist
Praying
Prostration of mind, mental exhaustion, brain-fag
Quarrelsome, scolding
  jealousy, from
Quiet disposition
  alternating with rage ●
Rage, fury
  day and night ●
  evening
  night
  alternating with repose ●
  convulsions, rage with
  epilepsy, rage with
  kill people, tries to
  love, after disappointed ●
  menses, during
  shining objects, from
  shrieking, with
  strength increased
  violent
  water, at sight of
Recognize anyone, does not
  relatives, does not recognize his
Refuses to take the medicine
Religious affections
  narrow-minded in religious questions
  talking on religious subjects ●
Remorse
Reproaches himself
  others
Reserved
Restlessness
  morning
  afternoon
  night
  bed, driving out of
  go from one bed to another,

Restlessness
> *wants to*
>> tossing about in
> busy
> driving about
> menses, during
> metrorrhagia, during
Reveals secrets
Reverence for those around him
Roving about naked •
> senseless, insane
Rudeness
Runs about
> room, in
Sadness, despondency, dejection,
> **mental depression, gloom,**
> **melancholy**
>> continence, from
>> eating, after
>> flowers, smell of •
>> *love, from disappointed*
>> urination amel.
Satyriasis
Senses, dull, blunted
> vanishing of
Sensitive, oversensitive
> morning
> noise, to
>> *chill, during*
> want of sensitiveness
Serious, earnest
Shamelessness
> **exposes the person**
Shining objects agg.
Shrieking, screaming, shouting
> anxiety, from
> brain cry
> chilldren sh., sleep, and sob, in ★
> convulsions, before
>> **during**
>> **epileptic**
>> *puerperal*
> delusions, with
> drunkenness, during
> plaintively, stupor, in, touch agg. ★
> *sleep, during*
> waking, on
>> without ★

Sighing
Singing
Sit, inclination to
Sits, erect
> *stiff, quite*
> still
Slander, disposition to
Slowness
Smiling
> foolish
> sleep, in
Solemn
Somnambulism
Speech :
> *affected*
> *babbling*
> *confused*
> *delirious*
> facile
> fine •
> **foolish**
> future, about •
> **hasty**
> **incoherent**
> **intoxicated, as if**
> *loud*
> **nonsensical**
> **prattling**
>> **lies naked in bed and**
>> **prattles •**
> **unintelligible**
> **vivacious**
> **wandering**
Spitting, faces of people, in
Spoken to, averse to being
> *chill, during* •
Starting, startled
> convulsive
> **fright, from and as from**
> **sleep, during**
>> **from**
Strange, crank
Striking
> *about him at imaginary objects*
> *bystanders, at*
> **desires to strike**
> drunkenness, during

327

Striking himself, knocking his head
    against wall and things
Stupefaction, as if intoxicated
    convulsions, between
    eating, agg. after
    sits motionless like a statue
Suicidal, disposition
    delusions, from
    despair, from
    drowning, by
        love, from disappointed •
    knife, with
    throwing himself from a height
Suppressed or receding skin diseases
    or haemorrhoids, mental symp-
    toms agg. after
Suspicious, mistrustful
Syphilophobia ★
Talk, indisposed to, desire to be silent,
    taciturn
    others agg., talk of
Talking, sleep, in
    confess themselves loud,
        they
    war, of •
Talks, dead people, with
    himself, to
Tastelessness in dressing
Tears things
Thinking, aversion to
Thoughts, persistent
    rapid, quick
    rush, flow of
    night
        partial, sleep, in •
    stagnation, of
    thoughtful
    wandering
Timidity
    bashful
Torpor
Touch everything, impelled to
Tranquillity, serenity, calmness
Truth, tell the plain

Unconsciousness
    morning
    alcoholic
    answers correctly when spoken
        to, but delirium and uncon-
        sciousness return at once
    apoplexy, in
    conduct, automatic
    fever, during
    frequent spells of u., absences
    hydrocephalus, in
    mental insensibility
    remains motionless like a statue
    twitching of limbs, with
Unfeeling, hard hearted
Violent, vehement
    beats the head ★
    deeds of violence, rage leading to
Vivacious
Wanders restlessly about
Weary of life
Weeping, tearful mood
    night
    aloud, wobbing
    alternating with laughter
    children, in
    convulsions, during
    menses, during
    sleep, in
    waking, on
    whimpering
        sleep, during
Well, says he is, when very sick
Wildness
Work, aversion to mental
    afternoon
    impossible

HYOSCYAMINUM
BROMATUM

Delirium
    giggling •
    laughing
    quiet

Delirium tremens, mania-a-potu
Excitement, excitable
    children, in
Gestures, grasping or reaching at some-
    thing, at flocks; carphologia
Irritability
Mania
Restlessness
    children, in
Starting, sleep, from

HYPERICUM PERFORATUM

Activity, mental, desire for
Ailments from :
    fright
    injuries, accidents; mental symp-
    toms from
Anxiety
    fever, during
Confusion of mind
    morning
        waking, on
    waking, on
Delirium
    aroused to answer questions, could
        be •
    raging, raving
    sleep, during
Delusions, bed, no lying on (on waking
    4h.) •
    spectres, ghosts, spirits, sees
    voices of dead people, hears
Despair, pains, with the
Dullness, morning
    injuries of head, after
Excitement, excitable
    evening
Fear, apprehension, dread
    downward motion, of
    falling, of
Frightened easily
    trifles, at
Hydrophobia
Ideas abundant, clearness of mind
Indolence, aversion to work
Industrious, mania for work
Insanity, pain, from intolerable

Irritability
Lascivious, lustful
Memory, loss of, aphasia, in
    concussion of the brain, after •
    injuries of head, after
Memory, weakness of
    say, for what is about to
Mistakes, speaking
    misplacing words
    spelling, in
    words, using wrong, putting
    right for left
        or vice versa
    writing, in
        omitting letters
        words
        wrong words
Prostration of mind, mental exhaus-
    tion, brain-fag
    injuries, from
Rage, fury
Religious affections
Restlessness
    morning
        waking, on
    night
    heat, during
    waking, on
Sadness, despondency, dejection, men-
    tal depression, gloom, melan-
    choly
    morning
    evening
    injuries, from •
Sensitive, pain, to
Shrieking, screaming, shouting
Singing, shrieking and weeping, fol-
    lowed by •
    sleep, in
Soberness
Speech, sharp
    wild in sleep •
Starting, startled
    easily
    fright, from and as from
    sleep, during

Strength increased, mental
Talking, sleep, in
Thoughts, sexual
Thunderstorm, mind symptoms before
Unbearable, pains ★
Unconsciousness, exertion, after
Weeping, evening
Work, aversion to mental

HYPOTHALAMUS

Affability
Anxiety
    dark, in
Discouraged
Fear, sleep, close the eyes lest he
    should never wake, fear to
Love with one of own sex, homosexual-
    ity, tribadism
Mildness
Sadness, despondency, dejection, mental
    depression, gloom, melancholy
    exertion, after
Sensitive, oversensitive
Weeping, alternating with laughter
    trifles, at
Will, loss of
Work, mental, fatigues

IBERIS AMARA

Activity, mental
Concentration, difficult
Confusion of mind
Discouraged
Dullness, sluggishness, difficulty of
    thinking and comprehending,
    torpor
Excitement, excitable
Face, with cold perspiration of λ
Fear, apprehension, dread
    medicine, of taking too much
    tremulous
Frightened easily
    evening
Grief
Irritability
    morning
Memory, active
Memory, weakness of
    heard, for what has just
Morose, cross, fretful, ill-humor, peevish
Restlessness
    night
Sadness, despondency, dejection, men-
    tal depression, gloom, melan-
    choly
Sighing
Weeping, tearful mood

ICHTHYOLUM

Concentration, difficult
Dipsomania, alcoholism
Memory, weakness of

ICTODES FOETIDA

Absent minded, unobserving
Abstraction of mind
Anger, violent
Anguish, stool, before
Anxiety
    sudden
Concentration, difficult
Contradict, disposition to
Contradiction, is intolerant of
Hysteria
Impetuous
Morose, cross, fretful, ill-humor, peevish
Quarrelsome, scolding
Violent, vehement

IGNATIA AMARA

Absent minded, unobserving
Absorbed, buried in thought
Abusive, insulting
Activity, restless
Admonition, kindly agg.
Affections, in general ★
Affectionate
Ailments from :
    anger, vexation
    anxiety, with
    fright, with
    silent grief, with
        suppressed
    **anticipation, foreboding, pre-
        sentiment**
    bad news
    cares, worries
    contradiction
    death of a child
        parents or friends, of
    disappointment
        new ●
    embarrassment
    excitement, emotional
        moral ★
    fear
    friendship, deceived
    fright
    grief
    homesickness
    honor, wounded

Ailments from :
    jealousy
    literary, scientific failure
    love, disappointed
        unhappy
    mortification
    pecuniary loss
    position, loss of
    punishment
    reproaches
    shame
    work, mental
Amativeness
Amorous
Amusement, averse to
Anger, irascibility
    alternating with cheerfulness
        hysteria ●
        jesting
    contradiction, from
    reproaches, from
    talk, indisposed to
    violent
Anguish, menses, during
Anorexia mentalis
Antics, plays
Anxiety
    morning
        waking, on
    night
        midnight on waking, after
    air, in open
    bed, in
    chill, during
    coffee, after
    conscience, as if guilty of a crime
    faintness, with
    fear, with
    fever, during
    fits, with
    flushes of heat, during
    fright, after
    head, with congestion to
    health, about
    house amel., in ●
    hypochondriacal
    menses, before
        during
            anger and anxiety

Anxiety,
  paroxysms, in ★
  pregnancy, in
  salvation, about
    scruples, excessive religious
    scrupulous as to their religious
      practices, too
  waking, on
  walking, while
  air, in open
Approach of persons agg.
Attention agg ★
Audacity
Aversion to women
Awkward ★
Benevolence
Beside oneself, being
Bite, desire to
Brooding
Busy
Capriciousness
  evening
Cares, worries, full of ★
  sleeplessness from ★
Carried, desires to be
Cautious
Censorious, critical
Chaotic, confused behavior
Cheerful, gay, mirthful
  alternating with anger
    bursts of indignation
    bursts of passion
    sadness
Childish, behavior
Climacteric period agg.
**Company, aversion to; presence of
  other people agg. the symp-
  toms; desire for solitude**
  loathing at company
*Company, desire for; aversion to soli-
  tude, company amel.*
Complaining
  sleep, in
Comprehension, easy
Concentration, difficult
  attention, cannot fix ★
Confidence, want of self

Confusion of mind
  morning
    rising and after, on
    waking, on
  beer, from
  dream, as if in
  heat, during
  intoxicated, as if
  motion, from
  waking, on
Conscientious about trifles
  eating, after ●
Consolation, kind words agg.
Contemptuous
Contradict, disposition to
Contradiction, is intolerant of
  agg.
Contrary
Conversation agg.
Courageous
Cowardice
  opinion, without courage of own
Dancing
  amel.
**Deception causes grief and morti-
  fication ★**
Defiant
Delirium
  anxious
  fever, during
  haemorrhage, after
  hysterical, almost
  laughing
  look fixed on one point, staring
  sleep, falling asleep, on
  sleeplessness, and ★
  trembling, with
Delirium tremens, mania-a-potu
**Delusions, imaginations, halluci-
  nations, illusions**
    evening in bed
  anxious
  crime, he had committed a
  criminal, he is a
  criticised, she is
  disease, has incurable

Delusions,

    doomed, being
        soul cannot be saved, cries and
        rages •
    falling asleep, on
    fancy, illusions of
    images, phantoms, sees
        night
        frightful
    insulted, he is
    laughed at, mocked, being
    married, he is •
    murdered, he will be
    neglected his duty, he has
    persecuted, he is
    pregnant, she is
    ruined, he is
    snakes, white ★
        in and around her
    spectres, ghosts, spirits, sees
        closing eyes, on
    stomach, has corrosion of; an
        ulcer
    troubles, broods over imaginary
    visions, has, evening
        closing the eyes, on
        horrible
        monsters on falling asleep and
            on waking, of •
    voices, hears
    vow, she is breaking her •
    walk, cannot, he
    water, of
    wrong, he has done
Dementia
    senilis
Desires, full of
Despair
    chill, during
    heat, during
    lost, thinks everything is
    recovery, of
    religious despair of salvation
    social position, of
Destructiveness, clothes, of
Dipsomania, alcoholism
Disconcerted

Discontented, displeased, dissatisfied
    evening
    everything, with
    headache, during
Discouraged
Doubtful, recovery, of
Dullness, sluggishness, difficulty of think-
    ing and comprehending, torpor
    morning
        waking, on
    evening
    chagrin, vexation, from
    heat, during
    mental exertion, from
Eat, refuses to
Ecstasy
Embittered, exasperated
Emptiness, sensation of ★
Ennui, tedium
Escape, attempts to
Excitement, excitable
    agg.
    bad news, after
    climacteric period, during
    hearing horrible things, after
    women, in
Exertion, agg. from mental
Exhilaration
Fancies, exaltation of
        evening in bed
        night
        going to bed, after
        sleeplessness, with
    lascivious
    sleep, falling asleep, on
    vivid, lively
    waking, on
Fear, apprehension, dread
    morning
    night
    midnight, after
    anorexia from fear •
    approaching him, of others
    away from home ★
    birds ★
    death, of

Fear,
    waking from afternoon sleep,
      on ★
  diarrhoea, from
  disease, of impending
    cancer, of ★
    incurable, being
  doctors, of ★
  insanity, losing his reason, of
  men, dread, fear of
  narrow places, in; claustrophobia ★
  noise, from
  people, of; anthropophobia
  poisoned, of being
  position, to lose his lucrative
  restlessness from fear
  robbers, of
    midnight on waking
  sleep again, he will never •
  stomach, of ulcer in
  trifles, of
  waking, on
Feigning sick
Fists, makes (after fright) •
Foolish behavior
Forgetful
  everything except dreams, of •
Fright, menses, during ★
Frightened easily
  night
  waking, on
    dream, from a
Gestures, convulsive
  ridiculous or foolish
  stamp the feet, children, during
    sleep •
Grief
  headache from grief
  losing objects, grief after •
  offences, grief from long past
  silent
  undemonstrative
Grimaces
Grunting
  sleep, during •
Hatred, men, of
Haughty
Heedless
Hide, desire to

Homesickness
Honor, wounded
Horrible things, sad stories, affect her
    profoundly
Howling
Hurry, haste
  mental work, in
  writing, in
Hypochondriasis
Hysteria
  climacteric period, at
  fainting, hysterical
  grief, from
  menses, during
Ideas abundant, clearness of mind
  deficiency of
Imbecility
  negativism
  shrieks on being engaged
Impatience
  menses, during ★
Impulsive
Inconstancy
Indifference, apathy
  chill, during
  everything, to
  music, which he loves, to
  weeping, with
  work, with aversion to
Indignation
Indiscretion
Indolence, aversion to work
  eating, after
Industrious, mania for work
  menses, before
Injustice, cannot support
Insanity, madness
  anger, from
  black insanity with despair and
    weary of life from fear of
    mortification or of loss of
    position
  cheerful, gay
  fortune, after losing
  fright, from
  melancholy
  menses, with copious ★
    with suppressed
  position, from fear to lose one's

Intolerance, noise, of
Introspection
Irresolution, indecision
   changeable
   marry, to
Irritability
   afternoon
   evening
   air, amel. in open
   chill, during
   consolation agg.
   contradiction, at slightest ●
   pain, during
   trifles, from
   warm room, in
Jealousy
Jesting
   alternating with anger
      weeping ●
Kicks with legs (in convulsions) ●
Lamenting, bemoaning, wailing
   perspiration, during ●
Lascivious, lustful
Laughing
   alternating with shrieking
   convulsions, before, during or after
   immoderately
   involuntarily
   sardonic
   serious matters, over
   spasmodic
Loquacity, alternating with silence
   sleep, during
   speeches, makes
Love, disappointed
   sadness from
   silent grief, with
Magnetized, desire to be, mesmerism
   amel.
Malicious, spiteful, vindictive
Mania
Meditation
Memory, weakness of
   expressing oneself, for
   labor, for mental
   music, for
Mental symptoms alternating with
   physical ★

Mildness
   complaining, bears suffering, even
      outrage without ●
Mistakes, speaking, in
   hurry, from ●
   writing, in
   hurry, from ●
Moaning, groaning, whining
   convulsions, in
   heat, during
   sleep, during
Mocking
   others are mocking at him, thinks
   sarcasm
Monomania
Mood, agreeable
   alternating
   changeable, variable
   repulsive
Morose, cross, fretful, ill-humor, peevish
   evening
   chill, during
   contradiction, by
   pain, after
   waking, on
Music agg.
   agreeable, is
Narrating her symptoms agg.
Nymphomania
Obstinate, headstrong
   evening
Occupation, diversion amel.
Offended, easily; takes everything in
   bad part
   offences, from past
Paradoxical ★
Passionate
Playful
Pregnancy, mental affections in
Prostration of mind, mental exhaustion, brain-fag
   evening
   night
   grief, from long ●

Punishment agg. mental symptoms •
Quarrelsome, scolding
Quick to act ★
Quiet disposition
Rage, fury
Religious affections
    very religious ★
Remorse
    menses, after •
Reproaches, himself
        others
Reserved
Restlessness
        night
    bed, tossing about in
    busy
    headache, during
    menses, during
    move, must constantly
Rudeness
Sadness, despondency, dejection,
    mental depression, gloom,
    melancholy
        morning on waking
        afternoon
            twilight, in
        evening
    anger, from
    chill, during
    climaxis, during
    grief, after
    heat, during
    labor, during
    love, from disappointed
    menses, during
    mortification, after
    perspiration, during
    quiet
    sighing, with
    sleeplessness from sadness
        with
    suicidal disposition, with
    talk, indisposed to
    waking, on
    weep, cannot
Searching on floor
Secretive

Self accusation, with anger ★
Selfishness, egoism
Senses, acute
    dull, blunted
Sensitive, oversensitive
    moral impressions, to
    music, to
    noise, to
        talking, of
    odors, to
    pain, to
    reprimands, to
Sentimental
Serious, earnest
Shrieking, screaming, shouting
    aid, for
    approaches bed, when anyone •
    brain cry
    children, in
        on waking with trembling ★
        sleep, during
    chorea, in
    convulsions, during epileptic
    drunkenness, during
    paroxysmal
    sleep, during
    waking, on
Sighing
        morning, 9.30 h. •
        night, 2h. •
    heat, during
    hysteria, in
    menses, before
        during
    perspiration, during
        weeping, continues long after •
Sit, inclination to
Slowness
Somnambulism
Speech, hasty
    incoherent on waking
    prattling
    wandering
Spoken to, averse to being
Staring ★

336

Starting, startled
frequently •
heat, during
menses, during
sleep, on falling
during
from
Striking
Starving ★
Stupefaction, as if intoxicated
Suicidal disposition
drowning, by
poison, by
sadness, from
thoughts
throwing himself from a height
Suppressed or receding skin diseases
or haemorrhoids, mental symptoms agg. after
Suspicious, mistrustful
Sympathy, compassion
Talk, indisposed to, desire to be silent,
taciturn
alternating with loquacity
fright, after •
mortification, after •
sadness, in
suffering, over his •
Talking, sleep, in
unpleasant things agg., of
Talks, himself, to
Tears things
Thoughts, persistent
evening
desires, of
music, in evening about •
unpleasant subjects, on waking
rapid, quick
rush, flow of
thoughtful
wandering
Timidity
bashful
Touched, aversion to being
Tranquillity, serenity, calmness
Travel, amel. ★

Trifles seem important
Unconsciousness, coma, stupor
morning
crowded room, in a
emotion, after
frequent spells of u. absences
menses, during
semi-consciousness
transient
Undertakes many things, perseveres in
nothing
Violent, vehement
deeds of violence, rage leading to
Walk, walking in open air agg. mental
symptoms
amel.
Wearisome
Weeping, tearful mood
night
sleep, in
admonition, from
aloud, wobbing
alternating with cheerfulness
jesting •
laughter
amel.
anxiety, after
caressing, from
children, in
chill, during
consolation agg.
contradiction, from
convulsions, during
heat, during
involuntary
menses, during
music, from
noise, at
offence, about former
pregnancy, during
refused, when anything
remonstrated, when
sleep, in
spasmodic
spoken to, when
trifles, at

Weeping, tearful mood
 vexations, from
  from old
 waking, on
 whimpering
  sleep, during
Wildness, trifles, at •
Will, weakness of
Work, mental, fatigues
 impossible
  evening •
Writing, inability for
 learning to as rapidly as she us.
 wishes, anxious behavior,
  makes mistakes •
Yielding disposition

INDIUM METALLICUM

Absent-minded, unobserving
Dullness, sluggishness, difficulty of thinking and comprehending, torpor
 pollutions, after
 reading, while
Excitement, mental work, from
Fear, work, dread of
Heedless
Indifference, apathy
Indolence, aversion to work
Irritability, headache, during
 menses, during
 sleepiness, with •
Love with one of the own sex, homosexuality tribodism perversity
Morose, cross, fretful, ill-humor, peevish
 menses, during
Prostration of mind, mental exhaustion, brain-fag
Restlessness
 night
 mental labor, during and after
 study, when attempting to
Sadness, despondency, dejection, mental
 depression, gloom, melancholy
Stupefaction, as if intoxicated
 waking, on
Weeping, tearful mood
 menses, during

Work, aversion to mental
 seems to drive him crazy, owing
 to the impotency of his mind

INDIGO TINCTORIA

Absorbed, buried in thought
Anger, irascibility
 epileptic attack before •
Anxiety
Confusion of mind
 motion, from
Delirium, maniacal
Delusions, fancy, illusions of
 goitre, he has a
Discontented, displeased, dissatisfied
Dullness, sluggishness, difficulty of think-
 ing and comprehending, torpor
Excitement, epilepsy, before
Hysteria
Indolence, aversion to work
 morning
 forenoon
Industrious, mania for work
Insanity, madness
Introspection
Irritability
 evening
Mania
Mildness
 epileptic attacks, after •
Morose, cross, fretful, ill-humor, peevish
 evening
Muttering, sleep, in
Reserved
Restlessness, night
Sadness, despondency, dejection, mental
 depression, gloom, melancholy
Senses, dull, blunted
Starting, night
 dreams, from a dream
 sleep, during
Talking, sleep, in
Wearisome
Weeping, night
 convulsions, during epileptic

INDOLUM

Concentration, difficult
Discontented, displeased, dissatisfied
Dullness, sluggishness, difficulty of think-
    ing and comprehending, torpor
Indifference, apathy
Irritability
Morose, cross, fretful, ill-humor, peevish
Sadness, despondency, dejection, mental
    depression, gloom, melancholy

INULA HELENIUM

Anxiety
    menses, during
Cheerful, gay, mirthful
Shrieking, children, during sleep
    sleep, during
Starting, startled
    sleep, during

IODIUM PURUM

Absorbed, buried in thought
Activity, amel.
Ailments from:
    anger, vexation
    fright
    love disappointed
    sexual excesses
    shock, mental
    work, mental
Amorous
Anger, irascibility
    touched, when
Answers, aversion to answer
    difficult
Anxiety
    cough, before
    driving from place to place
    eating amel.
    fasting, when •
    future, about
    hungry, when
    hypochondriacal
    manual labor, from •
    mental exertion, from
    rest, during
    sitting amel.
    walking in open air amel., while

Aversion to being approached
    his own mind, to ★
    members of family, to
Busy
Capriciousness
Cares, worries
Carefulness
    over - careful ★
Cheerful, gay, mirthful
    alternating with sadness
        weeping
Company, aversion to; presence of other
    people agg. the symptoms; de-
    sire for solitude
    avoids the sight of people
    friends, of intimate
    presence of strangers, aversion to
Concentration, difficult
    drawing, when
    studying, reading etc., while
Confidence, want of self
Confusion of mind
    morning
    evening
    mental exertion, from
    warm room, in
Conscientious about trifles
Conversation agg.
Cowardice
Cross, crossness (anger) ★
Delirium
    bed and escape, springs up sud-
        denly from
    congestion, with
    fever, during
    restless
Delusions, imaginations, hallucinations,
    illusions
    dead persons, sees
    fancy, illusions of
    fasting
        afternoon
    iodine, illusions of fumes of •
    sick, being
    water, of
    well, he is
Despair
Destructiveness
Discomfort, dinner, after

Discontented, displeased, dissatisfied
  everything, with
Discouraged
Dullness, sluggishness, difficulty of thinking and comprehending, torpor
  children, in
  eating, amel.
  reading, while
Eating, amel. of mental symptoms after
Ecstasy
  perspiration, during
Elated
Escape, attempts to
Excitement, excitable
  afternoon
  nervous
  wine, after
Exertion, agg. from mental
  physical exertion amel.
Exhilaration
Extravagance
Exuberance
Fancies, exaltation of
  perspiration, during
Fear, apprehension, dread
  accidents, of
  approaching him, of others
  death, of
  evil, of
  failure, of
  happen, something will
  imaginary things of
  insanity, losing his reason, of
      if he wants to repose, must
        always move
  labour after •
  manual labor, after •
  misfortune, of
  people, of; anthropophobia
  physician will not see her; he
    seems to terrify her
  restlessness from fear
  sitting amel. •
  touch, of
  warm room, in •
  water, of
Forgetful
  purchases, of; goes off and leaves
    them
*Forgotten something, feels constantly
  as if he had*

Frightened easily
Gestures, convulsive
  *grasping or reaching at something,
    at flocks; carphologia
  picks at bedclothes*
**Horrible things, sad stories, affect
  her profoundly**
Hurry, haste
  walking, while
Hydrophobia
Hypochondriasis
Hysteria
Ideas, deficiency of
Imbecility
Impatience
  runs about, never sits or sleeps at
    night •
Impulse, morbid
  run, to; dromomania
Indifference, apathy
  pain, to
Indolence, aversion to work
  physical
Industrious, mania for work
Initiative, lack of
Insanity, madness
  busy
Irresolution, indecision
Irritability
  afternoon
  eating, after
  headache, during
  noise, from
Jesting, joke, cannot take a
Kill, desire to
  herself, sudden impulse to ★
  rest desire to kill, during •
  *woman, irresistible, impulse to
    kill a* •
Looked at, cannot bear to be
Loquacity
  cheerful, exuberant
  headless
Magnetized, des. to be mesmerism amel.
Mania
Manual work, fine work, mind symptoms from
Memory, weakness of
  do, for what was about to
  say, for what is about to

Mildness
Misanthropy
Mood, alternating
  changeable, variable
Morose, cross, fretful, ill-humor, peevish
  eating, after
Nothing ails him, says ★
Occupation, diversion amel.
**Offended, easily, takes everything
  in bad part**
Prostration of mind, mental exhaustion, brain-fag
Restlessness
  morning
  night
  midnight, after 1.30-4.30h. •
    2h.
  anxious
  bed, in
    driving out
  move, must constantly
  room, in
  sitting, while
  warm bed agg.
Runs about
**Sadness, despondency, dejection,
  mental depression, gloom,
  melancholy**
  afternoon
  anxious
  coughing, after
  digestion, during •
  eating, after
Selfishness; egoism
Senses, dull, blunted
Sensitive, oversensitive
  external impressions, to all
  noise, to slightest ★
  sensual impressions, to
Serious, earnest
Shrieking, convulsions, after puerperal
Sit, inclination to
  head on hands and elbows on
    knees, with
Sitting, aversion to
Spoken to, averse to being
  alone, wants to be let
Starting, sleep, during

Stupefaction, as if intoxicated
Suicidal, disposition
  throwing himself from a height
Sympathy, compassion
Talk, indisposed to, desire to be silent,
  taciturn
Tears things
Thinking, complaints agg., of
  about his own wrong, agg. ★
Thoughts, frightful
  future, of the
  persistent
    homicide
    stagnation of
    vagueness of
    vanishing of
    wandering
Timidity
  bashful
Torpor
Touched, aversion to being
Travel, desires to
Unconsciousness, coma, stupor
  vertigo, during
Violent, vehement
  deeds of violence, rage leading to
Vivacious
Weeping, tearful mood
  alternating with cheerfulness
  eating, after
  spoken to, kindly (children)
Well, says he is, when very sick

IODOFORMIUM

Cheerful, gay, mirthful
Delirium
Eccentricity
Loquacity
Mania
Shrieking, screaming, shouting
  sleep, during
Suicidal, disposition
  throwing himself from a height
    window from
Violent, deeds of violence, rage leading
  to

IPECACUANHA

Absorbed, buried in thought
Abusive, insulting
Ailments from:
    anger, vexation
      indignation, with
    suppressed
    grief
    indignation
    scorn, being scorned
Anger, irascibility
    business, about •
    noise, at
    trifles, at
Anxiety
    morning
      waking, on
    fever, during
    sleep, during
    waking, on
Aversion, everything, to
Brooding
Capriciousness
Carried, desires to be
Cautious
Censorious, critical
Cheerful, gay, mirthful
Confusion of mind
    evening
    heat, during
Contemptuous
    everything, to
Contrary
Cowardice
Cursing, swearing
Delirium
Delusions, unfortunate, he is '
Desire, full of
    indefinite
    inexpressible, full of •
Dipsomania, alcoholism
Discontented, displeased, dissatisfied
    everything, with
Discouraged
Disgust
    everything, with

Dullness, sluggishness, difficulty of
    thinking and comprehending,
    torpor
Fear, apprehension, dread
    morning
    night
    death, of
    heat, during
    misfortune, of
    sighing, with
Forgetful
Forsaken, feeling
Gestures, covers mouth with hands
    **grasping, children put fingers
    in the mouth**
Gourmand
Greed, cupidity
Grief, silent
Haughty
Howling
Hurry, haste
Hypochondriasis
Hysteria
Ideas, deficiency of
Impatience
    heat, with
Indifference, apathy
    joyless
    pleasure, to
    sleepiness, with
Indignation
Indolence, aversion to work
    sleepiness, with
Industrious, mania for work
    menses, before
Insanity, gluttony alternating with re-
    fusal to eat
Introspection
Irresolution, indecision
Irritability
    daytime
    business, about
    children, in
    heat, during
    noise, from
Jealousy
    *appreciate anything, desires that
    others should not* •

Jesting
Lamenting, bemoaning, wailing
Loathing, general
Loquacity
Malicious, spiteful, vindictive
Meditation
Memory, weakness of
Moaning, groaning, whining
    heat, during
    sleep, during
Mocking
Mood, repulsive
Morose, cross, fretful, ill-humor, peevish
    daytime
    business does not proceed fast,
        when •
    fever, during
Morphinism
Obstinate, headstrong
Passionate
Prostration of mind, mental exhaustion, brain-fag
Quarrelsome, scolding
Quiet, disposition
Reserved
Restlessness
    bed, tossing about in
    busy
    children, in
    heat, during
    menses, during
Revelry, feasting
Sadness, despondency, dejection, mental depression, gloom, melancholy
    heat, during
Sensitive, oversensitive
    noise, to
Shrieking, screaming, shouting
    children with fist in mouth ★
    convulsions, before
        during ★
    please, hard to ★
    sleep, during

Sighing
    heat, during
    perspiration, during
Sit, inclination to
Slander, disposition to
Slowness
Starting, sleep, on falling
    during
Strange, crank
Stupefaction, as if intoxicated
    walking, when
Suspicious, mistrustful
Talk, indisposed to, desire to be silent, taciturn
Thoughts, thoughtful
    vanishing of
Timidity
Tranquillity, serenity, calmness
    anger, after •
Trifles, seem important
Unconsciousness, coma, stupor
    fever, during
Unfortunate, feels
Walk, walking in open air agg. mental symptoms
Wearisome
Weeping, tearful mood
    night
    children, babies, in
    convulsions, during
    coughing, during
    desire to weep, all the time
    heat, during
    sleep, in
    whimpering
    sleep, during
Will, weakness of
Work, aversion to mental

IRIDIUM METALLICUM

Concentration, difficult

IRIS VERSICOLOR

Activity
Ailments from :
    work, mental
Anger, irascibility
    easily
    waking, on
Anxiety, waking, on
Censorious, critical
Company, aversion to, alone, amel.
    when ★
Concentration, difficult
Delirium
    muttering
Discouraged
Dullness, sluggishness, difficulty of think-
    ing and comprehending, torpor
Exertion, agg. from mental
Fear, death, of
    disease, of impending
    waking, on
Frightened easily
Irritability
    daytime
    morning on waking
    waking, on
Laughing, actions, at his own
Memory, weakness of
Morose, cross, fretful, ill-humor, peevish
    daytime
Muttering
Restlessness
    night
Sadness, despondency, dejection, men-
    tal depression, gloom, melan-
    choly
    headache, during
    menses, before ★
Senses, dull, blunted
Starting, sleep, during
Suicidal disposition,
    menses, before ★
    thoughts ★
Thoughts wandering, writing, while
Unconsciousness, fever, during

IRIS FLORENTINA

Delirium

IRIS FOETIDISSIMA

Confusion of mind
    standing, amel. while ●
Delirium
Mistakes, speaking, in
    word, using wrong, putting right
      for left or vice versa
    writing, in
Restlessness, morning

IRIS TENAX

Homesickness
Mania

J

JABORANDI

Anxiety
Cheerful, alternating with dullness •
Confusion of mind
Delirium, night
Delusions, murder her family with a
    hatchet, she will •
Dullness alternating with hilarity and
    mirth
Restlessness
    evening
Talk, indisposed to, desire to be silent,
    taciturn

JACARANDA GUALANDAI

Restlessness, night

JACARANDA CAROBA

Sadness, despondency, dejection, mental
    depression, gloom, melancholy
Sit, inclination to
Starting, fright, from and as from

JALAPA

Anxiety
    stool, during
Irritability, children, good all day, cross
    all night •
Morose, night
Restlessness
    anxious
    children, in
Shrieking, screaming, shouting
    night
    children, in

Weeping, children, in
    babies
    *sleep, in, child good during the
        day, screaming and restless at
        night* •

JASMINUM OFFICINALE

Helplessness, feeling of
Unconsciousness, coma, stupor

JATROPHA CURCAS

Anguish
Answers, abruptly, shortry, curtly
Anxiety
    night
    **burning of stomach, with cold-
        ness of body** ★
    sleep, after
Confusion of mind
Delirium
    raging, raving
Ecstasy
Fear, apprehension, dread
    cholera, of
    water of
Indifference, apathy
    pain, to
Irritability
    morning on waking
    waking, on
Loathing, general
Morose, cross, fretful, ill-humor, peevish
    waking, on
Rage, fury
Restlessness
    night
Shrieking, cramps in abdomen, during
Stupefaction, as if intoxicated
Talk, indisposed to, desire to be silent,
    taciturn
Unconsciousness, coma, stupor
    vertigo, during

JATROPHA URENS

Unconsciousness, coma, stupor

JUGLANS CINEREA

Absent minded, unobserving
Company, aversion to; presence of
    other people agg. the symp-
    toms; desire for solitude
Concentration, difficult
Confusion of mind
Dullness, sluggishness, difficulty of think-
    ing and comprehending, torpor
Memory, weakness of
    do, for what was about to
    read, for what has
Restlessness, afternoon
    night
Sadness, despondency, dejection, mental
    depression, gloom, melancholy

JUGLANS REGIA

Concentration, difficult
Confusion of mind, morning
    eating amel.
Discontented, displeased, dissatisfied
Excitement, excitable
    evening in bed
    wine, as from
Indifference, apathy
Indolence, aversion to work
Irritability, evening
Morose, cross, fretful, ill-humor, peevish
Talk, indisposed to, desire to be silent,
    taciturn
Weeping, tearful mood

JUNCUS EFFUSUS

Anxiety, partial slumbering in the
    morning, during •
Laughing, sleep, during

JUNIPERUS COMMUNIS

Answers, aversion to
Delirium
    fever, during
    raging, raving
Dullness, sluggishness, difficulty of think-
    ing and comprehending, torpor
Frightened easily
Memory, weakness of
Moaning, groaning, whining
Unconsciousness, coma, stupor

JUSTICIA ADHATODA

Stupefaction, as if intoxicated

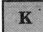

KALI ACETICUM

Anxiety
Dullness, pressing in hypogastrium,
    from •
Fear, disease, of impending,
        cancer, of ★
        heart, of disease of ★
Sadness, despondency, dejection, men-
    tal depression, gloom, melan-
    choly

KALI ARSENICOSUM

Anger, irascibility
Anguish
Answers, aversion to answer
    refuses to answer
Anxiety
        morning
            waking, on
        evening
            bed, in
        night
        causeless
        fear, with
        health, about
        stool, before
        waking, on
Bed, aversion to, shuns bed
Beside oneself, being
Business, averse to
Capriciousness
Censorious, critical
*Company, desire for; aversion to soli-
        tude, company amel.*
Concentration, difficult
Confusion of mind
        morning
        evening

Death, conviction of
    presentiment of
    thoughts of
Delirium
        night
Delusions, dead persons, sees
    enlarged, head is
    fancy, illusions of
    hearing, illusions of
    images, phantoms, sees
        frightful
Despair
    recovery, of
Discontented, displeased, dissatisfied
Excitement, excitable
Exertion, agg. from mental
Fancies, exaltation of
Fear, apprehension, dread
        evening
        night
        alone, of being
        bed, of the
        crowd, in a
        death, of
        evil, of
        happen, something will
        people, of; anthropophobia
Frightened, easily
        trifles, at
Hurry, haste
Hysteria
Impatience
Indifference, apathy
        everything, to
        pleasure, to
Indolence, aversion to work
Insanity, madness
        behaves like a crazy person
Irresolution, indecision
Irritability
        morning
            waking, on
        chill, during
        headache, during
Jealousy
        sadness, with •

347

Kill, desire to
    sudden impulse to kill
Lamenting, bemoaning, wailing
Memory, weakness of
Morose, cross, fretful, ill-humor, peevish
    morning waking, on
Quarrelsome, scolding
Restlessness
    evening
    night
    anxious
    bed, tossing about in
    chill, during
    heat, during
    menses, during
Sadness, despondency, dejection, mental
    depression, gloom, melancholy
    evening
    alone, when
    heat, during
    jealousy with sadness •
    periodical
        third day, every •
Sensitive, oversensitive
    noise, to
    voices, to
Shrieking, screaming, shouting
Sit, inclination to
Sits, still
Starting, startled
    noise, from
    sleep, on falling
    during
Suicidal, disposition
    thoughts
Suspicious, mistrustful
Talk, indisposed to, desire to be silent,
    taciturn
Talking, sleep, in
Thoughts, persistent
    night
    tormenting, night
Timidity
Violent, deeds of violence, rage leading
    to
    friends, to his •

Weeping, tearful mood
    night
    causeless
    sleep, in

KALI BICHROMICUM

Absent-minded, unobserving
Activity amel.
Anger, trifles, at
Antics, plays
Anxiety
    night
    conscience, as if guilty of a crime
    menses, before
    waking, on
Business, averse to
    incapacity for
Cheerful, gay, mirthful
Company, aversion to
Concentration difficult, studying, read-
    ing etc. while ★
Confusion of mind
    afternoon
    night, waking, on
Death, desires
    sensation of
Delirium
    delusions, with
    maniacal
Delirium tremens, delusions, with
Delusions, imagination, hallucination,
    illusions
    crime, about to commit a
    committed a, he had
    dead, child was, her
Dipsomania, alcoholism
Discomfort
Discouraged
Dullness, sluggishness, difficulty of think-
    ing and comprehending, torpor
Eating, amel. of mental symptoms
    while
Ennui, tedium
Excitement, excitable

Fear, crowd, in a
    dark, of
    death, of, menses, before
    insanity, losing his reason, of
    men, dread, fear of
    menses, before
    people, of; anthropophobia
    poisoned, of being
Forgetful
Gestures, convulsive
    covers mouth with hands
Grief
Imbecility
Impatience
Indifference, apathy
    business affairs, to
    external things, to
    vexation with distress in stomach,
        after least •
Indolence, aversion to work
    physical
Insanity, madness
    puerperal
Irritability
    eating amel.
Laughing
Loathing, general
Loathing, life, at
Mania
Memory, weakness of
    dates, for
Misanthropy
**Morose, cross, fretful, ill-humor,
    peevish**
Occupation, diversion amel.
Quarrelsome, scolding
Reading, aversion to
Rest, desire for
Restlessness
    night
Sadness, despondency, dejection, mental
    depression, gloom, melancholy
        evening
    eating amel.
    vexation, after
Sensitive, oversensitive

Shrieking, screaming, shouting
    convulsions, during epileptic
        between
Slowness
Speech, incoherent
    night
    sleep, during
        asleep, on falling •
Starting, evening, falling asleep, on
    sleep, on falling
        during
        from
Stupefaction, as if intoxicated
Sulky
Suspicious, mistrustful
Talk, indisposed to, desire to be silent,
    taciturn
Talking, sleep, in
    himself, to
Thoughts, vanishing of
Timidity
    bashful
Torpor
Unconsciousness, coma, stupor
    epilepsy, after
Violent, vehement
Weary of life
Weeping, tearful mood
Work, aversion to mental

KALI BROMATUM
Absent-minded, unobserving
Activity, fruitless ★
Ailments from:
    anger, vexation
    anticipation, foreboding, presen-
        timent
    business failure
    cares, worries
    death of a child
    embarrassment
    excitement, emotional
        sexual
    fright
    grief
    sexual excesses
    work, mental

Amativeness

Anger, irascibi' .y

Answers, disconnected

    monosyllable

    "no" to all questions

    repeats the question first

    slowly

Anxiety

    night, children, in

    alone, when

    dentition, during ●

    fright, after

    health, climacteric period, during

    pursued, as if

Aphasia ★

    amnestic ★

Business, averse to

Busy

Cares, worries, full of

Cheerful, gay, mirthful

Childish behavior

Climacteric period agg.

Company, aversion to; presence of other people agg. the symptoms; desire for solitude

    fear of being alone, yet

Company, desire for; aversion to solitude, company amel.

Complaining, climacteric period, during ●

Concentration, difficult

Confusion of mind

    identity, as to his

    waking, on

Death, desires

Delirium

    erotic

    muttering

    wild

Delirium tremens, mania-a-potu

Delusions, imaginations, hallucinations, illusions

    arrested, is about to be

    brother, fell over board in her sight ●

Delusions,

    conspiracies against her father, the landlord's bills are ●

    crime, about to commit a

    committed a, he had

    danger, impression of

    family, from his ●

    dead, child was, her

    persons, sees

    depressive ★

    deserted, forsaken, is

    destruction of all near her, impending ●

    devil, he is a

    doomed, being

    experienced before, thought everything had been ●

    fancy, illusions of

    floating in air

    God, vengeance, is the object of God's ●

    hearing, illusions of

    images, phantoms, sees

        night

        frightful

    injury; injured, is being

    insane, she will become

    insulted, he is

    boarders in hotel, by ●

    large, parts of body seem too, as if growing ●

    life, threatened, is ●

    melancholy

    money, sewed up in clothing, is ●

    murder her husband and child, she is about to ●

    murdered, he will be

    persecuted, he is

    place, he cannot pass a certain

    poisoned, he is about to be

    policeman come into house, he sees

    pursued by enemies

        he was

        police, by

        robbing a friend, for ●

Delusions,
> *religious*
> *spectres, ghosts, spirits, sees*
> thieves, accused of robbing, he
> > has been •
> violence, about •
> *visions, horrible*
> *voices, hears*
> wealth, of
> women, lewd, his mother's house
> > is invaded by •

Despair, recovery, of
Dipsomania, alcoholism
Dullness, sluggishness, difficulty
of thinking and compre-
hending, torpor
> *pollutions, with* •
> understands questions only after
> repetition

Escape, attempts to
Excitement, excitable
> night
> *alternating with sleepiness* •

Exertion, agg. from mental
> amel.

Exhilaration
Fancies, lascivious
> vivid, lively

Fear, apprehension, dread
> alone, of being
> apoplexy, of
> *corners, to walk past certain*
> *destruction to all near her, of*
> > *impending* •
> *ghosts, of*
> *happen, something will*
> insanity, losing his reason, of
> menses, before
> ordeals, of
> people, of; anthropophobia
> *piano, when at*
> *poisoned, of being*
> *sadness, with*
> spoken to, when

Fear,
> starting, with
> waking, on
> *wrong, of something* •

Forgetful
> morning, waking, on
> masturbation, after
> name, his own
> sexual excesses, after
> waking, on
> *words while speaking, of; word*
> > *hunting*

Forsaken feeling
Frightened easily
> waking, on

Gestures, grasping,
> picks at bed clothes
> hands, involuntary motion, of the
> > restlessly busy ★
> plays with his fingers
> violent
> wringing the hands

Grief
Ground gives way ★
Helplessness, feeling of
> afternoon •

Hesitates ★
Hypochondriasis
Hysteria, sleeplessness, with
Ideas, abundant, clearness of mind
> *deficiency of*

Imbecility
Inconsolable
Inconstancy
Indifference, apathy
> epilepsy, in

Indolence, aversion to work
Industrious, mania for work
Insanity, madness
> busy
> erotic
> > *menses, after* •
> *melancholy*
> paralysis, with
> puerperal
> *religious*

Irreligious *
Irresolution, indecision
Irritability
    grief, from
    sadness, with
    sleeplessness, with
Lamenting, bemoaning, wailing
Lascivious, lustful
Loathing, life, at
Looked at, cannot bear to be
Mania
    wild
Memory, weakness of
    dates, for
    expressing oneself, for
    names, for proper
    words, for
Mistakes, localities, in
    speaking, in
        misplacing words
        reverses words
        words, using wrong
            opposite, hot for cold e.g.
    writing, in
        omitting letters
        syllables
        words, repeating
Moaning, groaning, whining
    fate, about the •
    sleep, during
        grinding of teeth, with •
Moral feeling, want of
Morose, cross, fretful, ill-humor, peevish
Music: music lessons, cannot give her •
Muttering, sleep, in
Nymphomania
    menses, during
    puerperal
Occupation, diversion amel.
Prostration of mind, mental exhaus-
    tion, brain-fag
Recognize, friends, does not •
    relatives, does not recognize his
Religious affections
    melancholia
Remorse

Reproaches himself
Reputation, loss of, agg. ★
Restlessness   •
    daytime
    morning
    night
    climacteric period, at •
    move, must constantly
    women, in
**Sadness, despondency, dejection,
    mental depression, gloom,
    melancholy**
    anxious
    climaxis, during
    impotence, with
    pollutions, from
    sleepnessness from s.
Satyriasis
Senses, dull, blunted
Shrieking, screaming, shouting
    brain cry
    children, in
    convulsions, before
    sleep, during
    waking, on
Sits, bed, in, will not lie down ★
Slowness
Somnambulism
Speech, affected
    hesitating
    incoherent
    nonsensical
    slow
Starting, startled
    fright, from and as from
    sleep, during
        from
Stupefaction, as if intoxicated
Suicidal, disposition
    run over, to be
    thoughts
Sulky
Suspicious, mistrustful
Thoughts, sexual
    wandering
Timidity

Torpor
Tranquillity, serenity, calmness
Unconsciousness, coma, stupor
    alcoholic
    alternating with excitement •
    fever, during
    semi-consciousness
    vertigo, during
    waking, after
Wander, desires to
Weary of life
Weeping, tearful mood
    causeless
    easily
    involuntary
    paroxysmal
Work, mental, impossible
Writing, indistinctly, writes

KALI CARBONICUM

Absent-minded, unobserving
Absorbed, buried in thought
Abstraction of mind
Admonition agg.
Ailments, from:
    anticipation, foreboding, presen-
      timent
    bad news
    excitement, emotional
    fright
    love, disappointed
    sexual excesses
    work, mental
Anger, irascibility
    morning
      waking, on
    afternoon
    evening
    absent persons while thinking of
      them, at
    alternating with tranquillity
    dinner, during •
    violent
    waking, on
Anguish
    heat, during

Antagonism with herself
Anxiety
    evening
      bed, in
    night
    midnight, before
    alone, when
    bed, in
    breakfast, after
    children, in
    chill, after
    cramp in stomach, during •
    eating, after
    eructations amel.
    fear, with
    fever, during
    future, about
    health, about
    house, in
    hungry, when
    hypochondriacal
    lying, side, on
      right, from flatulence •
    menses, during
    sleep, during
    stool, before
      after
      bloody •
    waking, on
Aversion, husband, to
    members of family, to
Begging, entreating supplicating
Beside oneself, being
Business, averse to
Calculating, inability to
Capriciousness
Cares, evening
Carried, desires to be
Censorious, critical
Chaotic, confused behaviour
Cheerful, gay, mirthful
Closing eyes amel.
Company, aversion to; presence of
    other people agg. the symp-
    toms; desire for solitude

Company, desire for; aversion to solitude, company amel.
 evening
 alone agg., while
 treats them outrageously, yet •
Concentration, difficult
 headache, with
 studying, reading etc., while
Confidence, want of self
Confusion of mind
 morning
  rising and after, on
 afternoon
 evening
 chill, during
 intoxicated, as if
  as after being
 rising, after
 sitting, while
 sleeping, after long •
 waking, on
 walking, while
Consolation, kind words agg.
Contrary
Conversation agg.
Cowardice
Death, presentiment of
 thoughts of
Delirium
 night
 convulsions, after
 sopor, with
Delusions, imaginations, hallucinations, illusions
  day and night
  night
 abyss behind him •
 bed, sinking, is
 birds, sees
 calls, someone
 dead persons, sees
 devils, sees
 die, he was about to
 faces, sees
  hideous
 fancy, illusion of
  chill, during

Delusions,
 figures, sees, sleep, during •
 hollow, whole body is
 images, phantoms, sees
  night
  frightful
 masks, sees
 murdered, he will be
 neck is too large •
 people, sees
 pigeons flying in room which he tries to catch
 scream, obliging to
 sick, being
 sinking, to be
 spectres, ghosts, spirits, sees
 thieves, sees
 vermin, sees, crawl about
 visions, has
 water, of
 worms, creeping of
Despair, recovery, of
Dipsomania, alcoholism
Discomfort
Discontented, displeased, dissatisfied
 everything, with
 himself, with
Discouraged
 alternating with hope
Disgust
Doubtful, recovery, of
Dullness, sluggishness, difficulty of thinking and comprehending, torpor
 morning
  waking, on
 evening
 closing eyes, on, amel. •
 palpitation, with •
 speaking, while
Dwells on past disagreeable occurrences,
 night
Eccentricity
Emotions, feels her emotions in her epigastrium (predominated by the intelllect) ★

Emptiness, sensation of ★
  whole body were hollow, as if ★
Excitement, excitable
  alternating with prostration of
    mind •
  bad news, after
  heat, during
  hungry, when •
Exertion, agg. from mental
Fancies, exaltation of
    evening, bed, in
    night
  sleeplessness with
Fear, apprehension, dread
    evening
      bed, in
    night
    midnight, after,3h
  alone, of being
    evening
    lest he die
  bed, of the
  consumption, of
  crowd, in a
  death, of
    alone, when
      evening in bed
  disease, of impending
  eating, after, food
  evil, of
  falling, of
  ghosts, of
  hurt, of being
  lying in bed, while
  noise, from
  people, of; anthropophobia
  poverty, of
  solitude, of
  stomach, arising from
  stool, after ★
  touch, of
  trifles, of
  waking, on
  work, dread of
Foolish behavior

Forgetful
  words while speaking, of; word
    hunting
Forsaken feeling
Frightened easily
  touch, from
  trifles, at
  waking, on
Hatred
Heedless
Hopeful, alternating with despair
    sadness
Hurry, haste
  eating, while
  mental work, in
  movements, in
  occupation, in
Hypochondriasis
  imaginary illness
  weeping, with
Hysteria
  menses, before
Ideas, abundant, clearness of mind
    evening, bed, in
    night
Imbecility
Impatience
  children, about his •
Impetuous
Indifference, apathy
  company, society, while in
  money-making, to
  pleasure, to
Indiscretion
Indolence, aversion to work
  eating, after
Insanity
  anxiety, with
  puerperal
Irresolution, indecision
Irritability
  morning
    waking, on
  noon
  evening
  air, in open

Irritability,
> *coition, after*
> consolation agg.
> *eating, after*
> headache, during
> menses, before
>> during
> noise, from
> *sadness, with*
> *waking, on*

Jealousy
Kleptomania
Laughing agg.
Loathing, general
Loathing, work, at
Malicious, spiteful, vindictive
Mania
Mathematics, inapt for
Memory, weakness of
> business, for
> *expressing oneself, for*
> *words, of*

Menses, mental symptoms agg. before
Mildness
> alternating with anger •

Misanthropy
Mistakes, speaking, in
>> misplacing words
>> words, using wrong
> writing, in

Moaning, groaning, whining
>> **night, 3h •**

Mood, alternating
> *changeable, variable*
>> opinions, in
> repulsive

Morose, cross, fretful, ill-humor, peevish
> morning, bed, in
> afternoon
> evening
> alternating with cheerfulness
> eating, after
> sleepiness, with
> waking, on

Music agg.
> piano playing, from
> *violin playing agg.*
> cough, m. agg.
> piano, c. when playing
> violin, c. when playing on •

Nymphomania, menses, before
> during

Obstinate, headstrong
Optimistic, in spite of the weakness
Passionate
Prostration of mind, mental exhaustion, brain-fag
> night

Quarrelsome, scolding
> himself and his family, with ★

Quiet, wants to be, chill, during
Rage, fury
> morning in bed •

Reading agg. ★
Restlessness
> night
> **anxious**
> children, in
>> night •
> carried about, relieved by being
> eructations, from insufficient
> hunger, with •
> menses, before
>> during
>> suppressed, during
> pain, during

Revelry, feasting
Rocking amel.
Sadness, despondency, dejection, mental depression, gloom, melancholy
>> morning
>>> waking, on
>> evening
>>> amel.
>>> bed, in
>>> night, bed, in
> *air, in open*
> alone, when

Sadness,
    exertion in open air •
    headache, during
    sleeplessness, from
    waking, on
    walking in open air, while
Senses, dull, blunted
    vanishing of
Sensitive, oversensitive
    night •
    colors, to •
    noise, to
      voices, to
Shrieking, screaming, shouting
    aid, for
      sleep, in
    delusions, from
    imaginary appearances, about •
    sleep, during
    sudden
    touched, when
    trifles, at
Singing
Sit, inclination to
Somnambulism
Speech, hasty
    incoherent
    nonsensical, springing up while
      asleep, on •
    wandering
Starting, startled
    easily
    fright, from and as from
    noise, from
    sleep, on falling
      during
      from
    touched, when
      especially feet, ever so lightly ★
    waking, on
Striking
    about him at imaginary objects
Stupefaction, as if intoxicated
    head, with congestion of the •
Sulky

Talk, indisposed to, desire to be silent,
    taciturn
    evening
    others agg., talk of
Talking, sleep, in
Thoughts, persistent
    evening
    night
    alone
    lying, while
    unpleasant subjects, haunted by
    rush, flow of
      evening in bed
      night
    sleeplessness from
    tormenting, evening
    night
    vanishing of
Timidity
    evening in bed •
    night
    alternating with hope •
Touched, aversion to being
    ticklishness
Unconsciousness, coma, stupor
    morning
    chill, during
    cough, from •
    sudden
    transient
    vertigo, during
Unfortunate, feels
Violent, vehement
Wearisome
Weeping, tearful mood
    evening
    night
    admonition, from
    aloud, wobbing
    anxiety, after
    causeless
      without knowing why
    children, in
    chill, during
    consolation agg.
    desire to weep, all the time
    headache, with

Weeping, tearful mood
  pains, with the
  remonstrated, when
  sad thoughts, at
  sleep, in
  telling of her sickness, when
Will, weakness of
Work, aversion to mental
Writing, difficulty in expressing ideas
  when
  agg. mind symptoms ★

KALI CHLORICUM

Ailments from :
  quarrels
Anger, irascibility
  violent
Anxiety
  epistaxis amel. •
  hypochondriacal
Cheerful, gay, mirthful
  alternating with sadness
Confusion of mind,
  walking, while, air, in open
  wine, after
Death, desires, chill, during
Delirium, convulsions, after
Delusions, starve, he must •
Discomfort
Eat, refuses to
Hypochondriasis
  nosebleed amel. •
Indifference, apathy
  evening
Insanity, madness
Irritability
Loathing, life, at
  evening
Mania
Morose, cross, fretful, ill-humor, peevish
  alternating with cheerfulness
  epistaxis amel. •
Quarrelsome, scolding
Restlessness

Sadness, despondency, dejection, mental
  depression, gloom, melancholy
  evening
  chill, during
Stupefaction, as if intoxicated
Suicidal, evening
Unconsciousness, coma, stupor
Weary of life
  evening
Weeping, tearful mood
  evening

KALI CHLOROSUM

Unconsciousness, coma, stupor

KALI CYANATUM

Anger, irascibility
Censorious, critical
Cheerful, gay, mirthful
Confusion of mind, afternoon
Delirium, busy
  muttering
Indolence, aversion to work
Irritability, absent persons, with
Jesting
Memory, weakness of
Mildness
Moaning, groaning, whining
Restlessness
Sighing
Stupefaction, as if intoxicated
Unconsciousness, coma, stupor

KALI FLUORATUM

Irritability

KALI FERROCYANATUM

Fear, death, of
Sadness, despondency, dejection, mental depression, gloom, melancholy
Weeping, tearful mood

KALI IODATUM

Abrupt, harsh,
Abusive, insulting
    children and family, to ★
Ailments from :
    work, mental
Anger, irascibility
    violent
Anguish
Anxiety
    evening
    excitement, from
    fear, with
    menses, during
    motion, from
    sleep, during
        menses, after
    stool, after
    walking, air amel., in open
Business, averse to
Busy
Company, aversion to; presence of
    other people agg. the symp-
    toms; desire for solitude
Complaining
Concentration, difficult
Confusion of mind
Cruelty, inhumanity
Delirium
    raging, raving
Dementia
    syphilitics, of
Despair
Dipsomania, alcoholism
Discouraged
Disgust
    everything, with
Dullness, sluggishness, difficulty of think-
    ing and comprehending, torpor
Excitement, excitable
    wine, as from
Fear, apprehension, dread
    evening
        twilight
    dawn, of the return of ●
    death, of

Fear,
    evil, of
    misfortune, of
    sadness, with
    suffocation, of
Forgetful
Frightened, easily
    trifles, at
Harsh, with his family & children,
    abusive ★
Hatred
Haughty
Impetuous
Indifference, children, to her
Insanity, madness
    paroxysmal
Irritability
    children, towards ●
    eating, after
    sadness, with
Jesting
Lamenting, bemoaning, wailing
Loquacity
    cheerful, exuberant
    jesting, with
Malicious, spiteful, vindictive
    sadness, in ●
Mania
    night
Memory, weakness of
Moaning, groaning, whining
Morose, cross, fretful, ill-humor, peevish
Obstinate, headstrong
Passionate
Prostration of mind, mental exhaus-
    tion, brain-fag
Quarrelsome, scolding
Restlessness
    night
    anxious
    driving about
    headache, during
Sadness, despondency, dejection, mental
    depression, gloom, melancholy
    aversion, devoutly attached
    children become burden-
    some ●

Sensitive, oversensitive
  noise, to
Shrieking, brain cry
  hydrocephalus
Starting, startled
      evening, sleep, in
      midnight in sleep, before
  dream, from a
  easily
  noise, from
  sleep, during
      from
  sleepiness, with
Stupefaction, as if intoxicated
  loquacious
  restlessness, with
Thoughts, persistent
Touched, aversion to being
Unconsciousness, coma, stupor
Unfeeling, family, with his •
Violent, vehement
Weeping, tearful mood
      evening
      night
  alternating with ill-humor
  anxiety, after
  anxious
  evil impended, as if •
  sleep, in
  waking, on
Work, aversion to mental

KALI MURIATICUM

Anger, irascibility
  evening
Anxiety, evening
      bed, in
      night
  trifles, about
Cheerful, alternating with sadness
Delirium
  night
  convulsions, during
Delusions, eat, she must not •
  (starve, he must) ★
Discontented, displeased, dissatisfied

Discouraged
Dullness, sluggishness, difficulty of think-
      ing and comprehending, torpor
Excitement, excitable
Fear, evil, of
Imbecility
Indifference, chill, during
      pleasure, to
      sexual passion diminished •
Insanity, madness
Irresolution, indecision
Irritability, evening
Loathing, life, at
Mania
Moaning, groaning, whining
Obstinate, headstrong
Restlessness
*Sadness, despondency, dejection, mental
      depression, gloom, melancholy*
  chill, during
Sits, still
Slowness
Starving, he must (starve) ★
Talk, indisposed to, desire to be silent,
      taciturn
Talking, sleep, in
Unconsciousness, coma, stupor

KALI NITRICUM

Absent-minded, morning 11-16 h.
Anger, irascibility
Anxiety
      afternoon
        until, evening
      evening
        bed, in
      night
  bed, in
  congestion to chest, from
  fear, with
  headache, with
Beside oneself, being
Cares, worries, full of
Confidence, want of self

Confusion of mind
   morning
   evening
   intoxicated, as if
     as after being
   waking, on
Cowardice
Death, presentiment of
   sensation of
Delirium
Delusions, fire, visions of
   water, of
   wood, is made of •
Despair
Discontented, displeased, dissatisfied
Discouraged
Dullness, sluggishness, difficulty of think-
   ing and comprehending, torpor
     morning
       waking, on
Ennui, tedium
Exhilaration
Fancies, exaltation of
   night
   sleeplessness, with
   waking, on
Fear, apprehension, dread
   death, of
   perspiration, during •
Forgetful
   waking, on
Ideas abundant, clearness of mind
Indifference, apathy
   ennui, with
Indolence, aversion to work
   morning
Irritability
Love, with one of the own sex, homo-
   sexuality, tribadism perversity
Meditation
Memory, weakness of
   said, for what has
Morose, cross, fretful, ill-humor, peevish
Offended, easily; takes everything in
   bad part
Restlessness
   night
   anxious
   bed, tossing about in

Sadness, despondency, dejection, mental
   depression, gloom, melancholy
   alone, when
Sensitive, oversensitive
Shrieking, pains, with the
Starting, dream, from a
   sleep, during
Stupefaction, as if intoxicated
Sulky
Thinking, aversion to
   morning
Thoughts, rush, flow of
   night
   sleeplessness from
   thoughtful
Timidity
Unconsciousness, coma, stupor
   morning
Wearisome
Weeping, tearful mood
   music, from
Work, aversion to mental
   morning •

KALI OXALICUM

Insanity, madness
Weeping, tearful mood

KALI PHOSPHORICUM

Absent-minded, unobserving
Ailments from :
   anger, vexation
   anticipation, foreboding, presen-
     timent
   anxiety
   bad news
   cares, worries
   excitement, emotional
     sexual
   fear
   grief
   sexual excesses
   shock, mental
   work, mental
Anger, irascibility

Answer, aversion to answer
Anxiety
    evening,
       bed, in
    night
    children, in
    eating, after
    fear, with
    future, about
    health, about
    hypochondriacal
    salvation, about
    waking, on
Aversion, his own mind, to ★
    husband, to
    members of family, to
Brooding
Business, man, worn out
Cares, sleeplessness from ★
Cheerful, gay, mirthful
Clinging, held, wants to be
Company, aversion to; presence of
    other people agg. the symp-
    toms; desire for solitude
Company, desire for; aversion to soli-
    tude, company amel.
Concentration, difficult
    studying, reading, etc., while
Confusion of mind
    morning
    evening
Consolation, kind words agg.
Contrary
Cowardice
Cruelty, inhumanity
    family, to her
Delirium
    night
    quiet
Delirium tremens, mania-a-potu
    sleeplessness, with
Delusions, imaginations, hallucinations,
    illusions
    dead persons, sees
    doomed, being

Delusions,
    fancy, illusions of
    figures, sees
    images, phantoms, sees
       frightful
    strange, familiar things seem
Despair
    religious despair of salvation
Discontented, displeased, dissatisfied
Discouraged
Dullness, sluggishness, difficulty of think-
    ing and comprehending, torpor
    morning
Dwells on past disagreeable occur-
    rences
    night
Eat, refuses to
Excitement, excitable
    agg.
    bad news, after
    mental work, from
    nervous
Exertion, agg. from mental
    puberty, agg. from mental ex-
       ertion in
Fancies, exaltation of
Fear, apprehension, dread
    evening
    night, children, in ★
    alone, of being
    children, night
    crowd, in a
    public places, of; agoraphobia
    death, of
    diarrhoea from
    disease, of impending
    drunkards, in ●
    evil, of
    happen, something will
    people, of; anthropophobia
    places, building etc ★
    robbers, of
    weary of life, with
    work, dread
Forgetful
    words while speaking, 'of; word
       hunting
Frightened easily

Gestures, makes,
  fingers in the mouth, children
    put ★
  ridiculous or foolish
  wringing the hands
Homesickness
Hurry, haste
  occupation, in
Hypochondriasis
Hysteria
Ideas abundant, clearness of mind
Imbecility
Impatience
  trifles, about
Impetuous
Indifference, apathy
  business affairs, to
  joy, to
  relations, to
Indolence, aversion to work
Insanity, madness
  heat, with
  mental labor, from
  puerperal
Irresolution, indecision
Irritability
  morning
    waking, on
  evening
  coition, after
  headache, during
  menses, during
  spoken to, when
  waking, on
  weakness, with
Lamenting, bemoaning, wailing
Laughing
  alternating with shrieking
Loathing, life, at
Mania
Memory, active
  *past events, haunted by and long-
    ing for* •
Memory, weakness of
  expressing oneself, for
  words, for

Mildness
Mistakes, localities, in
  speaking, in
    misplacing words
  writing, in
Moaning, groaning, whining
  sleep, during
Mood, changeable, variable
Morose, cross, fretful, ill-humor, peevish
Nymphomania
Obstinate, headstrong
**Prostration of mind, mental ex-
    haustion, brain-fag**
Quarrelsome, scolding
  family, with her
Recognize surroundings, does not •
Refuses to take the medicines
Religious affections
  melancholia
Restlessness
  children, babies, in •
  menses, during
  mental labor, during and after
**Sadness, despondency, dejection,
    mental depression, gloom,
    melancholy**
  day and night
  morning
    waking, on
  evening
  night
  amenorrhoea, in
  menses, from delayed
  mental exertion, after
  waking, on
Senses, acute
  dull, blunted
Sensitive, oversentisive
  children
  colors, to •
  light, to
  noise, to
    menses, during •
  puberty, in

Shrieking, screaming, shouting
  children, in
    night
    waking, on
Sighing
  sleep, in
Sit, inclination to
Somnambulism
Speech, hasty
  incoherent
  slow
  wandering
Spoken to, averse to being
Starting, startled
  easily
  fright, from and as from
  noise, from
  sleep, during
  touched, when
Strange, everything seems
Stupefaction, as if intoxicated
Suspicious, mistrustful
Talk, indisposed to, desire to be silent,
  taciturn
Talking, sleep, in
Tears, things
  night-dress and bed clothes
Thoughts, ridiculous
  vanishing of
Timidity
  bashful
Violent, vehement
Weary of life
  fear of death, but
Weeping, tearful mood
  alternating with laughter
  hysterical
Work, mental, impossible
  seems to drive him crazy, owing to
    the impotency of his mind
Writing seems to drive him crazy,
  owing to the impotency of his
  mind

KALI PERMANGANICUM

Morphinism
Restlessness

KALI SULPHURICUM

Absent-minded, unobserving
Activity, mental
Ailments from :
  sexual excesses
Anger, irascibility
Anxiety
  evening
    bed, in
  night
  air, amel. in open
  fear, with
  waking, on
  walking, air amel., in open
  warmth, from
Business, averse to
Company, aversion to; presence of
  other people agg. the symptoms; desire for solitude
Concentration, difficult
Confidence, want of self
Confusion of mind
  morning
  evening
  air amel., in open
  warm room, in
Consolation, kind words agg.
Discontented, displeased, dissatisfied
  everything, with
Discouraged
Dullness, sluggishness, difficulty of think-
  ing and comprehending, torpor
Excitement, excitable
  evening
Exertion, agg. from mental
Fear, apprehension, dread
  night
  dark, of
  death, of
    night
  falling, of
  insanity, losing his reason, of
  people, of; anthropophobia
  work, dread of
Forgetful

Frightened, easily
    trifles, at
Hurry, haste
Hysteria
    evening
Ideas, abundant, clearness of mind
Impatience
Impetuous
Indifference, apathy
Indolence, aversion to work
Irresolution, indecision
Irritability
    morning
        waking, on
    evening
    menses, during
Memory, weakness of
    do, for what was about to
    say, for what is about to
Mistakes, speaking, in, misplacing
    words
    writing, in .
Mood, alternating
    changeable, variable
Obstinate, headstrong
Restlessness
    menses, during
    room, in
    warm bed agg.
Sadness, despondency, dejection, men-
    tal depression, gloom, melan-
    choly
        morning
        evening
Sensitive, oversensitive
    noise, to
Shrieking, screaming, shouting
    waking, on
Somnambulism
Starting, startled
    easily
    fright, from and as from
    sleep, on falling
        during
Talk, indisposed to, desire to be silent,
    taciturn
Talking, sleep, in

Timidity
Unconsciousness, coma, stupor
Weeping, tearful
Work, aversion to mental

KALI SILICICUM

Absent-minded, unobserving
Ailments from :
    sexual excesses
Anger, trifles, at
Anxiety,
    evening
        bed, in
    night
    eating, after
    fear, with
    health, about
    menses, during
    trifles, about
Capriciousness
Concentration, difficult
    studying, reading etc., while
Confidence, want of self
Confusion of mind,
    morning, rising and after, on
    evening
    mental exertion, from
    sitting, while
Consolation, kind words agg.
Contrary
Cowardice
Delusions, imaginations, hallucinations,
    illusions
    dead persons, sees
    fancy, illusions of
    images, sees
        night
        frightful
    spectres, ghosts, spirits, sees
    thieves, sees
Discontented, displeased, dissatisfied
Discouraged
Dullness, morning, waking, on
    reading, while
    writing, while

Excitement, excitable
Exertion, agg. from mental
Fear, work, dread of
Forgetful
Frightened eas··,
Heedless
Hysteria
Imbecility
Impatience
Indifference, apathy
      pleasure, to
Indolence, aversion to work
Irresolution, indecision
Irritability
      morning
      evening
      coition, after
      consolation agg.
Memory, weakness of
Mistakes, speaking, in
      misplacing words
      writing, in
Mood, changeable, variable
Obstinate, headstrong
Prostration of mind, mental exhaustion, brain-fag
Restlessness, night
Sadness, morning
Senses, vanishing of
Sensitive, noise, to
Sits, still
Starting, startled
      easily
      fright, from and as from
      noise, from
      sleep, on falling
      touched, when
Talk, indisposed to, desire to be silent, taciturn
Talking, sleep, in
Timidity
Weeping, tearful mood
      evening
      night
      sleep, in
Will, weakness of
Work, aversion to mental

KALI SULPHUROSUM

Restlessness

KALI TELLURICUM

Fear, disease, of impending

• KALMIA LATIFOLIA

Anxiety
      future, about
Busy
Concentration, difficult
Confusion of mind
      evening
Consolation, kind words agg.
Delirium
Excitement, morning
Fear, evil, of
Forgetful
Irritability
      morning
      evening
Memory, weakness of
Morose, cross, fretful, ill-humor, peevish
      morning
      evening and next forenoon •
Obstinate, headstrong
Remorse
Restlessness
Sadness, despondency, dejection, mental depression, gloom, melancholy
Somnambulism
Spoken to, averse to being
Talk, others agg., of
Talking, sleep, in
Thoughts, rapid, quick
Work, aversion to mental
      impossible

KEROSOLENUM

Cheerful, gay, mirthful
Delusions, floating, maze, in a wavy •
Ecstasy
Forsaken feeling

Laughing
Trance
Unconsciousness, coma, stupor
Vivacious

KISSINGEN AQUA

Absorbed, buried in thought
Anxiety
Brooding, unpleasant things •
Cheerful, gay, mirthful
Complaining
Dwells on past disagreeable occurrences
Ennui, tedium
Frightened, trifles, at
Indolence, aversion to work
Irresolution, indecision
Irritability
Memory, weakness of
    expressing oneself, for
Mistakes, speaking, in
Morose, cross, fretful, ill-humor, peevish
Restlessness, night
Starting, electric, as if
Thoughts, disagreeable
    frightful, night on waking
Weeping, tearful mood
    looked at, when
Work, mental, impossible
Yielding, disposition

KOLA

Dipsomania, alcoholism

KOUSSO (BRAYERA ANTHELMINTICA)

Thinking, himself, too little ★

KREOSOTUM

Absent-minded, unobserving
Abstraction, of mind
Ailments from :
    excitement, emotional

Anger, irascibility
    menses, during
    trifles, at
Anxiety
    night
    coition, during •
       thought of (in a woman) •
    fear, with
    menses, during
Capriciousness
Carried, desires to be
    caressed and, desires to be
Cheerful, gay, mirthful ★
    night
    sleep, during
Confusion of mind
Contrary
Cowardice ★
Death, desires
    despair, from •
Defiant
Delusions, fire, visions of
    longer, things seems
    motion, all parts being in (during
       rest) •
    tall, things grow taller
    well, he is
Despair
    recovery, of
Discontented, displeased, dissatisfied
    everything, with
Doubtful, recovery, of
Dullness, sluggishness, difficulty of
    thinking and comprehending,
    torpor
    sleepiness, with
Dwells on past disagreeable occurrences
Excitement, excitable
    menses, before
      during
    music, from
Fear, apprehension, dread
    coition, at thought of (in woman) •
    disease, of impending
    fasting, of •

Forgetful
    epistaxis, after •
Heedless
Ideas abundant, clearness of mind
    deficiency of
Impatience
Industrious, mania for work
    menses, before
Insanity, haemorrhage, after
Irritability
    daytime
    morning
    chill, during
    dentition, during
    headache, during
    menses, before
    during
Laughing
    night
    midnight
    sleep, during
Loathing, life, at
Memory, weakness of
    business, for
    do, for what was about to
Moaning, groaning, whining
    constant moaning and gasping for air
Morose, cross, fretful, ill-humor, peevish
    daytime
    morning
    forenoon
        10-22h. •
    chill, during
Music agg.
    cough, music agg.
        piano, c. when playing
    ear-ache from
Obstinate, headstrong
    children
Restlessness
    evening, 18-6 h. •
    night
    midnight, after, 3h.
        4h.
    bed, tossing about in

Restlessness
    chill, during
    menses, before
    move, must constantly
Sadness, despondency, dejection, mental
    depression gloom, melancholy
    morning
    • evening
    music, from
Senses, vanishing of
Sensitive, oversensitive
    music, to
Sentimental
Shrieking, screaming, shouting
    night
    children, in
        stool, during
    dentition, during
    involuntary ★
    night ★
    sleep, during
    stool, before ★
Slowness
Starting, fright, from and as from
    sleep, on falling
        during
Striking
Stupefaction, as if intoxicated
    vertigo, during
Suicidal, disposition
Thoughts, vanishing of
Throws things away
Unconsciousness, coma, stupor
    vertigo, during
Wearisome
Weary of life
Weeping, tearful mood
    morning
    causeless
    emotion, after slight
    headache, with
    music, from
    noise, at
    sleep, in
    whimpering
Well, says he is, when very sick
Work, mental, impossible

KRESOLUM

Absent-minded, unobserving
Anger, irascibility
Anguish, evening
Anxiety
Beside oneself, being, trifles, from
Cheerful, gay, mirthful
Childish behaviour
Confiding
Delusions, animals, beetles, worms etc.
   bells, hears ringing of
Ecstasy
Euphoria
Excitement, excitable
Fear, apprehension, dread
Gestures, makes
Indifference, apathy
Irritability
Kisses everyone
Loquacity
Mania
   alternating with depression
Restlessness
   driving about
Sadness, despondency, dejection, mental
    depression, gloom, melancholy
Schizophrenia
   hebephrenia
Speech, repeats same thing
Thoughts profound

LACTIS ACIDUM

Anxiety, night on waking
Business, averse to
Censorious, critical
Confusion of mind
   afternoon
Contemptuous
Dipsomania, alcoholism
Discouraged
Eccentricity
Fastidious
Hysteria
Ideas abundant, clearness of mind
Indolence, aversion to work
Memory, active
Memory, weakness of
Mistakes, speaking, spelling, in
   writing, in
Mocking, sarcasm
Reading, aversion to read
Restlessness
Sensitive, noise, to
Shrieking, midnight •
Talk, indisposed to, desire to be silent,
   taciturn
Thinking, aversion to
Thoughts, tormenting

LAC CANINUM

Absent-minded, unobserving
Ailments from :
   *anticipation, foreboding, presen-
   timent*
Anger, irascibility
   alternating with weeping
Antagonism with herself

Anxiety
> night
> health, about
> *success, from doubt about* •

Aversion, herself, to ★
Company, desire for; aversion to solitude, company amel.
Concentration, difficult
Confidence, want of self
Confusion of mind
Contemptuous, self, of
Cursing, swearing
Death, desires
> convalescence, during

Delirium
> anxious

Delusions, imaginations, hallucinations, illusions
> air, he is hovering in, like a spirit
> animals, of
> > creeping •
> bed, motion, in •
> birds, sees
> *clouds, heavy black, enveloped her*
> despised, is
> diminished, all is
> > short, he is •
> *dirty, he is*
> disease, incurable, has
> *eyes, of big*
> *faces, sees*
> > **dark, in the**
> > distorted •
> > hideous
> falling forward, to pieces •
> fancy, illusions of
> *floating in air*
> heart disease, is going to have, and die
> horrid ★
> identity, errors of personal
> images, phantoms, sees
> > *frightful*
> insane, she will become
> *insects, sees*
> insulted, he is
> lie, all she said is a •
> light, incorporeal, he is

Delusions,
> *looked down upon, she is* •
> mice, sees
> > mouse running from under a chair
> nose, someone else's, has ★
> sick, being
> *snakes in and around her*
> *spiders, sees* •
> swimming, air, in the •
> unreal, everything seems
> vermin, sees, crawl about
> visions, daytime
> > beautiful
> > horrible
> > monsters, of
> voices, hears

Despair, recovery, of
Dipsomania, alcoholism
Disgust
Doubtful, recovery, of
Dullness, sluggishness, difficulty of thinking and comprehending, torpor
> reading, while

Excitement, excitable
Fancies, exaltation of
> *frightful*

Fastidious
Fear, daytime, only
> *alone, of being*
> consumption, of
> **death, of**
> *disease, of impending*
> > incurable, of being
> downward motion, of
> *duties, she will become unable to perform her* •
> *failure, of*
> **fainting, of**
> *falling, of*
> > downstairs •
> *happen, something will*
> heart, of disease of
> *insanity, losing his reason, of*
> **snakes, of** ★
> *waking, on*

Forgetful
  *purchases, of : goes off and leaves
     them*
Gestures, makes, fingers spread apart ★
Grief, *waking, on*
Hatred
Hypochondriasis, evening
Hysteria, coition agg ●
Idiocy, shrill shrieking, with
Inconstancy
Indifference, apathy
Indolence, aversion to work
Insolence
Irresolution, indecision
Irritability
  night ★
  headache, during
Liar, lie, believes all she says is a ●
Light, desire for
Loathing, life, at
  oneself, at
Malicious, spiteful, vindictive
Memory, weakness of
  do, for what was about to
  done, for what has just
  expressing oneself, for
  read, for what has
  words, of
Mistakes, speaking, in
  misplacing words
  words, using wrong
     *name of object seen instead
        of one desired*
     names, calls things by wrong
  writing, in
     omitting letters
     repeating words
Mood, alternating
  changeable, variable
Moral feeling, want of
Morose, cross, fretful, ill humor, peevish
Persists in nothing
Poisoned, feeling ★
Rage, fury
  contradiction, from
Restlessness
  night
Rudeness

**Sadness, despondency, dejection,
  mental depression, gloom,
  melancholy**
  menses, before
     during
Sensitive, oversensitive
  external impressions, to all
  light, to
  noise, to
Shrieking, screaming, shouting
  children, in
  night
  sleep, during
Sit, inclination to
Starting, startled
Symptom, every, is a settled disease ★
Talking, sleep, in
Thinking, complaints agg., of
  himself too little ★
Thoughts, frightful
  in bed ●
  intrude and crowd around each
     other
  persistent, lying, while
  rapid, quick
  rush, flow of
  tormenting
  vanishing of
*Undertakes, many things, perseveres in
  nothing*
Washing always her hands
Weeping, tearful mood
  night
  anger, after
  children, night
  nervous, all day
  nursing, while
  paroxysmal
Writing, meannesses to her friends ●

LAC VACCINUM
DEFLORATUM

*Company, aversion to; presence of other
  people agg. the symptoms; desire for solitude
  avoids the sight of people*

Conscientious about trifles
Conversation amel. ★
Death, desires
    meditates on easiest way of self destruction ★
    presentiment of
    predicts the time
Delusions, convent, she will have to go to a •
    dead, all her friends are dead and she must go to a convent •
    die, he was about to
Fear, door, closed, lest the d. should be •
    narrow places, in; claustrophobia
Forsaken feeling
Hysteria, fainting, hysterical
Indifference, apathy
Indolence, aversion to work
Irresolution, indecision
Irritability
Loathing, life, at
Memory, weakness of
    read, for what has
Moaning, groaning, whining
Mood, changeable, variable
Prostration of mind, mental exhaustion, brain-fag
Restlessness
    nausea, with •
    sleeplessness, from
Sadness, despondency, dejection, mental depression, gloom, melancholy
    conversation amel. •
    menses, before
    during
Suicidal disposition
    meditates on easiest way ★
Talk, indisposed to, desire to be silent, taciturn
Unconsciousness, coma, stupor
    raising arms above head, on
Weary of life
Weeping, tearful mood
Work, aversion to mental

LAC FELINUM
Fear, pins, pointed things, of

LACERTA AGILIS
Delirium
Industrious, mania for work

LACHESIS MUTA
Abrupt, harsh
Absent-minded, unobserving
    epileptic attack, before •
    reading, while
Absorbed, buried in thought
Abusive, insulting
    husband insulting wife before children or vice versa
Activity
    mental
    night
Adulterous
Affections, in general ★
Affectionate
Ailments from :
    anger, vexation
    anticipation, foreboding, presentiment
    bad news
    death of a child
    debauchery ★
    dipsomania
    disappointment
    discords between chief and subordinates
      parents, friends
      servants ★
    excitement, emotional
    fright
    grief
    jealousy
    love, disappointed
    mortification
    reverses of fortune
    work, mental
Amativeness

Ambition
Amorous
Amusement, desire for
Anger, irascibility
    trifles, at
    violent
Anguish
Animation agg. ★
Answers, hastily
Anxiety
      morning
        waking, on
      evening, bed, in
      night
    air, in open
    conscience, as if guilty of a crime
      dream, anxiety of c. in
    eating, after
    fear, with
    fever, during
    future, about
    health, about
    hypochondriacal
    menses, during, anger and a.
    motion, from
    riding, while
    salvation, about
    sleep, on going to
    waking, on
    weary of life, with
Audacity
Avarice
    alternating with squandering
Aversion, everything, to
    women, to
Bed, aversion to, shuns bed
Bite, desire to
Boaster, braggart
    rich, wishes to be considered as
Brooding
Business, averse to
    desire for
Busy
Capriciousness
Carefulness
Cares, others, about
    relatives, about
Censorious, critical

Cheerful, gay, mirthful
    morning
    evening
    bed, in
    alternating with sadness
Clairvoyance
    clairvoyant dreams during drunk-
      enness ●
Climacteric period agg.
Clinging, held, wants to be
    held amel., being
Communicative, expansive
Company, aversion to; presence of other
    people agg. the symptoms; de-
    sire for solitude
    desire solitude to indulge her
    fancy ●
    perspiration, during
    pregnancy, during
Company, desire for, aversion to soli-
    tude, company; amel.
    alone agg., while
Complaining
    disease, of
    trifles, of ●
Comprehension, easy
Concentration, difficult
    children, in
    studying, reading etc., while
Confidence, want of self
Confusion of mind
      morning
        waking, on
    eating, after
      amel.
    epileptic attack, before
    identity, as to his
      duality, sense of
    intoxicated, as if
    sleeping, after
    time, of
    waking, on
    walking, while
Conscientious about trifles
Contemptuous
    hard for subordinates and agree-
      able pleasant to superiors or
      people he has to fear

Contradict, disposition to
Contradiction, is intolerant of
Contrary
Cowardice ★
Crawling, on floor
Cruelty, inhumanity
Death, desires
  presentiment of
  thoughts of
Deceitful, sly
Delirium
    noon, 12-24 h. •
    evening
    night
  answers abruptly
  changing subjects rapidly •
  closing the eyes, on
  constant
  erotic
  fatigue, over-exertion, study,
    from •
  fever, during
  haemorrhage, after
  laughing
  loquacious
  loss of fluids, from
  maniacal
  mental exertion, from •
  muttering
  persecution in delirium, delusions
    of
  raging, raving
  religious
  sepsis, from
  sleep, during
    after
  sleepiness, with
  violent
  waking, on
  watching, vigil, from
  wild
Delirium tremens, mania-a-potu
  delusions, with
  loquacity, with

**Delusions, imaginations, hallucina-
  tions, illusions**
    evening
  afternoon, it is always
  air, he is hovering in, like a spirit
  asylum, insane, sent to •
  beautiful
    landscape, of
  bed, sinking, is
  body, disintegrating •
    lighter than air, is
  *charmed and cannot break the
    spell* •
  conspiracies against him, there
    are
  crime, committed a, he had
  dead, he himself was
    mother is, his
    persons, sees
  devils, sees
  die, he was about to
    time has come to
  disease, incurable, has
  doomed, being
    drunkards, in •
  double, of being
  fancy, illusions of
  floating in air
    bed, resting in, is not
  flying, sensation of
  head, standing on ★
  heart disease, is going to have,
    and die
      large, too
  higher power ★
  home, away from, is
  house is full of people
  identity, errors of personal
    someone else, she is
  images, phantoms, sees
    alone, when
    frightful
    pleasant
  influence, is under a powerful
  injury, is about to receive
  injured, is being
    surroundings, by his

段ml

Delusions,
- *jealousy, with*
- journey, he is on a
- *lost, predestination, from* •
- loquacity, with
- mice, sees
- motion, up and down, of
- murder someone, he has to
- *music, he hears*
  - delightful
  - *sweetest and sublimest melody*
- people, behind him, someone is
  - converses, with absent
- *persecuted, he is* •
- *person, other, she is some*
- *poisoned, he has been*
  - he is about to be
  - medicine, being •
- proud
- *pursued by enemies*
  - he was
- religious
- rising, then falling ★
- smell, of
- snakes in and around her
- snakes, black ★
- *space, carried into, he was (while lying)*
- spectres, ghosts, spirits, sees
  - *closing eyes, on*
  - hovering in the air
- spied, being •
- stolen something, she has •
  - or somebody thinks it •
- *superhuman, control, is under*
- thieves, sees
  - *house, in*
  - *jump out of window, therefore wants to* •
- *visions, has*
  - beautiful
  - *closing the eyes, on*
  - clouds of colors •
  - fantastic
  - *horrible, behind him* •
  - wonderful

Delusions,
- *vivid*
- voices, hears, that he must follow
  - confess things she never did •
  - steal and kill, that she must •
- wills, possessed of two
- wrong, suffered, has

Dementia
- senilis

Desires, indefinite

Despair
- pains, with the
- recovery, of
- **religious despair of salvation**

Destructiveness

Dictatorial, domineering, dogmatical, despotic

Dipsomania, alcoholism
- hereditary •
- idleness, from

Discomfort

Discontented, displeased, dissatisfied
- always
- everything, with

Discouraged
- pain, from

Dishonest

Doubtful
- recovery, of
- **soul's welfare, of**

Dream, as if in a •

Duality, sense of ★

Dullness, sluggishness, difficulty of thinking and comprehending, torpor
- forenoon
- evening
- chagrin, vexation, from
- children, in
- *chill, during*
- mental exertion, from
- *reading, while*
- *says nothing*
- **waking, on**

Duty, no sense of duty

Eat, refuses to

Eccentricity
- political

Ecstasy
   joy, as after excessive ●
Egotism, self-esteem
   speaking about themselves in company, always
Ennui, tedium
Envy
   qualities of others, at
Escape, attempts to
Exaltation, politics ★
Excitement, excitable
   morning
   evening
     bed, in
   night
   bad news, after
   chill, during
   climacteric period, during
   hearing horrible things, after
   heat, during
     puerperal, during
   menses, before
   weeping, till
Exertion, agg. from mental
Exhilaration
Fancies, exaltation of
   night
   lascivious
   pleasant
   vivid, lively
   waking, on
Fear, apprehension, dread
   evening
   night
     waking, after
   apoplexy, of
   bed, of the
   behind him, someone is
   brilliant objects, looking glass or
   cannot endure, of
   cholera, of
   death, of
   die, fear he will, if he goes to sleep (after nightmare)
   impending death, of

Fear,
   disease, of impending
     contagious, epidemic disease, of
     incurable, of being
   eating food, after
   evil, of
   fit, of having a
   heart, of disease of
   infection, of
   insanity, losing his reason, of
   lighting, of
   men, dread, fear of
   misfortune, of
   narrow places, in; claustrophobia ★
   people, of; anthropophobia
   poisoned, of being
   riding in a carriage, when
   robbers, of
     night ●
   sleep, go to, fear to
   snakes, of
   strangers, of
   suffocation, of
   thunderstorm, of
   touch, of
   tremulous
   waking, on
   water, of
Firmness
Foolish behavior
Foppish
Forgetful
   climacteric period, during
   drunkards, forgetfulness in
   everything, occured for six years, that had ●
   mental exertion, from
   (-ness) old people, of
   streets, of well-known
   words while speaking, of; word hunting
Forsaken, feeling
   morning
   waking, on
Fright, menses, during ★

Frightened, easily
   trifles, at
   waking, on
Frivolous
Gestures
   covers mouth with hands
   plays with his fingers
   ridiculous or foolish
Gifts to his wife or son, husband making no •
Godless, want of religious feeling
Gossiping
Grief
   waking, on
Hard for inferiors and kind for superiors
Hatred
   revenge, h. and
Haughty
Heedless
Hide, desire to
Home, desires to go
   leave home, desire to
Homesickness
Honor, sense of, no
Horrible things, sad stories, affect her profoundly
Hurry, haste
   night •
   eating, while
   everybody must hurry
Hydrophobia
Hypochondriasis
   night
Hysteria
   climacteric period, at
   fainting, hysterical
   puberty, at
   sexual excesses, after
   suppression of discharges, after
Ideas abundant, clearness of mind evening
   compelling ★
   deficiency of
Idiocy
Idleness
Imbecility
Imitation, mimicry ★

Impatience
Impertinence
Impetuous
Impulse, morbid
Inconstancy
Indifference, apathy
   duties, to
   ennui, with
   morose
   perspiration, during
   puberty, in
   welfare of others, to
   work, with aversion to
Indolence, aversion to work
   morning
   forenoon
   children, in
   eating, after
Industrious, mania for work
   evening •
   menses, before
Initiative, lack of
Inquisitive
Insanity, madness
   anger, from
   behaves like a crazy person
   climacteric period, during
   crawls on the floor •
   domestic calamity, after •
   drunkards, in
   haughty
   loquacious
   megalomania
   menses during
   mental labor, from
   mortification, from
   paralysis, with
   persecution mania
   religious
   sexual excesses, from
Insolence
Intriguer
Irony, satire, desire for •
Irresolution, indecision
   marry, to

Irritability
    morning
    evening
    convulsions before
    epilepsy, before
    headache, during
    heat, during
    touch, by
    waking, on
Jealousy
    animal or an inanimate object, for
    brutal from, gentle husband be-
        coming
    crime, to a, driving ★
    drunkenness, during
    images, with frightful ●
    insane ★
    irresistible, as foolish as it is ●
    loquacity, with
    men, between
    quarrels, reproaches, scolds, with
    saying and doing what he wouldn't
        say and do
    strike his wife, driving to
    tearing the hair ●
Jesting
    fun of somebody, making ●
Jumping, bed, out of
Kill, desire to
    poison, impulse to
Lamenting, bemoaning, wailing
    pain, about
    sickness, about his
Lascivious, lustful
        daytime ●
    convulsions, before ★
    epilepsy, followed by ●
Laughing morning
    silly
Learns easily ★
Litigious
Loathing, general, waking, on
Loathing, life, at
        morning
        anxiety, with ●
    work, at

Loquacity
    evening
    busy
    **changing quickly from one
        subject to another**
    cheerful, exuberant
    drunkenness, during
    ecstasy, with ●
    excited
    heat, during
    heat and sweat, during, ★
    hoarseness, only kept in check by ●
    insane
    jesting, with
    menses, during
    mental exertion, after ●
    rambling ★
    selected expressions, in ●
    speeches, makes
    *sleeplessness with loquacity espe-
        cially before midnight* ●
*Love with one of own sex, homosexual-
    ity, tribadism*
Magnetized, desire to be
    easy to magnetize
Malicious, spiteful, vindictive
    dreams, in ●
Mania
    mental exertion, after ●
    rage, with
    shrieking, in
Marriage seemed unendurable, idea of
Mathematics, apt for
Meditation
Memory, active
    evening
    suppressing sexual desire, from ●
Memory, loss of: sunstroke, after
Memory, weakness of
    done, for what has just
    expressing oneself, for
    facts, past, for
        recent, for, old people, in
    happened, for what has
    heard, for what has
    names, for proper

Memory, weakness of
>   *orthography, for*
>   **read, for what has**
>   said, for what has
>   *time, for*
>   *words, of*

Menses, mental symptoms agg. before

Mental symptoms alternating with physical

Misanthropy

Mischievous

Mistakes, calculating, in
>   localities, in
>   reading, in
>   space and time, in
>   speaking, in
>>   misplacing words
>>   *spelling, in*
>   time, in
>>   afternoon, always, imagines it is
>   **writing, in**

Moaning, groaning, whining
>   children, in ★
>   heat, during
>   sleep, during

Mocking
>   *jealousy, with* ●
>   ridicule, passion to
>   *sarcasm*
>   *satire, desire for*

Mood, agreeable
>   changeable, variable

Moral feeling, want of,
>   criminal, disposition to become a; without remorse

Morose, cross, fretful, ill-humor, peevish
>   *morning*
>   drunkenness, during

Morphinism

Muttering

Nymphomania
>   climacteric period, at

Objective, reasonable

Obscene, lewd

Obstinate, headstrong

Offended, easily; takes everything in bad part

Orderly manner, cannot perform anything in ●

Partial, prejudiced

Persists in nothing

Pessimist

Philosophy, ability for

Play, dirty trick on others or their teachers, school boys play a

Playful

Poisoned feeling ★

Positiveness

Prejudice, traditional

Prostration of mind, mental exhaustion, brain-fag
>   **morning**
>   *eating, after*
>   sleeplessness, with

Pull one's hair, desire to

Quarrelsome, scolding
>   *alternating with gaiety and laughter*
>   *jealousy, from*

Quick to act

Quiet disposition

Rage, fury
>   evening
>   shrieking, with
>   touch, renewed by
>   water, at sight of

Reading, aversion to read

Recognize, relatives, does not r. his
>   streets, does not r. well known

Refuses to take the medicine
>   treatment, every

Religious affections
>   *children, in*
>   *melancholia*
>   *puberty, in*

Remorse

Reproaches himself
>   *others*

Reserved

Rest, desire for

Restlessness
  evening
  night
  air amel., in open
  anxious
  bed, tossing about in
  busy
  chill, at beginning of
  driving about
    air, in open
  eating, after
  headache, during
  warm bed agg.
Revelry, feasting
Rudeness
Sadness, despondency, dejection,
    mental depression, gloom,
    melancholy
        morning
            waking, on
        night
  children, in
  chill, during
  climaxis, during
  girls before puberty, in
  labor, during
  menses amel.
  pregnancy, in
  puberty, in
  respiration, with impeded
  sighing, with
    amel.
  waking, on
Self-control, want of
Selfishness, egoism
Senses, acute
  dull, blunted
  vanishing of
Sensitive, oversensitive
  external impressions to all
  mental exertion, after •
  noise, to
  odors, to
  reading, to
  touch, to
Sentimental
  drunkenness, weeping or being
    sentimental during

Serious, earnest
Shining objects agg.
Shrieking, screaming, shouting
  convulsions, before
    during epileptic
    puerperal
  urinating, before
Sighing
  shock from injuries, in •
Singing
  sleep, in
Sit, inclination to
Sitting, aversion to
Slander, disposition to
  denouncer
  sneak
Slowness
Sociability
Somnambulism
Speech, affected
  babbling
  bombast, worthless
  confused
  extravagant
  facile
  finish sentence, cannot
  foolish
  foreign tongue, in a
  hasty
  incoherent
  loud
  nonsensical
  prattling
  repeats same thing
  slow
  wandering
Starting, startled
    evening, asleep, on falling
  noise, from
  sleep, falling, on
      during
      from
  waking, on
      suffocated, as if
Strange, crank
Strength increased, mental

Stupefaction, as if intoxicated
    convulsions, between
    sleepiness, with
    warm, amel. when feet became •
Suicidal disposition
    night
    drowning, by
    intermittent fever, during
    pains, from
    run over, to be
    throwing himself from a height
Suppressed or receding skin diseases or
    haemorrhoids, mental symp-
    toms agg. after
Suspicious, mistrustful
    afternoon
    evening
Sympathy, compassion
Talk, anxious to talk in public
    indisposed to, desire to be silent,
        taciturn
        heat, during
Talking, sleep, in
Talks, when alone
    himself, to
        only when alone
Theorizing
Thinking, complaints agg., of
Thoughts, intrude, writing, while •
    persistent
        evil, of •
    rapid, quick
    ridiculous
    rush, flow of
        night
    thoughtful
    tormenting
    vanishing of
        chill, during
        reading, on
        speaking, while
        writing, while
    wandering
Thunderstorm, during, mind symptoms
Time, fritters away his
    passes too slowly, appears longer
Timidity, evening, going to bed, about
    appearing, talk in public, to

Torments those about him
Touched, aversion to being
Trance
Tranquillity, serenity, calmness
Travel, desire to
Unconsciousness, coma, stupor
    apoplexy, in
    chill, before
    conduct, automatic
    emotion, after
    fever, during
    looking upwards, on •
    menses, during
        after
    parturition, during
    raising arms above head, on
    sunstroke
    trance, as in a
    vertigo, during
    warm room, in
Undertakes many things, perseveres in
    nothing
Unfeeling, hard hearted
Ungrateful
Verses, makes
Violent
    deeds of violence, rage leading to
    touch, from •
Vivacious
Wearisome
Weary of life
    morning
    future, from solicitude about •
    heat, during
Weeping, tearful mood
    night
        sleep, in
    agg.
    amel.
    anecdotes, from •
    convulsions, during
        epileptic
    drunkenness, weeping or being
        sentimental during
    emotion, after slight
    involuntary
    joy, from

Weeping, tearful mood
  menses, during
  noise, at
  offence, former, about
  pains, with the
  poetry, at soothing ●
  pregnancy, during
  questioned, when ★
  reading, while
  sleep, in
  spasmodic
  vexation, from old
  waking, on
  whimpering, sleep, during
Whistling
Will, two wills, feels as if he had
    weakness of
Witty
Work, aversion to mental
  desires for
    evening
    easy at night ●
    fatigues
    impossible

LACHNANTHES TINCTORIA

Cheerful, gay, mirthful
  evening
Delirium
    night, 1-2 h. ●
  loquacious
Delusions, imaginations, hallucinations,
    illusions
  images, phantoms, sees
    dozing, during day, sees im-
      ages while ●
  snakes in and around her
Excitement, excitable
  trifles, over
Irritability
  headache, during
Loquacity
    night 1-2 h. ●
  stupid and irritable, then ●
Mistakes, writing, omitting words
Moaning, groaning, whining

Mood, changeable, variable
Morose, cross, fretful, ill-humor, peevish
Restlessness
  heat, during
  perspiration, during
Sadness, despondency, dejection, mental
    depression gloom, melancholy
  headache, during
Sensitive, noise, to
Singing
Touched, aversion to being
Weeping, tearful mood
Whistling

LACTUCA VIROSA

Anger, irascibility
Anguish
Antics, plays, delirium, during
Anxiety
    evening
    night
  cough, before
Concentration, difficult
Confusion of mind, morning, rising and
    after, on
Contrary
Delirium
  gay, cheerful
  jumping, with
  laughing
  singing
Delusions, ink stand, he saw one on bed
  light, incorporeal, he is
  murdered, he will be
  soldiers on his bed, sees ●
Dullness, sluggishness, difficulty of think-
    ing and comprehending, torpor
    morning
  sleepiness, with
  sleeplessness, with
Eccentricity
  fancies, in
Fancies, exaltation of
  vivid, lively
Fear, apprehension, dread

Foolish behavior
Forsaken feeling
Grief
Hysteria
Indolence, aversion to work
 morning
Irritability
Jumping
Memory, weak, expressing oneself, for
Mood, repulsive
Restlessness
 anxious
 internal
 sleepiness, with
Sadness, despondency, dejection, mental
 depression, gloom, melancholy
 evening
Senses, dull, blunted
Sighing
Singing
Stupefaction, as if intoxicated
Unconsciousness, coma, stupor
Weeping, tearful mood
 evening
Work, mental, impossible

LAMIUM ALBUM

Anxiety, chill, during
Concentration, difficult
Confusion of mind, intoxicated, as after
 being
Delusions, insane, she will become
Forsaken feeling
Restlessness
 chill, during
Sadness, despondency, dejection, mental
 depression, gloom, malancholy
Thoughts, disconnected
 persistent
  expression and words heard
 recur to his mind
Weeping, tearful mood

LAPIS ALBUS

Cretinism

LAPATHUM ACUTUM

Excitement, excitable
Sadness, despondency, dejection, mental
 depression, gloom, melancholy

LATRODECTUS HASSELTI

Delusions, imaginations, hallucinations,
 illusions

LATRODECTUS KATIPO

Delirium

LATRODECTUS MACTANS

Anguish
Anxiety
Death, agony before
 sensation of
 thoughts of
Fear, apprehension, dread
 death, of
 insanity, losing his reason, of
Moaning, groaning, whining
Prostration of mind, mental exhaus-
 tion, brain-fag
Restlessness
Sadness, despondency, dejection, mental
 depression, gloom, melancholy
Sensitive, oversensitive
 noise, to
Shrieking screaming, shouting
 anguish, from •
 pains, with the
Speech, hesitating
Weeping, tearful mood

LAUROCERASUS

Absorbed, buried in thought
Abstraction of mind
 ailments from:
  fright
Anger, irascibility

Anxiety
>> daytime
>> evening
>>> twilight, in the
>>> bed, in
>> midnight, before
>> air, amel. in open
>> bed, in
>> chill, during
>> fever, during
>> head, heat of, with
>> inactivity, with
>> stool, after
>> trifles, about

Business, averse to

Cheerful, gay, mirthful
>> evening
>>> bed, in
>> afternoon
>> heat, during

Concentration, difficult

Confusion of mind
>> afternoon
>> heat, during
>> intoxicated, as if
>>> as after being
>> mental exertion, from
>> rising, after
>> writing, while

Contented

Contrary

Cowardice

Delusions, accused, she is
> criticised, she is
> dead persons, sees
> enlarged
> faces, sees
>> distorted, on lying down, day time
> fire, visions of
> images, sees frightful
> man: old men with long beards and distorted faces, sees •
> old men, sees •

Dementia, epileptics, of •

Despair

Destructiveness

Dipsomania, alcoholism

Discontented, displeased, dissatisfied

Discouraged
> weeping, with

Disgust
> *everything, with*

Dullness, sluggishness, difficulty of thinking and comprehending, torpor
>> morning
>> afternoon

Ecstasy, heat, during

Ennui, tedium

Excitement, excitable
>> evening in bed
>> night

Exertion, agg. from mental

Exhilaration

Fancies, exaltation of
>> heat, during

Fear, apprehension, dread
> *evil, of*
> imaginary things, of
> insanity, losing his reason, of
> misfortune, of

Forgetful
>> afternoon
>> evening
>> motion, on •

Forsaken feeling

Grief

Heedless

Hurry, haste
>> mental work, in

Hydrophobia

Ideas abundant, clearness of mind
>> deficiency of

Imbecility

Impetuous

Indifference, apathy
>> sleepiness, with

Indiscretion

Indolence, aversion to work
>> sadness, from
>> sleepiness, with

Industrious, mania for work

Inquisitive

Irreligious ★
Irresolution, indecision
Irritability
    headache, during
Laughing agg.
Loathing, general
Loathing, life, at
Mania
Memory, weakness of
    pains, from, suddenly ★
    done, for what has just
    labor, for mental
    sudden and periodical
Mildness
Moaning, groaning, whining
Mood, repulsive
Moral feeling, want of
Morose, cross, fretful, ill-humor, peevish
    afternoon
Passionate
Prostration of mind, mental exhaus-
    tion, brain-fag
Restlessness
    evening
    air amel., in open
Sadness, despondency, dejection, mental
    depression, gloom, melancholy
    anxious
    house, driving out of ●
    respiration, with impeded
    work-shy, in
Senses, dull, blunted
    vanishing of
Sensitive, oversensitive
Sentimental
Shrieking, screaming, shouting
    aid, for
    convulsions, before
Sit, inclination to
Speech, hesitating
Starting, sleep, during
    from
Stupefaction, as if intoxicated
    vertigo, during
Thinking, complaint agg., of
Thoughts, persistent
    vanishing of

Timidity
Tranquillity, serenity, calmness
Unconsciousness, coma, stupor
    apoplexy, in
    fever, during
    mental insensibility
    prolonged ★
    semi-consciousness
    sudden
    trance, as in a
    vertigo, during
Unfeeling, hard hearted
Weary of life
Weeping, tearful mood
Will, weakness of
Work, aversion to mental
    desire for
    impossible
Writing agg. mind symptoms

LECITHINUM

Concentration, difficult
Confusion of mind
    dream, as if in a
Excitement, excitable
    company, in
Exertion, agg. from mental
Fear, disease, of impending
Forgetful
Irritability
Memory, weakness of
**Prostration of mind, mental exhaus-
    tion, brain-fag**
Restlessness
Sadness, despondency, dejection, mental
    depression, gloom, melancholy
Thinking, aversion to
Work, aversion to mental

LEDUM PALUSTRE

Absent-minded, unobserving
Activity, mental, desire for
Anger, irascibility
    violent
Answers
    refuses to answer

Anxiety
> morning
> conscience: dreams, anxiety of c. in

Aversion, friends, to
Capriciousness
Chaotic, confused behaviour
Cheerful, gay, mirthful
Company, aversion to; presence of other people agg. the symptoms; desire for solitude
> *avoids the sight of people*

Concentration, difficult
Confusion of mind
> eating, after
> intoxicated, as if

Contented, himself, with
Contrary
Cowardice
Death, desires
Delirium, closing the eyes, on
> maniacal

Delirium tremens, mania-a-potu
Delusions, imaginations, hallucinations, illusions
> fancy, illusions of
> eyes, on closing
> images, phantoms, sees
> night
> spectres, ghosts, spirits, sees, closing eyes, on
> visions, closing the eyes, on

Dipsomania, alcoholism
Discontented, displeased, dissatisfied
> daytime

Disgust
> *everything, with*

Dullness, sluggishness, difficulty of thinking and comprehending, torpor
> chill, during
> eating, after

Ennui, tedium
Exertion, agg. from mental
Exuberance
Fancies, exaltation of
> night, closing the eyes in bed
> sleeplessness, with

Fear, apprehension, dread
> crowd, in a
> death, of
>> die, fear he will, if he goes to sleep (after nightmare)
> *men, dread, fear of*
> *people, of; anthropophobia*
> *sleep, fear to go to*

Forgetful
Frightened, easily
> waking, on

Hatred
> men, of
> revenge, hatred and

Ideas abundant, closing the eyes, on
Impetuous
Inconstancy
Industrious, mania for work
Insanity, madness
Irresolution, indecision
> changeable

Irritability
Loathing, life, at
Malicious, spiteful, vindictive
Mania
Meditation
Memory, weakness of
Misanthropy
Moaning, sleep, during
Mood, repulsive
Morose, cross, fretful, ill-humor, peevish
Passionate
Prostration of mind, mental exhaustion, brain-fag
Restlessness
> night
> bed, tossing about in
> **move, must constantly** ★

Sadness, despondency, dejection, mental depression, gloom, melancholy
> *company, aversion to, desire for solitude*

Senses, dull, blunted
Serious, earnest

Starting, startled
    dream, from a
    sleep, falling, on
        during
        from
    wáking, on
Stupefaction, as if intoxicated
Talk, indisposed to, desire to be silent,
    taciturn
Talking, sleep, in
Tranquillity, serenity, calmness
Unconsciousness, coma, stupor
    morning
Violent
Walk, walking in open air agg. mental
    symptoms
Wearisome
Weary of life
Weeping, tearful mood

LEPIDIUM BONARIENSE

Cheerful, gay, mirthful
Delusions, alone, graveyard, she is
    alone in a
    grave, he is in his
    pursued by enemies
        ghosts by
    spectres ghosts, spirits, sees
        pursued by, is
Discontented, displeased, dissatisfied
Dullness, ˙sluggishness, difficulty of
    thinking and comprehending,
    torpor
Ideas, deficiency of
Indifference, apathy
    everything, to
Laughing
Quarrelsome, scolding
Restlessness
Sadness, despondency, dejection, mental
    depression, gloom, melancholy
    waking, on
Shrieking, screaming, shouting
Torpor
Unconsciousness, coma, stupor

LEPTANDRA VIRGINICA

Anxiety, waking, on
Delirium
Despair
Doubtful, recovery, of
Fear, waking, on
Irritability
**Sadness, despondency, dejection,
    mental depression, gloom,
    melancholy**
Sensitive, noise, to
Thoughts, disease, of

LEVOMEPROMAZINUM

Ailments from:
    anticipation, foreboding, presenti-
    ment
Anguish
    room with light and people, agg.
    in a •
Anorexia mentalis
Anxiety, anticipation, from
Concentration, difficult
Delusions, imaginations, hallucinations,
    illusions
    enlarged, eyes are
    faintness, of
Fear, crowd, in a
    public places, of; agoraphobia
    insanity, losing his reason, of
Indifference, apathy
    surroundings, to the
Malicious, spiteful, vindictive
    injure someone, desire to
Restlessness
Schizophrenia
Shrieking, aid, for
Weeping, tearful mood

LILIUM SUPERBUM

Concentration, difficult
Fear, insanity, losing his reason of
Indifference, apathy
Restlessness, night
    midnight, after, 2h.
    headache, during

Sadness, despondency, dejection, mental
    depression, gloom, melancholy
    morning
Fear, insanity, losing his reason, of

LILIUM TIGRINUM

Absorbed, buried in thought
    misfortune, imagines ★
Activity
    amel.
    fruitless ★
Affections, in general ★
Ailments, from:
    sexual excesses
Amorous ★
Amusement, averse to
Anger, irascibility
Answers: aversion to answer
Anxiety
        evening, bed, in
        night
        future, about
        salvation, about
Aversion to being approached
Awkward, drops things ★
Brooding, disease, imaginary, over ★
Business, averse to
Busy
    fruitlessly
Climacteric period agg.
Clinging, held amel., being
Company, aversion to; presence of other
        people agg. the symptoms; de-
        sire for solitude
*Company, desire for; aversion to soli-
        tude, company amel.*
    alone agg., while
Concentration, difficult
        crazy feeling on top of head, wild
        feeling in head with confusion
        of ideas ●
Confusion of mind
        night, lying down, on
        identity, duality, sense of
        lying, when
        reading, while
        writing, while

Conscientious, trifles, occupied with
Consolation, kind words agg.
Cursing, swearing
        evening ●
Death, desires
Delirium
Delusions, body, divided, is
        deserted, forsaken, is
        disease, incurable, has
        divided into two parts
        doomed, being
            expiate her sins and those of her
            family, to ●
        double, of being
        insane, she will become
        unreal, everything seems
Dementia
    senilis
Desires, beautiful things, finery ★
Despair
    pains, with the
    religious despair of salvation
        *alternating with sexual excite-
            ment* ●
Destructiveness
Discontented, displeased, dissatisfied
        everything, with
        his own things, with ★
Doubtful, recovery, of
        soul's welfare, of
Dream, as if in a
Dullness, sluggishness, difficulty of think-
        ing and comprehending, torpor
        afternoon
        words, with inability to find right ●
Ennui, entertainment amel.
Envy
Escape, attempts to
Excitement, excitable
        amel.
        palpitation, with violent
Exertion, agg. from mental
Fancies, confused
        exaltation of
        lascivious

Fear, apprehension, dread
    business, of
    death, of
    disaster, of
    disease, of impending
      incurable, of being
    downward motion, of
    evil, of
    falling, of
      room, agg. in ●
    happen, something will
    heart, of disease of
    insanity, losing his reason, of
    misfortune, of
    moral obliquity alternating with
      sexual excitement ●
    say something wrong, lest he
      should ●
    suffering, of
Forgetful
    thinking of something agg. forget-
      fulness,
      diversion amel. ●
    words while speaking, of; word
      hunting
Forsaken feeling
Gestures, makes, grasping ★
Grief, hunting for something to grieve
    oneself ●
Haughty
Hurry, haste
    aimless ★
    drives everyone, shouting "hurry,
      hurry" ★
    duties, as by imperative ●
    occupation, in
    . desires to do several things
      at once
    walks to and fro, cannot be amused
      by thinking or reading ●
Hysteria
Ideas, deficiency of
Impatience
Indifference, apathy
    done for her, about anything
      being ●

Indolence, aversion to work
    physical
Industrious, mania for work
Insanity, madness
    alternating mental with physical
      symptoms
    business, from failure in
    climacteric period, during
    erotic
    religious
    sexual excesses, from
Introspection
Irritability
    morning, waking, on
    forenoon
    afternoon
    evening
    consolation agg.
    pollutions, after
    prolapsus uteri, in ●
    spoken to, when
    waking, on
Jealousy
Lascivious, lustful
Laughing
    serious matters, over
Loquacity
Mania
Memory, weakness of
    expressing oneself, for
    say, for what is about to
    words, of
Mental symptoms alternating with
    physical
Mildness
Mistakes, speaking, in
    writing, in
Morose, cross, fretful, ill-humor, peevish
Nymphomania
Obscene, lewd
    talk
Occupation, diversion amel.
Profanity ★
Pull one's hair, desire to
Reading, aversion to read

Recognize, streets, does not recognize
well known
Religious affections
night tortured by religious ideas
alternating with sexual excitement
melancholia
Restlessness
anxious, compelling rapid walking
*Sadness, despondency, dejection, mental
depression, gloom, melancholy*
day and night, with diarrhoea
in the morning •
night
bed, in
alternating with sexual excitement •
climaxis, during
headache, during
Self-torture
Senses, confused
Sensitive, noise, to slightest ★
Shreiking, screaming, shouting
must shriek, feels as though she
Sighing
Sit, inclination to ★
Snappish
Speech, hasty
Spoken to, averse to being
alone, wants to be let
Starting, startled
Striking
desires to strike
Stupefaction, as if intoxicated
Suicidal disposition
poison, by
thoughts
Talk, desire to talk to someone
indisposed to, desire to be silent,
taciturn
Tears, hair, her
Throws things, persons, at
Timidity
Torments himself
Tranquillity, serenity, calmness
Unconsciousness, coma, stupor

**Undertakes many things, perse-
veres in nothing**
Unreasonable
Violent
deeds of violence, rage leading to
Weeping, tearful mood
anger, after
consolation agg.
Wild feeling in head ★
Will, muscles refuse to obey the will
when attention is turned away
Work, aversion to mental
impossible

LIMULUS CYCLOPS

Dullness, sluggishness, difficulty of thinking and comprehending, torpor

LINARIA VULGARIS

Dullness, sluggishness, difficulty of thinking and comprehending, torpor

LINUM CATHARTICUM

Asks for nothing
Dullness, sluggishness, difficulty of think-
ing and comprehending, torpor
Indifference, apathy
Indolence, aversion to work
Irritability
Memory, weakness of
Morose, cross, fretful, ill-humor, peevish
Perseverance, duties, in performing
irksome •

LIPPIA MEXICANA

Anxiety
Restlessness

LIPPSPRINGE AQUA

Anxiety
Fear, apprehension, dread
misfortune, of
Homesickness
Irritability

Memory, weakness of
Morose, cross, fretful, ill-humor, peevish
Restlessness
    sitting, while
Sadness, despondency, dejection, mental
    depression, gloom, melancholy
Writing, desire for

LITHIUM CARBONICUM

Anxiety
    night
Confusion of mind, standing, while
Despair
    all night ●
Discouraged
Emotion, slightest, causes palpitation ★
Excitement, excitable
    palpitation, with violent
Forgetful, names of objects ★
Forsaken feeling
Helplessness, feeling of, night ●
Memory weak, names, for proper
Sadness, despondency, dejection, mental
    depression, gloom, melancholy
Weeping, tearful mood
    lonely feeling, from ★

LOBELLIA INFLATA

Anguish
Anxiety
Confusion of mind
    eating, after
    motion, from
Death, presentiment of
    thoughts of
Delirium
    maniacal
    raging, raving
    waking, on
Dipsomania, alcoholism
Dullness, sluggishness, difficulty of think-
    ing and comprehending, torpor
    spoken to, when
Excitement, excitable
Fear, apprehension, dread
    death, of
    suffocation, of

Hysteria
Insanity, madness
Morphinism
Prostration of mind, mental exhaus-
    tion, brain-fag
Rage fury
Restlessness
    internal
Sadness, despondency, dejection, mental
    depression, gloom, melancholy
Stupefaction, as if intoxicated
Torpor
Weeping, tearful mood
    aloud wobbing

LOBELIA CARDINALIS

Ailments from :
    grief
Singing
Starting, sleep, during

LOBELIA PURPURASCENS

Hurry, haste
Restlessness

LOBELIA SYPHILITICA

Ailments from:
    grief
Sadness, despondency, dejection, mental
    depression, gloom, melancholy
Singing
Weeping, tearful mood
Wildness
Mistakes
    speaking, spelling in
    writing, in

LOLEUM TEMULENTUM

Anxiety
Concentration, difficult
Confusion of mind
Delirium
    raging, raving
Delirium tremens, mania-a-potu
Delusions, imaginations, hallucinations,
    illusions

Dullness, sluggishness, difficulty of think-
   ing and comprehending, torpor
Excitement, excitable
Fear, apprehension, dread
Imbecility
Insanity, madness
Mania, rage, with
Prostration of mind, mental exhaus-
   tion, brain-fag
Rage, fury
Restlessness
   anxious
Stupefaction, as if intoxicated

LONICERA CAPRIFOLIUM

Stupefaction, as if intoxicated

LONICERA PERICYLMENUM

Irritability

LONICERA XYLOSTEUM

Answers: unable to answer
Unconsciousness, coma, stupor

LUFFA OPERCULATA

Indifference, apathy
Irritability
Sadness, despondency, dejection, mental
   depression, gloom, melancholy
Vivacious

LUPULUS HUMULUS

Delirium
Delirium tremens, mania-a-potu
Dipsomania, alcoholism
Sadness, despondency, dejection, mental
   depression, gloom, melancholy
Starting, sleep, from
Stupefaction, as if intoxicated
Unconsciousness, coma, stupor
Weeping, night

LYCOPODIUM CLAVATUM

Abrupt, rough
   rough, yet affectionate
Absent-minded, unobserving
   old age, in
Abstraction of mind
Abusive, insulting
   children insulting parents
   fever, during typhoid •
Activity, mental
Affectation,
   words, in
Affections, in general ★
Affectionate
Ailments from:
   anger vexation
      anxiety with
      indignation with
      silent grief, with
      suppressed
   **anticipation, foreboding, pre-
      sentiment**
   anxiety
   continence ★
   disappointment
   egotism
   excitement, emotional
   fear
   fright
   grief
   literary, scientific failure
   mortification
   scorn, being scorned
   sexual excesses
   work, mental
Amativeness
   want of amativeness in men
      women
Ambition
   means, employed every possible
Amorous
Anger, irascibility
   morning, waking, on
   ·evening
   night
   absent persons while thinking of
      them, at

Anger,
> **contradiction, from**
> easily
> **former vexations, about**
> himself, with
> trembling, with
> trifles, at
> *violent*
> **waking, on**

Anguish

Answers, dictatorial ●
> *distracted* ●
> *hastily*
> slowly

Anticipation, complaints from

Anxiety
> *morning*
>> *waking, on*
> *forenoon*
> *afternoon, 16 h.*
> *evening*
>> *bed, in*
> night
>> waking, on
> *midnight, before*
>> after
>> on waking
> *air, in open, amel.*
> **anticipation, from, an engagement ★**
> **exaggerated ★**
> *bed, in*
>> turning in, when ●
> chagrin, after ●
> company, when in
> cramps, as from ●
> crowd, in a
> dreams, on waking from frightful
> *epilepsy, during intervals of*
> *fear, with*
> fever, intermittent, during
> *flatus, from*
> fright, after
> **house, in**
> **health, about ★**
> hypochondriacal
> pulsation in the abdomen, with ●

Anxiety,
> *salvation, about*
>> scruples, excessive religious
>> scrupulous as to their religious
>>> *practices, too*
> *sleep, on going to*
>> *during*
> *stormy weather, during* ●
> vexation, after
> waking, on
> **walking, air, in open**

Approach of persons agg.

Automatism, motions (automatic) ★

Avarice

Aversion to being approached
> *children, to her own*
> everything, to
> his own mind, to ★
> members of family, to
> *men, to*
> sex, to opposite, religious aversion
> **women, to**

Barking,
> growling like a dog, during sleep ●

Bed, aversion to, shuns bed

Beside oneself, being

Blasphemy, cursing and

Boaster, rich, wishes to be considered
> as

Brooding

Business, averse to

Calculating, inability for

Capriciousness

Carefulness

Cares, worries, full of

Carried, desires to be

Cautious, anxiously

Censorious, critical

Character, lack of ★

Cheerful, gay, mirthful
> afternoon
> evening, bed, in
> night
> alternating with sadness
> sleep, during
> thunders and at lightnings, when
> it

Children, flies from the own •
Company, aversion to; presence of other
people agg. the symptoms; de-
sire for solitude
alone, amel. when
fear of being alone, yet
loathing at company
perspiration, during
presence of strangers, aversion to
Company, desire for; aversion to
solitude, company amel.
alone agg., while
Complaining
Comprehension, easy
Concentration, difficult
aversion to
calculating, while
conversation, during
studying, reading etc., while
Confidence, want of self
Confusion of mind
morning
waking, on
evening
night
eating, after
daily affairs, about ★
identity, duality, sense of
intoxicated, as if
menses, during
mental exertion, from
reading, while
waking, on
walking, air, in open
amel.
warm room, in
Conscientious about trifles
16-20h •
Consolation, kind words agg.
Contemptuous
hard for subordinates and agreeable, pleasant to superiors or
people he has to fear
Contradict, disposition to

Contradiction, is intolerant of
agg.
Contradictory to speech, intentions are
Contrary
Coquettish, not enough
too much
Corrupt, venal
Cowardice
Cross, waking, on ★
Cursing, swearing
Cynical ★
Darkness agg.
Death, desires
presentiment of
thoughts of
morning
waking, on •
Deception causes grief and mortifi-
cation ★
Deceitful, sly
Defiant
Delirium
evening
night
envy, with •
exhaustion, with
haemorrhage, after
imperious •
maniacal
menses, before
during
murmuring
muttering
, **raging, raving**
reproachful
sleep, during
sleeplessness, and ★
sorrowful
Delirium tremens, mania-a-potu
Delusions, imaginations, hallucina-
tions, illusions
evening
night
animals, of
assembled things, swarms, crowds
etc.

Delusions,
  childish fantasies, has ●
  die, he was about to
  dogs, sees
  doomed, being
  double, of being
  faces, sees hideous
  fancy, illusions of
  flies, sees ●
  house is full of people
  images, phantoms, sees
      afternoon ●
      evening
      night
      frightful
    sleep, during ●
      hateful (afternoon) ●
      preventing
  wall, on the
  injury, is about to receive
  insulting, with ●
  murdered, he will be
  music, he hears
    evening, hears the music heard
      in the day ●
  neglected his duty, he has
  people, sees
    *day and evening (on entering
      the room)* ●
  person is in the room, another
  *places at a time, of being in
      different*
    *two at the same time,
      of being in*
  present, someone is
  presumptuous ●
  pursued by enemies
  religious
  room, sees people at bedside, en-
      tering, on ●
  sick, being
  sinking, to be
  spectres, ghosts, spirits, sees
  unfortunate, he is
  vanish, everything will ●
  visions, has
      daytime

Delusions, visions,
    closing the eyes, on
    horrible
    vivid
    voices, hears
    weeping, with
    wrong, he has done
Dementia ★
Despair
    perspiration, during
    recovery, of
    religious despair of salvation
*Dictatorial, domineering, dogmatical,
    despotic*
        command, talking with air of
    power, love of ●
Dipsomania, alcoholism
Discomfort forenoon
Discontented, displeased, dissatisfied
    morning
    himself, with
Discouraged
    children, in ●
    quiet, and ●
    weeping, with
Disobedience
Doubtful, recovery, of
    soul's welfare, of
**Dullness, sluggishness, difficulty of
    thinking and comprehend-
    ing, torpor**
    evening
    night on waking
air, in open, amel.
    after being in open air ●
    children, in
    menses, during
    mental exertion, from
    old people, of
    reading, while
    siesta, after
    sleepiness, with
    speaking, while
    walking, air amel., in open

Dwells on past disagreeable occur-
rences
    night
    recalls, disagreeable memories
Effeminate
Egotism, self-esteem
Ennui, tedium
Envy
    avidity, and
    qualities of others, at
Escape, attempts to
    family, children, from her
Estranged, being kind with strangers,
    but not with his family and
    entourage
    flies from her own children •
Excitement, excitable
    morning
    afternoon
    evening
      bed, in
    night
      sleep, during •
    children, in
    chill, during
    menses, before
    perspiration, during
    wine, as from
Exertion, agg. from mental
Exuberance
Fancies, exaltation of
    afternoon
    evening, bed, in
    night, closing the eyes in bed
    sleeplessness, with
    lascivious
    vivid, lively
Fear, apprehension, dread
    daytime, only
    morning
      bed, in
    evening
    night
      waking, after
    alone, of being
    appearing in public, of
    approaching him, of others
    bed, of the

Fear,
    children, in
    crowd, in a
    dark, of
    death, of
      morning
    destination, of being unable to
      reach his •
    disease, of impending
    door, in opening
    everything, constant of
    ringing of door bell, even at •
    evil, of
    ghosts, of
      evening
      night
    happen, something will
    heart, arising from
    imaginary things, of
    lifelong
    men, dread, fear of
    menses, suppressed, from
    narrow places, in; claustro-
      phobia
    new persons, of •
    noise, from
    door, of
    people, of; anthropophobia
    children, in
    yet agg. if alone ★
    pregnancy, during
    room, on entering
    solitude, of
    stomach, arising from
    stoppage of circulation, with sen-
    sation of (at night) •
    strangers, of
    suffocation, of, night
    thunderstorm, of
    trifles, of
    undertaking, anything
    waking, on
      dream, from a
    walking, while
      air, in open
    weary of life, with

Finance, aptitude for
    inaptitude for
Flatterer
Flattery, gives everything, when flat-
    tered
Foolish behavior
Forgetful
    evening
    (-ness) old people, of
        words while speaking, of; word
        hunting
Forsaken, beloved by his parents, wife,
    friends, feels of not being
Forsakes his own children •
Frightened, easily
    night
    trifles, at
    waking, on
        dream, from a
Frown, disposed to
Gamble (*see* Play)
Gestures, grasping or reaching at some-
    thing, at flocks; carphologia
    fingers in the mouth, children
        put
    fingers spread apart ★
    picks at bedclothes
    strange attitudes and positions
    talking, gesticulate while, head,
        with
Godless, want of religious feeling
Greed, cupidity
Grief
    silent
Hard for inferiors and kind for superiors
Hatred
    men, of
Haughty
    stiff and pretentious •
    stupid and haughty
Heedless
Helplessness, feeling of
Horrible things, sad stories, affect her
    profoundly

House, aversion to being kept in •
House-keeping, women unable to
Howling
Hurry, haste
    drinking, on
    eating, while
Hypochondriasis
    morning
    waking, on
Hypocrisy
Hysteria
Ideas abundant, clearness of mind
    evening
        bed, in
        night
    deficiency of
Idiocy
Imbecility
    rage, stamps the feet
Impatience
    heat, with
    waking, on •
    walking, while •
Impolite
    children •
Impulse, morbid
Inconsolable
Inconstancy
Indifference, apathy
    children, to her
    company, society, while in
    ennui, with
    everything, to
    external impressions, to
        things, to
    life, to
    sleepiness, with
Indolence, aversion to work
    afternoon
    eating, after
    physical
    sleepiness, with
Industrious, mania for work
Inquisitive

Insanity, madness
    anger, from
    dictatorial •
    envy, with •
    haughty
    malicious, malignant
    megalomania
    puerperal
    religious
    reproaches others •
Insolence
    servants to chiefs, of
Introspection
Irresolution, indecision
    acts, in
    trifles, about
    waking, on •
Irritability
    day time
    morning, waking, on
    evening
    night
        waking, on
    absent persons, with
    alternating with cheerfulness
    children, in
        cross all day, good all night •
        pushes nurse away
        sick, when •
    chill, during
    consolation agg.
    menses, before
        during
    noise, crackling of newspaper, even from
    sadness, with
    suspicious
    waking, on
Jealousy
Jesting
    joke, cannot take a
Kicks
    child is cross, kicks and scolds on waking •
Kill, desire to
    knife, with a

Kleptomania
Lamenting, bemoaning, wailing
    future, about •
Languages, unable for
Lascivious, lustful
Laughing
    night
    anxiety, after
    dream, during
    involuntarily
    joyless •
    looked at, when •
    ludicrous, everything seems
    serious matters, over
    silly
    sleep, during
    spasmodic
    trifles, at
    vexation, at •
    weeping and laughing at same time
Liar
Libertinism
Loathing, general
    waking, on
Loathing, life, at
    morning
Looked at, can't bear to be agg. mental symptoms
Loquacity; changing quickly from one subject to another
Malicious, spiteful, vindictive
    anger, with
Mania
    rage, with
Mathematics, inapt for
    horror of mathematics
Meddlesome, importunate
Memory, weakness of
    colors, for
    done, for what has just
    expressing oneself, for
    facts, past, for
    forms, for
    labor, for mental
    letters, for the names of the. •

Memory, weakness of
  music, for
  names, for proper
  orthography, for
  persons, for
  read, for what has
  words, of
Menses, mental symptoms agg. before
  at beginning of
  during
Mildness
Misanthropy
Mistakes, calculating, in
  reading, in
  speaking, in
    misplacing words
    spelling, in
    wrong syllables, gives
    words, using wrong
      says plums, when he means
      pears
    writing, in
      adds letters •
      confounding letters •
      omitting letters
      omitting syllables
      words
    transposing letters
    wrong words
Moaning, groaning, whining
  menses, during
  sleep, during
Mood, alternating
  changeable, variable
  opinions, in
  repulsive
Morose, cross, fretful, ill-humor, peevish
  daytime
    morning
      bed, in
  evening
  night
  fever, during
  menses, before
  during
  trifles, about
  waking, on

Music agg.
  organ agg., of
  wearisome from •
Muttering
Nagging ★
Nymphomania
Obscene, lewd
Obstinate, headstrong
  children
  simpleton, as a
Occupation, diversion amel.
Offended, easily; takes everything
  in bad part
Optimistic
Passionate
Perseverance
Play, aversion to play in children
  passion for gambling
  to make money
Pompous, important
Prejudice, traditional
Precocity ★
Presumptuous
Prostration of mind, mental ex-
  haustion, brain-fag
Pushed, down ★
Quarrelsome, scolding
    morning
    disputes with absent persons •
    waking, on •
Quiet, disposition
Rage, fury
    night
    headache, with
    malicious
    striking, with
    violent
Reading, unable, to read
    written, what he has •
Rebels against poultice
Recognize, relatives, does not, his
Reflecting, unable to reflect
Religious affections
    horror of the opposite sex
    melancholia
    very religious ★

Repeated ★
Reproaches himself
   others
Reserved
Resignation
Rest, desire for
Restlessness
   morning
      waking, on
   afternoon 16-18 h
   evening
      bed, in
   night
   midnight, after
   air amel., in open
   anxious
   bed, driving out of
      tossing about in
   headache, during
   heat, during
   internal
      beat about herself with hands
         and feet, as if would ●
   menses, before
   pain, during
      from
   room, in
   sitting, while
   walking, air. amel., in open
Rhythmic ★
Rudeness
   employees to the chiefs, of
   fever, during ●
Sadness, despondency, dejection,
   mental depression, gloom,
   melancholy
   morning
      waking, on
      evening
   alone, when
   anger, from
   anxious
   children, in
   chill, during
   company, agg. in
   diarrhoea, during

Sadness,
   heart sensations, from ●
   heat, during
   menses, before
      during
      delayed, from
   music, from
   perspiration, during
   respiration, with impeded
   waking, on
Secretive
Selfishness, egoism
Senses, dull, blunted
Sensitive, oversensitive
   heat, during
   menses, during
   mental impressions, to
   music, to
   noise, to
      crackling of paper, to
      slightest, to
   odors, to
   pain, to
   sensual impressions, to
   want of sensitiveness
Sentimental
Serious, earnest
Servile, obsequious, submissive
Shamelessness
Shrieking, screaming, shouting
   anxiety, from
   brain cry
   children, in
      sleep, during
   convulsions, before
      during epileptic
   cramps in abdomen, during
   fever, during
   hydrocephalus, in
   paroxysmal
   sleep, during
   urinating, before
   waking, on
Sighing
   menses, before

Singing
    involuntarily
    trilling
Sit, inclination to
Sits erect
    still
Slander, disposition to
Slowness
Smiling, involuntarily
Somnambulism
    climbing the roofs, the railing of
        bridge or balcony
Speech, affected
    babbling
    childish
    confused
    delirious, menses, before •
    hasty
    intoxicated, as if
    slow
    unintelligible
    wandering
    wild
Spit, desire to
Spoiled children
Spoken to, averse to being
Spying, everything
Squanders, order, from want of
Starting, startled
    night
    anxious
    feet, as if coming from the •
    fright, from and as from
    lying, while •
    noise, from
    pain agg.
    sleep, falling, on
        as from feet •
    during
    from
    trifles, at
    waking, on
Strangers, presence of strangers agg.
Striking
    about him at imaginary objects
    bystanders, at
    children, in

Stupefaction, as if intoxicated
    morning
    afternoon
    evening
    reading, on •
    rouses with difficulty
Suicidal disposition
    morning
    waking, on
Sulky
Suppressed or receding skin diseases or
    haemorrhoids, mental symp-
    toms agg. after
Suspicious, mistrustful
Sympathy, compassion
Talk, anxious to talk in public
    indisposed to, desire to be silent,
        taciturn
    heat, during
Talking, sleep, in
Talks, humming
    one subject, of nothing but
Tastelessness in dressing
Theorizing
Thinking, aversion to
    afternoon •
    evening •
Thoughts, disagreeable
    on waking •
    disconnected
    rush, flow of
        evening in bed
        sleeplessness from
    stagnation of
    thoughtful
    tormenting
    vacancy of
    vanishing of
    wandering
Time passes too slowly, appears longer
Timidity
    evening, going to bed, about
    appearing, talk, in public, to
        but capable to •
    bashful ★

Torpor
Touched, aversion to being
Traquillity, serenity, calmness
Unconsciousness, coma, stupor
    morning
    evening
    conduct, automatic
    crowded room, in a
    fever, during
    hydrocephalus, in
    jaw, dropping
    menses, after
        suppression of
    periodical
    scarlatina, in
    standing, while
    talking, while •
    vertigo, during
    warm room, in
Undertakes many things, perseveres in
    nothing
Unfortunate, feels
Ungrateful
Unreliable, promises, in his
Usurer
Vanity
Verses, makes
Violent
    deeds of violence, rage leading to
    pain, from
Wearisome
Weary of life
    morning, bed, in •
    waking, on
    company, in •
    syphilis, in •
    waking, on
Weeping, tearful mood
    daytime
    afternoon, 16-20 h. •
    evening
    night
        sleep, in
    admonition, from
    aloud, wobbing

Weeping, tearful mood
    alternating with laughter
    amel.
    anxiety, after
    causeless
    children, in
    chill, during
    consolation agg.
    convulsions, during
    coughing, during
    desire to weep, all the time
    easily
    emotion, after slight
    future, about the •
    heat, during
    joy, from
    laughing at same time, weeping
        and
    menses, before
        during
        after
    nervous, all day
    pains, with the
    past events, thinking of
    perspiration, during
    sleep, in
    thanked, when •
    trifles, children at the least worry
    ungratefulness, at •
    urination, before
    waking, on
    whimpering, sleep, during
Whistling
    involuntary
Will, loss of
    weakness of
Work, aversion to mental
    fatigues
    impossible
Writing;
    difficulty in, expressing ideas,
    when
    inability for
Yielding, disposition

LYCOPERSICUM ESCULENTUM

Anger, irascibility
Irritability
Morose, cross, fretful, ill-humor, peevish
Sensitive, noise, to

LYCOPUS VIRGINICUS

Activity, mental,
  5 h.
    evening
    restless
Concentration, difficult
Delusions, dirty, he is
Dullness, sluggishness, difficulty of thinking and comprehending, torpor
    menses, during
Excitement, excitable
    evening
Hurry, haste
Hypochondriasis
Ideas, abundant, evening
    deficiency of
      menses, during •
Irritability, diabetes, in
Restlessness, evening
    night
Sadness, despondency, dejection, mental depression, gloom, melancholy
Sighing, evening, 19h. •
Stupefaction, menses, during
Suspicious, mistrustful
Talk, indisposed to, desire to be silent, taciturn
Thinking, complaints agg., of
Thoughts, control of, lost
    vanishing of
    wandering
Touch everything, impelled to
Work, desire for mental
    evening

LYSSINUM

Abrupt, harsh
Absent-minded, unobserving
Abstraction of mind
Abusive, insulting
    husband insulting wife and children •
Ailments from:
    anticipation, foreboding, presentiment
    bad news
    excitement, emotional
    fright
    mortification
Anger, irascibility
    alternating with, repentance, quick
    trifles, at
    violent
    waking, on
Answers: aversion to answer
    offensive •
    rapidly
    refuses to answer
Anxiety
    anticipation, from, an engagement ★
    bed, in
      driving out of
    church bells, from hearing •
    headache, with
    noise of rushing water
Attack others, desire to
Aversion, water, to ★
Barking, growling like a dog
Bite, desire to
    convulsions, with
    delirium, during
    himself, bites
    pillow, bites
    spoon etc., bites
Cheerful, evening
Clairvoyance
Comprehension, easy
Concentration, difficult
Confusion of mind
Cruelty, inhumanity

Cursing, swearing
Cut, mutilate, slit others, desire to •
Death: dying, feels as if
    presentiment of
Delirium
        night
    loquacious
    rabid
Delusions, imaginations, hallucina-
        tions, illusions
    abused, being •
    animals, of
    attack and insults, defend them-
        selves against imaginary •
    bird, he is a, runs about, chirping
        and twittring, until he faints •
    deserted, forsaken, is
    dog: he is a dog, growls and barks
    engaged in some occupation, is
    falling, walls
    falling inward, epileptic fit, before ★
    fancy, illusions of
    fire, visions of
    great person, is a
    happen, something terrible is go
        ing to •
    hell, is in
        suffers the torments of, with-
            out being able to explain
    injure: injured, is being
    insulted, he is
    mouth, cannot open, lower jaw stiff
    and   painful •
    objects: immaterial o., in room.
    people, sees
    strange, familiar things seem
        notions seem •
    swallow, cannot •
    tormented, he is
    walls, falling
    wrong, suffered, has
Despair, shrieks of despair, paroxys-
        mal •
Discontented, displeased, dissatisfied
Drinking, mental symptoms after

Dullness, sluggishness, difficulty of think-
    ing and comprehending, torpor
        night on waking
Eccentricity
Ecstasy
Estranged, forgetful of relatives and
        friends •
Excitement, excitable
        agg.
        conversation, from hearing •
        convulsive
        water poured out, from hearing
Exhilaration
        daytime •
Fancies, lascivious
        strange, pregnancy, during •
Fear, apprehension, dread
    alone, of being
    approaching vehicles, of
    bad news, of hearing
    bitten, of being
    dogs, of
    evil, of
    falling, of
        evening •
        walking, when
    fit, of having a
    happen, something will
        terrible ★
    insanity, losing his reason, of
    knaves, of
    knives, of
    mirrors in room, of
    misfortune, of
    noise, rushing water, of
    ordeals, of
    pregnancy, during
    run over, of being (on going out)
    senses, with exalted state of, smell,
    taste, touch •
    waking, on
    water, of
Forgetful
    friends and relatives, of •
Forsaken feeling

Gestures, grasping, wrong things, at •
Hydrophobia
   hear the word "water" without shudder of fear, cannot •
   idea of water causes paroxysm •
Hypochondriasis, evening
Ideas abundant, clearness of mind
Impatience
   day time •
   headache, during
Impulse, stab his flesh with the knife he holds, to •
Indifference, apathy
   coition, during •
Injure: frenzy causing him to injure himself
Insanity, erotic
Insolence
Irresolution, indecision
   trifles, about
Irritability
   evening
   headache, during
   water, on hearing or seeing of •
Jumping, bed, out of
Kill, desire to
   injure with a knife, impulse to
   throw child into fire, sudden impulse to
   out of the window •
Lamenting, bemoaning, wailing
Lascivious, lustful
   afternoon •
   eating with feeling of weakness in parts, after •
   erections, with
   painful, with •
Loquacity
   night
Mania
Meditation
Memory, active
Memory, weakness of
   words, of

Mistakes, speaking, words, using wrong
Morose, cross, fretful, ill-humor, peevish
   evening
   night
   conversing amel. •
   waking, on
News, feels as if he had received joyful •
Obscene, lewd
Offended, easily; takes everything in bad part
Praying
   others to pray for him, begged •
Pregnancy, mental affections in
Prostration of mind, mental exhaustion, brain-fag
Quarrelsome, scolding
   afternoon, 16 h.
Rage, repentance, followed by
Reflecting
Restlessness
   forenoon
   noon
   night
   driving about
   headache, during
Roaming and roving ★
Rudeness
Sadness, despondency, dejection, mental depression, gloom, melancholy
   daytime
   evening
   anxious
Satyriasis
Senses, acute
Sensitive, oversensitive
   music, sacred music, to
   noise, to
     others eat apples, hawk or blow their noses, cannot bear to hear •
   water splashing, to
   singing, to
Shining objects agg.
   surface of water agg. •

Sighing
Singing
    involuntarily
Speech, hasty
    offensive •
    pathetic •
Spitting, directions, in all •
Starting, startled
    afternoon
    noise, from
Striking
Stupefaction, as if intoxicated
    night
Suicidal, throwing himself from
    height ★
Sympathy, felt same pain his brother
    complained of •
Talk: others agg., talk of
Thoughts, frightful
    insane •
    persistent
    strange
      pregnancy, in
    two trains of thoughts
Throws things away
    persons, at
Tranquillity, serenity, calmness
Unconsciousness, coma, stupor
    transient
Wander, desires to
Weeping, tearful mood
    evening
    aloud, sobbing
    headache, with
Wildness
Work, mental
    impossible

M

MAGNETIS POLUS ARCTICUS

Anger, irascibility
Anxiety
    evening
    night
    midnight, after
    conscience, as if guilty of a crime
    fear, with
    fever, during
    future, about
    hypochondriacal
    menses, before
Audacity
Capriciousness
Cautious
Censorious, critical
Cheerful, gay, mirthful
    alternating with sadness
      timidity •
Clairvoyance
Discouraged
    anxiety, with
    reproaches himself •
Dullness, sluggishness, difficulty of think-
    ing and comprehending, torpor
Fancies, exaltation of
    night
Fear, apprehension, dread
    disease, of impending
    evil, of
Heedless
Hurry, haste
Hypochondriasis, night
    morose
Ideas, deficiency of
Inconsolable
Industrious, mania for work

Irresolution, indecision
  evening
Irritability
  heat, during
    bemoaing, wailing
Lamenting, asleep, while
Loquacity, heat, during
Memory, weakness of
Mildness
Mistakes, writing, in
Mood, changeable, variable
Morose, cross, fretful, ill-humor, peevish
  night
Reproaches himself
Restlessness, anxious
  busy
  heat, during
Sadness, despondency, dejection, mental
  depression, gloom, melancholy
  evening
  anxious
Senses, dull, blunted
Sensitive, oversensitive
Singing
  night
  sleep, in
Slowness
  work, in
Somnambulism
Starting, dream, from a
  sleep, during
Stupefaction, sleepiness, with
Talk, indisposed to, desire to be silent,
  taciturn
Talks, himself, to
Thoughts, rush, flow of
  night
  waking, on
  stagnation of
Weeping, tearful mood
  evening
  night
  midnight, at
  sleep, in
Work, mental, impossible

MAGNETIS POLUS AUSTRALIS

Abusive, insulting
Anger, irascibility
  trembling, with
  violent
  work, aversion to
Capriciousness
Cheerful, evening in bed
Company, aversion to; presence of other
  people agg. the symptoms; desire
  for solitude
Discontented, displeased, dissatisfied
  himself, with
Disgust, exhilarations of others, at •
Dullness, sluggishness, difficulty of think-
  ing and comprehending, torpor
  evening, bed, in
Excitement, evening, bed in
Forsaken, feeling
Frightented easily
Hurry, haste
Inconstancy
Indolence, aversion to work
Irresolution, indecision
  changeable
  ideas, in
Irritability
  chill, during
  waking, on
Mood, changeable, variable
Morose, cross, fretful, ill-humor, peevish
  evening
  chill, during
  fever, during
  waking, on
Quarrelsome, scolding
Restlessness
  anxious
Sadness, despondency, dejection, mental
  depression, gloom, melancholy
  alone, when
Senses, dull, blunted
Starting, dream, from a
  sleep, during
Stupefaction, as if intoxicated
Talking, sleep, in

Violent, vehement
Weeping, tearful mood
    anger, after
Wildness

MACROTINUM

Anger, irascibility
Concentration, difficult
Dullness, sluggishness, difficulty of
    thinking and comprehending,
    torpor
Fear, apprehension, dread
    danger, of impending
Irritability
Memory, weakness of
Morphinism
Restlessness
Sadness, despondency, dejection, men-
    tal depression, gloom, melan-
    choly
    menses, agg. during
        amel. during
Starting, fright, from and as from
Suspicious, mistrustful

MAGNESIA CARBONICA

Absent-mindeded, unobserving
    writing, while •
Absorbed, buried in thought
Abstraction of mind
Abusive, insulting
Ailments from :
    anger, vexation
    friendship, deceived
    fright
    grief
    injuries, accidents; mental symp-
        toms from
Anger, irascibility
    violent
Anguish
    daytime
    bed, amel. after going to •
Anticipation, dentist, physician, before
    going to

Anxiety
    daytime
    morning
        rising, on and after
        waking, on
    noon
    afternoon
    evening
        bed, in
        amel. •
        uneasiness and anxiety,
            must uncover
    night
    midnight, before
    bed, in
    conscience, as if guilty of a crime
    dinner, after
    eating, while
        of warm food •
    fear, with
    fever, during
    head, heat of, with
    motion, from
    rising, after
    sleep, before
    soup, after
    stool, during
    supper, after
    waking, on
    warm bed, yet limbs cold if
    uncovered •
Aversion, everything, to
    women, to
Bad temper, morning ★
Beside oneself, anxiety, from
Capriciousness
Censorious, critical
Cheerful, afternoon
    evening
Company, aversion to; presence of other
        people agg. the symptoms; de-
        sire for solitude
    alone, amel. when
Concentration, difficult
    writing, while

Confusion of mind
    morning
        rising and after, on
    air, in open
    breakfast amel.
    intoxicated, as if
    mental exertion, from
    noise agg. •
    room, in
Contradict, disposition to
Contrary
Delirium, headache, during
Delusions, anxious
    dead persons, sees
    disease, incurable, has
    money, he is counting
    murdered, he will be
    people, sees
    thieves, sees
    water, of
Despair, pains, with the
    recovery, of
Dipsomania, alcoholism
Discomfort .
    morning
    forenoon
Discontented, displeased, dissatisfied
    everything, with
Disgust
    everything, with
Dullness, forenoon
    dinner, after
    mental exertion, from
    writing, while
Excitement, heat, during
    menses, before
Exertion, agg. from mental
Fear, apprehension, dread
    daytime, only
    morning
    afternoon
    evening
        amel.
        bed, in
            amel. •
    night
    accidents, of

Fear,
    death, vomiting,
    evil, of
    exposure night in bed, of •
    happen, something will ★
        evening in bed amel.
        warmth of bed amel.
    insanity, losing his reason, of
    menses, during
    misfortune, of
        evening in bed amel. •
    robbers, of
    tremulous
Forgetful
    eating, after
Forsaken feeling
    beloved by his parents, wife,
    friends, feels is not being
Frightened easily
Gourmand
Greed, cupidity
Homesickness
Hypochondriasis
Hysteria
Indifference, apathy
    morning
    afternoon
    pleasure, to
    sleepiness, with
Indolence, aversion to work
    morning
    forenoon
    afternoon
    evening
    dinner, after
    eating, after
    sleepiness, with
Industrious, mania for work
    menses, before
Irritability
    daytime
    morning
    forenoon
    afternoon
    evening
        amel.

Irritability,
  air, amel. in open
  children, in
  chill, during
  grief, from
  menses, during
  perspiration, during
  walking, amel., in open air
Jealousy, loquacity, with
Kleptomania, dainties, steals
Looked at, cannot bear to be
Loquacity
  drunkeness, during
Memory, weakness of
Menses, mental symptoms agg. during
Mistakes, writing, in
Moaning, groaning, whining
Mood, changeable, variable
  repulsive
Morose, cross, fretful, ill-humor, pee-
  vish
    morning
    forenoon
    afternoon amel. •
    evening
    house, agg. in; amel. on walking
      in open air
    menses, during
    perspiration, during •
Naked, wanis to be morning in bed
Nervous, worn-out
    women ★
Nibble, desire to ★
Prostration of mind, mental exhaus-
  tion, brain-fag
Quarrelsome, scolding
Reading: unable, to read, in children
Reserved
Restlessness
    evening
    night
    bed, driving out of
      tossing about in
    heat, during
    menses, after •
    sitting, while

Sadness, despondency, dejection, mental
  depression, gloom, melancholy
    evening
      amel.
    talk, indisposed to
Senses, dull, blunted
Sensitive, oversensitive
    noise, to
    sensual impressions, to
Shrieking, screaming, shouting
    night
    children, in
    pain, with the
    sleep, during
    waking, on
Sighing, sleep, in
Singing
    trilling
Sit, inclination to
Starting, noon
      sleep, in
    night
      midnight in sleep, about
    dream, from a
    fright, from and as from
    itching and biting, from •
    lying on back
      right side •
    noise, from
    sleep, on falling
      during
      from
    sleepiness, with
    touched, when
Striking, knocked his head against wall
  and things
Stupefaction, exertion agg., mental
Sulky
Talk, indisposed to, desire to be silent,
  taciturn
    sadness, in
Talking agg. all complaints
    sleep, in
Talks, himself, to
Thinking, complaints amel., of
Timidity
Touched, aversion to being

Travel, desire to
Unconsciousness, coma, stupor
    morning
    evening when lying down
    night, waking, on
    lying, while
    sensation, of •
    vertigo, during
    waking, on
Walk; walking in open air amel. mental
    symptoms
Wearisome, evening
Weeping, night
    midnight, at
    aloud, wobbing, in sleep •
    pregnancy, during
    sleep, in
    waking, on
    whimpering with toothache •
Work, mental, impossible

MAGNESIA FLUORATA

Anxiety
Indolence, aversion to work
Irritability
Sadness, despondency, dejection, mental depression, gloom, melancholy

MAGNESIA MURIATICA

Absorbed, buried in thought
Ailments from:
    anger, vexation
    friendship, deceived
    homsickness
    sexual excesses
Anger, irascibility
Anguish
Answers: aversion to answer
    morning •
Anxiety
    morning
        waking, on
    afternoon
        until evening
    evening

Anxiety, evening,
    bed, in
        closing the eyes, on •
    night
    midnight, before
    abdomen, with distension of •
    air, amel. in open
    bed, in
    closing eyes, on
    dinner, during •
        after
    eating, after
    eructations amel.
    fever, during
    health, about
    house, in
    menses, before
        during
    reading, while
    stool, before
Barking, growling like a dog
Busy
    himself, with
Capriciousness
Chaotic, confused behavior
Cheerful, gay, mirthful
    daytime
    morning
Company, aversion to; presence of other
    people agg. the symptoms; desire
    for solitude
Concentration, difficult
    morning
Confusion of mind
    morning
        rising and after, on
        waking, on
    air, amel. in open
    dinner, during •
        after •
    eating, after
    intoxicated, as if
    lying, when
    mental exertion, from
    wrapping up head amel. •
Contrary
Conversation agg.

Delusions, imaginations, hallucinations,
  illusions
  animals, of
  clouds, rocks and, looking over •
    sees
  dead, mutulated c.
    persons sees
  fancy, illusions of
    heat, during
  fire, visions of
  friendless, he is
  growling as of a bear, hears •
  hearing, illusions of
  horses, sees
  images, phantoms, sees
  journey, he is on a
  mutilated bodies, sees
  noise, hears
  people: behind him, someone is
    reading after her, which makes
    her read faster, someone is •
  rocks in air •
  strange, familiar things seem
  thieves, sees
  walks behind him, someone
  water, of
  wedding, of a
Discontented, displeased, dissatisfied
Discouraged
Disgust
  everything, with
Dullness, sluggishness, difficulty of think-
  ing and comprehending, torpor
    morning, rising, on
    evening
    air amel., in open
Ennui, tedium
  evening
Excitement, excitable
  menses, before
    during
Exertion, agg. from mental
Fancies, exaltation of
  reading, on
Fear, apprehension, dread
    morning
    evening

Fear,
    dinner, after
    eating food, after
    liver, in affections of the ★
    noise, from
    robbers, of
    waking, dream, from a
Forsaken feeling
Frightened easily
    waking, dream, from a
Gamble (*see* Play)
Grief
Homesickness
Hypochondriasis
Hysteria
    menses, during
                copious
Ideas, same, repeated ★
Indifference, apathy
    morning, waking, on
    pleasure, to
    sleepiness, with
Indolence, aversion to work
    evening
    sleepiness, with
Introspection
Irresolution, indecision
Irritability
    morning
      rising, after
      waking, on
    forenoon
    evening
    coition, after
    headache, during
    menses, before
      during
    waking, on
Loathing, general
    morning
Menses, mental symptoms, agg. before
      during
Mildness
Misanthropy
Mood, changeable, variable
    repulsive

Morose, cross, fretful, ill-humor, peevish
    morning
    evening
    alternating with cheerfulness
Nibble, desire to
Obstinate, headstrong
Patient
Play, passion for gambling, to make
    money
Reading, mental symptoms agg. from
Restlessness
    evening
    bed, in
    night
    midnight, after
        2 h.
        closing eyes, agg. on
    anxious
    bed, driving out of
        tossing about in
    closing eyes at night agg.
    heat, during
    waking, on
Sadness, despondency, dejection, mental
    depression, gloom, melancholy
        morning
    alone, when
    eating, before ●
        amel., after
    menses, during
Senses, dull, blunted
Sensitive, oversensitive
    noise, to
        voices, to
    pain, with the
    reading, to
    sleep, during
Shrieking, sleep, during
Sit, inclination to
Spoken to, averse to being
Starting, night
    midnight in sleep, before
    electric shocks through the body
        while wide awake
    sleep, on falling
        during
        from
Stupefaction, as if intoxicated

Sulky
Talk, indisposed to, desire to be silent,
    taciturn
    morning
    others agg., talk of
Talking, sleep, in
    anxious
Thoughts, thoughtful
Time passes too slowly, appears longer
Torpor
Unconsciousness, coma, stupor
        evening, when, lying down
    eating, after
    lying, while
Unfriendly humor ★
Weeping, tearful mood
    night
    dinner, after ●
    eating, after
    sleep, in
Work, aversion to mental
    impossble

MAGNESIA PHOSPHORICA

Ailments from:
    work, mental
Capriciousness
Concentration, difficult
    studying, learns with difficulty
Delusions, imaginations, hallucina-
    tions, illusions
    die, he was about to die
    tetanus, must die of, with pain in
        right leg ●
Discontented, displeased, dissatisfied
Dullness, sluggishness, difficulty of think-
    ing and comprehending, torpor
Fear, motion, of
    touch, of
Forgetful, heat, after
Irritability, headache, during
Lamenting, bemoaning, wailing
    pains, about
Restlessness
Sadness, despondency, dejection, mental
    depression, gloom, melancholy
        morning
        sleepiness, with

Shrieking, screaming, shouting
    cramps in abdomen
    pain, with the
Study agg. ★
Talking agg. all complaints
Talks, himself, to
    always about her pain ★
    troubles, of her ★
Weeping, tearful mood
    aloud, sobbing
    convulsions, during
Work, aversion to mental
    impossible
Writing agg. mental symptoms ★

MAGNESIA SULPHURICA

Anger, irascibility
    night
    violent
    waking, on
Anguish
Anxiety
    morning
        waking, on
    conscience, as if guilty of a crime
Beside oneself, being
Business, averse to
Cheerful, gay, mirthful
Company, aversions to;
    alone, amel. when
Confusion of mind
    morning
        rising and after, on
            after, amel.
        waking, on
    evening
    air amel., in open
    stool amel.
    waking, on
Contented
    himself, with
Delusions, fancy, illusions of
    mice, sees
    people, sees
    strangers, he sees
        knitting, she sees strangers,
            while ●
    visions, has

Discontented, displeased, dissatisfied
Dullness, sleepiness, with
Excitement, excitable
Fear, apprehension, dread
    morning
    accidents, of
    death, of
    evil, of
        morning, on waking ●
    misfortune, of
    morning
    waking, on
Indolence, aversion to work
    afternoon
Irritability
    menses, during
Morose, cross, fretful, ill-humor, pee-
    vish
    afternoon
Offended, easily; takes everything in
    bad part
Quarrelsome, scolding
Restlessness
Sadness, despondency, dejection, mental
    depression, gloom, melancholy
    morning
    evening
Sensitive, oversensitive
    pain, to
Starting, dream, from a
    fright, from and as from
    sleep, during
Talk, indisposed to, desire to be silent,
    taciturn
    afternoon
Thinking, complaints agg., of
Tranquillity, serenity, calmness
Violent, vehement
Weeping, tearful mood

MAGNOLIA GRANDIFLORA

Sadness, climaxis, during

MALANDRINUM

Dullness, sluggishness, difficulty of thinking and comprehending, torpor

MANCINELLA

Absent-minded, unobserving
Activity, business, in
    mental
Ailments from:
    anger, vexation
    joy, excessive
Anger, irascibility
Answers: aversion to answer
Anxiety
    cold, becoming, from
    fear, with
    walking, while
Cheerful, gay, mirthful
    desires to be cheerful, ineffectually
    •
Company, desire for; aversion to soli-
    tude, company amel.
Delirium
Delusions, devils: taken by the devil, he
    will be
    hearing, illusions of
    insane, she will become
    voices, hears
Discontented, displeased, dissatisfied
Dullness, sluggishness, difficulty of think-
    ing and comprehending, torpor
        morning
Ennui, tedium
Fear, apprehension, dread
    night
    midnight
    dark, of ★
    devil, of being taken by the
    ghosts, of
    insanity, losing his reason, of
Forgetful
    errand, of ★
Homesickness
Impatience
    headache, during

Indifference, apathy
    morning
        on waking
Indolence, aversion to work
Industrious, mania for work
Insanity, madness
    erotic
Irritability
Mania
Meditation
Memory, active
Memory, weakness of
    do, for what was about to
Mildness
Morose, cross, fretful, ill-humor, pee-
    vish
Nymphomania
    climacteric period, at
Puberty, mental affections in
Restlessness
    bed, tossing about in
*Sadness, despondency, dejection, mental
    depression, gloom, melancholy*
    morning
        midnight, after
    climaxis, during
    menses, before
    puberty, in
    sexual excitement, with
Sensitive, noise, to
Sentimental
Singing
Sympathy, compassion
Talk, indisposed to, desire to be silent,
    taciturn
Thoughts, thoughtful
    vanishing of
    wandering
Timidity
    bashful
Tranquillity, serenity, calmness
    morning on waking
Unconsciousness, coma, stupor
    fever, during
    vertigo, during
Weary of life

MANDRAGORA OFFICINARUM

Anxiety
Concentration, difficult
Confusion of mind
Delirium
Delusions, possessed, being
Discontented, displeased, dissatisfied
Discouraged
Euphoria, alternating with sadness
Excitement, excitable
Exhilaration
Hysteria
Indifference, apathy
Industrious, mania for work
Insanity, madness
Irresolution, indecision
Irritability
Kisses everyone
Mania
Memory, weakness of
Mood, alternating
Prostration of mind, mental exhaustion, brain-fag
Restlessness
Sadness, despondency, dejection, mental depression, gloom, melancholy
    urination, sadness followed by frequent •
Sensitive, oversensitive
    noise, to
    odors, to

MANGANUM ACETICUM AUT CARBONICUM

Absent- minded, unobserving
Absorbed, buried in thought
    afternoon •
Abstraction of mind
Anger, irascibility
    morning
    talk: of others, from talking
    trifles, at

Anxiety
    daytime
    night
    midnight,after
    fear, with
    future, about
    lying amel., while •
    menses, before
    mental exertion, from
    walking, while
Cares, worries, full of
Company, aversion to; presence of other people agg. the symptoms; desire for solitude
Concentration, difficult
Confusion of mind
    air, amel. in open
    sitting, while
Conversation agg.
Delusions, enlarged, body, parts of
    head is
    images, frightful, sees
Discomfort, afternoon
Discontented, displeased, dissatisfied
    himself, with
Discouraged
Dullness, sluggishness, difficulty of thinking and comprehending, torpor
Embittered, exasperated
Excitement, excitable
    morning
Exertion, agg. from mental
Fear, apprehension, dread
    midnight, after
    happen, something will
    menses, before
    misfortune, of
Frown, disposed to
Grief, future, for the
Hatred
    persons who had offended him, of
    revenge, h. and
Hysteria
Imbecility
Irresolution, indecision

Irritability
> *morning*
> *forenoon*
> afternoon
> headache, during
> *music, during*
> sitting, while
> talking, while

Laughing agg.
Malicious, spiteful, vindictive
Meditation
Memory, weakness of
Menses, mental symptoms agg. before
Mildness
Mistakes, speaking, in
> words, using wrong

Moaning, groaning, whining
> constant moaning and gasping for air

Morose, cross, fretful, ill-humor, peevish
> morning
> forenoon
> afternoon
> *music, during sad ●*
> > amel. ●

Music amel.
> aversion to joyous, but immediately affected by saddest ●

Prostration of mind, mental exhaustion, brain fag
Quiet disposition
Reading agg. ★
Reserved
> afternoon

Restlessness
> night
> midnight, after, 1h
> anxious
> bed, tossing about in
> menses, before

Sadness, despondency, dejection, mental depression, gloom, melancholy
> afternoon
> music amel., sad ●

Senses, confused
> dull, blunted

Sensitive, oversensitive
> noise, to
> pain, to

Stupefaction, afternoon
Sulky
Talk, indisposed to, desire to be silent, taciturn
> others agg., talk of

Thoughts, thoughtful
> afternoon

Timidity, bashful
Violent, vehement
> talk of others, from

Wearisome
Weeping, tearful mood
Work, mental, impossible

MATÉ

Contented
Pleasure
Sensitive, oversensitive

MEDORRHINUM

Abrupt, harsh
Ailments from:
> **anticipation, foreboding, presentiment**
> *bad news*
> reproaches
> work, mental

Answers, slowly
> *repeats the question, first ★*

Anticipation, complaints from
Anxiety
> **anticipation, from, an engagement, of**
> *conscience, as if guilty of a crime*
> *salvation, about*
> time is set, if a

Bites
> fingers, ★

Cares, worries, full of
Cheerful, evening
     alternating with sadness
Clairvoyance
Concentration, difficult
Confidence, want of self ★
Confusion of mind
     identity, as to his
Conscientious about trifles
Contradiction, is intolerant of
Cruelty, inhumanity ★
Death, presentiment of
Delusions, imaginations, hallucinations,
     illusions
     animals, of
     persons are rats, mice, insects etc.
     doomed, being
     dream, as if in a
     faces, sees
          wherever he turns his eyes,
               or looking out from corners
     hands, felt a delicate hand, smoo-
          thing her head●
     head caressed on, by someone ★
     hearing, illusions of
     insane, she will become
     people, sees
          behind him, someone is
          say "come" ●
     pursued, he was
     rats, sees
          running across the room
     religious
     strange, familiar things seem
     talking, someone, behind him ★
     time, exaggeration of, passes too
          slowly
     touched her head, someone ★
     unreal, everything seems
     voices, hears
     walks behind him, someone
     whispering him anything, some-
          one ●

Despair
     critique, after a light ●
     recovery, of
     religious despair of salvation
Dream, as if in a
Dullness, sluggishness, difficulty of think-
     ing and comprehending, torpor
     children, in
     understands questions only after
          repetition
     waking, on
Egotism, self-esteem
Excitement, anticipating events, when
     mental work, from
     reading, while
     trifles, over
     writing, while ●
Exertion, agg. from mental
Exhilaration
     evening
     night ●
Far off ★
Fear, apprehension, dread
     alone, of being, night ★
     behind him, someone is
     cats, of ★
     creeping out of every corner, of
          something
     dark, of
     death, of
     ghosts, of
     insanity, losing his reason, of
     misfortune, of
     noise, from
     sensation, of making ●
     suffocation of, night
     waking, on
Fishy ★
Forgetful, name, his own
     errand, of ★
     *words while speaking, of; word
          hunting*
Frightened, waking, on
Gestures, makes, fingers spread apart ★
Hurry, haste
     always, accomplishes nothing, but ★
     everybody moves too slowly ●

Ideas, many, uncertain in execution, but ● ★
    persistent ★
Idiocy, masturbation, with
Imbecility
Impatience
    trifles, about
Impulsive ★
Insanity, madness
Irritability
    daytime ★
    reading, while
    trifles, from
Jealousy
Kicks animals ★
Mania
Marriage seemed unendurable, idea of
Memory, weakness of
    dates, for
    heard, for what has
    names, for proper
    read, for what has
    said, for what has
    say, for what is about to
    thought, for what has just
    words, of
    write, for what is about to
Mistakes, speaking, spelling, in
    words, using wrong
    time, in
        present with the past
    writing, in
Mood, alternating
    changeable, variable
Morose, cross, fretful, ill-humor, peevish
    daytime
Music agg.
Play, desire to, night
Postponing everything to next day (Procrastination)
Praying, vomiting, constantly during paroxysms of ●
Prophesying, disagreeable events, of ●
Pull one's hair, desires to

Rage, pulls hair ★
    reading and writing, by ●
Reading, mental symptoms agg. from
Religious affections
Remorse
Reproaches himself
Responsibility, aversion to
Restlessness
    night
Sadness, despondency, dejection, mental depression, gloom, melancholy
    pollutions, from
    suicidal disposition, with
    weeping amel.
Schizophrenia, paranoid
Selfishness, egoism
Sensitive, oversensitive
    noise, to
    reprimands, to
        children, even mild scolding ★
Speech, confused
    finish sentence, cannot
Starting, startled
    noise, from
    sleep, during
    from
Stupefaction, as if intoxicated
Suicidal disposition
    sadness, from
    shooting, by
Superstitious ★
Suspicious, mistrustful ★
Talk, cannot, weeping, without ★
    same, over and over again ★
Thinking, complaints agg., of
Thoughts, vanishing of
    speaking, while
Time passes too slowly, appears longer
Touched, aversion to being
Unconsciousness, transient
Washing always her hands
Weeping, tearful mood
    amel.
    speaking, when ●
    spoken to, when
    telling of her sickness, when

Wild feeling in head ★
Wildness
Work, aversion to mental
    impossible
    seems to drive him crazy, owing
        to the impotency of his mind
Writing, agg. mental symptoms

MEDUSA

Anxiety

MELILOTUS OFFICINALIS

Anger, irascibility
    violent
Avarice
Confusion of mind
Delirium
    headache, during
    loquacious
Delusions, arrested, is about to be
    devils: possessed of a devil, every-
        one is •
    doomed, being
    home, away from, is
    looking at her, everyone is
    mesmerised by her absent pastor,
        she is •
    pursued by enemies
        police
Dullness, sluggishness, difficulty of think-
    ing and comprehending, torpor
Escape, attempts to
Fear, apprehension, dread
    people, of; anthropophobia
    poverty, of
    talking loud, as if it would kill
        her •
Forgetful
Hide, run away, and (children) ★
Homesickness
Imbecility
Indifference, apathy
Indolence, aversion to work

Insanity, madness
    eats refuse, only •
Irritability
Kill herself, sudden impulse to ★
    threatens to kill ★
Memory, weakness of
Mistakes, work, in
    writing, omitting letters in
        omitting words
Prostration of mind, mental exhaus-
    tion, brain-fag
Rage, fury
Recognize own house, does not
    relatives, does not recognize his
Religious affections
    melancholia
Sadness, despondency, dejection, men-
    tal depression, gloom, melancholy
Stupefaction, as if intoxicated
Suicidal disposition
Suspicious, mistrustful
Thoughts, persistent
Timidity
Unconsciousness, coma, stupor
    fever, during
Weeping, tearful mood
Work, mental, impossible

MENISPERMUM
CANADENSE

Absent minded, unobserving
Indolence, physical
Irritability
Morose, cross, fretful, ill-humor, peevish
Obstinate, headstrong
Prostration of mind, mental exhaus-
    tion, brain-fag
Restlessness
    night
Sadness, despondency, dejection, men-
    tal depression, gloom, melancholy
Starting, sleep, from
Sulky

MENTHA PIPERITA

Ideas abundant, clearness of mind
Industrious, mania for work
Unconsciousness, coma, stupor

MENTHA PULEGIUM

Restlessness
    night

MENYANTHES TRIFOLIATA

Amusement, averse to
Anxiety
    fear, with
Chaotic, confused behavior
Cheerful, gay, mirthful
Company, aversion to; presence of other
    people agg. the symptoms;
    desire for solitude
    desire for headache, during •
    headache, during •
Confusion of mind
    air amel., in open
    eating, after
Contented
    himself, with
Delirium
Delusions, imaginations, hallucinations,
    illusions
    night
Discontented, displeased, dissatisfied
    everything, with
    himself, with
    surroundings, with
Dullness, sluggishness, difficulty of think-
    ing and comprehending, torpor
    air in open, amel.
    eating, after
    painful
    room, in a •
Dwells on past disagreeable occur-
    rences
Exertion, agg. from mental
Fear, apprehension, dread
    alone, headache, with •

Fear,
    driving him from place to place •
    evil, of
    heart, arising from
    misfortune, of
Forsaken feeling
    headache, during •
Grief
Hurry, haste
    movements, in
Ideas, deficiency of
Indifference, apathy
    alternating with cheerfulness
        jesting •
    joyless
Indiscretion
Indolence, aversion to work –
Introspection
Jesting
    alternating with indifference •
    indifference, jesting, after
Meditation
Mood, agreeable
    changeable, variable
Morose, cross, fretful, ill-humor, pee-
    vish
Playful
Prostration of mind, mental exhaus-
    tion, brain-fag
Rashness
Reflecting
Reserved
Restlessness
    anxious
    driving about
Sadness, despondency, dejection, mental
    depression, gloom, melancholy
Senses, dull, blunted
Sensitive, touch, to
Shrieking, waking, on
Suspicious, mistrustful
Talk, indisposed to, desire to be silent,
    taciturn
Thoughts, disagreeable
    past, of the·
Tranquillity, serenity, calmness
Weeping, tearful mood

MEPHITIS PUTORIUS

Anger, irascibility
  easily
  trifles, at
Anguish, morning
Cheerful, followed by melancholy
Company, aversion to; presence of other
  people agg. the symptoms; desire
  for solitude
Comprehension, easy
Concentration, difficult
Delusions, imaginations, hallucinations,
  illusions
  head, large, seems too
  unfit for work •
  water, of
Dipsomania, alcoholism
Dullness, head as if enlarged, with ill
  humor and nausea •
Excitement, excitable
  head, with heat of •
Exertion, agg. from mental
Fancies, exaltation of
  vivid, lively
Frightened, waking, on, dream, from a
Gestures, angry, in night walking •
Ideas abundant, clearness of mind
Indifference, apathy
  pleasure, to
Indolence, aversion to work
Irritability
  headache, during
Loquacity
  drunk, as if
Memory, active
Moonlight, mental symptoms from
Morose, cross, fretful, ill-humor, peevish
  trifles, about
Quarrelsome, scolding
Restlessness
  morning
  evening
Sadness, despondency, dejection, mental
  depression, gloom, melancholy
  alternating with euphoria
Sensitive, oversensitive
Slowness

Somnambulism
Speech, intoxicated, as if
Stupefaction, as if intoxicated
  loquacious
Thoughts, rush, flow of
Work, aversion to mental

MERCURIUS SOLUBILIS

Absent-minded, unobserving
Absorbed, buried in thought
Abstraction of mind
Abusive, insulting
Ailments from:
  ambition, deceived
  anger, vexation
    indignation, with
  anticipation, foreboding, presen
    timent
  disappointment
  discords between chiefs and subordinates
    parents, friends
  egotism
  fright
  mortification
  sexual excesses
  surprise, pleasant
Amativeness
Amorous
Anarchist, revolutionary •
Anger, irascibility
  contradiction, from
  stabbed anyone, so that he could
    have
  trembling, with
  weeping from pain, with
Anguish, daytime
  menses, during
  stool, before
    during
Answers: aversion to answer
  incorrectly
  monosyllable
  slowly
Antics, plays
Anxiety
    daytime
    evening
    night

Anxiety,
>   midnight, before
>   *conscience, as if guilty of a crime*
>   driving from place to place
>   eating, after
>   exaggerated ★
>   *fear, with*
>   fever, during
>   fright, after
>   future, about
>   health of relatives, about
>   inactivity, with
>   menses, before
>   during
>   salvation, faith, about loss of his
>   sleep, on going to
>   during
>   *stool, before*
>   during
>   after
>   *suicidal disposition, with*
>   weary of life, with

Audacity
Avarice, alternating with squandering
Aversion, everything, to
>   *members of family, to*
>   *persons, to all*
Bed, aversion to, shuns bed
>   remain in, desires to
Beside oneself, being
Boaster, braggart
Busy
Calculating, inability for
Capriciousness
Carried, desires to be
Censorious, critical
Chaotic, confused behavior
Cheerful, gay, mirthful
>   *evening, bed, in*
>   alternating with want of sympa-
>   thy ●
>   foolish, and
Company, aversion to, bear anybody,
>   cannot
Company, desire for; aversion to soli-
>   tude, company amel.
>   *alone agg., while*

Complaining
>   *relations and surroundings, of* ●
Concentration, difficult
>   *calculating, while*
>   studying, reading etc., while
>   writing, while
Confidence, want of self
Confusion of mind
>   morning
>   rising and after, on
>   waking, on
>   air amel., in open
>   bed, jump out of, makes him
>   *eating, after*
>   loses his way in well-known streets
>   lying, when
>   rising, after
>   sitting, while
>   waking, on
>   working, while ●
Consolation, kind words agg.
Contemptuous
Contradict, disposition to
Contradiction, is intolerant of
Contrary
Country, desire for ★
Courageous
>   alternating with discouragement
Cowardice
Dancing
Death, desires
>   **presentiment of**
>   thoughts of
>   fear, without
Deceitful, sly
>   fraudulent
Deception causes grief and mortifica-
>   *tion* ★
Delirium
>   morning
>   *night*
>   crying, with
>   foolish, silly
>   jumping, with
>   maniacal
>   mouth, puts stones in ●
>   murmuring, himself, to

Delirium
> *muttering*
> naked in delirium, wants to be
> persecution in delirium, delusions
> > of
> *raging, raving*
> recognizes no one
> scolding
> sleep, during
> > falling asleep, on
> > waking, on

Delirium tremens, mania-a-potu

Delusions, imaginations, hallucina-
tions, illusions
> evening, bed, in
> > *night*
> animals, of
> > *jumping at her* •
> assembled things, swarms, crowds,
> etc.
> body, sweets, is made of •
> crime, committed a, he had
> *criminal, he is a*
> criminals, about
> dead, multilated corpse
> die, he was about to
> dogs, sees
> *enemy, everyone is an*
> > *surrounded by enemies*
> faces, sees
> > hideous
> fail, everything will
> falling asleep, on
> *fancy, illusions of*
> > heat, during
> foolish
> hearing, illusions of
> hell, is in
> > *suffers the torments of, without*
> > *being able to explain*
> house is full of people
> *images, phantoms, sees*
> > *night*
> > all over, sees
> > *frightful*
> > sleep, before
> injury, is about to recieve

Delusions,
> insane, she will become
> insects, sees
> men are on the bed at night •
> mouth, living things are creeping
> > into (at night) •
> murdered, he will he
> music, he hears
> mutilated bodies, sees
> needles, sees
> nose, takes people by
> people, sees
> persecuted
> pursued by enemies
> religious
> shoot with a cane, tries to
> spectres, ghosts, spirits, sees
> > night, sees at
> stove, heats, in heat of summer,
> > the •
> strange, familiar things seem
> thieves, sees
> > house, in
> vagina, living things creep into
> > (at night) •
> visions, has
> > horrible
> waking, on
> *water, flowing, sees* •
> weeping, with
> well, he is
> wrong, he has done

Dementia
> syphilitics, of

Despair
> chill, during
> *recovery, of*

Dictatorial, domineering, dogmatical,
despotic

Dipsomania, alcoholism

Dirtiness

Discontented, displeased, dissatis-
fied
> **always**
> **everything, with**
> > **revolutionary ★**
> himself, with
> surroundings, with

Discouraged
    alternating with courage
        hope
    future, about
Disgust
    everything, with
    himself, with; has no courage to
       live •
Disobedience
Doubtful, recovery, of
Dream, as if in a
Dress, unable to •
Dullness, sluggishness, difficulty of think-
    ing and comprehending, torpor
    daytime
      morning
        waking, on
    children, in
    damp air, from
    heat, during
    injuries of head, after
    sleepiness, with
Duty, no sense of duty
    stimulate sense of, to ★
Egotism, self-esteem
Enemy, considers everybody •
Enuui, tedium
Escape, attempts to
    night •
    anxiety at night, with •
    crime, for fear of having commit-
    ted a •
    run away, to
Estranged, ignores his relatives
Excitement, excitable
    evening, bed, in
    feverish
    lascivious, with painful nocturnal
      erections •
    suppression of excretions, from
    talking, while
    waking, frightened, as if •
Faces, made strange
Fancies, exaltation of
    evening, bed, in
    frightful
    sleeplessness, with

Fear, apprehension, dread
    evening
      bed, in
      night
    alone, of being
    bed, of the
    death, of
    impending death, of
    disease, of impending
    epilepsy, of
    escape, with desire to
    evil, of
    fit, of having a
    faith, to lose his religious ★
    health of loved persons, about
    health, ruined, that she has, of
      those she loves ★
    imaginary things, of
    insanity, losing his reason, of
      night
    men, dread, fear of
    misfortune, of
    palpitation, with
    people, of; anthropophobia
    pins, pointed things, sharp things,
      of
    restlessness, from fear
    robbers, of
      waking, on
    sleep, to go to
    suffocation, of
    suicide, of
    syphillis, of
    thunderstorm, of
Feces, licks up cow-dung, mud, saliva •
    swallows his own
Fight, wants to
Foolish behavior
Forgetful
    drunkards, forgetfulness in
    going, forgets where she is
Forsaken feeling
Frightened easily
    evening
    trifles, at
Frivolous
Fur, wraps up in summer
Gamble (*see* Play)

Gestures, convulsive
    grasping, children put everythig
        in the mouth
    genitals, delirium, during ★
    hands, motions, involuntary, of
      the
    ridiculous or foolish
    strange attitudes and positions
Gluttony
Godless; want of religious feeling
Gourmand
Greed, cupidity
Grief
     fear at night, with ●
Grimaces, strange faces, makes
Hatred, persons who had offended him,
    of
Haughty
Heedless
Home; leave home, desire to
Homesickness
Howling
Hurry, haste
    movements, in
Hydrophobia
Hypochondriasis
Hypocrisy
Hysteria
    menses, during
Ideas abundant, clearness of mind
    deficiency of
Idiocy
Imbecility
Impatience
    always
    trifles, about
Impolite
Impulse, morbid
    walk, to ★
Impulsive
Inconsolable, thoughts, of
Indifference, apathy
    daytime
    agreeable things, to
    duties, to
    eating, to
    everything, to

Indifference,
    life, to
    loved ones, to
    money-making, to
    reprimands, to all ●
    surroundings, to the
Indiscretion
Indolence, aversion to work
    morning ★
Injure himself, fears to be left alone, lest
    he should
Insanity, madness
    drunkards, in
    eats dung ●
    face, with pale
    foolish, ridiculous
    religious
    restlessness, with
    wantonness, with
    weeping, with
Intolerance
Irresolution, indecision
Irritability
    daytime
    alternating with cheerfulness
    chill, during
    consolation agg.
    eating, after
      to satiety ●
    headache, during
    perspiration, during
    stool, before
    suspicious
Jesting
    aversion to
Jumping, bed, out of
Kill, desire to
    beloved ones
    child, her own
    contradicts her, desire to kill the
      person that ●
    husband, impulse to kill her be
      loved
      menses, agg.during ●
      razor, therefore in
      plores him to hide his ●
    knife, with a
      at sight of a

Kill,
>   *menses, during*
>   *offence, sudden impulse to kill for*
>   *a slight*

Lamenting, bemoaning, wailing
>   others, about •
>   waking, on

Lascivious, lustful

Laughing, silly

Liar

Libertinism

Loathing, general

Loathing, life, at
>   work, at

Looked at, can't bear to be agg. mental
>   symptoms

Malicious, spiteful, vindictive
>   insulting

Mania
>   *rage, with*

Memory, loss of ; injuries of head, after
>   *insanity, in*

Memory, weakness of
>   dates, for
>   names, for proper
>   persons, for
>   places, for
>   *read, for what has*
>   said, for what has
>   say, for what is about to
>   time, for

Menses, mental symptoms agg. during

Misanthropy

Mischievous
>   *imbacility, in* •

Mistakes, calculating, in
>   localities, in
>   reading, in
>   *speaking, in*
>   misplacing words
>   words, using wrong

Moaning, groaning, whining
>   constant moaning and gasping for
>   air
>   *perspiration, during*
>   sleep, during

Mood, alternating
>   changeable, variable
>   *repulsive*

Moral feeling,want of; criminal, disposition to become a; without remorse

Morose, cross, fretful, ill-humor, peevish
>   daytime
>   eating, after

Morphinism

Music agg.
>   aversion to

Muttering
>   sleep, in

Naked, wants to be
>   delirium, in
>   sleep, in

Noise, inclined to make a

Nymphomania

Objective, reasonable

Obscene, lewd

Obstinate, headstrong

Offended, easily; takes everything in
>   bad part

Play, aversion to play in children
>   inability to
>   *passion for gambling*
>   to make money

Positiveness

Precocity

Prostration of mind, mental exhaustion, brain-fag

Pull, nose in the street, one's •

Quarrelsome, scolding
>   herself, with •
>   sleep, in

Rage, fury
>   evening
>   night
>   water, at sight of

Reading, unable, to read

Rebels against poultice

Recognizes own house, does not
>   *relatives, does not recognize his*

Religious affections

Remorse

Reproaches himself
>   others

Repugnance, everything, to ★

Restlessness
  afternoon
  evening
    20 h.
  night
  midnight, after
  anxious
  bed, driving out of
    go from one bed to another,
  wants to
  children, in
  conscience, of
  driving, about
  exertion, agg. after least ★
  sitting, while
  sleepiness, with
  waking, on
  walking, while
Sadness, despondency, dejection, mental depression, gloom, melancholy
  anxious
  chill, during
  menses, during
  sunshine, in ★
Satyriasis
Selfishness, egoism
Senses, dull, blunted
  vanishing of
Sensitive, oversensitive
  evening
  noise, to
  odors, to
  reading, to
Serious, earnest
Shrieking, screaming, shouting
  brain cry
  hydrocephalus, in
  touched, when
Sit, inclination to
Slander, disposition to
Slowness
Smiling, foolish
Speech, affected
  embarrassed
  hasty
  hesitating
  incoherent

Speech,
  nonsensical
  slow
  unintelligible
  wandering
Spit, desire to
  faces of people, in
  floor and licks it up, on the ●
Squanders
Starting, startled
  easily
  fright, from and as from
  noise, from
  sleep, on falling
    during
    from
  sleepiness, with
  tossing of arms, from ●
Stupefaction, as if intoxicated
  air, amel. in open
  knows not where he is
Succeeds, never
Suicidal, disposition
  fear of an open window or a knife, with
  knife, with
  menses, during
  seeing cutting instruments, on ●
  starving, by ●
  thoughts
  weeping amel. ★
Sulky
Suspicious, mistrustful
  daytime ●
  insulting ●
Talk, indisposed to, desire to be silent, taciturn
  perspiration, during
Talking, sleep, in
Talks, himself, to
Tears things
Thinking, complaints agg., of
Thoughts, disease, of some incurable ●
  intrude and crowd around each other
  persistent
  rush, flow of
  vanishing of
  wandering

Time passes too slowly, appears longer
Timidity
    bashful
Touch everything, impelled to
Touched, aversion to being
Travel, desire to
Unconsciousness, coma, stupor
    morning
    dream, as in a, does not know
       where he is
    meningitis, in
    vertigo, during
Unreliable, promises, in his
Vanity
Violent, vehement
Wander, desires to
Wearisome
Weary of life
    perspiration, during
Weeping, tearful mood
    night
    midnight, before
    aloud, wobbing
    alternating with laughter
    amel.
    chill, during
    consolation agg.
    convulsions, during
    desire to weep, all the time
    involuntary
    pains, with the
    sleep, in
    waking, on
    whimpering
    sleep, during
Well, says he is, when very sick
Will, loss of
    weakness of
Work, mental, impossible
Writing; indistinctly, writes

MERCURIUS ACETICUS

Weeping, night

MERCURIUS AURATUS

Death, desires
Sadness, despondency, dejection, mental
    depression, gloom, melancholy
    suicidal disposition, with
Suicidal disposition
    sadness, from

MERCURIUS BROMATUS

Fear, pains, during •
    suffering, of

MERCURIUS CORROSIVUS

Anxiety
    night
    coughing, from
    sleep, during
    menses, after
Cheerful, gay, mirthful
    alternating with moroseness
Complaining
Concentration, difficult
    talking, while
Confusion of mind
Delirium
    night
    bed and escapes, springs up sud-
      denly from
    maniacal
Discontented, displeased, dissatisfied
    everything, with
Discouraged
Dullness, sluggishness, difficulty of think-
    ing and comprehending, torpor
Escape, attempts to
Excitement, excitable
    feverish
      evening •
Fancies, exaltation of
Fear, apprehension, dread
    heart, arising from
    misfortune, of

Ideas, deficiency of
Imbecility
Insanity, madness
Irritability •
   daytime
   afternoon
   alternating with cheerfulness
Jumping, bed, out of
Mania
Memory, weakness of
Moaning, groaning, whining
Morose, cross, fretful, ill-humor, peevish
   daytime
   afternoon
   alternating with cheerfulness
Naked, wants to be
Prostration of mind, mental exhaustion, brain-fag
   evening
Restlessness
   night
   heat, during
Sadness, despondency, dejection, mental depression, gloom, melancholy
Sensitive, oversensitive
Shamelessness
Shrieking, brain cry
Sighing
Speech, incoherent
Staring, thoughtless
Starting, evening on falling asleep
   night
   fright, from and as from
   sleep, on falling
     during
     from
Stupefaction, as if intoxicated
Thoughts, disconnected,
   talking while •
   wandering
Torpor
Unconsciousness, coma, stupor
Violent, vehement
Weeping, desires to weep, all the time
   pains, with the

MERCURIUS CYANATUS

Anger, irascibility
Delirium
   night
   loquacious
   raging, raving
Loquacity
Morose, eating, after
Restlessness
   night
Unconsciousness, frequent spells of u., absences

MERCURIUS DULCIS

Excitement, excitable
Hypochondriasis
Restlessness

MERCURIUS IODATUS FLAVUS

Capriciousness
Cares: symptoms disappear during cares •
Cheerful, gay, mirthful
   afternoon ★
   evening
   air, in open
Confusion of mind, morning, waking, on
   night, waking, on
   waking, on
   walking, air amel., in open
   warm room, in
Delusions, men: perforate his throat with a gimlet, man in the room intending to •
Destructiveness
Excitement amel.
Fear, suffocation, goitre, in •
Indifference, apathy
Loquacity
Occupation, diversion amel.

Sadness, despondency, dejection, mental depression, gloom, melancholy
Sensitive, odors, to
Singing
    sadness, after •
Whistling

MERCURIUS IODATUS RUBER

Cheerful, gay, mirthful
    afternoon, 16-18 h. •
    evening
Confusion of mind: walking, air amel.,
    in open
Delirium
    fever, during
Dullness, sluggishness, difficulty of thinking and comprehending, torpor
Fear, apprehension, dread
Irritability
    morning
        waking, on
    waking, on
Morose, cross, fretful, ill-humor, peevish
    morning
        waking, on
    trifles, about
Restlessness
    midnight, after
Sadness, despondency, dejection, mental depression, gloom, melancholy
Weeping, tearful mood

MERCURIUS METHYLENUS

Delirium, bed and escapes, springs up
    suddenly from
Jumping, bed, out of
Laughing, idiotic
Restlessness
    night
Shrieking, screaming, shouting
Speech, incoherent
Starting, bed, in
Weeping, idiotic •

MERCURIUS NITROSUS

Anxiety
Delirium
Unconsciousness, coma, stupor

MERCURIUS PRAECIPITATUS RUBER

Unconsciousness, coma, stupor

MERCURIUS SULPHOCYANATUS

Anxiety

MERCURIUS SULPHURICUS

Delirium
    night
    restless
Irritability, eating, after
Morose, eating, after
Restlessness
    afternoon
    night
    chill, during

MERCURIALIS PERENNIS

Anger, irascibility
Cheerful, gay, mirthful
Concentration, difficult
Confusion of mind,
    morning, rising and after, on
Delirium
Delusions, imaginations, hallucinations,
    illusions
    double, nose is
    noses, has two •
Dullness, sluggishness, difficulty of thinking and comprehending, torpor
Excitement, excitable
Fear, insanity, losing his reason, of
Hurry, haste
    movements, in
Indifference, everything, to
    external things, to

Indolence, aversion to work
Irritability
Jesting
Laughing
Morose, cross, fretful, ill-humor, peevish
Quarrelsome, scolding
Restlessness
Sadness, despondency, dejection, mental
    depression, gloom, melancholy
      headache, during
Singing
Speech, foolish
Stupefaction, as if intoxicated
    evening
    warm room, in
Tranquillity, serenity, calmness
Unconsciousness, coma, stupor
    evening
Violent, vehement
Weeping, tearful mood
Work, aversion to mental

METHYLIUM
AETHYLOAETHEREUM

Excitement, excitable
Restlessness
Shrieking, screaming, shouting
Unconsciousness, coma, stupor

METHYSERGIDUM

Delusions, visions, has
Memory, weakness of
Sadness, despondency, dejection, men-
    tal depression, gloom, melancholy
Weeping, tearful mood

MEZEREUM

Absent-minded, unobserving
Absorbed, buried in thought
Abstraction of mind
Activity
Affectation ★
    gestures and acts, in
Ailments from:
      anger, vexation
      bad news

Anger, irascibility
    alternating with quick repentance
    causeless
    trifles, at
    violent
Anguish, lie down, must
Anxiety
    noon
    evening
    bed, in
    alone, when
    chill, during
    eating, before
      while
      amel.
    eructations amel.
    fear, with
    pains, from the abdomen
    salvation, about
    stool, before
Asks for nothing
Audacity
Aversion, everything, to
Brooding
Censorious, critical
Chaotic, confused behavior
Cheerful, gay, mirthful ★
    evening, bed, in
    eating, after
Company, desire for; aversion to soli-
    tude, company amel.
    alone agg., while
Concentration, difficult
      interrupted, if
    on attempting to concentrate, has
      a vacant feeling
Confusion of mind
    evening
    night, waking, on
    coition, after
    concentrate the mind, on attempt-
      ing to
    dream, as if in
    eating, after
      amel.
    interruption, from
    intoxicated, as if
    knows not where she is nor when-
      ever came to objects around her

Confusion of mind
    mental exertion, from
    waking, on
    walking, while
Conscientious about trifles
Contented
Contradiction, is intolerant of
Conversation agg.
Courageous
Death, desires
Delirium
Delusions, imaginations, hallucinations,
    illusions
    brain, hard, is •
    dead, everything is •
    fire, visions of
    light, incorporeal, he is
    poor, he is
    warts, he has •
Desires, vexatious things, to say •
Despair
    religious despair of salvation
Dipsomania, alcoholism
Discomfort, noon •
Discontented, displeased, dissatisfied
    everything, with
    himself, with
    surroundings, with
Disgust
Dullness, sluggishness, difficulty of
    thinking and comprehending,
    torpor
        morning
        evening
    eating amel.
    looking out the window lasting for
        hours •
    reading, while
    sleep, after sound
    speaking, while
Dwells on past disagreeable occur-
    rences
Eating, after, amel.
Ennui, tedium
Escape, attempts to
    run away, to

Excitement, excitable
    evening
        bed, in
    night
Exhilaration
Fear, apprehension, dread
    alone, of being
    exertion, of
    heart, arising from
    misfortune, of
    stomach, arising from
Forgetful
Frightened easily
    trifles, at
Grief
Heedless
Hurry, haste
Hypochondriasis
    weeping, with
Hysteria
Ideas abundant, clearness of mind
    deficiency of
        over exertion, from
Imbecility
Impatience, perspiration, during
Impulse, run, to; dromomania
Inconstancy, thoughts, of
Indifference, apathy
    dead, everything seems to
        him •
    everything, to
    pleasure, to
    reading, while •
    window, looked hours at •
Indolence, aversion to work
    sadness, from
    sleep, after
Industrious, mania for work
    menses, before
Insanity, madness
    cheerful, gay
    wantonness, with
Introspection
Irresolution, indecision

Irritability
    morning, waking, on
    afternoon, 14h. •
    alternating with remorse
    chill, during
    headache, during
    waking, on
Laughing agg.
Loathing, general
Loathing, life, at
Meditation
Melancholy, financial ★
    religious ★
Memory, weakness of
    heard, for what has
    said, for what has
    say, for what is about to
Moaning, groaning, whining
Mood, changeable, variable
Morose, cross, fretful, ill-humor, peevish
    morning, bed, in
    chill, during
    waking, on
Occupation, diversion amel.
Prostration of mind, mental exhaustion, brain-fag
Pull one's hair, desires to
Quarrelsome, scolding
Reflecting, unable to reflect
Religious affections
    melancholia
Reproaches others
Rest, desire for
    afternoon •
Restlessness
    alone, when
    bed, go from one bed to another, wants to
    chill, during
    coition, after
    company, in ★
Sadness, despondency, dejection, mental depression, gloom, melancholy
    alone, when
    trifles, about
    work - shy, in

Senses, dull, blunted
    vanishing of
Sensitive, oversensitive
Singing
Sit, inclination to
Speech, inconsiderate
    slow
    vexatious things, desire to say •
Starting, dream, from a
    easily
    falling, as if
    sleep, during
    from
Stupefaction, as if intoxicated
Suicidal disposition
Suspicious, mistrustful
Talk, indisposed to, desire to be silent, taciturn
    eating, after
    others agg., talk of
Thoughts, disagreeable
    persistent
    thoughtful
    tormenting
    vanishing of
        mental exertion, on
        speaking, while
Timidity, bashful
Touched, aversion to being
Tranquillity, serenity, calmness
Unconsciousness, coma, stupor
    vertigo, during
    waking, on
Violent, vehement
Wearisome
Weary of life
Weeping, tearful mood
    daytime
    evening
    pains, with the
Will, weakness of
Window, looks hours at •
Work, aversion to mental
    impossible

MILLEFOLIUM

Anxiety
    rising from a seat, amel. on
Asks for nothing
Confusion of mind, morning
           evening
    coffee, after
    eating, after
    wine, after
Delirium
Dullness, evening
    wine, after
Excitement, excitable
Forgetful
Forgotten something, feels constantly
    as if he had
Hypochondriasis
Hysteria
Indolence, aversion to work
Irritability
    evening
    dinner, after
Memory, weakness of
Moaning, groaning, whining
    children, in ★
Restlessness
Sadness, despondency, dejection, mental
    depression, gloom, melancholy
Sighing
Stupefaction, as if intoxicated
    vertigo, during
Unconsciousness, vertigo, during
Violent, evening ●
       supper, after ●

MIMOSA PUDICA

Delusions, enlarged, body is ●
    large, parts of body seem too
Irritability
    medicine, at thought to take the ●

MITCHELLA REPENS

Business, incapicity for
Cheerful, gay, mirthful
Dullness, sluggishness, difficulty of think-
    ing and comprehending, torpor

Frightened, waking, on
Memory, weakness of
Sadness, despondency, dejection, men-
    tal depression, gloom, melancholy
Sighing
Thoughts, wandering, morning ●

MOLYBDAENUM
METALLICUM

Company, aversion to; presence of other
    people agg. the symptoms; desire
    for solitude
Confusion of mind
Discontented, displeased, dissatisfied
Discouraged
Indifference, apathy
Sadness, despondency, dejection, men-
    tal depression, gloom, melancholy
Talk, indisposed to, desire to be silent,
    taciturn

MORBILLINUM

Fear, sea, of ★

(BACILLUS) MORGAN

Fear, narrow places, in; claustrophobia
Idiocy
Irritability, menses, before

MORPHINUM ACETICUM

Activity, mental
Ailments from:
       fright
Anxiety
    coffee amel. ●
Censorious, critical
Concentration, difficult
Confusion of mind
    intoxicated, as after being
Contradiction, is intolerant of
Death, sensation of

Delirium
  bed and escapes, springs up sud-
    denly from
  fever, during
  raging, raving
Delusions, imaginations, hallucinations,
  illusions
    bed, hard, too
Despair
Discomfort
Dullness, sluggishness, difficulty of think-
  ing and comprehending, torpor
Emotions, easily excited ★
Excitement, excitable
  trifles, over
Fancies, vivid, lively
Forgetful
Frightened easily
Gestures, convulsive
Hurry, haste
Hysteria
Ideas abundant, clearness of mind
Indifference, apathy
Irritability
Jumping, bed, during fever, out of
Lamenting, bemoaning, wailing
Liar
    lies, never speaks the truth, does
    not know what she is saying
Memory, weakness of
  expressing oneself, for
Mistakes, writing, in
Mood, changeable, variable
Moral feeling, want of
Morose, cross, fretful, ill-humor, peevish
Muttering
Prostration of mind, mental exhaus-
  tion, brain-fag
Rest, desire for
Restlessness
    night
    headache, during
Runs, room, in
Sadness, despondency, dejection, mental
  depression, gloom, melancholy
Senses, acute
  dull, blunted

Sensitive, oversensitive
Sighing
Speech, embarassed
  excited
  hasty
  hesitating
  incoherent
  slow
Starting, night
  sleep, during
Stupefaction, as if intoxicated
  eating, agg. after
Suicidal disposition
Suspicious, mistrustful
Thoughts, control of thoughts lost, while
  undressing •
  rapid, quick
  rush, flow of
Tranquillity, incomprehensible
Unconsciousness, coma, stupor
  incomplete
Weeping, involuntary
Work, mental, impossible

MOSCHUS

Absent - minded, unobserving
    noon •
Absorbed, buried in thought
Abusive, insulting
    scolds until the lips are blue and
    eyes stare and she falls down
    fainting •
Activity
Ailments from :
  anticipation, foreboding, presen-
    timent
Anger, irascibility
  stabbed anyone, so that he could
    have
  violent
Anguish
  palpitation, with
Answers; aversion to answer
  confused as though thinking of
    something else

Anxiety
    anticipation, from
    cough, during whooping
    fear, with
    hypochondriacal
    work, anxiety preventing •
Awkward, drops things ★
Busy
    week-end, in the •
Censorious, critical
Chaotic, confused behavior
Cheerful, gay, mirthful
    heat, during
Complaining
    pain, of
    pregnancy, during •
Concentration, difficult
Confusion of mind
            morning
        intoxicated, as after being
        motion, from
Death, presentiment of
Delirium
    convulsions, during
    headache, during
    raging, raving
Delusions, imaginations, hallucination,
    illusions
    animals, of
    blind, he is
    dead, he himself was
    double, of being
    faintness, of
    falling forward, he is
    figures, large black, about to spring
        on him, sees •
    finger cut off •
    hear, he cannot
    identity, errors of personal
        someone else, she is
    injury: fingers and toes are being
        cut off, his •
    opposed by everyone •
    sick, being
    strange, familiar things seem
    toes cut off •
Destructiveness
Dipsomania, alcoholism

Discomfort
Dullness, sluggishness, difficulty of think-
    ing and comprehending, torpor
Excitement, excitable
    night
    heat, during
    wine, as from
Fancies, exaltation of
Fear, apprehension, dread
    death, of
    heat, during
    lying down, on •
    evil, of
    happen, something will
    insanity, losing his reason, of
    noise, from
    suffocation, lying, while
    tremulous
Foolish behavior
Forgetful
Frightened easily
Gestures, makes
    crossing the hands •
    grasping or reaching at some-
        thing, at flocks; carphologia
    hands, motions, involuntary, of
        the throwing about
            overhead
    plays, buttons of his clothes, with
        the •
    ridiculous or foolish
Hurry, haste
    awkward from
    walking, while
Hypochondriasis
    sexual abstinence, from
Hysteria
    fainting, hysterical
    lascivious
    menses, before
        during
    sleeplessness, with
Ideas, imaginary disease, of ★
Idiocy
Imbecility
Impatience
    convulsions, before attack, in •

Industrious, mania for work
    menses, before
Insanity, madness
Irritability
    heat, during
    sleeplessness, with
Lamenting, bemoaning, wailing
Lascivious, lustful
Laughing, alternating with shrieking
    immoderately
    nervous ★
Loquacity
    drunk, as if
Malicious, spiteful, vindictive
Memory, weakness of
Mildness
Mood, changeable, variable
Morose, cross, fretful,, ill-humor, peevish
    fever, during
    hypochondriasis, in
Nymphomania
    metrorrhagia, during
Obstinate, headstrong
Play, desire to, buttons of his clothes, with the •
Prostration of mind, mental exhaustion, brain-fag
Quarrelsome, scolding
    face, with heat of •
        pale, with •
    staring of eyes, heat of face, bluish lips, dry mouth, with •
Rage, fury
    malicious
    paroxysms, in
Restlessness
    night
    bed, tossing about in
    busy
    heat, during
Sadness, despondency, dejection, mental depression, gloom, melancholy
    eating, after

Self-control
Selfishness, egoism
Senses, dull, blunted
    vanishing of
Sensitive, noise, to
Shamelessness
Shrieking, screaming, shouting
Somnambulism
Speech, confused
    hasty
Spoiled, children
Starting, startled
    door is opened, when a
    fright, from and as from
    noise, from
    sleep, during
Striking
    about him at imaginary objects
Stupefaction, as if intoxicated
    air, amel. in open
    vertigo, during
Talk, indisposed to, desire to be silent, taciturn
Talks, himself, to
    excitedly ★
    herself, to, and gesticulates ★
Thinking, complaints agg., of
Tranquillity, serenity, calmness
Unconciousness, coma, stupor
    air, in open
    emotion, after
    sitting, while
    transient
    vertigo, during
Violent, vehement
    deeds of violence, rage leading to
Weeping, tearful mood
    alternating with laughter
    anger, after
    convulsions, during
    involuntary
    pains, with the
    spasmodic
Wildness

MURIATICUM ACIDUM

Absorbed, buried in thought
    menses, during •
Activity
    amel.
Ailments from:
    anger, vexation with indignation
Anger, irascibility
    afternoon, air, in open •
    dreams, after •
    weakness, anger followed by •
Anguish
    evening
Answers abruptly, shortly, curtly
    monosyllable
Anxiety
    evening
        20 h.
        bed, in
    night, midnight, before
    dreams, on waking from frightful
    fever, during
    future, about
Brooding
Cares, worries, full of
Cheerful, daytime
    dreams, after •
Concentration difficult,
    studying, reading etc., while ★
Confidence, want of self
Confiding
Confusion of mind
    night
Conscientious about trifles
Contradiction, is intolerant of
Cowardice
Delirium
    fever, during
    muttering
    raging, raving
    sepsis, from
    sleep, during
    watching, vigil, from
Delusions, imaginations, hallucinations,
    illusions
    images, everchanging past to
        present •

Delusions,
        frightful
    vermin, sees crawl about
    worms, creeping of
Discontented, displeased, dissatisfied
    afternoon
    air, in open •
    everything, with
    himself, with
Discouraged
Dullness, sluggishness, difficulty of think-
    ing and comprehending, torpor
    forenoon
    evening
Emptiness, sensation of ★
Excitement, excitable
    working, when
Fancies, exaltation of
        working, while
Fear, apprehension, dread
    daytime only
    morning
    evil, of
    misfortune, of
Frightened easily
Gestures, grasping, pick, at bed clothes
Grief
Ideas abundant, clearness of mind
Imbecility
Indifference, apathy
    air, in open
    pleasure, to
Indolence, aversion to work
Industrious, mania for work
    menses, before
Introspection
Irresolution, indecision
Irritability
    afternoon
    evening
    air, in open
    weakness, from •
Laughing agg.
Loquacity
Meditation
Memory, weak, said, for what has
Menses, mental symptoms agg. during

Mildness
Moaning, groaning, whining
   heat, during
     loud, persistently ★
   sleep, during
Morose, cross, fretful, ill-humor, peevish
   afternoon
     evening
   air, in open
Morphinism
Muttering
   sleep, in
Obstinate, headstrong
   evening
Occupation, diversion amel.
Prostration of mind, mental exhaustion, brain-fag
Quiet disposition
   menses, during
Rebels against poultice
Reserved
   menses, during
Restlessness
   evening
   night
     midnight, before
   bed, tossing about in
   heat, during
   waking, on
Sadness, despondency, dejection, mental
   depression, gloom, melancholy
     morning
     afternoon
   air, in open
   menses, during
Senses, acute
Sensitive, oversensitive
   noise, to
     voices, to
     slightest, to ★
Serious, earnest
Sighing
Sit, inclination to
Speech, abrupt
   merry
     sleep, in ●
   unintelligible, sleep, in

Starting, startled
   fright, from and as from
   sleep, from
   uneasiness, from
Stupefaction, as if intoxicated
   vertigo, during ●
Succeeds, never
Sulky
Suspicious, mistrustful
Talk, indisposed to, desire to be silent,
   taciturn
       die, as if he would ●
     menses, during
     perspiration, during
Talking, sleep, in
Talks, himself, to
Thoughts, intrude and crowd around
   each other
   work, while at
   persistent
   profound
   rush, working, during
Timidity
Tranquillity, serenity, calmness
Unconsciousness, coma, stupor
   face, with red
   fever, during
   scarlatina, in
Walk; walking in open air agg. mental
   symptoms
Wearisome
Weary of life
   afternoon
   air, in open
Weeping, sleep, in
Work, aversion to mental

MURURE LEITE

Eccentricity

MUREX PURPUREA

Anguish
   daytime
   menses, before

Anxiety
    fear, with
Clinging, held amel., being
Company, aversion to; presence of other
    people agg. the symptoms; desire
    for solitude
Confusion of mind
        morning
        evening
Conversation, aversion to
Delusions, imaginations, hallucinations,
    illusions
        melancholy
        sick, being
Fear, apprehension, dread
Impatience
    pain, from
Industrious, mania for work
Insanity, madness
    erotic
Irritability
Lascivious, lustful
    women at every touch •
Mania
Memory, weakness of
    expressing oneself, for
    words, of
Mental symptoms alternating with
    leucorrhoea •
        physical ★
Mildness
Mistakes, speaking, in
Nymphomania
    climacteric period, at
    menses, after suppressed
    metrorrhagia, during
**Sadness, despondency, dejection,
    mental depression, gloom,
    melancholy**
        evening
        leucorrhoea amel. •
        menses, before
        during
        sleepiness, with
Sensitive, oversensitive

Shamelessness
Starting, dream, from a
        sleep, from
Talk, indisposed to, desire to be silent,
    taciturn
Thoughts, disease, of
Unconsciousness, menses, before
Weeping: desire to weep, all the time

MYGALE LASIODORA

Anxiety
Business, talks of
Delirium
    evening 20h. •
Excitement, excitable
Fear, death, of
Hatred: revenge, h. and
Hysteria
Restlessness
        morning on waking
        night
*Sadness, despondency, dejection, mental
        depression, gloom, melancholy*
Sensitive, oversensitive

MYRICA CERIFERA

Anger, irascibility
Censorious, critical
Concentration, difficult
Confusion of mind
Delusions, better than others, he is •
    die, he cannot ★
Dullness, sluggishness, difficulty of think-
        ing and comprehending, torpor
        forenoon
        evening
Excitement, excitable
Exhilaration
Indifference, business affairs, to
Irritability
        morning
Loathing, general
Morose, cross, fretful, ill-humor, peevish

Restlessness
    morning
    night
    midnight, 2h. after
Sadness, despondency, dejection, men-
    tal depression, gloom, melancholy
    morning
    afternoon
    exhilaration, after
Spoken to, averse to being
Talk, indisposed to, desire to be silent,
    taciturn
Unconciousness, coma, stupor

MYRISTICA SEBIFERA

Concentration, difficult
    afternoon
Heedless, business, about
Starting, sleep, during
Stupefaction, as if intoxicated
Thoughts, persistent in evening about
    music, song, since 16 h. •

MYRTUS COMMUNIS

Discouraged

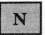

NABALUS SERPENTARIA

Anticipation, morning
Cheerful, gay, mirthful
Clairvoyance
Irritability
    evening
Sadness, despondency, dejection, mental
    depression, gloom, melancholy
    evening

NAJA TRIPUDIANS

Absent-minded, unobserving
Activity, mental
Ailments from:
    anticipation, foreboding, presenti-
    ment
    grief
Anguish
Anxiety
    motion amel.
    others, for
Brooding
    disease, imaginary, over ★
    over wrongs and misfortunes and
        makes himself miserable ★
Censorious, critical
Cheerful, gay, mirthful
    night
Company, desire for; aversion to soli-
    tude, company amel.
Confidence, want of self   ·
    failure, feels himself a
Confusion of mind
    morning on waking
    identity: duality, sense of
    waking, on
Delirium
    loquacious
    meningitis, cerebrospinalis
    paroxysmal

Delusions, hearing, illusions of
    injury: injured, head is ●
        surroundings, by his
    neglected his duty, he has
        he is
    starved, being ●
    superhuman, control, is under
    troubles, broods over imaginary
    visions, has
    wrong, has suffered
Despair
Duality, sense of ★
Dullness, sluggishness, difficulty of
    thinking and comprehending,
    torpor
    evening
Excitement, excitable
    wine, as from
Exertion, agg. from mental
Failure, feels himself a ★
Fancies, exaltation of
    evening
    vivid lively
Fear, death, of
    heart symptoms, during
    failure, of
    misfortune, of
    rain, of
Fire, desire to be near to ●
Forgetful
    evening
Impulse, walk, to ★
Indifference, apathy
Insanity, madness
    split his head in two, will ●
    suicidal ★
Irresolution, indecision
Irritability
Loathing, life, at
Meditation
Memory, confused
Memory, weakness of
    labor, for mental
Moaning, groaning, whining
Mood, alternating
Morose, cross, fretful, ill-humor, peevish
Occupation, desire for
Playful

Poisoned, feeling ★
Prostration of mind, mental exhaustion,
    brain-fag
Restlessness
    afternoon
    headache, during
Sadness, despondency, dejection, mental
    depression, gloom, melancholy
    morning
    evening
    headache, during
    suicidal disposition, with
    superfluous, feeling ●
    wrong way, as if having done
        everything in ●
Self-deception
Serious, earnest
Speech, unintelligible
Suicidal disposition
    axe, with an ●
    sadness, from
    thoughts
Talk, indisposed to, desire to be silent,
    taciturn
Thoughts, wandering
Timidity
Tranquillity, serenity, calmness
Unconsciousness, coma, stupor
Unsuccessful, thinks himself ★
Weary of life
Weeping, tearful mood
    emotions, after slight
Will, contradiction of
    loss of
    two wills, feels as if he had
Work, desire for mental
    impossible
Wrong, everything seems

NAPHTA

Starting, fright, from and as from
Unconsciousness, coma, stupor

NARCEINUM

Stupefaction, as if intoxicated

NARCOTINUM

Concentration, difficult
Confusion of mind
Conversation, desire for
Reading: unable, to read

NARZAN AQUA

Indifference, apathy

NATRUM ACETICUM

Anxiety, future, about
Cowardice
Dullness, sluggishness, difficulty of thinking and comprehending, torpor

NATRUM ARSENICOSUM

Absent-minded, unobserving
Activity, mental
Ailments from :
    anger, vexation
Anger, irascibility
    agg.
    contradiction, from
    trifles, at
Anguish
Anxiety
    evening
        bed, in
        night
    bed, in
    fear, with
    fever, during
    future, about
    waking, on
Business, averse to
Cheerful, gay, mirthful
Concentration, difficult
    air, amel. in open. •
    studying, reading etc., while
Confusion of mind
    evening
Conscientious about trifles

Delusion, neglected his duty, he has wrong, he has done
Despair
Discontented, displeased, dissatisfied
Discouraged
Dullness, sluggishness, difficulty of thinking and comprehending, torpor
    daytime
    morning
    forenoon
    air, in open
    walking, air amel., in open
Excitement, excitable
Exertion, agg. from mental
Fear, apprehension, dread
    evening
    crowd, in a
    disease, of impending
    evil, of
    happen, something will
    people, of; anthropophobia
Forgetful
Frightened easily
    roused, when
Hurry, haste
Hysteria
Ideas abundant, clearness of mind
Imbecility
Impatience
Indifference, apathy
    air, in open, amel. •
    business affairs, to
    joy, to
    pleasure, to
Indolence, aversion to work
Irritability
Lamenting, bemoaning, wailing
Laughing
Loathing, life, at
Loquacity
Memory, weakness of
    names, for proper
Mildness
Morose, cross, fretful, ill-humor, peevish
Prostration of mind, mental exhaustion, brain-fag

Quarrelsome, scolding
Reading: aversion to read
Reproaches himself
    others
Restlessness
    night
    midnight, after, 1h.
        3h.
    anxious
    bed, tossing about in
Sadness, despondency, dejection, mental depression, gloom, melancholy
    evening
    heat, during
Sensitive, oversensitive
    noise, to
Sit, inclination to
Starting, startled
    fright, from and as from
    noise, from
    sleep, on falling
        from
Suspicious, mistrustful
Talk, indisposed to, desire to be silent, taciturn
        alternating with headache
    others agg., talk of
Thinking, aversion to
Timidity
Weeping, tearful mood
Work, aversion to mental
    afternoon
    impossible
    air, in open •

NATRUM BROMATUM

Sadness, despondency, dejection, mental depression, gloom, melancholy
Unconsciousness, waking, on
Will, loss of

NATRUM CARBONICUM

Absent-minded, unobserving
    morning
Absorbed, buried in thought
    morning
Abstraction of mind
Abusive, insulting
Affections, in general ★
Ailments from :
    anger, vexation
    anxiety, with
    fright, with
    silent grief, with
    anticipation, foreboding, presentiment
    excitement, emotional
    fright
    joy, excessive
    sexual excesses
    work, mental
Anger, irascibility
    forenoon
    evening
    contradiction, from
    trifles, at
Anguish
    daytime
Anxiety
    daytime
    afternoon
        until evening
    evening
        bed, in
    night
        waking, on
        midnight, before
    bathing the feet, after •
    bed, in
    daily
    eating, after
    fear, with
    fever, during
    flushes of heat, during
    future, about
    health, about

Anxiety,
> hypochondriacal
> menses, during
> mental exertion, from
> motion, from
> *music, from*
> noise, from
> *pains, from the*
> paroxysms, in
> periodical
> *playing piano, while* •
> shuddering, with
> sleep, before
>> *during*
> speaking, when
> stool, after
> *thunderstorm, before*
>> *during*
> waking, on

Audacity

Avarice

Aversion, husband, to
> *members of family, to*
> **persons, to certain**
> society, to ★

Bed, aversion to; shuns bed

Beside oneself, being

Blasphemy
> cursing, and

Business, averse to

Calculating, inability for

Capriciousness

Cares, worries, full of

Chaotic, confused behavior

Cheerful, gay, mirthful
> evening
> alternating with moroseness
>> sadness
> fearful, but ★
> stool, after

Company, aversion to; presence of other
> *people agg. the symptoms; desire*
> *for solitude*
> *alone, amel. when*
> *avoids the sight of people*
> **fear of being alone, yet**
> *friends, of intimate*

Company, desire for; aversion to solitude, company amel.
> alone agg., while

Concentration, difficult
> morning
> evening
> *studying, reading, etc., while*

Confidence, want of self

Confusion of mind, morning
> evening
> air amel., in open
> bed amel., while in •
> chill, during
> concentrate the mind, on attempting to ★
> eating, after
> heat, during
> **mental exertion, from**
> motion, from
> sitting, while
> *sun, in*
> waking, on
> walking, while
>> air amel., in open
> writing, while

Conscientious about trifles

Contented

Contradict, disposition to

Contradiction, is intolerant of
> forenoon •

Courageous

Cursing, swearing

Death, desires
> morning on waking

Delirium, morning on waking
> sleeplessness, and ★
> waking, on

Delirium tremens, mania-a-potu

Delusions, imaginations, hallucinations, illusions
> morning, bed, in
> evening, bed, in
> assembled things, swarms, crowd etc.
> body, heavy and thick, has become (at night) •
>> thick, is •

Delusions,
    criminals, about
    dead persons, sees
    deserted, forsaken, is
    devils, sees
    division between himself and others
    enlarged
    fancy, illusions of
    figures, sees
        marching in the air (evening while half asleep)
    heart disease, having
    heavy, is
    images, phantoms, sees
        frightful
    journey, he is on a
    music, he hears
    pursued by enemies
        soldiers, by
    right, does nothing
    sick, being
    small, things appear
    soldiers, sees
        in half asleep •
        march, air, in the (evening, while half asleep) •
        surrounded by •
    spectres, ghosts, spirits, sees •
    succeed, he cannot; does every thing wrong
    thieves, sees
    waking, on
    water, of
    wedding, of a
Despair
Dipsomania, alcoholism
Discomfort
Discontented, displeased, dissatisfied
    everything, with
Discouraged
Dream, as if in a, night •
Dullness, sluggishness, difficulty of thinking and comprehending, torpor
    morning
    eating amel.

Dullness,
    heat, during
    mental exertion, from
    painful
    pollutions, after
    reading, while
    waking, on
Elegance, want of
Ennui, tedium
Envy
    hate, and
Estranged from her family
    friends, from •
Excitement, excitable
    morning
    bad news, after
    hearing horrible things, after
    menses, during
Exertion, agg. from mental
    amel.
Fancies, exaltation of, evening in bed
    sleeplessness with
    lascivious
Fear, apprehension, dread
    afternoon
    evening
    night
    alone, of being
    apoplexy, of
    bed, of the
    cold, of taking
    crowd, in a
    death, of
    disease, of impending
    everything, constant of
    evil, of
    men, dread, fear of
    misfortune, of
    music, from
    noise, from
    people, of; anthropophobia
    recurrent
    robbers, of
    sleep, before
    thunderstorm, of
    tremulous
    trifles, of
    waking, on

Foolish behavior
Forgetful
 mental exertion, from
Forsaken feeling
Frightened easily
 noon nap, after
Gamble (*see* Play)
Gestures, awkward, in
 hand, motions, involuntary, throwing about
Gourmand
Greed, cupidity
Grief
 future, for the
Heedless
Horrible-things, sad stories, affect her
 profoundly
Hurry, haste
Hypochondriasis
 eating, after
Hysteria
Ideas abundant, clearness of mind
 deficiency of
Imbecility
Impatience
 reading, while •
Impetuous
Inconsolable
 weeping from consolation, continuous •
Inconstancy
Indifference, apathy
 children, to her
 company, society, while in
 eating, to
 ennui, with
 everything, to
 money-making, to
 pleasure, to
 relations, to
 sleepiness, with
Indignation
Indolence, aversion to work
 morning, rising, on
 coition, after •
 physical
 pollutions, after
 sitting, while
 sleepiness, with

Industrious, mania for work
 menses, before
Insanity, madness
 anxiety, with
 drunkards, in
 religious
Introspection, morning •
Irresolution, indecision
 morning
 acts, in
Irritability
 daytime
 morning
 noon
 evening
 alternating with cheerfulness
 chill, during
 coition, after
 dinner, after
 eating, after
 heat, during
 menses, during
 music, during
 noise, crackling of newspaper, even from
 pollutions, after
 reading, while
 stool, after
 supper, after
 thunderstorm, before
 trifles, from
Kicks, sleep, in
Kelptomania: dainties, steals
Lamenting, bemoaning, wailing
Laughing
 alternating with sadness
 spasmodic
Loathing, general life, at waking on
 morning
Loquacity
 cheerful, exuberant
 exhausted, until •
 vivacious
Magnetized, desires to be,
 mesmerism amel.

Malicious, spiteful, vindictive
Meditation
Memory, loss of :
   mental exertion, from •
Memory, weakness of
  labor, for mental
    fatigue, from
    read, for what has
    studies, w. of m. of young people in
      their •
Mildness
Misanthropy
Mistakes, speaking, in
    misplacing words
    work, in
    writing, in
Moaning, groaning, whining
Mood, alternating
    changeable, variable
Morose, cross, fretful, ill-humor, peevish
    afternoon
    evening
    coition, after
    eating, after
    pollutions, after
Music agg.
   piano playing, from
    trembling from
Nibble, desire to
Nymphomania
Occupation, diversion amel.
Offended, easily; takes everything in
    bad part
Passionate
Perseverance
*Play, passion for gambling to make
   money*
Prostration of mind, mental exhaustion, brain-fag
Quarrelsome, scolding
    pugnacious
Rage, night
Reflecting, unable to reflect
    studying, from •
Remorse

Restlessness
    daytime
    forenoon
    evening
    night
  anxious
    bed, driving out of
      tossing about in
    busy
    chill, during
    dinner, after
    driving about
    internal
    menses, during
    mental labor, during and after
     amel. from •
    music, from
    reading, while
    storm, during
Revelry, feasting
Sadness, despondency, dejection, mental depression, gloom, melancholy
    evening
    night
    coition, aversion to coition, desire
      for solitude
    dinner, after
    eating, after
  errors of diet, from •
    flushes of heat, during •
    headache, during
    heat, during
    menses, during
    music, from
    noise, from
    pollution (seminal emission),
      from ★
Senses, dull, blunted
Sensitive, oversensitive
    forenoon •
  certain persons, to
    chill, during
    mental impressions, to
  music, to
    piano, to

Sensitive,
> *noise, to*
>> crackling of paper, to
>> slightest, to
> *sensual impressions, to*

Sentimental ★
Serious, earnest
Sighing
Singing
> *supper, after* •
> trilling

Sit, inclination to
Slander, disposition to, denouncer
> sneak

Sociability
Speech, affected
> *awkward* •
> excited
> slow
> *violent*

Starting, startled
> noon
>> sleep, in
>> evening, asleep, on falling
> dream, from a
> **easily**
> **noise, from**
> sleep, on falling
>> during
>> *from*
> *trifles, at*

Striking
> about him at imaginary objects
> *anger, from* •
> desire to strike

Stupefaction, as if intoxicated
> morning
>> waking, on
> waking, on

Succeeds, never
Suicidal disposition, morning
> music, from •
> waking, on

Suspicious, mistrustful
> *fear of company*

Sympathy, compassion

Talk, indisposed to, desire to be silent,
> taciturn
> *others agg., talk of*

Talks, verses, in ★
Talking, sleep, in
Thoughts, disconnected
> *read, cannot*
> sexual
> thoughtful
> wandering

Thunderstorm, mind symptoms before
> during

Time, fritters away his
> passes too slowly, appears longer

Timidity
> evening •
>> going to bed, about
> awkward, and
> *bashful*

Tranquillity, serenity, calmness
Unconsciousness, coma, stupor
> morning
>> waking, on
> crowded room, in a
> incomplete
> vertigo, during
> waking, on

Violent, vehement
> deeds of violence, rage leading to
> **exhaustion, to** •
> *trifles, at*

Vivacious
Wearisome
Weary of life
> morning,
> waking, on

Weeping, tearful mood
> *night*
> aloud, wobbing
> consolation agg.
> *music, from*
>> *piano, of*
> *sleep, in*

Will, loss of
> weakness of

Work, aversion to mental
> **fatigues**
> **impossible**

NATRUM FLUORATUM

Restlessness
Sadness, despondency, dejection, mental depression,   g l o o m ,
    melancholy
Unconsciousness, coma, stupor

NATRUM HYPOCHLOROSUM

Foolish, behavior
Hysteria
Indolence, aversion to work
Laughing, sleep, during
Sadness, despondency, dejection, mental depression, gloom, melancholy
Stupefaction, as if intoxicated
Unconsciousness, coma, stupor

NATRUM IODATUM

Dementia, senilis
Imbecility

NATRUM MURIATICUM

Abrupt, rough
    harsh
Absent-minded, unobserving
Absorbed, buried in thought
    as to what would become of him •
Abstraction of mind
Abusive: children insulting parents
Affectation
Affections, in general ✶
Affectionate
Ailments from:
    anger, vexation
        anxiety, with
        indignation, with
        silent grief, with
        suppressed
    anticipation, foreboding, presentiment
    bad news
    business failure
    cares, worries

Ailments from:
    disappointment
        old
    discords between chief and subordinates
        parents, friends
        servants ★
    excitement, emotional
    fright
    grief
    love, disappointed
    mortification
    rudeness of others
    scorn, being scorned
    sexual excesses
        excitement ★
    work, mental
Amativeness
Anger, irascibility
    evening
    alternating with cheerfulness
        vivacity
    answer, when obliged to
    consoled, when
    face, with pale, livid
    talk, indisposed to
    trifles, at
    violent
    work, about •
Answers: aversion to answer
Anxiety
    morning
        waking, on
    forenoon
    evening
        bed, in
        uneasiness and anxiety, must
            uncover
    night
        waking, on
        midnight, before
        after, 2h.
        5h •
    alternating with indifference •
    anticipation
    bed, in
        driving out of
    chill, during

451

Anxiety
  conscience, as if guilty of a crime
  dark, in
  dinner, after
  dreams, on waking from frightful
  eating, after
  fear, with
  fever, during
  fright, after
  future, about
  hypochondriacal
  hurry, with •
  menses, before
    during
  periodical
  salvation, about
  sleep, on going to
    during
  sudden
  thunderstorm, during
  waking, on
Avarice
  generosity towards strangers, ava-
        rice as regards his family
Aversion:
  fuss, to ★
  husband, to
  members of family, to
  men (females), to ★
  persons to certain
  school, to ★
  sex, to opposite
  women, to
Awkward ★
Blasphemy
  cursing, and
Boaster, braggart
Calculating, inability for
Cares, worries, full of
  company, with aversion to
  daily cares, affected by
Censorious, critical
Cheerful, gay, mirthful
  forenoon
  evening
    bed, in

Cheerful,
  alternating with irritability
    moroseness
    sadness
    vexation
  coition, after •
  dancing, laughing, singing, with
Company, aversion to; presence of
    other people agg. the symp-
    toms; desire for solitude
  alone, amel. when
  fond of solitude ★
  pregnancy, during
  presence of people intolerable
    during urination •
Company, desire for, alone agg., while
Concentration, active
Concentration, difficult
  on attempting to concentrate, has
    a vacant feeling
  studying, learns with difficulty
  talking, while
Confidence, want of self
Confusion of mind
  morning
    rising and after, on
    waking, on
  afternoon
  evening
  calculating, when
  concentrate the mind, on attempt-
    ing to
  eating, after
  headache, with
  identity, as to his
    duality, sense of
  intoxicated, as after being
  lying amel. •
  menses, after
  mental exertion, from
  reading, while
  rising, after
  sitting, while
  stooping, when
  talking, while
  walking, while
    after
  warm room, in

Consolation, kind words agg.
    sympathy agg.
Contemptuous
Contented
Contradiction, is intolerant of
Conversation agg.
Cowardice
Cursing, swearing
    headache, during ★
Dancing
      evening ●
    amel.
Darkness agg.
Death, desires
    presentiment of
Deceitful, sly
    perjured
Deception causes grief and mortifi-
      cation ★
Delirium
      morning, waking, on
      chill, during
      fever, during
      frightful
      maniacal
      muttering
      persecution in delirium, delusion
        of
      raging, raving
      rambling
      trembling, with
Delirium tremens, mania-a-potu
Delusions, imaginations, hallucinations,
    illusions
    conversing, delirium with
    dead, mother is, his
      persons, sees
    doomed, being
    double, of being
    emaciation, of
    faces when stooping, sees ●
    fire, visions of
    floating in air ★
    head belongs to another
    house is full of people
    identity, errors of personal

Delusions,
    images, phantoms, sees
      night
      closing eyes, on
      sleep, going to, on
    insane, she will become
    objects, different ●
    people, sees
      closing eyes, sees p. on
    persecuted, he is
    pitied on account of his misfortune
      and he wept, he is ●
    sick, being
    spectres, ghosts, spirits, sees
      closing eyes, on
      conversing with, he is
    talking, dead people, with
      spirits, with
    thieves, sees
      and, will not believe the con-
        trary until the search is made
        (after a dream) ●
      house, in
    visions, has
      daytime
      closing the eyes, on
    voices, hears
      dead people of
      distant
    wretched, she looks (when looking
      in a mirror) ●
Dementia, senilis
Despair
    future, about ●
    pregnancy, during ●
    religious despair of salvation
Dipsomania, alcoholism
Dirtiness, dirtying everything
Discontented, displeased, dissatis-
    fied
    afternoon
    everything, with
Discouraged
Dream, as if in a
Dullness, sluggishness, difficulty of
    thinking and comprehending,
    torpor
    forenoon

Dullness,
    afternoon
    evening
    mental exertion, from
    sleepiness, with
    walking, rapidly, after
Duty, no sense of
Dwells on past disagreeable occurrences
    night
    grieve therefor, to ●
    recalls disagreeable memories
Elegance, want of
Envy, hate and
Estranged from her family
Excitement, excitable
    morning
    evening, bed, in
    night
    bad news, after
    chill, during
    menses, before
        during
    sleep, before
    waking, on
    walking, after
Exclusive, too
Exertion, agg. from mental
    amel.
Extravagance
Fancies, lascivious
    vivid, lively
    falling asleep, when ●
Fastidious ★
    schedules of time (of punctuality) ★
Fear, apprehension, dread
    evening
    night
    bed, of the
    crowd, in a
    dark, of
    death, of
        evening in bed ●
    disease, of impending
    doctors, of ★
    dogs, of ★

Fear,
    evil, of
    failure, of
    falling when walking, of
    ghosts, conversing with, thinks he is ★
    happen, something will
    heart, of disease of ★
    insanity, losing his reason, of
        evening in bed ●
    insects, of ★
    men, dread, fear of
    menses, during
    misfortune, of
        evening
    narrow places, in; claustrophobia ★
    palpitation, with
    people, of; anthropophobia
    pins, pointed things, of
    poisoned, of being
    recurrent
    robbers, of
        midnight, waking, on
        waking, on
    sadness, with
    sleep, go to f. to
    throat, fear from sensation of swelling of
    thunderstorm, of
    trifles, of
    waking, on
    walking, of ●
    work, dread of
Forgetful
    evening
    eating, after
    mental exertion, from
    periodical
    purchases, of; goes off and leaves them
    words while speaking, of; word hunting
Frightened, easily
    night
    waking, on
Generous, strangers, for

Gestures, awkward, in
  grasping, picks at bed clothes
  fingers in the mouth, children put ★
  hands, motions, involuntary, of the
Grief
  cry, cannot
  future, for the
  headache from grief
  prolonged ★
  silent
Hatred
  persons who had offended him, of
  revenge, h. and
Haughty
Heedless
Homesickness
Hopeful
Howling
Hurry, haste
  awkward from
Hypochondriasis
  night
  suicide, driving to
Hysteria
  fainting, hysterical
  menses, before
  during
  scanty ●
Ideas, deficiency of
  fixed ★
Idleness
Imbecility
Impatience
  heat, with
  trifles, about
Impertinence
Impetuous
  perspiration, with
Improvident
Inconsolable
Indifference, apathy
  alternating with anxiety and rest-
    lessness
  company, society, while in
  duties, to
  eating, to

Indifference,
  everything, to
  exertion, after ●.
  joyless
  mental exertion, after ●
  pleasure, to
  welfare of others, to
  women, to ●
Indignation, pregnant, while ●
Indiscretion
Indolence, aversion to work
  morning
  forenoon
  afternoon
  evening
  eating, after
  physical
  postpones the work ●
Industrious, mania for work
Insanity, madness
  neuralgia, with disappearance of
  paroxysmal
  puerperal
Insolence
  servants to chiefs, of
Irresolution, indecision
  ideas, in
  marry, to
Irritability
  daytime
  morning
    waking, on
  forenoon
  noon
  afternoon
  evening
    amel.
  alternating with cheerfulness
  business, about
  chill, during
  coition, after
  consolation, agg.
  eating, after
  headache, during
  heat, during

Irritability
>   menses, before
>   during
>   after
>   music, during
>   noise, from
>   perspiration, during
>   questioned, when
>   sadness, with
>   sitting, while
>   sleeplessness, with
>   snapping, amel. ★
>   spoken to, when
>   takes everything in bad part
>   waking, on

Jealousy, children, between
>   women, between

Jesting
>   aversion to
>   joke, cannot take a

Kleptomania
Lamenting, bemoaning, wailing
Lascivious, lustful
>   evening, bed, in ●

Laughing
>   evening
>   agg.
>   immoderately
>   involuntarily
>   serious matters, over
>   spasmodic

Liar
>   charlatan, and

Libertinism
Light, desire for
Loathing, life, at
>   work, at

Looked at, cannot bear to be
>   agg. mental symptoms ★

Loquacity
Love with one of the own sex, homo-
>   sexuality, tribadism
>   married man, with ●

Love, disappointed
>   jealousy, anger and incoherent
>   talk, with
>   sadness from
>   **silent grief, with**

Ludicrous, things seem
Malicious, spiteful, vindictive
>   anger, with

Mania
Mannish habits of girls
Mathematics, horror of
Memory, active
Memory, weakness of
>   do, for what was about to
>   expressing oneself, for
>   facts, for recent
>   happened, for what has
>   heard, for what has
>   **labor, for mental**
>   fatigue, from
>   names, for proper
>   occurrences of the day, for
>   periodical
>   read, for what has
>   say, for what is about to
>   thought, for what has just
>   words, of
>   write, for what is about to

**Menses, mental symptoms agg. be-
fore**
>   at beginning of
>   during
>   after

Mildness
Misanthropy
Mistakes, localities, in
>   **speaking, in**
>   intend, what he does not
>   misplacing words
>   wrong answers, gives
>   words, using wrong
>   headache, during ★
>   writing, in

Moaning, chill, during
>   sleep, during

Mood, alternating
>   changeable, variable

Moral feeling, want of
Morose, cross, fretful, ill-humor, peevish
>   daytime
>   morning
>   waking, on

Morose,
    forenoon
    afternoon
    evening
    alternating with cheerfulness
    causeless
    children, spoken to, when ●
    chill, during
    coition, after
    questioned, when ●
    women, in
Music, amel.
Muttering
Nymphomania
Objective, reasonable
Obscene, lewd
Offended, easily; takes everything in
    bad part
Passionate
    trifle, at every
Pregnancy, mental affections in
Prostration of mind, mental exhaustion,
    brain-fag
    afternoon
    evening
    eating, after
    talking, from
Puberty, mental affections in
Quarrelsome, scolding
    evening
Quiet disposition
Rage, fury
    night
    consolation, from ●
    headache, with
Reading: unable to read
Religious affections
Remorse
Reproaches, himself
    others
Reserved
Resignation
Restlessness
    daytime
    morning
    night
    midnight, before
        at ●

Restlessness, midnight
    after, 3h.
    alternating with indifference ●
    anxious
    bed, driving out of
        tossing about in
    chill, during
    internal
    sitting, while
    storm, during
    waking, on
    walking amel.
    warm bed agg.
Reverence for those around him
Rudeness
    employees to the chiefs, of
Sadness, despondency, dejection,
    mental depression, gloom, mel-
    ancholy
    daytime
    evening
    night
        bed, in
    alone, when
    canine hunger, with ●
    chill, during
    climaxis, during
    coition, after
        aversion to coition, desire for
        solitude
    drunkards, in
    grief, after
    headache, during
    heat, during
    labor, during
    love, from disappointed
    masturbation, from
    menses, before
        during
        suppressed
    perspiration, during
    pollutions, from
    pregnancy, in
    puberty, in
    puerperal
    stool, amel. after
    suicidal disposition, with
    weep, cannot

Satyriasis
Searching thieves after having dream of
   them •
Senses, dull, blunted
Sensitive, oversensitive
   evening
   heat, during
   music, to
   noise, to
   rudeness, to
   steel points directed toward her
Sentimental ★
Shamelessness
   bed, in •
Shrieking, sleep, during
Sighing
Singing
   evening •
   hilarious, joyously
Sit, inclination to
Slander, disposition to; denouncer
Slowness
Somnambulism
   do day-labor, to
   **strike sleepers, from vengeance,
      to**
Speech, affected
   confused
   embarrassed
   intoxicated, as if
   slow
Spoken to, averse to being
Starting, startled
   easily
   *electric shock through the body
      during sleep*
   wakening her
   fright, from and as from
   heat, during
   noise, from
   sleep, on falling
   during
   from
   trifles, at
Strange, crank
Stranger, sensation as if one were a
   presence of stranges agg.

Stupefaction, as if intoxicated
   dinner, after
Suicidal disposition
   hypochondriasis
   sadness, from
   shooting, by
   thoughts
Sympathy, compassion
   agg.
*Talk, indisposed to, desires to be silent,
   taciturn*
   forenoon
   others agg., talk of
   slow learning to
Talking amel., prolonged •
   pleasure in his own
   sleep, in
Talks, dead people, with
Tastelessness in dressing
Testament, refuses to make a
Thinking, aversion to
   complaints agg., of
Thoughts, control of thoughts lost,
   evening •
   disagreeable
   disease, of
   past, of the
   persistent
      evening
      **unpleasant subjects, haunted
         by**
   rush, flow of
   night
   tormenting
   vanishing of
      mental exertion, on
   wandering
Thunderstorm, mind symptoms before
   during
Time, fritters away his
Timidity
   awkward, and
   bashful ★
Torments himself
Torpor
Tranquillity, serenity, calmness

Trifles seem important
Unconsciousness, coma, stupor
    morning
    night
    chill, during
    conduct, automatic
    crowded room, in a
    diphtheria, in
    fever, during
    frequent spells of unconsciousness,
        absences
    head, on moving
    hydrocephalus, in
    sitting, while
    transient
    vertigo, during
Ungrateful
Unsympathetic, unscrupulous
Verses, makes
    asleep, on falling •
Violent, vehement
    trifles, at ★
Washing, always, her hands ★
Wearisome
Weary of life
Weeping, tearful mood
    evening
    night
        sleep, in
    anger, with ★
    admonition, from
      agg.
    alone, when
    aloud, wobbing
    alternating with laughter
    anxiety, with
    anxious
    bitter ★
    causeless
    chill, during
    consolation agg.
    easily
    hysterical
    impossible, though sad ★
    involuntary

Weeping, tearful mood
    looked at, when
    menses, during
    music, from
    past events, thinking of
    pitied, if he believes he is •
    pregnancy, during
    sleep, in
    spasmodic
    spoken to, when
    trifles, at
    whimpering during sleep
Will, loss of
    weakness of
Work, aversion to mental
    desire for
    impossible
      exertion, from •

NATRUM NITRICUM

Capriciousness
Dipsomania, alcoholism
Indolence, aversion to work
Sadness, despondency, dejection, mental depression, gloom, melancholy
Work, aversion to mental

NATRUM PHOSPHORICUM

Absent-minded, unobserving
Absorbed, buried in thought
Ailments from:
    anger, vexation
    bad news
    sexual excesses
    work, mental
Ambition, loss of
Anger, irascibility
    trifles, at
Anxiety
    evening
    night
    midnight, before
    bed, in

Anxiety,
- eating, after
- fear, with
- fever, during
- *future, about*
- health, about
- home, about •
- waking, on

Cheerful, gay, mirthful

Company, aversion to; presence of other people agg. the symptoms; desire for solitude

Concentration, difficult
- studying, reading etc., while

Confusion of mind
- morning
- evening
- eating, after
- *mental exertion, after*
- waking, on

Conversation agg.

Delusions, imaginations, hallucinations, illusions
- dead persons, sees
- footsteps, hears
  - next room, in •
- furniture, imagines it to be persons (night on waking) •
- hearing, illusions of
- images, phantoms, sees frightful
- inanimate objects are persons
- sick, he is going to be
- typhoid fever, he will have •

Discontented, displeased, dissatisfied

Discouraged

Dullness, sluggishness, difficulty of thinking and comprehending, torpor
- reading, while

Excitement, excitable
- mental work, from ★

Fear, apprehension, dread
- *night*
- bad news, of hearing
- disease, of impending
- *happen, something will*
- night
- misfortune, of

Fear,
- waking, on
- work, dread of
  - mental of

Forgetful
- *sexual excesses, after*

Frightened easily

Heedless

Hurry, haste
- everybody must hurry

Hysteria

Ideas abundant, clearness of mind
- evening
- deficiency of

Imbecility

Impatience

Indifference, apathy
- everything, to
- loved ones, to
- relations, to

Indolence, aversion to work

Irritability
- morning
- forenoon
- breakfast, before •
- menses, during

Memory, active

Memory, weakness of

Morose, forenoon

Morphinism

Music agg.

Prostration of mind, mental exhaustion, brain-fag

Restlessness
- evening
- night
- anxious

Sadness, despondency, dejection, mental depression, gloom, melancholy
- evening
- heat, during
- masturbation, from
- music, from
- pollutions, from

Sensitive, oversensitive
- music, to
- noise, to

Serious, earnest
Sighing
> menses, before
>> during, amel. •
> after
Sit, inclination to
> still
Starting, startled
> **easily**
> electric shock through the body
>> while wide awake
> fright, from and as from
> **noise, from**
> sleep, on falling
>> during
>> from
Stupefaction, as if intoxicated
Suspicious, mistrustful
Talk, indisposed to, desire to be silent,
> taciturn
Thoughts, disease, of
> wandering
Timidity
> bashful
Tranquillity, serenity, calmness
Unconsciousness, coma, stupor
Weeping, tearful mood
Work, desire for mental
> evening
> impossible

NATRUM SALICYLICUM

Delirium, wild
Delusions, imaginations, hallucinations,
> illusions
Dementia
Memory, weakness of
Sadness, despondency, dejection, mental
> depression, gloom, melancholy
Unconsciousness, coma, stupor

NATRUM SILICICUM

Anger, contradiction, from
Anxiety, evening
> night
> midnight, before
> bed, in
> eating, after
> waking, on
Concentration, difficult
Confidence, want of self
Confusion of mind, morning
> evening
> eating, after
> **mental exertion, after**
> waking, on
Conscientious, about trifles
Despair
Discouraged
Dullness, mental exertion, from
> reading, while
> waking, on
Excitement, excitable
Exertion, agg. from mental
Fear, waking, on
Forgetful
Frightened easily
Hysteria
Imbecility
Indifference, loved ones, to
> surroundings, to the
Indolence, aversion to work
Irresolution, indecision
Irritability, evening
> coition, after
> waking, on
Loathing, life, at
Memory, weakness of
Prostration of mind, mental exhaustion,
> brain-fag
Reading, mental symptoms agg. from
Restlessness, night
> anxious
> bed, driving out of
Sadness, menses, during
Sensitive, noise, to

Starting, fright, from and as from
    noise, from
    sleep, from
Talk, indisposed to, desire to be silent,
    taciturn
Weeping, tearful mood

NATRUM SULPHURICUM

Activity, mental, desire for
Ailments from:
    anger, vexation
    injuries, accidents; mental
      symptoms from
Anger, irascibility
    morning
    evening amel.
    violent
Anguish, night
    waking, on
Anxiety
    morning
    evening, bed, in
    midnight, before
    fever, during
    future, about
    paroxysms, in ★
    stool, after
    waking, on
Aversion, wife, to his ★
Cheerful, gay, mirthful
    morning
    forenoon
    afternoon
    followed by irritability
    stool, after
Clinging, held, wants to be
Company, aversion to; presence of other
    people agg. the symptoms; de-
    sire for solitude
Confusion of mind
    morning
    injury to head, after ●
    rising, after
    stools amel.
.Death, desires
Delirium
    meningitis, cerebrospinalis

Despair
    recovery, of
Dipsomania, alcoholism
Discouraged
Doubtful, recovery, of
Dullness, sluggishness, difficulty of think-
    ing and comprehending, torpor
    morning
Estranged from her family
    wife, from his
Excitement, excitable
    morning
Exertion, agg. from mental
Fastidious ★
Fear, apprehension, dread
    crowd, in a
    evil, of
    misfortune, of
    music, from
    noise, from
      night
    people, of; anthropophobia
    suicide, of
Forgetful
Frightened, easily
Hysteria
Indolence, aversion to work
    morning
    breakfast, after ●
Industrious, mania for work
Injure himself, fear to be left alone, lest
    he should
    shooting himself from satiety, must
      use self control to prevent ●
Insanity, madness
    injuries to the head, from
Irritability
    morning
    rising, after
    waking, on
    eating, amel. after
    spoken to, when
    waking, on
Kill herself, sudden impulse to
Loathing, life, at
    injury, must restrain herself
      to prevent doing herself ●
Mania, alternating with depression
    periodical

Morose, cross, fretful, ill-humor, peevish
    morning
Music agg.
Passionate
    morning ●
Praying
    kneeling and
Prostration of mind, mental exhaustion,
    brain-fag
Qualmishness ★
Quarrelsome, scolding
Restlessness
    night
Sadness, despondency, dejection,
mental depression, gloom, mel-
ancholy
    morning
    heat, during
    injuries of the head, from
    music, from
    suicidal disposition, with
Self-control
Sensitive, oversensitive
    morning
    music, to
    noise, to
      slightest, to
    pain, to
    reprimands, to, children, even mild
    scolding ★
Spoken to, averse to being
    morning
Starting, night
    dream, from a
    fright, from and as from
    noise, from
    sleep, on falling
      during
Stupefaction, as if intoxicated
Succeeds, never
Suicidal disposition
    hanging, by
    sadness, from
    shooting, by
Suspicious, mistrustful
Talk, indisposed to, desire to be silent,
    taciturn
      morning
      others agg., talk of

Violent, vehement
    morning
Wearisome
Weary of life
Weeping, tearful mood
    air, amel. in open
    delirium, after ●
    music, from
Wildness
Work, mental, impossible

NEPENTHES DISTILLATORIA

Activity
Anguish
Delusions, animals
    beetles, worms etc.
Excitement, excitable
Hypochondriasis
Impatience
Indifference, apathy
Irritability
Optimistic
Restlessness
Sadness, despondency, dejection, mental
    depression, gloom, melancholy
Strength increased, mental
Weary of life

NICCOLUM CARBONICUM AUT METALLICUM

Anger, irascibility
    evening
    contradiction, from
Anguish, forenoon
Anxiety
    dreams, on waking from frightful
    fear, with
    fever, during
    motion, from
    waking, on
Asks for nothing
Cheerful, gay, mirthful
Company, aversion to; presence of other
    people agg. the symptoms; de-
    sire for solitude

Confusion of mind
    morning
Contradict, disposition to
        evening •
        amel. •
Contradiction, is intolerant of
        evening amel. •
Contrary, evening •
Cruelty, inhumanity
Discomfort
    night
Dullness, sluggishness, difficulty of think-
    ing and comprehending, torpor
Fear, apprehension, dread
    morning
    forenoon
    afternoon
    evil, of
    happen, something will
    misfortune, of
    tremulous
Impatience
Irritability
    morning
    evening
        amel.
    talking, while
Loquacity
Malicious, spiteful, vindictive
    anger, with
Morose, cross, fretful, ill-humor, peevish
    forenoon
Quarrelsome, scolding
    evening
    pugnacious
Restlessness
    afternoon
        15 h.
    evening
    night
    midnight, 3h after, everything
    feels sore, must move about •
    bed, driving out of
    menses, suppressed, during
    walking amel.

Sadness, despondency, dejection, mental
    depression, gloom, melancholy
    morning
    afternoon
        amel.
Starting, afternoon
    dream, from a
    sleep, during
Stupefaction, as if intoxicated
    stooping, on
Talk, indisposed to, desire to be silent,
    taciturn
Violent, deeds of violence, rage leading
    to
Weeping, tearful mood
    night
    sleep, in
    waking, on

NICOTINUM

Concentration, difficult
Delirium
Delusions, visions, horrible, sees
Restlessness
    night
Stupefaction, as if intoxicated
Thoughts, wandering

NIDUS EDULIS

Cheerful, alternating with sadness
Impatience
Indifference, apathy
    alternating with anger
Indolence, aversion to work
Irritability
    alternating with tolerance •
Laughing, alternating with sadness
Memory, weakness of
Mood, alternating
    changeable, variable
Prostration of mind, mental exhaustion,
    brain-fag
Sadness alternating with euphoria
Weeping, tearful mood
Will, loss of

NITRI ACIDUM
(NITRIC ACID)

Abrupt, rough
Absent-minded, unobserving
Absorbed, buried in thought
Abusive, insulting
Admonition agg.
Affectionate
Ailments from :
    discords between chief and subor
        dinates, parents, friends
      servants ★
    excitement, emotional
    fright
    grief
    hurry
    sexual excesses
Amorous
Anger, irascibility
    contradiction, from
    mistakes, about his
    trembling, with
    trifles, at
    violent
Anguish
    loss of his friend, from •
    menses, during
Anxiety
    daytime
    morning
        waking, on
    afternoon
    evening
        bed, in
    night
        waking, on
    alone, when
    ascending steps, on
    bed, in
        driving out of
    congestion to heart, from •
    conscience, as if guilty of a crime
    contraction in heart region, from •
    coughing, from
    eating, after
    fear, with
    fever, during
    future, about

Anxiety,
    headache, with
    health, about
    hypochondriacal
    menses, before
        during
    mental exertion, from
    night watching, from
    paroxysms, in
    sitting, while
    sleep, during
        loss of
    stool, after
    thinking about it, from
    thunderstorm, during
    waking, on
    walking rapidly, when
Avarice
Aversion, persons, to certain
Barking
Beside oneself, being
        pain, by little •
Bite, desire to
Blasphemy
    cursing, and
Capriciousness
    morning
Caressed, aversion to being
Cheerful, gay, mirthful
    evening, bed, in
    alternating with sadness
    never
Company, desire for; aversion to soli-
    tude, company amel.
Complaining
Concentration, difficult
    on attempting to concentrate has a
        vacant feeling
Confidence, want of self
Confusion of mind
    air, in open
    concentrate the mind, on attempt-
        ing to
    eating, after
    mental exertion, from
    sitting, while
    stooping, when
    walking, while

Conscientious, trifles, occupied with
Consolation, kind words agg.
    refuses, for his own misfortunes ★
Contemptuous
Contradict, disposition to
Contradiction, is intolerant of
Contrary
Cowardice
Cruelty, inhumanity
Cursing, swearing
    evening, when home
    rage, in
Cynical ★
Death, desires
    presentiment of
Deceitful, perjured
Delirium
    night
    **bed and escapes, springs up
      suddenly from**
    raging, raving
*Delusions, imaginations, hallucinations,
    illusions*
    evening, bed, in
    night
    criminals, about
    dead persons, sees
    die, he was about to
    disease, incurable, has
    elevated in air •
    fancy, illusions of
      chill, during
    figures, sees
    images, phantoms, sees
      evening
        in bed •
      night
      disappearing and reappearing,
        sees •
      frightful
      increasing and decreasing, sees •
      running, sees •
      sleep, before
    lawsuit, being engaged in a •
    longer, things seem
    offended people, he has
    sick, being
    small: things grow smaller
    soul, body was too small for soul or
      separated from

Delusions,
    spectres, ghosts, spirits, sees
      chill, during •
    strangers, sees
      surrounded by
    talking insane •
      irrationally •
    tall: things grow taller
    visions, has
      fantastic
      horrible, night
    voices, hears
    wealth, of
Dementia, syphilitics, of
Despair
    **rage, cursing and impreca-
      tions, with** •
    recovery, of
Discontented, displeased, dissatisfied
    always
    everything, with
    himself, with
    weeping amel.
Discouraged
    cursing, with •
    rage, with
    weeping amel. •
Disobedience
Doubtful, recovery, of
Driving amel. mental symptoms •
*Dullnesss, sluggishness, difficulty of think-
    ing and comprehending, torpor*
Dwells on past disagreeable occurrences
    recalls disagreeable memories
Ecstasy, perspiration, during
Embittered, exasperated
Envy, avidity, and
    hate, and
Estranged from her family
Excitement, excitable
    evening, bed, in
    night
    debate, during
    palpitation, with violent
    trifles, over
Exertion, agg. from mental

Fancies, exaltation of
    night
    perspiration, during
Fear, apprehension, dread
    morning
    evening
    night
    alone, of being
    ascending, of
    cholera, of
    death, of
      heat, during
    disease, of impending
      cancer, of ★
    eating food, after
    evil, of
    noise, from
    palpitation, with
    process (legal) of a ●
    starting, with
    thunderstorm, of
    touch, of
    waking, on
    weariness of life, with
Forgetful
Frightened, easily
       noon, nap, after
    falling asleep, on
    trifles, at
    waking, on
Greed, cupidity
Grief
Gristly ★
Hatred
    persons who had offended him, of
    unmoved by apologies ●
    revenge, and
Heedless
Homesickness
    silent ill-humor, with
Horrible things, sad stories, affect her
    profoundly
Hurry, haste
Hypochondriasis
Hysteria

Ideas abundant, clearness of mind
    compelling ★
    deficiency of
Imbecility
Impatience
    afternoon
    supper, after ●
Impertinence
Impetuous
    daytime ●
Indifference, apathy
    everything, to
    family, to his
    joyless
    pleasure, to
Indolence, aversion to work
    burning in the right lumbar-
      region ●
    sitting, while
    walking, while
Insolence
Irresolution, indecision
Irritability
    morning
      waking, on
    afternoon
    burning in right lumbarregion,
      from ●
    chill, during
    coition, after
    consolation agg.
    sadness, with
    spoken to, when
    stool, after
    waking, on
Lamenting, bemoaning, wailing
Lascivious, lustful
Laughing, involuntarily
Loathing, life, at
Malicious, spiteful, vindictive
Mania
Memory, weakness of
Menses, mental symptoms agg. before
Mildness
Misanthropy

Moaning, groaning, whining
  sleep, during
Mood, changeable, variable
  repulsive
Moral feeling, want of
Morose, cross, fretful, ill-humor, peevish
  morning
    bed, in
    waking, on
  afternoon
  waking, on
  weeping amel.
Music, aversion to
Objective, reasonable
Obstinate, headstrong
Offended, easily; takes everything in
  bad part
Perseverance
Philosophy, ability for
Pities herself
Profanity ★
Prostration of mind, mental exhaustion, brain-fag
  nursing, after
Quarrelsome, scolding
Rage, fury
  evening
  night
  cursing, with
Rebels against poultice
Remorse
Reserved
Resignation
Restlessness
    midnight, after, 4 h., until •
    morning, waking, on
    evening
    night
    midnight, after
  anxious
  bed, in
    driving out of
    tossing about in
  internal
  menses, during
Rudeness

Sadness, despondency, dejection, mental depression, gloom, melancholy
  morning
  waking, on
    after
  evening
  anger, from
  anxious
  burning in right lumbar region, from
  chill, during
  menses, before
    during
  mercury, after abuse of
  perspiration, during
  talk, indisposed to
  waking, on
Secretive
Senses, acute
  dull, blunted
  vanishing of
Sensitive, oversensitive
  external impressions, to all
  heat, during
  menses, before
  mental impressions, to
  noise, to
    shrill sounds, to
    stepping, of
    voices, to
      male, to
  water splashing, to
  pain, to
  sensual impressions, to
Sentimental
Shrieking, screaming, shouting
  convulsions, before
    during epileptic
  sleep, during
Sighing
Sit, inclination to
Slander, disposition to
Somnambulism, strike sleepers, from
  vengeance, to
Spoken to, averse to being

Starting, startled
    noon
       sleep, in
    night
    dream, from a
    easily
    fright, from and as from
    lying on back
    noise, from
    sleep, on falling
       during
       from
    waking, on
Stupefaction, as if intoxicated
    daytime •
Suicidal disposition
    courage, but lacks
    fear of death, with
Suspicious, mistrustful
Sympathy, compassion
Talk, indisposed to, desire to be silent,
    taciturn
    sadness, in
    others agg., talk of
Talking, sleep, in
    unpleasant things agg., of
Thinking, complaints agg., of
Thoughts, disagreeable
    persistent
    thoughtful
    tormenting
    vanishing of
       exertion, on •
       mental exertion, on
    wandering
Thunderstorm, mind symptoms during
Timidity
    bashful
Touched
    caressed, aversion to being
Unconsciousness, coma, stupor
Unsympathetic, unscrupulous
Violent, vehement
    deeds of violence, rage leading to
Vivacious
Wearisome

Weary of life
    fear of death, but
Weeping, tearful mood
    night
       sleep, in
    admonition, from
    agg.
    amel.
    causeless
    children, in
    consolation agg.
    remonstrated, when
    sleep, in
    trifles: children at the least worry
    whimpering
       sleep, during
Work, aversion to mental
    impossible
       burning in right lumbar re-
       gion, from •

NITROMURIATICUM ACIDUM

Restlessness

NITRI SPIRITUS DULCIS

Anger, irascibility
Anxiety
Confusion of mind
Delirium
    sleep, during
Excitement agg.
Indifference, apathy
    everything, to
    fever, during
    sleeplessness, with •
    taciturn
    typhoid, in
Irritability
Morose, cross, fretful, ill-humor, pee-
    vish
Muttering, sleep, in
Prostration of mind, fever, in
Quarrelsome, scolding
Unconsciousness, coma, stupor
    fever, during

NITROGENIUM OXYGENATUM

Activity, mental
    night
Anxiety
Cheerful, gay, mirthful
    night
Confidence, want of self
Confusion of mind
Dancing
Delirium
Despair
Discrimination, lack of
Dullness, sluggishness, difficulty of
    thinking and com-
    prehending, torpor
Eccentricity
Ecstasy
Excitement, nervous
    trembling, with
Gestures, enthusiastic ●
    sublime
Haughty
Hysteria
Indolence, aversion to work
Irritability
Laughing, desire to laugh
    immoderately
Memory, weakness of
Restlessness
Sadness, shock, from ●
Thoughts, rush, flow of
    tormenting
    vagueness of
Unconsciousness, coma, stupor
    incomplete
Violent, vehement
Weeping, tearful mood

NUPHAR LUTEUM

Anger, irascibility
Contradiction, is intolerant of
Fancies, lascivious
Impatience
    contradiction, at slightest
Lascivious, lustful
Restlessness
Sympathy, compassion

NUX JUGLANS

Confusion of mind, morning
Talk, indisposed to, desire to be silent,
    taciturn

NUX MOSCHATA

Absent minded, unobserving
    periodical attacks of, short lasting
    reading, while
    standing in one place, never ac-
        complishes what he under-
        takes ●
    waking, on; does not know where
        he is or what to answer ●
Absorbed, buried in thought
Abstraction of mind
Ailments from :
    anger, vexation
    excitement, emotional
    fright
    love, disappointed
    work, mental
Anger, irascibility
    pregnancy, during
Answers, incorrectly
    irrelevantly
    reflects long
    refuses to answer
    slowly
Anxiety
    evening
    fear, with
    health, about
    walking, cool air, in ●
Automatism
Barking
Bellowing
Blood, or knife, cannot look at ★
Capriciousness
Cheerful, gay, mirthful
    morning, waking, on
    evening
    air, in open
    alternating with sadness
    chill, during
Childish, behavior
Clairvoyance

Clinging, held, wants to be
Company, aversion to, pregnancy, during
Concentration, difficult
Confusion of mind
    evening
    chill, during
    identity: duality, sense of
    intoxicated, as if
    loses his way in well-known streets
    mental exertion, from
    pregnancy, during •
    reading, while
    waking, on
    walking, while
      air, in open
Contradictory to speech, intentions are
Conversation agg.
Cowardice
Delirium
    maniacal
    menses, during
    raging, raving
Delirium tremens, mania-a-potu
Delusions, imaginations, hallucinations, illusions
    brain, cracking, is •
    changed, thinks everything is ★
    diminished, shrunken, parts are
    distances, of
    double, of being
    dream, as if in a
    enlarged, distances are
      head is
    fancy, illusions of
    figures, sees
    floating in air
    heads, having two
    hearing, illusions of
    images, phantoms, sees
      dwells upon
    large, parts of body seem too
    ludicrous
    persons, three, that he is ★
    space, expansion of

Delusions,
    strange, everything is
      familiar things seem
        ludicrous, are
    three persons, he is
    time, exaggeration of, passed too slowly
    visions, has
Dipsomania, alcoholism
Distances, inaccurate judgement of
    exaggerated, are
Dream, as if in a
Dullness, sluggishness, difficulty of thinking and comprehending, torpor
    chill, during
    reading while
    sleepiness, with
    waking, on
    writing, while
Ecstasy
Excitement confusion, as from •
    pregnancy, during
Exertion, agg. from mental
Fancies, exaltation of
Fear, dark, of
    death, of
      morning 17-30h. •
    fit, of having a
    heart, of disease of
    heat, during
    menses, suppressed from fear
    pregnancy, during
    sleep, go to sleep, fear to
      lest he die •
    touch, of
Foolish behavior
    air, in open •
Forgetful
    house was, on which side of the street his
    streets, of well known
Gestures, makes
    automatic
    ridiculous or foolish
      air, in open •
      standing on the street, while •
    strange attitudes and positions

Grimaces
Heedless
Hurry, everybody must hurry
Hypochondriasis
    forenoon •
    fever, during •
Hysteria
    fainting, hysterical
    menses, before
        during
    scanty
Ideas abundant, clearness of mind
    deficiency of ★
    vanishing of ★
Idiocy
Imbecility
Imitation, mimicry ★
Impatience
Indifference, apathy
    everything, to
Indolence, eating, after
Insanity, madnesss
    behaves like a crazy person
    foolish, ridiculous
    sleeplessness, with
Irresolution, indecision
    acts, in
Irritability
    aroused, when
Jesting
Lamenting, bemoaning, wailing
Laughing
    forenoon
    air, in open
    alternating with seriousness
        shrieking
    everything, at ★
    hysterical
    immoderately
    ludicrous, everything seems
    menses, before
    sardonic
    serious matters, over
    silly
    spasmodic
    stupid expression, with
Loquacity
Ludicrous, things seem

Mania
    singing, with
Memory, active
Memory, weakness of
    do, for what was about to
    done, for what has just
    facts, for past
    happened, for what has
    heard, for what has
    pains, from, sudden ★
    places, for
    read, for what has
    said, for what has
    say, for what is about to
    words, of
    write, for what is about to
    written, for what he has
Menses, mental symptoms agg. after
    suppressed
Mental symptoms, alternating with
    physical ★
Mistakes, localities, in
    space and time, in
    speaking, in
        misplacing words
    spelling, in
    words, using wrong
        opposite, e.g. hot for cold
    time, in
        present with the past
    writing, in
        omitting letters
        wrong words during headache •
Mocking
Monomania
Mood, alternating
    changeable, variable
        heat, during •
Morose, cross, fretful, ill-humor, peevish
Pregnancy, mental affections in
Prophesying
Prostration of mind, mental exhaustion, brain-fag
    alternating with laughing •
Quiet disposition, alternating with laughing •

Rage, fury
Recognize: relatives, does not recognize
    his
    **streets, does not recognize well
    known**
Restlessness
    night
    eating, after
    headache, during
    pregnancy, during
Rudeness
Sadness, despondency, dejection, mental depression, gloom, melancholy
    morning after waking
    forenoon
    heat, during
    menses, from suppressed
    pregnancy, in
Senses, dull, blunted
    vanishing of
Sensitive, noise, to
Serious, earnest
    alternating with laughing •
Shamelessness
Shrieking, locomotive, like a •
    sleep, during
Sighing
Singing
Slowness
Speech, affected
    confused
    extravagant
    foolish
    hesitating
    incoherent
    loud
    nonsensical
    slow
    wandering
Starting, startled
    afternoon
    consciousness, recovering
    easily
    electric shock through the body
      during sleep
      wakening her
    sleep, during
    trifles, at

Stupefaction, as if intoxicated
    chill, during
    menses, during
    remains fixed in one spot •
    sleepiness, with
Talk: desire to talk to someone
    indisposed to, desire to be silent, taciturn
    heat, during
    slow learning to
Talks, himself, to
    loudly ★
Thinking, complaints agg., of
Thoughts, control of thoughts lost, 14 h. •
    persistent
      humorous •
    rush, flow of
    vanishing of
      menses, before •
      reading, on
      speaking, while
      writing, while
      wandering, writing, while
Time, passes too slowly, appears longer
Torpor
Touched, aversion to being
Unconsciousness, coma, stupor
    noon, 14 h. •
    evening
    blood, sight of •
    conduct, automatic
    crowded room, in a
    dream, as in a
      does not know where he is
    emotions, after
    excitement, after
    fever, during
    menses, before
      during
      suppression of
    mental insensibility
    pain, from
    pregnancy, during
    remains fixed on one spot •
    standing, while
      having dress fitted •
    vertigo, during

*Undertakes many things, perseveres in
      nothing*
Walk, walking in open air agg. mental
      symptoms
Weeping, tearful mood
      alternating with laughter
Work, mental, impossible
Writing agg. mind symptoms

NUX VOMICA

Abrupt, rough
      harsh
      rough yet affectionate
Absent-minded, unobserving
      inadvertence
      spoken to, when
Absorbed, buried in thought
      morning
Abstraction of mind
Abusive, insulting
      drunkenness, during
      husband, insulting wife before chil-
            dren or vice versa
Activity, mental ★
      restless
Admonition agg.
      kindly agg.
Affections, in general ★
Affectionate
Ailments from:
      ambition, deceived
      anger vexation
            anxiety, with
            fright, with
            indignation, with
            silent grief, with
      anticipation, foreboding, presen-
            timent
      business failure
      cares, worries
      death of a child
            parents or friends, of
      debauchery
      dipsomania
      disappointment
      discords between chief & subordi-
            nates
      discords between parents, friends ★

Ailments from:
      excitement, emotional
      friendship, deceived
      fright
      grief
      hurry
      honor, wounded
      indignation
      jealousy
      literary, scientific failure
      love, disappointed
      mortification
      rudeness of others
      scorn, being scorned
      sexual excesses
      work, mental
Ambition
Amorous
Anger, irascibility
      morning
      answer, when obliged to
      contradiction, from
      delusions during climaxis, with
      easily
      face, with red
      himself, with
      interruption, from
      mistakes, about his
      stabbed anyone, so that he could
            have
      trembling, with
      trifles, at
      violent
Anguish
      morning
      afternoon
      night
            4h.
      waking, on
Answers, aversion to answer
      incorrectly
      refuses to answer
Anxiety
      morning
            rising, amel. on
            waking, on
      afternoon
      evening
      twilight, in the

Anxiety,
> *bed, in*
>> night
>> midnight, before
>>> **after**

bed, in
business, about
chill, during
clothes and open windows, must
> loosen

cold becoming, from
coffee after
conscience, as if guilty of a crime
eating, after
exaggerated ★
faintness, with
fear, with
fever, during
flatus, from
future, about
head, perspiration on forehead,
with
> cold

health, about
hypochondriacal
> *mania to read medical books*

lying, while
menses, before
> during
> anger and anxiety

mental exertion, from
others, for
perspiration, with cold
salvation, about
> faith, about loss of his
> scruples, excessive religious

sleep, during
suicidal disposition, with
supper, after
waking, on
walking, while
> air, in open

weary of life, with
Ardent
Avarice
> *anxiety about future, from a.*
> generosity towards strangers, a.
>> as regards his family
> squandering on oneself, but

Aversion, persons, to all
Benevolence
Beside oneself, being
Blasphemy, cursing, and
Blood, wounds, cannot look at
Boaster, braggart
> squander through ostentation

Break things, desire to
Brooding
Brutality, drunkenness, during
Buoyancy, alternating with despon-
> *dency ●*

Business, averse to
> **-man, worn out**

Capriciousness
Carefulness
Cares, worries, full of
> daily cares, affected by

Cautious
Censorious, critical
Chaotic, confused behavior
Cheerful, gay, mirthful
> evening
> sad in morning, and ●
>> *bed, in*

> *alternating with sadness*

Childish behavior
Clinging, held, wants to be
Company, aversion to; presence of
> **other people agg. the symp-**
> **toms; desires for solitude**

> bear anybody, cannot
> loathing at company
> menses, during, desires to be let
>> alone

Company, desire for; aversion to soli-
> *tude, company*
> *amel.*

Complaining
> night in sleep ●
> *disease, of*
> *pain, of*
> sleep, in

Concentration, active
Concentration, difficult
> aversion to ★
> **calculating, while**
> conversation, during
> **studying, reading, etc., while**

Confidence, want of self
Confounding, objects and ideas
Confusion of mind
    morning
    afternoon
    evening
    air, in open
    calculating, when
    carousal, after
    dinner, after
    eating, after
    intoxicated, as if
      as after being
    loses his way in well known streets
    mental exertion, from
    mixes subjective and objective
    motion, from
    spirituous liquors, from
    sun, in
    vexation, after ●
Conscientious about trifles
    trifles, occupied with
Consolation, kind words agg.
Contemptuous
Contradict, disposition to
Contradiction, is intolerant of
    agg.
Contrary
Conversation agg.
Coquettish, too much
Cowardice
Cruelty, inhumanity
Cursing, swearing
Death, desires
    presentiment of
    sensation of
    spasm, during ●
Deceitful, sly
**Deception causes grief and mortifi-
    cation ★**
Defiant
Delirium
    evening, nap, during
    night
    anxious
    bed and escapes, springs up sud-
      denly from
    chill, during

Delirium,
    frightful
    headache, during
    muttering
    raging, raving
    recognizes no one
    sleeplessness, and ★
**Delirium tremens, mania-a-potu
oversensitiveness, with**
    sleeplessness, with
Delusions, imaginations, hallucinations,
    illusions
    evening, bed, in
    night
    animals, of
    frightful
    bed, evening someone gets into
      and no room in it,
        someone has sold it ●
    someone is in bed with him
    body, headless, is ●
    threads, inside is made of ●
    crime, committed a, he had
    criminals, about
    dead, corpse, mutilated c.
      persons, sees
    die, he was about to
    dying, he is
    enlarged
    faces, sees
      hideous
    fail, everything will
    fancy, illusions of
    fire, visions of; baby, desires to
      throw, in ★
    foolish
    happened, anything, of, having
    head: deceased acquaintances
      without bodies, h. of (at night)
    home, away from, is
    house is full of people
    images, phantoms, sees
      night
      frightful
    injury, is about to receive
    insane, she will become
    insulted, he is
    journey, he is on a

Delusions,
    laughed at, mocked, being
    melancholy
        night, while half awake at
    mortification, after
    murdered, her mother had been ●
    mutilated bodies, sees
    people, beside him, are
        **pranks with him, carry on
        all sorts of ●
        questions and he must an-
        swer, ply with him ●**
    persecuted, he is
    poor, he is
    pregnant, she is
    pursued by enemies
    religious
    sick: work, and for this reason will
        not
    sold: bed, someone has s. his ●
    strangers, he sees
    study, after
    time, exaggeration of, passes too
        slowly
    vermin, sees, crawl, about
    visions, has
        horrible
    worms, creeping of
Dementia
    senilis
Despair
    chill, during
    pains, with the
    recovery, of
Destructiveness
    clothes, of
Dipsomania, alcoholism
    hypochondriasis, with ●
    idleness, from
    irritability, with ●
    pregnancy, during or after ●
Dirtiness
Discontented, displeased, dissatisfied
    morning
    everything, with
    himself, with
Discouraged
    moaning, with
    pain, from
    weeping, with

Disgust
    everything, with
Distances, exaggerated, time, during
    sleepiness, and ●
Doubful, recovery, of
    soul's welfare, of
Dream, as if in a
*Dullness, sluggishness, difficulty of think-
    ing and comprehending, torpor*
    morning
    loss of fluids, after
    mental exertion, from
    reading, while
Eccentricity
Egotism, self-esteem
Elegance, want of
Ennui, tedium
Envy
    avidity, and
Escape, attempts to
    family, children, from her
    run away, to
    springs up suddenly from bed
Estranged from her family
    being kind with strangers, but not
    with his family and entourage
Excitement, excitable
    morning
    evening
        bed in
    night
    agg.
    chill, during
    hearing horrible things, after
    menses, before
    perspiration, during
    trembling, with
Exertion, agg. from mental
Fancies, exaltation of
    morning
    evening, bed, in
    night
    sleeplessness, with
    lascivious
    vivid, lively

Fastidious
Fear, apprehension, dread
  morning
   bed, in
  afternoon
   17 h. •
  evening
   walking, while •
 air, in open
 alone, of being
 approaching him, of others
 blind, of going
 crowd, in a
  public places, of; agoraphobia
 death, of
  impending, of
 disease, of impending
 dreams, of terrible
 eating: after e. food
 evil, of
 faith, to lose his religious ★
 falling, of
  afternoon •
 get talked about, to
 happen, something will
 insanity, losing his reason, of
 killing, of
  knife, with a
 misfortune, of
 music, from
 narrow places, in; claustrophobia
 noise, from
 opinion of others, of
 overpowering
 physician, of ★
  will not see her, he seems to
   terrify her
 poverty, of
  spending in order to not being
  short of money in future, fear of
 rage, to fly into a
 rags, of ★
 sleep, go to s., fear to
 suffocation of
 suicide of
 touch, of
 waking, on

Fear,
 walking, while
 water, of
 work, dread of
  daily, of
  literary, of
Flatterer
Foolish behavior
Foppish
Forgetful
 drunkards, forgetfulness in
 house was, on which side of the
  street his
 loss of fluids, from
 mental exertion, from
 words while speaking, of; word
 hunting
Fright, menses, during ★
Frightened easily
 falling asleep, on
 trifles, at
 wakens in a fright from least
  noise •
 waking, on
Frown, disposed to
Gamble (*see* Play)
Generous, too much
 strangers, for
Gestures, makes
 awkward in
 convulsive
 grasping, sides of the bed, at •
 plays with his fingers, counting
  money, as if
 ridiculous or foolish
 strange attitudes and positions
  gait, in
 talking, gesticulates while
Greed, cupidity
Grief
 morning
 evening amel.
 cry, cannot
Hatred, persons who had offended him,
 of
Haughty
Heedless
Honor wounded

Horrible things, sad stories, affect her
    profoundly
House-keeping, women unable to
Howling
Hurry, haste
    always in
Hypochondriasis
    evening
    drunkards, in ●
    eating, after
Hysteria
    fainting, hysterical
    menses, during
        copious
Ideas abundant, clearness of mind
    evening
        bed, in
    night
    deficiency of
Imbecility
    rage, stamps the feet
Impatience
    coryza, with ●
    heat, with
    spoken to, when ●
    working, in
Impertinence
Impetuous
Impulse, rash
Impulsive
Inconsolable
Inconstancy
Independent ★
Indifference, apathy
    ennui, with
    everything, to
    welfare of others, to
Indignation
    bad effects following ★
Indiscretion
Indolence, aversion to work
      morning
    anger, after
    business, when transacting
    eating, after
    physical
Industrious, mania for work

Injustice, cannot support
Insanity, madness
    drunkards, in
    erotic
    escape, desire to
    foolish, ridiculous
    melancholy
    mental labor, from
    mortification, from
    obstinate in
    puerperal
    purchases, makes useless
    religious
    restlessness, with
    travel, with desire to
Insolence
Intolerance, ailment, of ●
Introspection
Irresolution, indecision
    changeable
    marry, to
Irritability
      morning
        waking, on
      night ★
    after - pains, in ●
    air, in open
    anxiety, with ●
    chill, during
    coition, after
    consolation agg.
    eating, after
    hemorrhoids, with
    headache, during
    heat, during
    liver trouble, in
    menses, before
      during
    music, during
    pollutions, after
    questioned, when
    remorseful, after ★
    sexual excitement, from (in a
    woman) ●
    spoken to, when
    stool, before
    waking, on

Jealousy
- animal or an inanimate objects, for
- brutal from, gentle husband becoming
- children, between
- drunkenness, during
- impotence, with
- *insult, driving to* •
- *quarrels, reproaches, scolds, with*
- sexual excitement, with
- strike his wife, driving to
- weeping, with
- women, between

Jesting, aversion to
- erotic
- joke, cannot take a

Jumping
- *wild leaps in mania puerperal* •

Kicks, animals ★

Kill, desire to
- *beloved ones*
- *herself, sudden impulse to*
- *husband, impulse to kill her beloved*
- *knife, with a*
  - at sight of a
- *offence, sudden impulse to kill for a slight*
- poison, impulse to
- *sudden impulse to kill*
- *throw child into fire, sudden impulse to*

Kleptomania

Lamenting, bemoaning, wailing
- *pain, about*
- sickness, about his

Laughing
- agg.
- *immoderately*

Liar

Libertinism

Litigious

Loathing, life, at

Longing, repose and tranquillity, for

Looked at, cannot bear to be

Loquacity
- *afternoon* •
- evening
- **health, about his** •

Love, with one of the own sex, homosexuality tribodism, perversity

Magnetized desires to be, mesmerism amel.

Malicious, spiteful, vindictive

Mania
- rage, with
- tears clothes

Marriage seemed unendurable, idea of

Mathematics, apt for

Memory, active

Memory, weakness of
- dates, for
- *expressing oneself, for*
- facts, recent, for
- labour, fatigue, from
- names, for proper
- persons, for
- sudden and periodical
- verses, to learn
- *words, for*

Mildness

Mischievous

Mistakes, calculating, in
- differentiating of objects, in
- localities, in
- measures and weights, in •
- speaking, in
  - *misplacing words*
  - omitting, words
  - spelling, in
  - wrong answers, gives
  - *words, using wrong*
- time, in
- writing, in
- writing, omitting letters
  - syllables
  - words

Moaning, groaning, whining
- heat, during
- *honor, from wounded* •
- *pain, from*
- *sleep, during*

Mocking
> others are mocking at him, thinks
> ridicule, passion to
> sarcasm

Mood, changeable, variable
> repulsive

Moral feeling, want of

Morose, cross, fretful, ill-humor, peevish
> *morning*
>> bed, in
> drunkenness, during
> eating, after
> *menses, before*
> sleep, in
> waking, on
> women, in

Morphinism

Music agg.
> aversion to
> headache from

Muttering
> *unintelligible*

Nagging ★

Nymphomania

Obscene, lewd
> *talk*

Obstinate, headstrong
> *menorrhagia, in* ●
> **resists wishes of others**

Occupation, diversion amel.

Offended, easily; takes everything in bad part

Optimistic

Passionate

Persevere, cannot ★

Perseverance

Pessimist

Plans, making many

Play: passion for gambling

Positiveness

Postponing everything to next day

Prostration of mind, mental exhaustion, brain fag
> night

Quarrelsome, scolding
> **disturbed, if** ●
> jealousy, from
> pains, during

Quiet disposition

Quiet, wants to be, repose and tranquillity, desires
> amel. ★

Rage, fury

Reading, aversion to read
> *passion to read medical books*

Rebels against poultice

Refuses treatment, in spite of being very sick

Religious affections
> very religious ★

Remorse

Reproaches others
> pains, during ●

Reserved

Rest, desire for

Restlessness
> night
> anxious
> bed, driving out of
>> *tossing about in*
> busy
> chest, from heat rising up into the mouth from chest ●
> children, roving, wandering
> driving about
> eating, after
> lying, while
> menses, before
>> *during*
> suppressed, during

Revelry, feasting

Revengeful ★

Reverence for those around him

Roaming and roving ★

Roving, senseless, insane

Rudeness

Runs about

Sadness, despondency, dejection, mental depression, gloom, melancholy
> *morning*
>> but cheerful in evening
> chill, during

Sadness,
    dinner, after
    drunkards, in
    drunkenness, during
    eating, after
    loss, place, after l. of •
    masturbation, from
    perspiration, during
    pollutions, from
    quiet
    sighing, with
    stool, amel. after
    supper, after •
    walking, air, in open
    weep, cannot
Selfishness, egotism
Senses, acute
    dull, blunted
    vanishing of
Sensitive, oversensitive
    ailment, to the most trifling •
    eating, after
    external impressions, to all
    light, to
    menses, before
        during
    moral impressions, to
    music, to
    noise, to
        painful sensitiveness to
        slightest, to
        stepping, of
        voices, to
    odors, to
    pain, to
    rudeness, to
    sensual impressions, to
    singing, to
Sentimental
Shamelessness
Shrieking, screaming, shouting
    anger, in
    children, in
        colic, with
        weeping and
        convulsions, before
            during epileptic
    drinking, while •
    must shriek, feels as though she

Sighing
    causeless •
    heat, during
    honor, from wounded •
    perspiration, during
Singing, trilling
Sit, inclination to
    still
Slander, disposition to
Speech, affected
    anxious, in sleep
    bombast, worthless
    confused
    hasty
    intoxicated, as if
    low
    monosyllabic
    phrases, in high-sounding •
    prattling
    sleep, in •
    unintelligible
        midnight, before •
    unsuitable •
    wandering
        afternoon and especially
            evening •
Spitting, desires to •
Spoken to, aversion to being
Squanders
    boasting, from
Starting, startled
    daytime •
    noon
    easily
    noise, from
    sleep, falling, on
        during
        from
    trifles, at
Steals money, without necessity ★
Striking
    about him at imaginary objects
    desires to strike
    drunkenness, during
Stupefaction, as if intoxicated
    air, in open
    dinner, after
    sleepiness, with
    sun, agg. in •

Succeeds, never
Suicidal disposition
>night
>>midnight, after
>anxiety, from
>**courage, but lacks**
>drowning, by
>drunkenness, during
>gassing, by
>heat, during
>*pain, from*
>shooting, by
>stabbing, by
>**talks always of suicide, but does not commit •**
>*throwing himself from a height*
>>window, from
Sulky
Suppressed or receding skin diseases or haemorrhoids, mental symptoms agg. after
Suspicious
Sympathy, compassion
Talk, indisposed to, desire to be silent, taciturn
>heat, during
>**others agg., talk of**
Talking, sleep, in
>comatose sleep, in
>excited
Talks, when alone
>**anxious about his condition**
>*himself, to, only when alone*
>humming
>troubles, of her ★
Tastelessness in dressing
Tears things
Teasing
Thinking, complaints agg., of
Thoughts, disconnected
>**read, cannot**
>*persistent*
>*rush, flow of*
>>morning
>>>after rising •

Thoughts, rush
>*evening, in bed*
>*night*
>*sleeplessness from*
>thoughtful
>vanishing
Time, fritters away his
>*passes too slowly, appears longer*
>>night •
Timidity
>awkward, and
>bashful
Touched, aversion to being
Trifles seem important
Ugly (in behavior) ★
Unconsciousness, coma, stupor
>**morning**
>air, in open
>*answers correctly when spoken to but delirium and unconsciousness return at once*
>chill, during
>**delirium tremens, in •**
>*eating, after*
>fever, during
>menses, during
>>suppression of
>**odors, from**
>**parturition, during**
>*pregnancy, during*
>vertigo, during
Undertakes nothing, lest he fail
Ungrateful
Vanity
Violent, vehement
>*deeds of violence, rage leading to*
Vivacious
Wanders, restlessely about
Wearisome
Weary of life
>night
Weeping, tearful mood
>night
>>sleep, in
>>>midnight, before
>>aloud, wobbing

Weeping, tearful mood
> alternating with cheerfulness
>> laughter
> anger, after
> causeless
> consolation agg.
> *contradiction, from*
> *convulsions, during*
> drinking, after
> *music, from*
> opposition, at least •
> *pains, with the*
> perspiration, during
> *sad thoughts; though sad, is impossible to weep •*
> *sleep, in*
> trifles, at
> vexation, from
> waking, on
> whimpering
>> *sleep, during*

Well, before an attack, feels ★
Will, weakness of
Work, aversion to mental
> *fatigues*
> *impossible*

Writing, inability for
Wrong, everything seems
Yielding disposition
Zealous ★

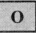

OCIMUM CANUM

Irritability

OCIMUM SANCTUM

Anxiety
Concentration, difficult
Confusion of mind

OENANTHE CROCATA

Abstraction of mind
Anguish
Anxiety
Confusion of mind
Cursing, swearing
Delirium
> loquacious
> *maniacal*
> *moves constantly from place to place •*
> *raging, raving*

Delirium tremens, mania-a-potu
Delusions, imaginations, hallucinations, illusions
> elevated: carried to an elevation •
> flying, sensation of
> objects, try to seize

Dementia, epileptics, of
Destructiveness
Dream, as if in a
Escape, attempts to
Excitement, excitable
Fear, menses, during
Gestures, grasping or reaching at something, at flocks; carphologia
Insanity, madness
> drunk, as if •

Irritability
Laughing, sardonic
> spasmodic

Loquacity

Magnetized: mesmerized, seem, as if ★
Mania
Memory, weakness of
Moaning, groaning, whining
Morose, alternating with cheerfulness
Rage, fury
    paroxysms, in
Recognize: relatives, does not recognize
    his
Restlessness
    convulsions, after •
    paroxysms, after •
Sadness, despondency, dejection, men-
    tal depression, gloom, melan-
    choly
Shrieking, convulsions, before
Stupefaction, convulsions, between
Talks, himself, to
Tears things
Thoughts, control of thoughts lost
    vacancy of
Unconsciousness, coma, stupor
    evening
    apoplexy, in
    conduct, automatic
    convulsions, after
    mental insensibility
    sudden
Violent, crossed, agg. during menses
    when •

OENOTHERA BIENNIS

Unconsciousness, coma, stupor

OKOUBAKA AUBREVILLEI

Concentration, difficult, studying, learns
    with difficulty, while
Memory, weakness of

OLEUM ANIMALE
AETHEREUM DIPPELI

Absent minded, unobserving
Absorbed, buried in thought
Abstraction of mind

Ailments from :
    anger, vexation
    sexual excesses
Anger, irascibility
Anxiety
    fever, during
    heart ★
    soup, after
Cheerful, gay, mirthful
    afternoon, 17 h. •
    evening
    followed by irritability
Concentration, difficult
Confusion of mind, concentrate the
    mind, on attempting to
Cowardice ★
Discomfort, eating, dinner, after
Discontented, displeased, dissatisfied
Dream, as if in a
Dullness, sluggishness, difficulty of think-
    ing and comprehending, torpor
Fishy ★
Frightened easily, evening
Hypochondriasis
Hysteria
Ideas, vanishing of ★
Indolence, aversion to work
    eating, after
Introspection
Irritability
    sexual excesses, from •
Meditation
Menses, mental symptoms agg. during
Morose, cross, fretful, ill-humor, peevish
    alternating with cheerfulness
    eating, after
    sleepiness, with
Prostration of mind, mental exhaus-
    tion, brain-fag
Reflecting
Restlessness
Sadness, despondency, dejection, men-
    tal depression,
    gloom, melancholy
    morning
    afternoon
    chill, during
    eating, after
    headache, during

Senses, dull, blunted
    vanishing of
Starting, sleep, during
Stupefaction, as if intoxicated
Talk, indisposed to, desire to be silent,
    taciturn
Thoughts, vanishing of
Unconsciousness, coma, stupor
        noon, 13 h. •
        evening
        transient

OLEUM JECORIS ASELLI

Anxiety
Excitement, excitable
Fear, insanity, losing his reason, of

OLEANDER (NERIUM OLEANDER)

Absent minded, unobserving
    dreamy
Abstraction of mind
Ailments from :
    anger, vexation
    scorn, being scorned
Amusement, averse to
Anger, irascibility
    alternating with quick repentance
    contradiction, from
    violent
Answers: stupor returns quickly after
    answer
Anxiety
Brooding
Concentration, active
Concentration, difficult
    on attempting to concentrate, has
        a vacant feeling
    studying, reading, etc. while
        learns with difficulty
Confidence, want of self
Confusion of mind
    concentrate the mind, on attempt-
        ing to
    eating, after

Confusion of mind
    mental exertion, from
    reading, if he attempts to under-
        stand it •
    thinking of it agg.
Contradict, disposition to
Contradiction, is intolerant of
    agg.
Cowardice
Delusions, beautiful, things look
    visions, has beautiful
Discomfort, eating, after
Discontented, displeased, dissatisfied
Discouraged
Dream, as if in a
    future: poetical future •
Dullness, sluggishness, difficulty of
    thinking and comprehending, tor-
    por
    mental exertion, from
    reading, while
Ecstasy
Emptiness, sensation of ★
Excitement, working, when
Exertion, agg. from mental
Fancies, exaltation of
    working, while
Forgetful
Grimaces
Heedless
Hurry, eating, while
Ideas abundant, clearness of mind
    deficiency of
    overexertion, from
Idiocy
Imbecility
Impetuous
Indifference, apathy
Indolence, aversion to work
Insanity, madness
Introspection
Irritability
Languages, unable for
Memory, weakness of
    names, for proper
    read, for what has
Morose, cross, fretful, ill-humor, peevish

Passionate
Plans, making many
Prostration of mind, mental exhaustion, brain-fag
Quarrelsome, scolding
Rage, contradiction, from
Reading, mental symptoms agg. from
Remorse
    repents, quickly
Reserved
Restlessness
Sadness, despondency, dejection, mental depression, gloom, melancholy
Senses, dull, blunted
Sensitive, oversensitive
Serious, earnest
Shrieking, screaming, shouting
Sit, inclination to
Slowness
Stupefaction, as if intoxicated
Thinking, complaints agg., of
Thoughts, persistent
    rush, flow of
      reading, while
      working, during
    vanishing of, on mental exertion
    wandering
Unconsciousness, coma, stupor
Violent, vehement
Wearisome
Weeping, involuntary, from weakness
Work, aversion to mental
    impossible

ONOPORDON ACANTHIUM

Anguish
Concentration, difficult
Irritability
Mistakes, speaking, in, reverses words
    wrong syllables, gives
Restlessness
Sadness, despondency, dejection, mental depression, gloom, melancholy
    alternating with euphoria
Sensitive, oversensitive
Slowness
Tranquillity, serenity, calmness

ONOSMODIUM VIRGINIANUM

Absent-minded, unobserving
Absorbed, buried in thought
Abstraction of mind
Ailments from :
    sexual excesses
Anxiety, fear, with
Confusion of mind
Delusions, time, exaggeration of, passes too slowly
Fear, apprehension, dread
    evil, of
    falling, of
    happen, something will
Forgetful, words while speaking, of;
    word hunting
Impatience
Indifference, apathy
Irresolution, indecision
    acts, in
Loquacity
    rambling ★
Memory, weakness of
    do, for what was about to
    done, for what has just
    read, for what has
    say, for what is about to
Mistakes, speaking, in
    writing, in
      omitting letters
Proportion, sense of, disturbed ★
Prostration of mind, mental exhaustion, brain fag
Restlessness
Sensitive, noise, to
Slowness
Talk, indisposed to, desire to be silent, taciturn
Thoughts, rapid, quick
Time passes too slowly, appears longer

OPIUM

Absent-minded, unobserving
Absorbed, buried in thought
Abstraction of mind

Activity
   mental
   perspiration, during ●
Affections, in general ★
Ailments from :
   anger, vexation
     anxiety, with
     fright, with
   dipsomania
   disappointment
   embarrassment from
   fear
   fright
   accident, from sight of an
   grief
   homesickness ★
   injuries, accidents, mental symp-
     toms from
   joy, excessive
   mortification
   reproaches
   shame
   shock, mental
   surprise, pleasant
Alert ●
Anger, irascibility
   evening
   alternating with playing antics ●
     cheerfulness
     exhilaration ●
   contradiction, from
   pains, about
   seizes the hands of those about
     him ●
   weeping from pains, with
Anguish
   oppression, with
   shock from injury, in ●
Answers: aversion to answer
   incorrectly
   slowly
   stupor returns quickly after an-
     swer
Antics, plays
   delirium, during

Anxiety
   fever, during
   flushes of heat, during
   fright, after
     remains, if the fear of the
       fright ●
   menses, during, anger and anxiety
   sleep, during
Asks for nothing
Audacity
Benevolence
Bite, desires to
   arms, bites own ●
   fingers, bites
   hands, bites
   himself, bites
Blasphemy, cursing and
Blissful feeling
Brooding
Business, neglects his
   talks of
Busy
Capriciousness
Cares, worries, full of
   alternating with exhilaration ●
Cautious
Cheerful, gay, mirthful
   night
   alternating with grief
     sadness
   drunkenness, during
   followed by irritability
   heat, during
Childish behavior
Clairvoyance
Clinging, grasps at others
Company, aversion to; presence of
     others people agg. the symp-
     toms; desires for solitude
Complaining
   sleep, in comatose
Comprehension, easy
Concentration, active
Concentration, difficult
Confidence, want of self
Confiding

Confusion of mind
    morning
    afternoon
  eating, after
  heat, during
  intoxicated, as after being
  sitting, while
  sleeping, after
  waking, on
Contented
    night •
    forgets all his ailments and
      pains •
    quiet, and •
Contradiction, is intolerant of
Courageous
    alternating with discouragement
Cowardice
Crawling, rolling on the floor
Cruelty, inhumanity
Cursing, swearing
    afternoon •
    evening, when home
Death, contempt of •
  desires
  sensation of
  thoughts of
Deceitful, sly
Deception causes grief and mortifica-
    tion ★
Delirium
    day and night
    night
    answers correctly when spoken to,
      but delirium and unconscious-
      ness return at once
    anxious
      bed and escapes, springs up
      suddenly from
  blames himself for his folly •
  business, talks of
  cold, after catching •
  convulsions, before
  delusions, with
  devils, sees ★
  epilepsy, during •
  face, with red
  fantastic

Delirium
  fever, during
  foolish, silly
  frightful
  gay, cheerful
  injuries to head, after
  laughing
  loquacious
    indistinct
  maniacal
  muttering
  nonsense, with eyes open
  quiet
  raging, raving
  recognises no one
  rolls on floor •
  sleep, during
  sleepiness, with
  sleeplessness, and ★
  sopor, with
  spectres ★
  trembling, with
  violent
  watching, vigil, from
  wild
Delirium tremens, mania-a-potu
  delusions, with
  old emaciated persons, in •
  small quantity of alcoholic
    stimulants, from •
  sopor with snoring •
Delusions, imaginations, hallucina-
  tions, illusions
  night
  absurd figures are present
  animals, of
    frightful
  assembled things, swarms, crowds
    etc.
  bed, someone is in bed with him
  body, lighter than air, is
  business, is doing
  cats, sees
  criminal, he is a
    executed, to be •
  dead, corpse, he himself was
    persons, sees

Delusions,
- *devils, sees*
  - present, are
- disorder, objects appear in
- doomed, being
- double, of being
- dragons, of •
- *enlarged*
  - body, parts of
  - distances are
  - eyes are
  - objects are
  - tall, is very
- *execute him, people want to* •
- eyes, of big
- **faces, sees**
  - *closing eyes, on*
  - **hideous**
  - mask-like
- *fancy, illusions of* •
- fighting, people are
- *figures, sees*
- **floating in air ★**
- flying, sensation of
- *grimaces, sees*
- heaven, is in
- home, away from, is
  - *away from, must get there*
- *images, phantoms, sees*
  - night
  - black
  - *frightful*
  - sleep, preventing
- *injury, is about to receive*
- journey, he is on a
- large, himself seems too
  - parts of body seem too
- laughter, with
- legs don't belong to her
- light, incorporeal, he is
- loquacity, with
- *masks, sees*
- mice, sees
- *murdered, he will be*
- past, of events long
- people, sees
  - converses with absent
- pleasing

Delusions,
- possessed, being
- *pregnant, she is*
- rats, sees
- scorpions, sees •
- skeletons, sees
- *smell, of*
- snakes in and around her
- soldiers, sees
- *spectres, ghosts, spirits, sees*
- strange, familiar things seem
- superhuman control, is under
- swollen, he is
- *tactile hallucinations*
- tall, she is very
- unpleasant, distinct from surrounding objects
- visions, has
  - beautiful
  - fantastic
  - *horrible*
  - **monsters**
  - vivid
- weight, has no
- well, he is

Dementia
- senilis, talking, with foolish

Desires, unattainable things

Despair
- masturbation, in •

Destructiveness

Dipsomania, alcoholism

Discomfort

Discontented, displeased, dissatisfied
- afternoon

Discouraged
- alternating with courage
  - *hope*
- morose, and •

Distances, inaccurate judgement of

Dream, as if in a

Dullness, sluggishness, difficulty of thinking and comprehending, torpor
- *diabetes, in*
- *drunken, as if*

Dullness,
    drunkenness, during
    emotions, from
    reading, while
    waking, on
Dwells on past disagreeable, occurrences
Eat, refuses to
Eccentricity
    all night •
Ecstasy
    amorous
Elevation, mental •
Eloquent
Escape, attempts to
    fever, during
    run away, to
Excitement, excitable
    heat, during
Exertion, agg. from mental
Exhilaration
    alternating with grief •
    blissful •
    perspiration, during •
Fancies, exaltation of
    night
    frightful
    sleeplessness, with
    lascivious
    impotency, with
    pleasant
    sleep, preventing
    unpleasant
    vivid lively
Fear, apprehension, dread
    night
    abortion from f., threatening
    amenorrhoea from fear •
    approaching him, of others
    death, of
    impending, of
    diarrhoea from
    eating, of
    extravagance, of •
    fright, of ★
    ghosts, of
    labor, during

Fear,
    long-lasting ★
    murdered, of being
    palpitation
    starting, with
    tremulous
    urine from f., retention of •
Foolish behavior
Forgetful
    connection of consecutive thoughts, of (after apoplexy) •
    drunkards, forgetfulness in
    emotions, from
Fright, menses, during ★
Frightened, eyes, on closing •
    waking, on
Generous, too much
Gestures, convulsive
    grasping or reaching at something, at flocks; carphologia
    picks at bed clothes
    hands, motion, involuntary, sleep, during
    waving in the air
    ridiculous or foolish
    strange attitudes and positions
Gluttony
Grief
    offences, grief from long past
Groping as if in the dark
Hatred
    revenge, hatred and
Heedless
High-spirited
Home, desires to go
Homesickness
Howling
Hurry, haste
    occupation, in
    work, in
Hypochondriasis
Hysteria
Ideas abundant, clearness of mind
    night
    heat, during
    deficiency of
Idiocy

Imbecility
    rage, stamps the feet
Impatience
Inconstancy
Indifference, apathy
    agreeable things, to
    chill, during
    complain, does not
    epilepsy, in
    everything, to
    external things, to
    fever, during
    fine feeling, to •
    irritating, disagreeable things, to
    joy, to
        and suffering, to
    joyless
    pain, to
    pleasure, to
    stoic ★
    suffering, to
Indignation, discomfort, from general •
Indiscretion
Indolence, aversion to work
    morning, rising, on
    afternoon
Industrious, mania for work
    heat, during
Insanity, madness
    alternating with stupor •
    anger, from
    drunkards, in
    escape, desire to
    face, red, with
    laughing, with
    sleeplessness, with
Introspection
Irresolution, indecision
    changeable
Irritability
    afternoon
    aroused, when
    disturbed, when
    headache, during
    pain, during

Jealousy
    people around, of •
Jesting
Joy, headache from excessive joy
Jumping, bed, out of
Kill, desire to
Lamenting, bemoaning, wailing
    asleep, while
Lascivious, lustful
    erections with
    impotence, with
Laughing
    night
    involuntarily
    loudly
    spasmodic
Liar
    lies, never speaks the truth,
        does not know what she
        is saying
Loathing, life, at
Loquacity
    sleep, during
Malicious, spiteful, vindictive
Mania
    demoniac
    rage, with
Meditation, night •
Memory, active
    fever, during •
Memory, confused
Memory, weakness of
    persons, for
    read, for what has
    words, of
Mildness
Mistakes, time, in
    writing, omitting letters, in
Moaning, groaning, whining
    sleep, during
Mood, alternating
    changeable
Moral feeling, want of
Morose, cross, fretful, ill-humor, peevish
    afternoon
    dreams, by •

Morphinism
Muttering
Neglects business
Noise, inclined to make a
Nothing ails him, says ★
    wants ★
Nymphomania
Obscene, lewd
    songs
Offended, easily; offences, from past
Overactive
Plans, making many
    gigantic •
Praying
    morning •
Prostration of mind, mental exhaustion, brain-fag
    waking, on
Quarrelsome, scolding
    evening
Quiet disposition
Rage, fury
    evening
    epilepsy, rage with
        rage after
    touch, renewed by
*Recognize: relatives, does not recognize
    his*
Reproaches himself
Reserved
Rest, desires for
Restlessness
    evening
    bed, in
    night
    anxious
    bed, heat of, from •
        tossing about in
    heat, during
    internal
    menses, during
Rolling on the floor
Rudeness

Sadness, despondency, dejection, mental depression, gloom, melancholy
    morning
    afternoon
    alternating with playing antics •
    heat, during
    suicidal disposition, with
    waking, on
Self, accusation ★
Senses, acute
    dull, blunted
Sensitive, oversensitive
    noise, to
        slightest, to
    pain, to
    touch, to
Serious, earnest
Shamelessness
Shrieking, screaming, shouting
    convulsions, before
    during epileptic
    pains, with the
    sleep, during
Sighing
    sleep, in
Singing
    fever, during •
    hilarious, joyously
    monotonous •
Sit, inclination to
Slowness
Somnambulism
Speech, confused
    convincing •
    delirious
    hasty
    incoherent
        dozing, after •
        waking, on
    nonsensical
    prattling
    slow
    terse •
    wandering
        night

Spoiled children
Spoken to, averse to being
Staring ★
Starting, easily
    fright, from and as from
    heat, during
    noise, from
    sleep, falling, on
        during
        from
    waking, on, suffocated, as if
Strength increased, mental
Striking, about him at imaginary objects
Stupefaction, as if intoxicated
    convulsions, between
    rouses with difficulty
    vertigo, during
    waking, on
Suicidal disposition
    poison, by
    sadness, from
    shooting, by
Sulky
Superstitious
Suspicious
Talk, indisposed to, desire to be silent, taciturn
    perspiration, during
Talking, sleep, in
    comatose sleep, in
Talks, himself, to
Tears things
Temerity
Theorizing
Thoughts persistent
    homicide
    rapid, quick
    rush, flow of
        night
        sleeplessness from
    thoughtful, all night ●
    vanishing of
    wandering
Time passes too quickly, appears shorter

Timidity
    business, in transacting ●
Torpor
Trance
Tranquillity, serenity, calmness
Unconsciousness, coma, stupor
    answers correctly when spoken to,
        but delirium and unconscious-
        ness return at once
    apoplexy, in
    chill, during
    emotion, after
    epilepsy, after
    fever, during
    incomplete
    jaw dropping
    menses, suppression of, from fright●
    mental insensibility
    rising up, on
    snoring, involuntary urination
        and stool, with
    sun stroke, in
    uraemic coma
    vertigo, during
Unfeeling, hard hearted
Unreliable, promises, in his
Unsympathetic, unscrupulous
Violent, sleep, before ●
Weary of life
Weeping, tearful mood
        night
    aloud, sobbing
    convulsions, during
    coughing, after
    desires to weep, all the time
    easily
    pains, with the
    perspiration, during
    sleep, in
    taking cold, after ●
    waking, on
    whimpering, sleep, during
        comatose
Well, says he is, when very sick
Wildness
Will, loss of
    weakness of
Witty

Work, aversion to mental
    impossible
Writing, talent for easier •

OPERCULINA TURPENTHUM

Delirium
    bed and escapes, springs up sud-
        denly from
    loquacious
Escape, attempts to
    springs up, to, suddenly from bed

OPUNTIA VULGARIS

Anger, afternoon, 12-14 h.
Business, averse to
Ideas abundant, clearness of mind
Indolence, business, when transacting
Insanity, madness
Mistakes, writing, in
        transposing letters
Morose, cross, fretful, ill-humor, pee-
    vish
Praying

ORIGANUM MAJORANA

Anxiety
Cheerful, gay, mirthful
Concentration, difficult
Desire, exercise, for
Despair
Discontented, displeased, dissatisfied
Fancies, lascivious
Fear, apprehension, dread
Frightened easily
Hysteria
Idiocy, masturbation, with
Impulse to run; dromomania
Insanity, erotic
Irritability
Lascivious, lustful
Libertinism
Mania
Marriage, idea of, amel. ★
Morose, cross, fretful, ill-humor, peevish

Nymphomania
    young girl, in a •
Obscene, lewd
Occupation, diversion amel.
Restlessness
Runs about
Sadness, despondency, dejection, mental
    depression, gloom, melancholy
Serious, earnest
Suicidal disposition
    throwing himself from a height
Talk, indisposed to, desire to be silent,
    taciturn
Thoughts, intrude, sexual
    rush, flow of
    sexual ★
Unconsciousness, sexual excitement,
    with

ORIGANUM VULGARE

Delusions, imaginations, hallucinations,
    illusions
    despised, is
Delusions, hell, is in
    chains of, in •

OSMIUM METALLICUM

Anger, irascibility
Anxiety
Confusion of mind
Fear, respiration, of •
Impatience
    itching, from
Indolence, aversion to work
Irritability
Malicious, injure someone, desire to
Mistakes, speaking, in
    misplacing words
    reverses words
    words: using wrong
Morose, cross, fretful, ill-humor, peevish
Prostration of mind, evening
Restlessness
    night
Thoughts, persistent
    injury to others, of doing •
Weeping, coughing, during

OSTRYA VIRGINICA

Restlessness-night

OXALICUM ACIDUM

Affectionate
Ailments from :
    anticipation, foreboding, presen-
    timent
Answers, slowly
Anxiety
        evening, from violent exercise •
    ascending steps, on
    hypochondriacal
Cheerful, gay, mirthful
    afternoon
    stools, after
Children, desires to beget and to have
        children •
Comprehension, easy
Concentraction, active
Concentration, difficult
    studying, reading, etc., while
Confusion of mind, morning
    mental exertion, from
    wine, after
Conversation, aversion to
Delirium
    fever, during
Delusions, imaginations, hallucinations,
    illusions
Desires, beat children, to ★
Distances, exaggerated, are
Dullness, sluggishness, difficulty of think-
        ing and comprehending, torpor
    morning
    rising from bed •
Excitement, excitable
    evening
    alternating with sadness
    palpitation, with violent
Exhilaration
    alternating with sadness
    diarrhoea, during •
Fancies, exaltation of
Fear, apprehension, dread
    bed, when he raised himself in •
    death, of
Hurry, haste
Ideas abundant, forenoon •

Indolence, aversion to work
    morning
Insanity, madness
Irritability
    afternoon
    evening
Mania
Memory, active
Moaning, groaning, whining
Morose, afternoon
    evening
Morphinism
Occupation, diversion amel.
Playful
Reading, aversion to read
    walking in open air amel. •
Restlessness
    night
Sensitive, noise, to
Slowness
Starting, door slams, when a
    noise, from
    sleep, during
Stupefaction, as if intoxicated
Talk, indisposed to, desire to be silent,
    taciturm
    headache, during
Thinking, complaints agg., of
Thoughts, rapid, quick
Unconsciousness, coma, stupor
    stool, during
Violent, vehement
Vivacious, afternoon
Work, aversion to mental

OXYTROPIS LAMBERTI

*Company, aversion to; presence of other
        people agg. the symptoms; de-
        sire for solitude*
Delusions, imaginations, hallucinations,
    illusions
    hollow in organs, being
Imbecility
Sadness, despondency, dejection, mental
        depression, gloom, melancholy
Talk, indisposed to, desire to be silent,
    taciturm
Thinking, complaints agg., of

PAEONIA OFFICINALIS

Ailments from:
bad news
Anxiety
forenoon
evening
Delirium
Excitement, excitable
Fear, forenoon
evening
Gestures, grasping or reaching at some-
thing, at flocks; carphologia
Irritability
afternoon, 17h. •
Morose, cross, fretful, ill-humor, peevish
Restlessness, walking, while
Senses, dull, blunted
Sensitive, oversensitive
Somnambulism
Starting, sleep, on falling
Uunconsciousness, warm room, in

PALLADIUM METALLICUM

Abusive, insulting
Ailments from:
bad news
egotism
excitement, emotional
mortification
Ambition
Anger, irascibility
trembling, with
violent
Anxiety
menses, after
*Company, aversion to; presence of other
people agg.
the symptoms; desire for solitude*

*Company, desires for; aversions to soli-
tude, company amel.
alone agg., while*
Confidence, want of self
Contemptuous
Contradiction, is intolerant of
Cursing, swearing
Delusions, appreciated, she is not
criticised, she is
deserted, forsaken, is
enlarged: tall, is very
hollow, whole body is
insulted, he is
neglected, he is
tall, walking, had grown, while •
Discontented, displeased, dissatisfied
everything, with
Eccentricity
fancies, in
Egotism, self-esteem
Excitement, excitable
company, in
music, from
Faces, made strange
Fear, evil, of
happen, something will
menses, after
Flattery, desires •
Forsaken feeling
Grimaces
strange faces, makes
Haughty
**wounded, wishes to be flat
tered •**
Hysteria
Impatience
headache, during
Impertinence
Indolence, aversion to work
morning
evening
Insolence
Irresolution, indecision
morning
Irritability
evening
headache, during
takes everything in bad part
waking, on

Longing for good opinion of others •
Memory, weakness of
    pains, from, suddenly ★
Misanthropy
Mistakes, time, in
Mocking, sarcasm
Morose, cross, fretful, ill-humor, peevish
    evening
Music agg.
Obstinate, headstrong
    amiable, tries to appear •
Occupation, diversion amel.
Offended, easily; takes everything in
    bad part
Prostration of mind, mental exhaus-
    tion, brain-fag
Quarrelsome, scolding
Rudeness
Selfishness, egoism
Sensitive, music, to
Society, social functions agg. ★
Speech, embarrassed
    forcible •
Starting, afternoon
      night
    waking, on
Thinking, complaints amel., of
Time passes too slowly, appears longer
Weeping, tearful mood
    mortification, after
Work, aversion to mental

PALOONDO

Euphoria
Excitement, excitable
Irritability
Morose, cross, fretful, ill-humor, peevish
Sadness, despondency, dejection, men-
    tal depression, gloom, melancholy
Sensitive, noise, to

PANACEA ARVENSIS

Company, aversion to; presence of
    other people agg. the symp-
    toms; desire for solitude

Discontented, displeased, dissatisfied
    himself, with

PARIS QUADRIFOLIA

Affectionate
Ailments from:
    scorn, being scorned
Anger, irascibility
Anxiety
    fever, during
Capriciousness
Censorious, critical
Cheerful, gay, mirthful ★
    foolish, and
Childish behavior
Confusion of mind
    air amel., in open
    walking, air amel., in open
Contemptuous
Delirium
    loquacious
    raging, raving
    waking, on
Delusions,, imaginations, hallucina-
    tions, illusions
    enlarged, distances are
      head is
      objects are
    fancy, illusions of
    home, is away from
    places, strange and solitary, find-
      ing himself in (at night on
      waking) •
    smell, of
    strange land, as if in a
    waking, on
Discomfort
Discontented, displeased, dissatisfied
    surroundings, with
Dulllness, sluggishness, difficulty of
    thinking and comprehending, tor-
    por
Egotism, self-esteem
    speaking about themselves in
      company, always

Excitement, excitable
Exertion, agg from mental
Foolish behavior
Frivolous
Gossiping
Haughty
Hysteria
Imbecility
Indolence, aversion to work
Insanity, madness
      loquacious
Irritability
Laughing, silly
Loquacity
      changing quickly from one sub-
         ject to another
      cheerful, exuberant
      foolish •
      insane
      self-satisfied •
      vivacious
Malicious, spiteful, vindictive
Mania
Mistakes, localities, in
Mocking
Morose, cross, fretful, ill-humor pee-
      vish
Prostration of mind, mental exhaus-
      tion, brain-fag
Rage, fury
Reproaches others
Restlessness, night
      bed, tossing about in
      internal ⬎
         night, on waking, with head-
         ache •
Rudeness
Slander, disposition to
Speech, foolish
      incoherent
      wandering
Stupefaction, as if intoxicated
Talking, pleasure in his own
Thinking agg. ★
Unconsciousness, coma, stupor

Vivacious
Walk, walking in open air agg. mental
      symptoms
      amel.
Work, aversion to mental

PARATHYROIDINUM

Confusion of mind
Sadness, despondency, dejection, men-
      tal depression gloom, melancholy

PARONYCHIA ILLECEBRUM

Confusion of mind, identity, duality,
      sense of
Delusions, persons: two personalities
      opposing to each other in him-
      self, who are discussing their
      disease, there are •
Thoughts, two trains of thought
Tranquillity, serenity, calmness

PARTHENIUM
HYSTEROPHORUS

Loquacity

PASSIFLORA INCARNATA

Delirium tremens, mania-a-potu
Delusions, imaginations, hallucinations,
      illusions
Dipsomania, alcoholism
Insanity, madnes
Mania
Morphinism
**Restlessness, working, while,
      tedious •**

PASTINACA SATIVA

Delirium, bed and escapes, springs up
      suddenly from
      quiet
Delirium tremens, mania-a-potu
Delusions, imaginations, hallucinations,
      illusions

Jumping, bed, out of
Loquacity
Rejects everything offered to him •
Restlessness
Speech, delirious
    incoherent
Unconciousness, coma, stupor

PAULLINIA PINNATA

Delusions, dead persons, sees
Ennui, tedium
Fear, consumption, of
    disease, of impending
Indolence, aversion to work
Loathing, general
Retirement, desire for
Sadness, despondency, dejection, mental
    depression, gloom, melancholy
        daytime
Weeping, waking, on

PEDICULUS CAPITIS

Ailments from :
    joy, excessive
Anger, irascibility
    causeless
Cheerful, gay, mirthful
    afternoon, 15h. •
Dullness, sluggishness, difficulty of
    thinking and comprehending, tor-
    por
Gestures, live
Heedless
Hurry, writing, in
Industrious, mania for work
Irritability
Malicious, spiteful, vindictive
Mocking
Moral feeling, want of
Restlessness, night
Sadness, causeless
Speech, fluent
Starting, evening
Suicidal, drowning, by
Thoughts, rapid, quick
Work, desire for mental

PENTHORUM SEDOIDES

Delusions, floating in air, on closing
    eyes •
Discouraged
Dullness, sluggishness, difficulty of think-
    ing and comprehending, torpor
Sadness, despondency, dejection, men-
    tal depression, gloom, melancholy

PENICILLINUM

Activity, mental
Dullness, sluggishness, difficulty of think-
    ing and comprehending, torpor
Insanity, madness
Sadness, despondency, dejection, mental
    depression, gloom, melancholy
    climaxis, during

PERHEXILINUM

Anguish
Anorexia mentalis
Anxiety, others, for
Fear, accidents, of
    water, of
Memory, weakness of
    names, for proper
    occurrences of the day, for
    read, for what has
Restlessness
Sadness, despondency, dejection, men-
    tal depression, gloom, melancholy
Slowness

PERSEA AMERICANA

Ailments from:
    position, loss of
Irritability
Pessimist

PETIVERIA TETRANDRA

Cheerful, gay, mirthful
Confusion of mind
Delusions, feet touching scarcely the
    ground, when walking •

Jesting
Laughing
      daytime •
Memory, weakness of
Retirement, desire for
Sadness, despondency, dejection, mental
    depression, gloom, melancholy
Singing
Starting from a dream
Thoughts, wandering
Vivacious
Weeping, tearful mood
      morning
      involuntary

PETROLEUM

Absent-minded, unobserving
Absorbed, buried in thought
Abusive, insulting
    drunkeness, during
Affectation
Ailments from :
    anger vexation
      anxiety, with
      fright, with
    anticipation, foreboding, presen-
      timent
    fright
    sexual excesses
Ambition, loss of
Anger, irascibility
      morning
        waking, on
      evening
    contradiction, from
    face, with pale, livid
    talk, indisposed to
    trembling, with
    trifles, at
    violent
    waking, on
Answers, aversion to answer
    refuses to answer

Anxiety
      evening
      twilight, in the
        19 h.
     night
company, when in
crowd, in a
    dreams, on waking from frightful
    family, about his
fever, during
    future, about
    noise, from
    pollutions, after
    sleep, during
    tabacco, from smoking
Avarice
Cares, worries, causeless ★
Censorious, critical
Cheerful, gay, mirthful
      alternating with sadness
      followed by melancholy
Company, aversion to; presence of
      others people agg. the symp-
      toms; desire for solitude
    alone, amel. when
    presence of strangers, aversion to
Complaining
Concentration, difficult
Confidence, want of self
Confusion of mind
      morning
      afternoon
    dinner, after
    eating, after
    headache, with
    identity, as to his
      duality, sense of
    loses his way in well-known
      streets
    mental exertion, from
    smoking, after
    spirituous liquors, from
    waking, on
    walking, while
      air, in open
    wine, after

Conscientious, trifles, occupied with
Contradiction, is intolerant of
      agg.
Contrary
Cowardice, opinion, without courage of
  own
Cursing, swearing
Death, presentiment of
Delirium
  delusions, with
  loquacious
  same subject, all the time •
  sleep, after
**Delusions, imaginations, halluci-
  nations, illusions**
  arms, three, she has •
  babies are in bed, two •
  bed, occupied by another person •
    someone is in bed with him
  body, divided, is
    scattered about bed, tossed
    about to get the pieces
    together
      threefold, has a
  die, he was about to
  divided into two parts
  double, of being
    limb is, one •
  head, cold breeze blows on •
  identity, errors of personal
  images, sees, dark, in the
    frightful
  legs, three, has
  lying near him, someone is •
  people, sees
    beside him, are
  sick, being
  strange, everything is
    familiar things seem
  thieves, sees
  three persons, he is
  visions, horrible
    dark, in the
  voices, hears
    confused (swallowing or walk-
      ing in open air agg.)
  walks beside him, someone

Despair
  heat, during
Dipsomania, alcoholism
  weak of character, from
Dirtiness
Discomfort
    night
  eating supper, after
Discontented, displeased, dissatisfied
  everythig, with
Discouraged
  alternating with exaltation
    exuberance •
Disgust
  everything, with
Disobedience
Doubtful
*Dullness, sluggishness, difficulty of
  thinking and comprehending, torpor*
  fog, as enveloped in a •
  wine, after
Eating, after, amel.
Eccentricity alternating with sadness
Ennui, tedium
Excitement, excitable
  agg.
  heat, during
  trembling, with
    inward •
Exertion, agg. from mental
Extravagance
Exuberance
  alternating with sadness •
Fancies, exaltation of •
    night
  sleeplessness with
Fear, apprehension, dread
    evening
  approaching him, of others
  crowd, in a
  death, of
  evil, of
  life long
  work, dread of
Flatterer
Foolish, talking foolishly during
  drunkeness •

Forgetful
> *house was, on which side of the*
> *street, his*
> *streets, of well-known*

Frightened easily

Gestures, convulsive

Grief ★

Helplessness, feeling of

Homesickness

Hypochondriasis
> air, in open
> morose

Ideas, deficiency of

Imbecility

Inconsolable
> *anxiety about his family while a*
> *short journey, from* •

Inconstancy

Indifference, apathy
> morning on waking
> conscience, to the dictates of
> ennui, with
> pleasure, to

Indolence, aversion to work
> intelligent, although very

Insanity, melancholy
> *puerperal*

Insolence

Irresolution, indecision

Irritability
> daytime
> *morning*
> waking, on
> coition, after
> heat, during
> menses, during
> trifles, at
> waking, on

Jealousy, loquacity, with
> weeping, with

Kill, desire to

Lamenting, bemoaning, wailing

Loathing, work, at

Loquacity
> drunkness during

Malicious, spiteful, vindictive
> anger, with

Mania

Mannish habits of girls

Memory confused

Memory, weakness of

Mistakes, localities, in
> time, in

Moaning, groaning, whining

Mood, changeable, variable
> opinions, in
> repulsive

Morose, cross, fretful, ill-humor, peevish
> morning, bed, in
> coition, after
> fever, during
> waking, on

Nibble, desire to ★

Obstinate, headstrong

Offended, easily; takes everything in
> *bad part*

Passionate

Prostration of mind, mental exhaustion, brain-fag

Quarrelsome, scolding
> morning
> intoxicated, when •

Quiet disposition

Rage, fury
> malicious

Recognize, streets, does not recognize
> well known

Reserved
> morning

Restlessness
> night
> bed, tossing about in
> chill, during
> coition, after
> eating, when
> after
> *sleepiness, with*

Sadness, despondency, dejection, mental
> depression, gloom, melancholy
> morning
> air, in open
> alternating with eccentricity •
> exuberance

Sadness,
>anger, after
>*heat, during*
>*menses, during*
>walking, air, in open

Senses, dull, blunted
Sensitive, chill, during
Sit, inclination to
Slander, disposition to
Somnambulism
Speech, slow
Starting, startled
>evening, sleep, in
>dreams, in
>>from a dream
>sleep, falling, on
>>during
>*trifles, at*

Strangers, presence of strangers agg.
Stupefaction, as if intoxicated
>exertion agg., mental

Sulky
Talk, desires to talk to someone
>inapt to talk in public
>indisposed to, desire to be silent,
>taciturn
>others agg., talk of

Talks, one subject, of nothing but
Thinking, aversion to
Thoughts, persistent
>night
>unpleasant subjects, haunted
>by

Thunderstorm, mind symptoms before
>during, mind symptoms

Time, passes too slowly, appears longer
Timidity
>alternating with exaltation
>*bashful*

Tranquillity, serenity, calmness
Unconsciousness, coma, stupor
>*dream, does not know where he is*

Undertakes, many things, perseveres
in nothing
Violent, vehement
>morning

Vivacious
Wearisome

Weeping, tearful mood
>*chill, during*
>drinking, after
>*heat, during*
>*menses, during*
>*perspiration, during*
>trifles, at
>vexation, from

Wildness
>children, in •

Will, loss of
>*weakness of*

Work, aversion to mental
>*impossible*

Yielding disposition

PHOSPHORICUM ACIDUM

Absent-minded, unobserving
>morning
>reading, while

Abstraction of mind
Affectionate '
Affections, in general ★
Ailments from :
>*anger, vexation*
>>*silent grief, with*
>*anticipation, foreboding, presen-*
>>*timent*
>anxiety
>bad news
>business failure
>*cares, worries*
>death of a child
>dipsomania
>**disappointment**
>embarrassment
>**excitement, emotional**
>>**moral ★**   -
>friendship, deceived
>**fright**
>**grief**
>**homesickness**
>**love, disappointed**
>>unhappy
>**mortification**
>reproaches
>rudeness of others
>**sexual excesses**
>*work, mental*

504

Amativeness
Amorous
Anger, irascibility
　　answer, when obliged to
　　violent
Anguish, afternoon
　　lie down, must
Anorexia mentalis
Answers, abruptly, shortly, curtly
　　aversion to answer
　　difficult
　　inappropriate
　　incoherently
　　incorrectly
　　irrelevantly
　　monosyllable
　　reflects long
　　refuses to answer
　　slowly
　　stupor returns quickly after answer
　　unintelligibly
Anticipation, complaints from
Anxiety
　　afternoon
　　　midnight after, on waking
　　anticipation, from, an engagement ★
　　children, about his
　　conscience, as if guilty of a crime
　　dreams, on waking from frightful
　　eating, after
　　fever, during
　　future, about
　　health, about
　　hypochondriacal
　　menses, anger and anxiety during
　　motion, amel. from
　　others, for
　　pressure on the chest, from
　　salvation, about
　　　scrupulous as to their religious
　　　　practices, too
　　sitting, while
　　standing, while
　　urination, before
　　waking, on

Avarice
　　anxiety about future, a. from
Beside oneself, being
Brooding
　　condition, over one's •
　　corner or moping, brooding in a
　　disappointment, over •
　　disease, over his •
Business, averse to
Calculating, inability for
Capriciousness
Cares, worries, full of
Chaotic, confused behavior
Cheerful, gay, mirthful
　　night
　　sleep, during
Company, aversion to; presence of
　　　other people agg. the symptoms; desire for solitude
　　alone, amel. when
Company, desire for; aversion to solitude, company amel.
　　alone agg., while
Complaining
　　disease, of
Concentration, difficult
　　aversion to ★
　　children, in
　　studying, learns with difficulty
Confusion of mind
　　morning
　　　rising and after, on
　　evening
　　carousal, as after a •
　　coition, after
　　eating, after
　　intoxicated, as if
　　　as after being
　　mental exertion, from
　　reading, while
　　waking, on
　　warm room, in
Conscientious about trifles
Conversation agg.
Cowardice
Culpability after masturbation, distressed by •

Dancing
    unconscious •
Deception causes grief and mortification ★
Defiant
Delirium
    answers correctly when spoken to, but delirium and unconsciousness return at once
    apathetic
    haemorrhage, after
    mild
    murmuring
        slowly •
    muttering
        slowly •
    quiet
    sleep, on falling asleep
    sleeplessness, and ★
Delusions, imaginations, hallucinations, illusions
    evening in bed
    bell, hears ringing of
    ciphers, sees
    clock, hears strike •
    dead persons, sees
    falling asleep, on
    fancy, illusions of
    figures, sees
    forehead, she must look out under •
    head, standing on ★
    hearing, illusions of
    hears objects moving •
    images, phantoms, sees
        frightful
    laughed at, mocked, being
    move, hears invisible things
    noise, hears
    rain, he hears (at night)
    tilted as if, and she were standing on her head ★
    visions, has
    waking, on
Dementia
Despair

Disomania, alcoholism
Discomfort, eating, after
Discontented, displeased, dissatisfied
    himself, with
Discouraged
    air, in open •
    walking, while
Doubtful, recovery, of
Dream, as if in a
Dullness, sluggishness, difficulty of thinking and comprehending, torpor
    morning
    alone, when •
    cares for his business, from •
    emotions, from
    impotency, with •
    masturbation, from
    mental exertion, from
    pollutions, after
    reading, while
    think long, unable to
    walking, while
Dwells on disappointments •
Eat, refuses to
Ecstasy
Envy, avidity, and
Excitement, excitable
    agg.
    perspiration, during
    reading, while
Exertion, agg. from mental
Extravagance
Exuberance
Fancies, exaltation of
    evening in bed
        night
    sleeplessness, with
    reading, on
Fear, apprehension, dread
    night
    cholera, of
    death, of
    pressure in hypogastrium, with •

Fear,

> *disease, of impending*
> exertion, of
> *happen, something will*
> poisoned, of being
> touch, of
> waking, on
>> dream, from a

Foolish behavior

Forgetful

> morning
> emotions, from
> *(-ness) old people, of*
> *sexual excesses, after*
> **words while speaking, of;
> word hunting**

Fright, menses, during ★

Frightened easily

Gestures, grasping or reaching at something, at flocks; carphologia

> *picks at bed clothes*

Greed, cupidity

Grief

> night in bed
> *headache from grief*
> prolonged ★
> waking, on

Hatred

> *revenge, and*

Heedless

Homesickness

> *silent ill humor, with*

Hurry, haste

Hypochondriasis

> pollutions, after
> *sexual excesses, from*

Hysteria

> *climacteric period, at*
> menses, before
> *sexual excesses, after*

Ideas abundant, clearness of mind

> **deficiency of**
>> *brain-fag, in* ●

Idiocy

Imbecility

Impatience

Indifference, apathy

> morning
>> *waking, on*
>> *business affairs, to*
> **chill, during**
> **everything, to**
> **fever, during**
> puberty, in
> *typhoid, in*

Indolence, aversion to work

> eating, after

Insanity, madness

> dancing, with
> haemorrhage, after
> melancholy

Irritability

> morning on waking
> coition, after
> heat, during
> menses, during
> *questioned, when*
> *waking, on*

Jealousy

Lamenting, bemoaning, wailing

> asleep, while
> sickness, about his

Lascivious, lustful

Laughing, sleep, during

Libertinism

Loathing, life, at

Loquacity, heat, during

Love, disappointed,

> **silent grief, with**

Malicious, spiteful, vindictive

Mania

> rage, with
> wild

Memory, weakness of

> *expressing oneself, for*
> *labor, for mental*
>> fatigue, from
> names, for proper
> *occurrences of the day, for*
> *read, for what has*
>> for what has just
> say, for what is about to
> *words, of*

Mildness
Mistakes, speaking, in
        words, using wrong
Moaning, sleep, during
Mocking, others are mocking at him,
        thinks
Moral feeling, want of
Morose, cross, fretful, ill-humor, peevish
        morning
           bed, in
        puberty, in
        sleepiness, with
        waking, on
Music agg.
        cough, music agg.
           piano, c. when playing
        earache from
        headache from
Muttering
Nymphomania
Obstinate, headstrong
Passionate
        trifle, at every
Prostration of mind, mental exhaustion, brain fag
        morning
        cares, from
        pollutions, after
        sleeplessness, with
Quarrelsome, scolding
Quiet disposition
Quiet, repose and tranquillity on walking in open air, desires
Rage, fury
Reading, mental symptoms agg. from
Religious affections
Remorse
Reproaches himself
        others, morning •
Reserved
        walking in open air, while
Resignation
Rest, desire for
Restlessness
        morning
           bed, in
        evening
        night

Restlessness,
        anxious
        eating, after
        heat, after
        internal
        urination, before
        waking, on
        walking in open air, amel. while
Sadness, despondency, dejection, mental depression,
        gloom, melancholy
           morning on waking
           night after midnight
        air, in open
        grief, after
        heat, during
        masturbation, from
        menses, from suppressed
        misfortune, as if from
        pollutions, from
        quiet
        talk, indisposed to
        waking, on
        walking in open air, while and after
           only while, the longer he walks the worse he
           gets •
Senses, dull, blunted
        vanishing of
Sensitive, oversensitive
        afternoon
        evening
        external impressions, to all
        music, to
        noise, to
        rudeness, to
        want of sensitiveness
Serious,, earnest
Sighing
Singing
        night
        sleep, in
Sit, inclination to
Slowness
Smiling, sleep, in

Speech, hasty
   hesitating
   incoherent
   monosyllabic
   slow
   unintelligible
Spoken to, averse to being
Starting, falling, as if
   sleep, during
     from
Stupefaction, as if intoxicated
Sulky
Suspicious, mistrustful
Talk, indisposed to, desire to be
   silent, taciturn
    evening
   air, in open
   heat, during
   sadness, in
   others agg., talk of
   slow learning to
Talking, sleep, in
Talks, himself, to
Thinking, aversion to
Thoughts, disconnected
   disease, of
   intrude and crowd around each
     other
    reading, while •
   persistent
   rush, flow of
    night
    reading, while
    waking, on
   stagnation of
   vanishing of
    morning •
    reading, on
   wandering
Timidity in company
Tranquillity, serenity, calmness
Unconsciousness, coma, stupor
   morning
   alone, when •
   answers correctly when spoken to,
    but delirium and unconscious-
    ness return at once

Unconsciousness,
   eating, after
   emotion, after
   fever, during
   mental insensibility
   somnolency, without snoring, eyes
    being closed, with •
Violent, vehement
Vivacious
Wearisome
Weary of life
Weeping, tearful mood
    night
   coughing, during
   sad news, at •
   sleep, in
   whimpering during sleep
Wildness
   vexation, from •
Work, aversion to mental
   impossible
    morning
   sexual excesses, after

PHASEOLUS NANUS

Fear, death, of

PHELLANDRIUM
AQUATICUM

Absorbed, buried in thought
Anger, irascibility
Anguish, lie down, must
Anxiety
   afternoon
   night
   eating, after
   fear, with
   health, about ★
   waking, on
Cheerful, gay, mirthful
   evening
   air, in open
Confusion of mind
   afternoon
   intoxicated, as if

Excitement, evening
Exhilaration
    air, in open •
Extravagance
Exuberance
Fear, dinner, after
    behind him, someone is ★
    eating, after, food
    misfortune, of
        daytime •
    water, of
Gestures, light
Hydrophobia
Introspection
Irritability
    daytime
Loathing, general
Meditation
Mood, changeable, variable
Morose, cross, fretful, ill-humor, peevish
    daytime
Obstinate, headstrong
Sadness, despondency, dejection, mental depression,
    gloom, melancholy
        daytime
        morning after waking
        forenoon
    misfortune, as if from
Sensitive, noise, to
Stupefaction, as if intoxicated
Weeping, tearful mood
    sad thoughts, at

PHENOBARBITALUM

Embittered, exasperated
Excitement, alternating with sadness
Indifference, alternating with excitement
Memory, weakness of
Sadness, despondency, dejection, mental depression, gloom, melancholy
Sensitive, oversensitive

PHOSPHORUS

Absent - minded, unobserving
    morning
Absorbed, buried in thought
Abstraction of mind
Activity, mental
Adulterous
Affection, child accepts and returns ★
    craving for, in children ★
Affections, in general ★
Affectionate
    returns affection •
Ailments from:
    ambition, deceived
    anger, vexation
        anxiety, with
        fright with
        silent grief, with
    anticipation, foreboding, presentiment
    bad news
    cares, worries
    celibacy ★
    excitement, emotional
        moral ★
    fear
    fright
    grief
    jealousy ★
    love, disappointed
    music •
    scorn, being scorned
    sexual excesses
    work, mental
Amativeness
Amorous
Anger, irascibility
    morning, waking, on
    forenoon
    children, in
    coffee agg.
    easily
    trembling, with
    trifles, at
    violent
    waking, on

Anguish
  evening
  alone, when •
  menses, during
  stormy weather, in •
Answers, abruptly, shortly, curtly
  aversion to answer
  difficult
  disconnected
  incoherently
  incorrectly
  reflects long
  refuses to answer
  slowly
  stupor returns quickly after
    answer
  unintelligibly
  unsatisfactory •
Anticipation, dentist, physician, before
    going to
Antics, plays
  delirium, during
Anxiety
    morning
      waking, on
    afternoon
    evening
      twilight, in the
      bed, in
    night
      waking, on
    midnight, before
  alone, when
  bed, in
  causeless
  chill, during
  conscience, as if guilty of a crime
    no rest night or day, prevents
    lying down •
  dark, in
  dinner, after
  eating, after
  excitement, from
  fear, with
  fever, during
  flushes of heat, during
  friends at home, about
  future, about

Anxiety,
  head, heat of, with
    perspiration on forehead, with
  health, about
  heart ★
  hypochondriacal
  lying, side, on
    left
  menses, during
    after
  mental exertion, from
  others, for
  pain, from the, anus •
  paroxysms, in
  periodical
  pollutions, after
  sitting, while
  sleep, during
  standing amel.
  thoughts, from disagreeable
  thunderstorm, before
    during
  vexation, after
  waking, on
  warmth amel.
Automatism ★
Aversion, children, to her own ★
  everything, to
  his own mind, to ★
  members of family, to
  persons, to all
Awkward ★
Barking, growling like a dog
Beside oneself, being
Bite, desire to
  about him, bites •
  paroxysmally, bites •
  pillow, bites
Borrowing of everyone
Business, talks of
Busy
Capriciousness
Censorious, critical
Chaotic, confused behavior

Cheerful, gay, mirthful
>> forenoon
>> afternoon
>> *evening, bed, in*
>> *alternating with sadness*
>> weeping
>> chill, during
Children, watchful who are on the look
>> out for every gesture •
Clairvoyance
Clinging, grasps at others
Company, aversion to; presence of
>> other people agg. the symp-
>> toms; desire for solitude
>> alone amel., when
Company, desire for: aversion to
>> **solitude, company amel.**
>> alone agg., while
Complaining
Comprehension, easy
Concentration, active
Concentration, difficult
>> morning
>> *studying, learns with difficulty*
Confidence, want of self
Confounding, objects and ideas ★
Confusion of mind
>> morning
>>> rising and after, on
>>>> after amel.
>> *waking, on*
>> *evening*
>> night
>>> waking, on
>> air, in open, amel.
>> bed, while in
>> chill, during
>> coition, after
>> *cold bath amel.*
>>> after taking cold •
>> dinner, after
>> *dream, as if in*
>> *eating, after*
>>> amel.
>> headache, with

Confusion of mind
>> heat, during
>> identity, as to his
>>> duality, sense of
>> menses, during
>> *mental exertion, from*
>> motion, from
>> rising, after
>> sitting, while
>> sleeping, siesta, after a
>> stooping, when
>> **waking, on**
>> warm room, in
>> *washing the face amel.*
Consolation amel.
Contented
Contradiction, is intolerant of
Contradictory, actions are c. to inten-
>> tion
Contrary
Courageous
Cowardice
Cursing, swearing
Darkness agg.
Death, desires
>> *presentiment of*
>> *sensation of*
Delirium
>> evening
>>> 18h. •
>> *alternating with consciousness*
>> answers correctly when spoken
>>> to, but delirium and uncon
>>> sciousness return at once
>> anxious
>> aroused, on being
>> bed and escapes, spring up sud-
>>> denly from
>> business, talks of
>> crying, with
>> *erotic*
>> frightful
>> haemorrhage, after
>> *loquacious*

Delirium

    maniacal, love, from disappoin-
        ted •
    murmuring
    muttering
    naked in delirium, wants to be
    paroxysmal
    quiet
    raging, raving
    restless
    sleep, falling asleep, on
    sleeplessness, and ★
    violent
    watching, vigil, from
Delirium tremens, mania-a-potu
Delusions, imaginations, hallucina-
    tions, illusions
        evening, falling asleep, on
    accidents of relatives •
    animals, of
    anxious
    assembled things, swarms, crowds
        etc.
    body, scattered about bed, tossed
        about to get the pieces together
    business, is doing
    chair is rising up •
    choked by forms, being •
    choked, he is about to be (night on
        waking)
    ciphers, sees
    corners, sees something coming
        out of •
    criminal, he is a
    dead, he himself was
        persons, sees •
    devils, present, are
    distinguished, is
    double, of being
    faces, sees
        wherever he turns his eyes, or
            looking out
    from corners
    falling asleep, on
    fancy, illusions of
        chill, during
        heat, during
    fire, visions of

Delusions,

    flame of fire seems passing
        through him, a •
    floating in air
    great person, is a
    hanging or standing high, seems
        as if •
    hearing, illusions of
    hydrothorax, he has a
    identity, errors of personal
        someone else, she is
    images, phantoms, sees
        night
        frightful
    injury: injured, is being
    insects, sees
    island, is on a distant •
    light, incorporeal, he is
    move, hears invisible things
    murdered, he will be
        someone, he had (all night)
    noble, being
    objects, sees, motion, in
    obscene action of which she had
        not been guilty, accuses her-
        self of •
    person, other, she is some
    pursued, police, by
    rank, he is a person of
    rich, as if he is ★
    seized, as if
    sick, being
    spectres, ghosts, spirits, sees
    strange, familiar things seem
    thieves, sees
    thumbs, fingers are •
    vermin, sees crawl about
    visions, has
        evening
        horrible
        night
    vivid
    voices, hears
        confused (swallowing or walk-
            ing in open air agg.).

Delusions,
>   wealth, of
>   work, hard at w. is
>   worms, creeping of

Dementia
>   senilis

Desire, exercise, for
>   numerous, various things

Despair

Destructiveness

Development of children arrested

Dictatorial, domineering, dogmatical,
>   despotic
>   *command, talking with air of*

Dipsomania, alcoholism

Discontented, displeased, dissatisfied
>   health, about •

Discouraged

Disgust
>   everything, with

Disobedience

Doubtful, recovery, of

Dream, as if in a

**Dullness, sluggishness, difficulty
>   of thinking and compre-
>   hending, torpor**
>   morning
>   rising, on
>   night on waking
>   chill, during
>   *eating amel.*
>   painful
>   *sleepiness, with*
>   **think long, unable to**
>   *understand questions only after
>   repetition*
>   *waking, on*

Dwells on past disagreeable occur-
>   rences
>   recalls, disagreeable memories

Eating, after, amel.

Ecstasy
>   amorous, sleep, during •

Escape, attempts to
>   family, children, from her

Estranged from her family

Excitement, excitable
>   afternoon
>   evening
>   *bed, in*
>   **agg.**
>   bad news, after
>   chill, during
>   feverish
>   nervous
>   trifles, over
>   *weakness, with*

Exertion, agg. from mental

Exhilaration
>   evening

Fancies, confused
>   *exaltation of*
>   *evening*
>   bed, in
>   night
>   *going to bed, after*
>   sleeplessness, with
>   sleep preventing
>   unpleasant, bed, after going to •
>   *vivid, lively*
>   heat, followed by •

Fastidious, occasionally ★

Fear, apprehension, dread
>   morning
>   *evening*
>   *twilight*
>   night
>   waking, after
>   **alone, of being**
>   *lest he die*
>   apoplexy, of
>   approaching him, of others
>   vehicles, of
>   *cockroaches* ★
>   *creeping out of every corner, of
>   something*
>   crowd, in a
>   *dark, of*
>   **death, of**
>   *evening*
>   *night*
>   *alone, when*
>   *evening in bed*

Fear,
   disease, of impending
      cancer, of ★
   doctors, of ★
   evil, of
   exertion, of
   failure, of
   fit, of having a
   ghosts, of
   grief, as from
   happen, something will
   heart, of disease of ★
   imaginary things, of
   insanity, losing his reason, of
   lightning of
   men, dread, fear of
   menses, during
      after
   misfortune, of
   murdered, of being
   noise, from
   overpowering
   people, of; anthropophobia
   piano, when at
   poisoned, of being
   recurrent
   robbers, of
   runover, of being (on going out)
   starting, with
   stomach, arising from
   suffocation, of
   thinking of disagreeable things,
      when ●
   thunderstorm, of
   touch, of
   tremulous
   waking, dream, from a, on
   water, of
   weeping amel.
   work, dread of
Fire, wants to set things on
Foolish behavior
Foppish
Forgetful
   morning
Fright, menses, during ★

Frightened easily
   falling asleep, on
   trifles, at
   weeping amel. ●
Gestures, automatic
    sleep, during ●
   awkward in ★
   grasping or reaching at some-
      thing, at flocks; carphologia
      by standers, at
    picks at bed clothes
   hands, motions, involuntary, of
     the, head, to the ★
   sleep, during
   throwing about
   slow
   uncertian
   wringing the hands
Grief
   morning
   headache from grief
   undermining the constitution ●
Hatred
   men, of
   revenge, hatred and
Haughty
Heedless
Helplessness, feeling of
Homesickness
Horrible things, sad stories, affect her
    profoundly
Howling
Hurry, haste
Hydrophobia
Hypochondriasis
   evening
   morose
Hypocrisy
Hysteria
   menses, before
Ideas abundant, clearness of mind
   evening
   deficiency of
   wander ★
Idiocy

Imbecility
    sexual excitement, with
Impertinence
Impetuous
    perspiration, with
Impressionable
Inconsolable
Indifference, apathy
    evening
    alternating with weeping •
    children, to her
    chill, during
    dearest friends, even towards •
       (in chronic alcoholism)
    everything, to
    exposure of her person, to
    fever, during
    his own, to ★
    life, to
    loved ones, to
    relations, to
    surroundings, to the
Indolence, aversion to work
    daytime
    eating, after
Industrious, mania for work
    menses, before
Insanity, madness
    erotic
    megalomania
    mental labor, from
    paralysis, with
    paroxysmal
    puerperal
    sexual excesses, from
Insolence
Introspection, forenoon •
Irresolution, indecision
    marry, to
Irritability
    daytime
    morning
       rising, after
       waking, on
    forenoon
    evening
    night

Irritability
    alone, when
    chill, during
    coition, after
    dinner, before •
    eating, amel. after
    headache, during
    heat, during
    noise, from
    puberty, in •
Jealousy, sexual excitement, with
Jumping, bed, out of
Kicks, sleep, in
Kill, desire to
Kisses everyone
Lamenting, bemoaning, wailing
    asleep, while
Lascivious, lustful
Laughing
    morning
    agg.
    alternating with sadness
    involuntarily
    sad, when •
    serious matters, over
    spasmodic
Learns, easily ★
    poorly ★
Libertinism
Light, desire for
Loathing, life, at
Loquacity
Love, with one of own sex, homosexu-
    ality, tribadism
Love, disappointed,
    silent grief, with
Magnetized, desire to be
    mesmerism amel.
Malicious, spiteful, vindictive
Mania
    erotic ★
    rage, with
    sexual mania in men
       women, in
Meditation
Memory, active

Memory, weakness of
    business, for
    do, for what was about to
    read, for what has
Menses, mental symptoms agg. before
    during
Mildness
Misanthropy
Mistakes, localities, in
    speaking, wrong answers, gives
    work, in
    writing, in
Moaning, groaning, whining
    pain, from
    perspiration, after
    sleep, during
Mood, alternating
    changeable, variable
    repulsive
Morose, cross, fretful, ill-humor, peevish
    daytime
    morning
    forenoon
    afternoon, twilight, in
    evening
    night
    eating, after
    waking, on
Morphinism
Music agg.
    piano playing, from
    headache, during
Muttering
    evening
Naked, wants to be
    morning in bed
    delirium, in
Nymphomania
    menses, before
    suppressed, after
    pregnancy, during
Obscene, lewd
    man searching for little girls
    talk
Obstinate, headstrong
Offended, easily; takes everything in
    bad part

Passionate
    trifle, at every
Patient
Perseverance
Pompous, important
Precocity ★
Prostration of mind, mental exhaustion, brain-fag
    morning
    noon
    pollutions, after
    trifles, from ●
Quarrelsome, scolding
Rage, fury
    evening
    aroused, when ●
    sleep, in ●
Rebels against poultice
Recognize, relatives, does not r.
    his
Reflecting
Remorse
Reserved
Restlessness
    forenoon
    noon
    evening
        bed, in
    night
    midnight, after, 1h.
    alone, when
    anxious
    bed, in
        driving out of
        tossing about in
    chill, at beginning of
    eating, after
    feverish
    heat, during
    internal
    menses, during
    nausea, from
    sleep, before
    storm, during
    thunderstorm, during ●
    waking, on
Rudeness

*Sadness, despondency, dejection, mental
  depression, gloom, melancholy*
   morning
    waking, on
   afternoon
    twilight, in
   evening
    21h.
   night
    midnight, after
  alone, when
  anger, after
  causeless
  chill, during
  cold, from becoming
  darkness, in
  dream, from
  headache, during
  heat, during
  laughing, with involuntary •
  menses, before
   suppressed
  misfortune, as if from
  music, from
  noise, from
  weeping amel.
Satyriasis
Secretive
Senses, acute
 dull, blunted
Sensitive, oversensitive
 children
 chill, during
 crying of children, to
 external impressions, to all
 light, to
 menses, during
 mental impressions, to
 music, to
 noise, to
  slightest, to
 odors, to
 puberty, in
 sensual impressions, to
 touch, to
 want of sensitiveness

Sentimental
Shamelessness
 exposes the person
Shining objects agg.
Shrieking, screaming, shouting
 brain cry
 convulsions, before
 sleep, during
 waking, on
Sighing, perspiration, during
Singing
 trilling
Sit, inclination to
Slander, disposition to, hypocritical,
  and
Slowness
 motion, in
 old people, of
Somnambulism
 climbing the roofs, the railing of
  bridge or balcony
 do mental work, to
Speech, affected
 delirious, asleep, on falling •
 foolish
 incoherent
  sleep, during
 slow
 wandering
Spitting, faces of people, in
Starting, startled
 morning, after waking
 door is opened, when a
 easily
 fright, from and as from
 sleep, falling, on
  during
  from
Strangers, presence of s. agg.
 child coughs at sight of strangers
Striking
 about him at imaginary objects
  while dreaming •

Stupefaction, as if intoxicated
    morning
        waking, on
    rising, amel. after •
    vertigo, during
    waking, on
    warm room, in
Suicidal disposition
    night
    courage, but lacks
    weeping amel.
Suppressed or receding skin diseases
    or haemorrhoids, mental
    symptoms agg. after
Suspicious, mistrustful
Sympathy, compassion
    desires for •
Talk,
    indisposed to, desires to be silent,
        taciturn
    slow learning to
Talking, sleep, in
Tears things
    pillow with teeth
Thinking, aversion to
    complaints agg., of
    disagreeable things agg., of •
Thoughts, disease, of
    frightful
        night •
    intrude and crowd around each
        other
        sexual
    persistent
        homicide
    rapid, quick
    rush, flow of
        evening
        thoughtful
    tormenting
    vacancy of
    wandering
Thunderstorm, during, mind symp-
    toms
Timidity
    afternoon, twilight, in the
    bashful

Traquillity, serenity, calmness
Twilight agg. mental symptoms
Unconsciousness, coma, stupor
    morning
    night, waking, on
    answers correctly when spoken
        to, but delirium and uncon-
        sciousness return at once
    apoplexy, in
    conduct, automatic
    crowded room, in a
    delirium, after
    dream, as in a
    fever, during
    frequent spells of unconscious-
        ness, absences
    mental, insensibility
    muttering
    odors, from
    pneumonia, in
    stool, after
    vertigo, during, of drunkards •
    waking, on
Undertakes, lacks will power to under-
    take anything
    things opposed to his intentions
Violent, vehement
    deeds of violence, rage leading to
Walk: walking in open air agg. mental
    symptoms
Wearisome
Weary of life
Weeping, tearful mood
    morning
    afternoon
    night
    aloud, sobbing
    alternating with laughter
    amel.
    anxiety, after
    causeless
    cough, before ★
    headache, with
    involuntary
    menses, before
        during
        after

Weeping,
> palpitation, during
> paroxysmal
> perspiration, during
> sleep, in
> *spasmodic*
> stool, before
>> during
> waking, on
> whimpering
>> night •
> sleep, during
Well before an attack, feels ★
Wildness
Will, loss of
Work, aversion to mental
> *impossible*

PHOSPHORUS HYDROGENATUS

Sensitive, oversensitive

PHYSOSTIGMA VENENOSOM

Activity, mental
Ailments from:
> excitement, emotional
> grief
Anxiety, friends at home, about
> sleep, during
Cheerful, gay, mirthful
Concentration, difficult
Confusion of mind
> forenoon
Counting, continually
Delirium, trembling, with
Delusions, alone, being a castaway •
> insane, she will become
> objects, numerous objects in room,
>> too •
> snakes in and around her
> spectres, ghosts, spirits, sees
Discomfort, bathing, after •
Dream, as if in a

Dullness, sluggishness, difficulty of think-
> ing and comprehending, torpor
>> morning
>> forenoon
> walking, while
Excitement, climacteric period, during
Exhilaration, morning
Fear, insanity, losing his reason, of
> night
> lightning, of
> *mischief, he might do (night on*
>> *waking)* •
Foolish behavior
Forgetful, climacteric period, during
Gestures, nervous
Hysteria
Ideas abundant, clearness of mind
> chill, during
Impulse to run; dromomania
Indifference to business affairs ★
Insanity, madness
Irritability
Loquacity
> *climacteric period, during* •
Memory, active
Memory, weakness of
> expressing oneself, for
Moaning, groaning, whining
Music agg.
Nothing seems right ★
Prostration of mind, mental exhaus-
> tion, brain-fag
Reading, aversion to read
Restlessness
> morning
> evening
> night
>> 22h. •
>> heart, from uneasiness
>>> about •
Sadness, noon
Sighing
Size, frame seems lessened, of •
Smaller, things appear
Speech, slow

Starting, startled
    consciousness, recovering
    easily
    sleep, on falling
Stupefaction, as if intoxicated
    afternoon
Talk, indisposed to, desire to be silent,
    taciturn
Thoughts, frightful
    night on waking
    persistent
    rapid, quick
    wandering
    studying, while
Weeping, night ★
Will, muscles obey, feebly ★

PHYSALIS ALKEKENGI

Loquacity

PHYTOLACCA DECANDRA

Anxiety, daytime
Bite, desire to
Business, averse to
Confusion of mind, air amel., in open
    sitting, while
Death, conviction of
    desires
    morning on waking
Delusion
    naked in delirium, wants to be
    snakes in and around her
Eat, refuses to
Fear, apprehension, dread
    death, of
    exertion, of
Indifference, apathy
    morning on waking
    business affairs, to
    exposure of her person, to
    life, to
    surroundings, to the
Indolence, morning
Insanity, chilliness, with
Irritability
Killed, desires to be

Laughing, sardonic
Loathing, general
    morning
        waking, on ●
    pain, from
Moaning, groaning, whining
    night
    children, in
    constant moaning and gasping
        for air
    dentition, in
Naked, wants to be
        delirium, in
Restlessness
    night
        midnight on waking, before
Sadness, despondency, dejection, mental
        depression gloom, melancholy
Sensitive, pain, to
Shamelessness
    exposes the person
Stupefaction, vertigo, during
Unbearable, pains ★
Unconsciousness, coma, stupor
    pain, from
Weary of life
    morning on waking
    pains, from the ●
Weeping, night
    children from difficult dentition ●
    menses, during
Work, aversion to mental

PICRICUM (PICRONITRICUM) ACIDUM

Ailments from:
    cares, worries
    continence ★
    debauchery
    grief
    shock, mental
    work, mental
Cares, worries, full of

Company, aversion to; presence of
    other people agg. the symp-
    toms; desire for solitude
Comprehension, easy
Concentration, difficult
    studying, reading, etc., while
*Confusion of mind, mental exertion,
    from*
Delusions, arms reach the clouds (when
    going to sleep) •
    enlarged
        body, parts of
    faces, sees, reaching the clouds
        (when going to sleep) •
    large, parts of body seem too
    tongue seems to reach the clouds
        (when going to sleep) •
Dementia
Despair
**Dullness, sluggishness, difficulty
    of thinking and compre-
    hending, torpor**
    mental exertion, from
    think long, unable to
    waking,on
Ecstasy, amorous
Exertion, agg. from mental
Fancies, exaltation of
    vivid, lively
Fear, examination, of ★
Forgetful
Ideas abundant, clearness of mind
    night
Imbecility
Indifference, apathy
Indolence, aversion to work
Industrious, mania for work
Insanity, erotic
Irresolution, indecision
Irritability
    night
    exertion, from mental •
    impotency, with •
    sexual weakness, with •
Lascivious, lustful

Libertinism
Loathing, general, noon •
Mania
Marriage seemed unendurable, idea of
*Memory, weakness of
    labor, for mental*
Mood, changeable, variable
Moral feeling, want of
Morose, cross, fretful, ill-humor, peevish
Obscene, lewd
**Prostration of mind, mental ex-
    haustion, brain-fag**
    cares, from
    sleep, from loss of •
    writing, after
Resignation
Restlessness, night, midnight, before
Sadness, despondency, dejection, men-
    tal depression, gloom, melan-
    choly
Satyriasis
Sit, inclination to
Sits, still
Stupefaction, as if intoxicated
*Talk, indisposed to, desire to be silent,
    taciturn*
Thoughts, intrude, sexual
    rapid, quick
    vanishing of
    wandering
Undertakes: lacks will power to under-
    take anything
Weary of life
*Will, loss of
    weakness of
        exertion, from mental* •
*Work, aversion to mental
    fatigues*
    impossible
    sexual excesses, after

PICROTOXINUM

Sadness, despondency, dejection, men-
    tal depression, gloom, melan-
    choly

PILOCARPINUM

Unconsciousness, coma, stupor

PINUS SILVESTRIS

Anxiety
Dullness, sluggishness, difficulty of thinking and comprehending, torpor
Excitement, excitable
Sadness, despondency, dejection, mental depression, gloom, melancholy
Undertakes many things, perseveres in nothing

PIPER METHYSTICUM

Ailments from :
    work, mental
Amusement, desire for
Cheerful, gay, mirthful
    forenoon
    evening
    pollutions, after •
Comprehension, easy
Confusion of mind, sleepiness, with
Dancing
Delusions, enlarged, head is
Dullness, sluggishness, difficulty of thinking and comprehending, torpor
    afternoon
    evening
Ennui, tedium
    entertainment amel.
Exacting, too, disease, in ★
Excitement, excitable
    agreeable •
    amel.
Exertion, agg. from mental
Exhilaration
Fancies, exaltation of
Fear, apprehension, dread
    daytime, only
    pains, of
    suffering, of
Gestures, cautious •
Hurry, eating, while

Ideas abundant, clearness of mind
Indolence, aversion to work
    sleep, after
    waking, on
Industrious, mania for work
Irritability, noise, from
Jumping
Memory, active
Memory, weakness of
Occupation, diversion amel.
Prostration of mind, mental exhaustion, brain-fag
Restlesness, daytime
    night
Sensitive, pain, to
Strength increased, mental
Talk, indisposed to, desire to be silent, taciturn
Thinking, complaints agg., of
Timidity, daytime
Unbearable, pains ★
Work, desire for mental

PIPER NIGRUM

Occupation, diversion amel.
Thinking, complaints agg., of

PISCIDIA ERYTHRINA

Industrious, mania for work
Mania

PITUITARIUM POSTERIUM

Anxiety
    night
Fear, impotency, of •
    urine, of involuntary loss of •
Indifference, everything, to ★
Weary of life ★

PITUITRINUM

Concentration, difficult

PLANTAGO MAJOR

Anguish
    night
Anxiety
    night
    fever, during
    mental exertion, from
Confusion of mind
    dinner, after
    eating, after
Contradiction, is intolerant of
Dullness, sluggishness, difficulty of thinking and comprehending, torpor
    afternoon
    walking, air amel., in open
Excitement, excitable
Exertion, agg. from mental
Fancies, exaltation of
Forgetful
Home, desire to go
Homesickness
Hurry, occupation, in, desire to do several things at once
Impatience
Inconstancy
Indolence, aversion to work
    daytime
Industrious, mania for work
Irritability
    evening
    chill, during
    working, when •
Memory, weakness of
Mood, changeable, variable
Morose, cross, fretful, ill-humor, peevish
Persists in nothing
Prostration of mind, mental exhaustion, brain-fag
Restlessness
    daytime
    night
    bed, tossing about in
    chill, during
    heat, during
    pacing back and forwards •
    sitting, while

Sadness, despondency, dejection, mental depression, gloom, melancholy
Sensitive, noise, to
Spoken to, averse to being
Stupefaction, as if intoxicated
    dinner, after
Thinking, aversion to
    complaints agg., of
Thoughts, thoughtful
    vanishing of
Undertakes many things, perseveres in nothing
Weeping, sleep, in
    waking, on
Work, aversion to mental

PLATINUM METALLICUM

Abrupt, rough
Absent-minded, unobserving
    air, in open •
Absorbed, buried in thought
Abstraction of mind
Abusive, insulting ★
    children insulting parents
Admonition agg.
    kindly agg.
Adulterous
Affectation
    words, in
Affections, in general ★
Affectionate
Ailments from :
    ambition, deceived
    anger, vexation
    anxiety, with
    fright, with
    indignation, with
    silent grief, with
    bereavement ★
    continence ★
    death of a child
    parents or friends, of
    disappointment
    embarrassment
    excitement, emotional
    sexual
    fright

Ailments from :
  grief
  indignation
  mortification
  position, loss of
  scorn, being scorned
  sexual excesses
  excitement ★
  shock, mental
Amativeness
Ambition
  means, employed every possible
Amorous
Anger, irascibility
  activity, with great physical ●
  easily
  face, with pale, livid
  laughing and weeping alternate ●
  trembling, with
  trifles, at
  violent
Anguish
  amenorrhoea, in
  anger, from ●
  menses, during
  walking in open air
Answers, unconscious, as if ●
Anxiety
      daytime
      morning
        waking, on
      forenoon
      evening
      night
        waking, on
    air, in open
    chill, during
    company, when in
    conscience, as if guilty of a crime
    conversation, from
    crowd, in a
    excitement, from
    fear, with
    fever, during
      puerperal, during ●
    flushes of heat, during
    headache, with
    house, in

Anxiety,
  hypochondriacal
  joyful things, by most ●
  menses, during
  paroxysms, in ★
  periodical
  pressure on the chest, from
  salvation, about
    hell, of ●
  shuddering, with
  speaking, when
    company, in ●
  stool, during
  sudden
  suicidal disposition, with
  waking, on
  walking, while
    air, in open
  weary of life, with
Attitudes, assume strange ★
Audacity
Avarice
Aversion, children, to
      her, own
    everything, to
    his own, mind, to ★
    members of family, to
    wife, to his ★
    women, to, homosexuality, with ●
Begging, entreating supplicating
Blood or knife, cannot look at ★
Boaster, braggart
    squanders through ostentation
Borrowing of everyone
Brooding
Capriciousness
**Casting off of people against her
    will** ●
Censorious, critical
Charlatan
Cheerful, gay, mirthful.
    morning
      air, in open ●
    evening
    air, in open

Cheerful,
>   alternating with moroseness
>   pain
>   physical suffering ●
>   sadness
>   seriousness
>   weeping
>   dancing, laughing, singing, with
>   followed by melancholy

Childbed, mental symptoms during

Company, aversion to; presence of other people agg. the symptoms; desire for solitude
>   menses, during

Complaining

Comprehension, easy

Concentration, difficult

Confounding objects and ideas

Confusion of mind
>   night, waking, on
>   mixes subjective and objective
>   *waking, on*

Conscientious about trifles
>   eating, during

Consolation, kind words agg.

Contemptuous
>   air or when sun shines into room, in open ●
>   **everything, to**
>   *paroxysms against her will, in ●*
>   *ravenous hunger and greedy, hasty eating, contemptuous with sudden ●*
>   hard for subordinates and agreeable-pleasant to superiors or people he has to fear

Contradiction, is intolerant of

Conversation agg.

Cowardice

Cruelty, inhumanity

Dancing

Darkness agg.

Death, desires
>   *presentiment of*
>   *sensation of*
>   thoughts of

Deceitful, sly

Delirium, erotic ★
>   *fear of men, with*
>   *loquacious*
>   sleeplessness, and ★
>   trembling, with

Delusions, imaginations, hallucinations, illusions
>   *alone, she is alone in the world*
>   appreciated, she is not
>   *belong to her own family, does not ●*
>   black objects and people, sees
>   *body, greatness of, as to*
>   *changed, everything is*
>   *choked, he is about to be*
>   cut, in two
>   *dead persons, sees*
>   *deserted, forsaken, is*
>   *devils, sees*
>   **all persons are**
>   possessed of a devil, is
>   **present, are**
>   *die, he was about to*
>   diminished, everything in room is, while she is tall and elevated ●
>   disgraced, she is
>   divided, cut in two parts, or
>   *doomed, being*
>   enemy, everyone is an
>   *enlarged*
>   tall, is very
>   *family, does not belong to her own*
>   *fancy, illusions of* ●
>   air amel., in open
>   fire, visions of
>   fright, after
>   *great person, is a*
>   help, calling for ●
>   *horrible, everything seems ●*
>   humility and lowness of others, while he is great
>   images, phantoms, sees
>   black
>   inferior, people seem mentally and physically (on entering house after a walk) ●

Delusions,
> injury, injured, of being, sleep, during •
> insane, she will become
> large, entering the house after walking, on •
> melancholy
> narrow, everything seems too
> noble, being
> *places, none in the world, she has* •
> possessed, being
> proud
> pursued, ghosts, by
> rags, body torn into, as if ★
> religious
> rich, as if he is ★
> scream, obliging to
> *small, things appear*
>> things grow smaller
> spectres, ghosts, spirits, sees
>> conversing with, he is
>> pursued by, is
> *strange, everything is*
>> *familiar things seem*
>>> horrible, are •
>> land, as if in a
>> places seemed
> *superhuman control, is under*
> superiorty, of •
> surroundings, strange ★
> swollen, he is
> *talking, spirits, with*
> tall, she is very
> *vexation, after*
> visions, has
> war, being at
> *wealth, of*
Despair
> religious despair of salvation
Destructiveness
Dictatorial, domineering, dogmatical, despotic
Dipsomania, alcoholism
Dirtiness ★
Discontented, displeased, dissatisfied
> *everything, with*
> surroundings, with

Discouraged
> morning
Dullness, sluggishness, difficulty of thinking and comprehending, torpor
> morning
>> waking, on
>> night on waking
> air, in open
> company, in •
> waking, on
Dwells on past disagreeable occurrences
>> *night*
Eat, refuses to
Eccentricity
> alternating with sadness
> fancies, in
Ecstasy
Effeminate
Egotism self - esteem
Embraces anything, in morning, agg. in the open air
> companions, his
Ennui, tedium
Envy
Estranged from her family
> wife, from his
Excitement, excitable
> *palpitation, with violent*
Exclusive, too
Exertion, agg. from mental
Extravangance
Exuberance
Fancies, exaltation of
>> night
>> sleeplessness, with
> lascivous
> waking, on
Fastidious, occasionally ★
Fear, apprehension, dread
> evening
> air, in open amel.
> crowd, in a
> **death, of**
> *alternate, laughing and weeping, with·(after anger)* •

Fear,

amenorrhoea, in •
anger, from •
heart symptoms, during
labor, during
menses, before
  during
sadness, with
disease, of impending
fainting, of
ghosts, of
conversing with, thinks he is ★
hanged, to be •
happen, something will
husband: that he would never return, that something would happen to him •
insanity, losing his reason, of
knives, of ★
labor, during
men, dread, fear of
menses, before
  during
murdered, of being
overpowering
people, of; anthropophobia
pins, pointed things, sharp things, of
recurrent
room, on entering
sadness, with
serious thoughts, of
strangled, to be •
suicide, of
tremulous
weary of life, with
Flatterer
Foppish
Forgetful
Forsaken feeling
  isolation, sensation of
Frightened easily
Gamble (*see* Play)
Gestures, makes
  grasping or reaching at something, at flocks; carphologia
  wringing the hands

Godless, want of religious feeling
Grief, past events, about •
Grimaces
Hard for inferiors and kind for superiors
Haughty
  religious haughtiness •
  stupid and haughty
Heedless
Horror ★
Hurry, haste
  eating, while
Hypochondriasis
  weeping, with
Hysteria
  lascivious
  menses, before
Ideas abundant, clearness of mind
  deficiency of
Imbecility
Impatience
  room, in a warm crowded •
Impolite
Inconsolable
Inconstancy
Indifference, apathy
  air, in open
  company, society, while in
  everything, to
  external things, to
  loved ones, to
  others, towards
  relations, to
  taciturn
  weeping, with
  welfare of others, to
Indiscretion
Indolence, aversion to work
  morning
  eating, after
Insanity, madness
  alternating mental with physical symptoms
  anger, from
  erotic
  fright, from

Insanity,
    grief, from
    megalomania
    menses, during
    mortification, from
    periodical
    puerperal
    religious
Insolence
Irresolution, indecision
    changeable
    marry, to
Irritability
    daytime
    morning
        waking, on
    air, in open
    alternating with cheerfulness
        tenderness •
    chill, during
    consolation agg.
    eating, after
    headache, during
    menses, during
    sadness, with
    sleeplessness, with
    trifles, at
    waking, on
Jesting
    alternating with seriousness •
        taciturnity •
    gravity, jesting after •
Kill, desire to
    beloved ones
    child, her own
    husband, impulse to kill her be-loved
    knife, with a
        at sight of a
    sudden impulse to kill
Kisses everyone
Lamenting, bemoaning, wailing
Lascivious, lustful
Late, always too

Laughing
    morning
    air, in open
    alternating with anguish and
        fear of
        death after anger •
        seriousness
        taciturnity •
    convulsions, before, during or after
    immoderately
    serious matters, over
        air, in open •
    spasmodic
    wrong places, at ★
Learns, easily ★
Libertinism
Loathing, general
Loathing, life, at
Love, with one of own sex.
    homosexuality, tribadism
    anal-coition with a woman
    perversity
Ludicrous, things seem
Malicious, spiteful, vindictive
Mania
    demoniac
    lochia, from suppressed
    singing, puerperal mania, in •
    violence, with deeds of
Mannish habits of girls
Marriage, obsessed by idea of mar-riage, excited sexual girls are
Memory active
Memory, weakness of
    heard, for what has
    labor, fatigue, from
Menses, mental symptoms agg. during
Mental symptoms alternating with physical
Misanthropy
Mistakes, in differentiating of objects localities, in
Moaning, groaning, whining, night menses, during
Mocking

529

Mood, aggreable
  alternating
    changeable, variable
    opinions, in
Moral feeling, want of
Morose, cross, fretful, ill-humor, peevish
    daytime
    morning
      bed, in
    air, in open
    alternating with tenderness •
    chill, during
    menses, during
    waking, on
    weeping, amel.
    women, in
Morphinism
Music, desire to playing piano
Nagging ★
Nymphomania
    menses, during
      suppressed, after
    metrorrhagia, during
    puerperal
Objective, reasonable
Obscene, lewd
    man searching for little girls
    talk
Obstinate, headstrong
    simpleton, as a
Offended, easily; takes everything in
    bad part
Passionate
Play, passion for gambling, to make
    money
Pompous, important
Postponing everything to next day
Praying
    loud, in sadness •
Prejudices, traditional
Presumptuous
Prim ★
Proportion, sense of, disturbed ★
Prostration of mind, mental exhaus-
    tion, brain-fag
Quarrelsome, scolding
Quiet, disposition

Rage, evening
Recognize, streets, does not r. well
    known
Reflecting, sadness, in
Refuses, treatment, every
Religious, affections
    alternating with sexual excite-
      ment
    melancholia
    penance, desire to do •
    taciturnity, haughtiness, volup
      tuousness, cruelty, religious
      affections, with •
Remorse
Reserved
    air, in open
Restlessness
    midnight, before
      on waking
    anxious
    bed, tossing about in
    chill, during
    driving about
    menses, during
    sadness, with •
    tremulous
Reverence for those around him
Runs, room, in
Sadness, despondency, dejection,
    mental depression, gloom,
    melancholy
    morning
      waking, on
    afternoon
    evening
    night
    midnight •
    air, in open, amel.
    alternating with exuberance
      tenderness •
    anger, after
    anxious
    chill, during
    darkness, in
    dream, from

Sadness,
exhilaration, after
heat, during
house, in
  entering, on
laughing, after •
masturbation, from
menses, during
periodical
pregnancy, in
puerperal
sunshine amel. •
vexation, after
waking, on
walking, air, in open, amel.
warm room, in
Satyriasis
Selfishness, egoism
Senses, vanishing of ★
Sensitive, oversensitive
afternoon
evening
menses, during
noise, to
Sentimental
Serious, earnest
alternating with jesting •
Shamelessness
Shrieking, screaming, shouting
aid, for
delusions, from
pain, with the
sleep, during
Sighing
hysteria, in
menses, during
Singing
Sit, inclination to
Sits still
Smaller, things appear
Solemn
Somnambulism
Speech: repeats same thing
wandering
Spoken to, averse to being
being, agg. mental symptoms •

Squanders, boasting, from
order, from want of
Starting, startled
evening
asleep, on falling
sleep, during
from
sleepiness, with
Strange, everything seems
Striking
about him at imaginary objects
anger, his friends from
Striking himself
Stupefaction, as if intoxicated
headache, before •
Suicidal disposition
courage, but lacks
fear of death, with
Sulky
Suspicious, mistrustful
Talk, indisposed to, desire to be silent, taciturn
evening
air, in open
alternating with jesting •
laughing •
Thoughts, frightful
intrude, sexual
persistent
midnight, at •
unpleasant subjects, on waking
rush, flow of
night
sleeplessness, from
waking, on
sexual
Timidity
Tranquillity, serenity, calmness
Travel, desire to
Twilight agg. mental symptoms
Unconsciousness, coma, stupor
dream, as in a, does not know where he is
pain, from
Unfeeling, hard hearted
Unfriendly humour ★

Ungrateful
Unsympathetic, unscrupulous
Vanity
Violent, vehement
    activity, with bodily •
    deeds of violence, rage leading to
Walk, walking in open air agg. mental
    symptoms
Wearisome
Weary of life
    fear of death, but
Weeping, tearful mood
    morning
    evening
    night
    admonition, from
    air, in open, amel.
    aloud, sobbing
    alternating with cheerfulness
    laughter
    amel.
    anger, after
    chill, during
    consolation agg.
    headache, during
    heat, during
    involuntary
    joy, from
    menses, during
    pains, with the
    palpitation, during
    remonstrated, when
    reproaches, from
    room, in •
    sad thoughts, at
    sleep, in
    spoken to, when
    trifles, at
Whistling
Work, aversion to mental

PLATINUM MURIATICUM

Delusions, poisoned, he has been

PLUMBUM METALLICUM

Absent-minded, unobserving
Absorbed, buried in thought
Abstraction of mind
Abusive, insulting
Activity, mental
Ailments from :
    anticipation, foreboding, pre-
        sentiment
    sexual excesses
Amorous ★
Anger, irascibility
Anguish
Answers abruptly, shortly, curtly
    imaginary questions
    monosyllable
    slowly
Antics, plays
    delirium, during
Anxiety
    night
    faintness, with
    fever, during
    perspiration, with cold
    salvation, about
Attitudes, assumes strange ★
Aversion, everything, to
    members of family, to ★
Beside oneself, being
Bite, desire to
    clothes, bites •
    fingers, bites
    himself, bites
Brooding
    forbidden things, over •
Business, talks of
Capriciousness
Censorious, critical
Cheerful, gay, mirthful
    forenoon
    afternoon
    air, in open
    alternating with lachrymose mood
    walking in open air and after, on
Company aversion to; presence of other
    people agg. the symptoms;
    desire for solitude
    alone amel., when

Company desire for; aversion to soli-
      tude, company amel.
          evening
   alone agg., while
   friend, of a •
Concentration, difficult, aversion to ★
Confidence, want of self
Confusion of mind
      morning, rising and after, on
   chill, during
   epileptic attack, before
      after
   identity, as to his
      duality, sense of
   loses his way in well-known
      streets
   standing, while
Contrary
Conversation, aversion to
Cowardice
Cursing, swearing
Death, desires
Deceitful, sly
Delirium
      evening
      night
   aternating with colic •
      coma
      sopor
   anxious
   bed and escapes, springs up sud-
      denly from
   convulsions, during
   delusions, with
   epilepsy, after
   face, with distorted •
   frightful
   groping as if in dark •
   laughing
   loquacious
   maniacal
   paroxysmal
   quiet
   raging, raving
   rambling

Delirium
   restless
   urinate on the floor, tries to •
   violent
   wild
   night
Delirium tremens, mania-a-potu
Delusions, imaginations, hallucinations,
      illusions
      night
   animals, bed, on
   ants, bed is full of •
   arrested, is about to be
   assembled things, swarms, crowds
      etc.
   business, ordinary, they are pur
      suing
   calls, someone
   castles and palaces, sees •
   conspiracies against him, there
      are
   criticised, she is
   danger, life, to his •
   dead, brother and child, corpse of
      husband, corpse of •
      persons, sees
   devils, all persons are
   disease, incurable, has
   dolls, people appeared like •
   double, of being
   engaged in some occupation, is
      ordinary occupation, in
   fancy, illusions of
   figures, sees
   grotesque
   home, away from, is
   identily, errors of personal
      someone else, she is
   insects, sees
   lost, she is (salvation)
   machine, he is working a •
   motion, up and down, of
   murder him, others conspire to
   murdered, he will be
   murderer, everyone around him is
      a •

Delusions,
>   music, he hears
>   delightful
>   people, sees
>   person, other, she is some
>   places at a time, of being in
>   different
>   poisoned, he is about to be
>   pursued by enemies
>   fiends, by
>   he was
>   police, by
>   soldiers, by
>   *strange, everything is*
>   visions, sees, closing the eyes, on
>   vivid
>   voices, hears

Dementia, senilis, talking, with foolish

Despair
>   religious despair of salvation

Destructiveness
>   clothes, of

Dipsomania, alcoholism

Discontented, displeased, dissatisfied
>   morning

Discouraged

Disgust

**Dullness, sluggishness, difficulty
of thinking and compre-
hending, torpor**
>   chill, during
>   sleepiness, with

Ecstasy

Ennui, tedium
>   afternoon •
>   *silent* •

Escape, attempts to

Exaggerates her symptoms ★

Excitement, alternating with sadness

Exertion, agg. from mental

Fancies, exaltation of
>   night

Fear, apprehension, dread
>   alone, of being
>   crowd, in a
>   happened, something will
>   murdered, of being

Fear,
>   narrow places, in; claustrophobia
>   poisoned, of being
>   *sadness, with*
>   solitude, of
>   *touch, of*
>   water, of
>   work, dread of

Feigning sick

Foolish behavior

Forgetful
>   *words while speaking, of; word
>   hunting*

Frightened easily
>   cause, without ★

Gestures, makes
>   convulsive
>   hands, motion, involuntary, fold-
>   ing hands,
>   unfolding coverings, and •
>   head, to the
>   slow
>   strange attitudes and positions
>   usual vocation, of his
>   violent

Groping, as if in the dark

Homesickness

Hurry, haste

Hypochondriasis

Hysteria

Ideas, deficiency of

Idiocy

Imbecility

Indifference, apathy
>   *ennui, with*

Indolence, aversion to work
>   evening
>   eating, after

Industrious, mania for work

Insanity, madness
>   *masturbation, form*
>   **strength, increased, with ★**

Introspection

Irresolution, indecision

Irritability
>   morning, waking, on
>   afternoon
>   waking, on

Jumping, bed, out of
Lamenting, bemoaning, wailing
    anxious
Lascivious, lustful
Laughing
    agg.
    involuntarily
    sardonic
Light, desire for
Loathing, general
Loathing, life, at
Loquacity
    night
Mania
    rage, with
Meddlesome
Meditation
Memory, active
Memory, loss of
    apoplexy, after
Memory, weakness of
    expressing oneself, for
    occurrences of the day, for
    words, of
Mildness
Mistakes, reading, in
    time, in
Moaning, groaning, whining
    anxious
Mood, changeable, variable
    repulsive
Morose, cross, fretful, ill-humor, peevish
    morning, bed, in
    waking, on
Muttering
    evening
Nymphomania
Obstinate, headstrong
Prostration of mind, mental exhaustion, brain-fag
Quarrelsome, scolding
Quiet, disposition
Rage, fury
    night
    epilepsy, rage with
    shrieking, with

Recognize: relatives, does not recognize
    his
Religious mania
    melancholy
Reserved
    eating, after •
Restlessness
    night
    anxious
    bed, go from one bed to another, wants to
    internal
    pain, during
    paroxysms, during •
Rocking amel.
Runs about
Sadness, despondency, dejection, mental depression, gloom, melancholy
    morning
    headache, during
    menses, during
    waking, on
Searching on floor
Secretive
Self-torture
Senses, acute
    dull, blunted
    vanishing of
    pain, from ★
Sensitive, oversensitive
Sentimental
Serious, earnest
Shrieking, screaming, shouting
    convulsions, before
    after
    cramps in abdomen, from
    pain, with the
    sudden ★
Sighing
    epileptic attacks, before
Sit, inclination to
Slowness
Speech, abrupt
    babbling
    delirious
    extravagant

535

Speech,
 hasty
 incoherent
  night
  epileptic attack, after
 nonsensical
 prattling
 random at night, at •
 slow
 unintelligible
 wandering
 wild
Spitting, faces of people, in
Spoken to, aversion to being
Starting, fright, from and as from
 sleep, during
  from
Strange, everything seems
Striking
Stupefaction, as if intoxicated
 convulsions, between
 sleepiness, with
Suicidal disposition
Suspicious, mistrustful
Talk, indisposed to, desires to be silent,
 taciturn
  eating, after
Talking, sleep, in
Talks, himself, to
Tears himself
Thinking, complaints agg., of
Thoughts, thoughful
 wandering
Time, passes too slowly, appears longer
Timidity
 appearing in public, about
Torments, himself
Torpor
Touched, aversion to being
Tranquillity, serenity, calmness
Unconsciousness, coma, stupor
 apoplexy, in
 convulsions, after
 epilepsy, after
 menses, during
 sudden

Violent, vehement
Weary of life
Weeping, tearful mood
 aloud, sobbing
 convulsions, during
 involuntary
 spasmodic
Work, aversion to mental

PLUMBUM ACETICUM

Amorous
Sadness, despondency, dejection, mental
 depression, gloom, melancholy

PLUMBUM CHROMICUM

Confusion of mind
Restlessness
Shrieking, screaming, shouting

PLECTRANTHUS FRUTICOSOS

Answers, distracted
Concentration, difficult
 working, while •
Discomfort
 morning on waking
Dullness, sluggishness, difficulty of think-
 ing and comprehending, torpor
Excitement, excitable
 night
Hurry, eating, while
Indolence, aversion to work
Irritability
 forenoon
 conversation, from
 noise, from
Loathing, general, when rising •
Moaning, sleep, during
Morose, cross, fretful, ill-humor, peevish
Sadness, despondency, dejection, mental
 depression, gloom, melancholy
Thoughts, wandering
Weeping, aloud, sobbing

PLUMBAGO LITTERALIS

Aversion, everything, to
Sadness, despondency, dejection, mental
    depression gloom, melancholy
Talk, indisposed to, desire to be silent,
    taciturn

PNEUMOCOCCINUM

Anguish
Delusions, walk, he cannot
Fear, death, of
    disease, of impending
    going out, of
Loathing,, life, at
Memory, weakness of
Sadness, despondency, dejection, mental
    depression, gloom, melancholy

PODOPHYLLUM PELTATUM

Anxiety
    evening
        twilight, in the
    health, about
    salvation, about
Bite, desire to
Carried, desire to be
    shoulder, over
Confusion of mind, morning
Death, presentiment of
Delirium
Delusions, die, he was about to
    heart disease, having
        is going to have, and die
    sick, being
        he is going to be
Despair
    religious despair of salvation
Discouraged
Dullness, sluggishness, difficulty of think-
    ing and comprehending, torpor
Excitement, excitable
Fear, apprehension, dread
    death, of
    disease, of impending

Forgetful, chill, during
    heat, after
    words while speaking, of; word
    hunting
Hypochondriasis
Irritability
    liver trouble, in
Loathing, life, at
Loquacity
    alternating with chill and heat ★
    chill, during
    heat, during
    rambling ★
Memory, weakness of,
    say, for what is about to
    words, of
Moaning, groaning, whining
    night
    children, in
    cough, during
    dentition, in
    heat, during
    sleep, during
        eyelids half closed, rolling of
        head, with
Music, headache from
Prostration of mind, mental exhaus-
    tion, brain-fag
Restlessness, night
Sadness, despondency, dejection, mental
    depression, gloom, melancholy
    eating, after
Shrieking, screaming, shouting
    pain, with the
Stupefaction, as if intoxicated
Talking, sleep, in
Weeping, sleep, in
Whining, whimpering, sleep, in ★

POLYGONUM HYDROPIPEROIDES AUT PUNCTATUM

Hysteria
Irritability, sadness, with
Sadness, despondency, dejection, mental
    depression, gloom, melancholy
Torpor

POLYPORUS PINICOLA

Restlessness, night
    midnight, 3h. after
Retirement, desire for
Sadness, despondency, dejection, mental
    depression, gloom, melancholy

POPULUS CANDICANS

Discusses her symptoms with everyone •

POTHOS FOETIDUS

Anguish, stool, before
Concentration, difficult
Contradict, disposition to

(BACILLUS) PROTEUS

Anger, contradiction, from
Company, aversion to; presence of
    other people agg. the symp-
    toms; desire for solitude
Crawling, rolling on the floor
Irritability
Kicks
Rolling on the floor
Sadness, despondency, dejection, men-
    tal depression, gloom, melan-
    choly
Suicidal, thoughts
Throws thing away

PRUNUS SPINOSA

Cheerful, gay, mirthful
    evening in bed
Complaining, morning in bed •
    pain on waking, on
Discontented, displeased, dissatisfied
Excitement, excitable
    evening in bed
Hurry, walking, while
Indifference, apathy
    pleasure, to
Indolence, sadness, from

Irritability
Memory, weakness of,
    pains, from, suddenly ★
Morose, cross, fretful, ill-humor, peevish
Restlessness
    driving about
Sadness, despondency, dejection, men-
    tal depression, gloom, melan-
    choly
    work-shy, in
Thinking, complaints amel., of
Weeping, morning

PSILOCYBE CAERULESCENS

Absent-minded, unobserving
    conversing, when
Delusions, imaginations, hallucinations,
    illusions
    visions, has
Dullness, sluggishness, difficulty of think-
    ing and comprehending, torpor
Indifference, apathy
    everything, to
Memory, weakness of
    do, for what was about to
Moral feeling, want of
Nymphomania
Sadness, despondency, dejection, men-
    tal depression, gloom, melan-
    choly
Schizophrenia
Time passes too quickly, appears shorter
Tranquillity, serenity, calmness
Weeping, tearful mood

PSORINUM

Absent-minded, unobserving
Ailments from:
    anticipation, foreboding, pre-
    sentiment
    excitement, emotional
    sexual ★
    work, mental

Anger, irascibility
    easily
Anguish
    daytime
       5-17 h. •
Anxiety
    daytime
       5-17 h. •
    business, about
    closing eyes, on
    conscience, as if guilty of a crime
    eating, after
    fear, with
    future, about
    health, about
    hypochondriacal
    motion, from downward ★
    pregnancy, in
    pressure on the chest, from
    riding, while
       down hill
    salvation, about
       morning •
Bed, remain in, desire to
Cares, worries, full of
    night •
Cheerful, gay, mirthful
    morning
    alternating with lachrymose mood
       sadness
    constipated, when
Company, aversion to; presence of other people agg. the symptoms; desire for solitude
Concentration, difficult •
    calculating, while
Confusion of mind
    evening
    night
       waking, on
    air, in open, amel.
    calculating, when
    identity: duality, sense of
    head separated from body, as if
    intoxicated, as after being
    waking, on

Death, conviction of
    after fever, epistaxis amel. •
    desires
    thoughts of
Delirium
    fever, during
Delusions, imaginations, hallucinations, illusions
    doomed, being
    double, of being
    fortune, he was going to lose his
    head, separated from body, is
    poor, he is
    sick, being
    spectres, ghosts, spirits, sees
       throng upon him
Desire, uncontrollable, itching, for ★
Despair
    itching of the skin, from •
    recovery, of
       convalescence, during •
    religious despair of salvation
    typhus, after; nose bleed amel. •
Dipsomania, alcoholism
Dirtiness
Discontended, displeased, dissatisfied
Discouraged
Doubtful, recovery, of
Dullness, sluggishness, difficulty of thinking and comprehending, torpor
    forenoon
    waking, on
Dwells on past disaggreeable occurrences
Emotions, trembling, after ★
Estranged from her family
Excitement, excitable
    sleep, before
    trembling, while
Exertion, agg. from mental
Fancies, exaltation of
    lascivious
Fear, apprehension, dread
    busy streets ★
    death, of
       heart symptoms, during

Fear,
>   disaster of
>   disease, of impending
>   cancer, of •
>   **evil, of**
>   *failure, business, in* •
>   **misfortune, of**
>   *poverty, of*
>   *riding in a carriage, when*
>   thunderstorm, of
>   waking, on
Forgetful
Forsaken feeling
Fur, wraps up in summer
Gestures, grasping or reaching at some-
>   *thing at flocks; carphologia*
>   *picks at bed clothes*
>   *wringing the hands*
Impatience
Impulse, wash, to ★
Indifference, apathy
Indolence, aversion to work
Insanity, madness
Insolence
Intolerance
Irresolution, indecision
Irritability
>   morning
>   evening
>   night ★
>   *babies, in sick* •
>   *waking, on*
>   children, sleepless day and night •
>   *climacteric period, during*
>   *easily* •
>   *heat, during*
>   sleeplessness, with
>   children, in •
>   talking, while
>   *waking, on*
Jesting
Laughing, morning
Loquacity
Mania
>   alternating with depression

Melancholy, financial ★
>   religious ★
Memory, weakness of
>   heard, for what has
>   places, for
>   read, for what has
>   *said, for what has*
Mistakes, localities, in
>   time, in
Moaning, groaning, whining
Mood, changeable, variable
>   *repulsive*
Morose, cross, fretful, ill-humor, peevish
>   *night*
>   children, in
>   climacteric period, at •
Obstinate, headstrong
>   *children, annoy those about them* •
>   eruptions, during •
Passionate
Pessimist
Playful, alternating with sadness •
Prostration of mind, mental exhaus-
>   tion, brain-fag
Pushed, down ★
Quarrelsome, scolding
>   morning
>   evening
Recognize own house, does not
Religious affections
>   melancholia
Remorse
Restlessness
>   night
>   anxious
>   *children, night, but morning fresh*
>   *and lively* •
>   *eruptions, with* •
>   **eruptions, with ★**
>   *storm, before*
>   during
>   thunderstorm, before •
Riding in a carriage, averse to •
>   wants to •

Sadness, despondency, dejection, mental depression, gloom, melancholy
  alternating with vivacity
  climaxis, during
  eruptions, suppressed, with
  itching, from •
  menses, before
  suicidal disposition, with
Sensitive, oversensitive
  moral impressions, to
  pain, to
Sentimental
Shrieking, children, in, night
  sleep, during
  sleep, during
Starting, startled
  easily
  fright, from and as from
  sleep, from
  trifles,· at
Stupefaction, as if intoxicated
  night, waking must rise, on •
  debauchery, as after •
  vertigo, during
  waking, on
Suicidal disposition
  sadness, from
  thoughts
Talking, sleep, in
  children, in
Thoughts, disagreeable
  persistent
    ideas, of, which first appeared in his dreams •
    unpleasant subjects, on walking
  vanishing of
    overlifting, after •
Torments everyone with his complaints
Unconsciousness, coma, stupor
  morning
Violent, morning
Washing always her hands
Weary of life
Weeping, tearful mood
  night
  children, in, night

Well before an attack, feels ★
  feels very well before being worse ★
Work, aversion to mental

PTELEA TRIFOLIATA

Absent-minded, starts when spoken to
Anger, irascibility
Anxiety
Company, aversion to; presence of other people agg. the symptoms; desire for solitude
Concentration, difficult
  morning
  forenoon
Confusion of mind
  evening
  night
  ascending agg.
Conversation, aversion to
Delusions, neglected his duty, he has
Dullness, sluggishness, difficulty of thinking and comprehending, torpor
Forgetful
  waking, on
Hurry, haste
  writing, in
Indifference, apathy
  duties, to
Intolerance of noise
Irritability
  noise, from
  sadness, with
  trifles, from
Memory, weakness of
  names, for proper
Mistakes, writing, in
Morose, trifles, about
Prostration of mind, mental exhaustion, brain fag
Restlessness
  night
  rising, on

Sadness, despondency, dejection, mental
    depression, gloom, melancholy
      morning after waking
    eating, after
    headache, during
Sensitive, noise, to
Starting, startled
    noise, from
    spoken to, when
Stupefaction, as if intoxicated
Talk, indisposed to, desire to be silent,
    taciturn
Thinking, aversion to
Thoughts, rush, flow of
Will, loss of
Work, aversion to mental
    impossible

PULSATILLA PRATENSIS

Abrupt, rough
    rough, yet affectionate
Absent-minded, unobserving
Absorbed, buried in thought
Adulterous
Affection, craving for, in children ★
Affections, in general ★
Affectionate (see Kiss)
Ailments from :
    ambition, deceived
    anger, vexation
      anxiety, with
      fright, with
      silent grief, with
    **anticipation, foreboding, pre-
      sentiment**
    bad news
    business failure
    disappointment
    excitement, emotional
    fear
    fright
    grief
    hurry
    jealousy
    joy, excessive
    literary, scientific failure
    mortification
    sexual excesses

Ambition
Amorous
Anger, irascibility
    answer, when obliged to
    conversation, from
    face, with red
    talk, indisposed to
Anguish
    daytime
    morning
    night
    air amel., open
    palpitation, with
    *tremulous a., rest agg., motion
      amel.* •
Anorexia mentalis ★
Answers: aversion to answer
    monosyllable
    nods, by ★
Anxiety
    daytime
    morning
      waking, on
    afternoon
    evening
      bed, in
      *uneasiness and anxiety,
        must uncover*
    night
      waking, on
      midnight, before
    air, in open, amel.
    bed, in
      driving out of
    business, about
    chill, during
    climacteric period, during
    clothes and open windows, must
      loosen
    conscience, as if guilty of a crime
    dark, in
    dreams, on waking from frightful
    drinking, when, after •
    exaggerated ★
    fear, with
    fever, during
    flushes of heat, during

Anxiety,
  future, about
  head, with congestion to
  health, about
  hot air, as if in •
  house, in
  house hold matters, about (in
      morning) •
  hypochondriacal
    mania to read medical books
  lying, while
    side, on
        left
  menses, before
  mental exertion, from
  motion, from, amel.
  noise, from
  salvation, about
    scruples, excessive religious
  shuddering, with
  sitting, while
  sleep, on going to
        during
  suicidal disposition, with
  waking, on
  walking, air, in open, amel.
  warmth, from
  weary of life, with
Asks for nothing
Audacity
Avarice
Aversion, everything, to
  sex, religious aversion to opposite
  women, to
Bargaining
Bed, remain in, desires to
Begging, entreating, supplicating
Beside oneself, being
Bite, spoon etc., bites
Boaster, squander through ostentation
Business, averse to
Capriciousness
Carefulness
Cares, worries, full of
        morning
    business, about his
    domestic affairs, about

Carried, desires to be
  caressed and, desires to be
  fondled, and ★
    slowly •
Cautious
  anxious
Censorious, critical
Change, desire for
Chaotic, confused behavior
Cheerful, gay, mirthful
        evening, bed, in
    chill, during
Childbed, mental symptoms during
Childish behavior
Climacteric period agg.
Company, aversion to; presence of other
        people agg. the symptoms; de-
        sire for solitude
    heat, during
    perspiration, during
Company, desires for; aversion to soli-
        tude, company amel.
        evening
Complaints, can't describe properly ★
Complaining
Comprehension easy
Concentration, difficult
Confidence, want of self
Confusion of mind
        morning, waking, on
        evening
        night, waking, on
        eating, after
        heat, during
        identity, duality, sense of
        intoxicated, as after being
        loses his way in well-known
            streets
        mental exertion, from
        motion, from
        sitting, while
        waking, on
        walking, air, in open, amel.
        warm room, in
Conscientious about trifles
        eating, during

Consolation amel.
Contemptuous
Contradiction, is intolerant of
Contradictory, actions are c. to intention
Contrary
Conversation agg.
Coquettish, not enough
too much
Corrupt, venal
Courageous
Cowardice
Credulous
Cursing, swearing
Darkness agg.
Death, agony before
desires
presentiment of
thoughts of
**Deception causes grief and morti-
fication ★**
Deceitful, sly
Delirium
night
anxious
bed and escapes, springs up suddenly from
chill, during
encephalitis
frightful
menses, during
mild
raging, raving
sad
sleep, comatose, during
sleepiness, with
sleeplessness, and ★
sorrowful
trembling, with
violent
Delirium tremens, mania-a potu
*Delusions, imaginations, hallucina-
tions, illusions*
night
alone, she is always
world, she is alone in the
animals, of
anxious

Delusions,
body looks odious ●
*bed, naked man is wrapped in the
bed clothes with her* ●
someone is in bed with him
bees, sees ●
black objects and people, sees
cats, sees
black
clouds, heavy black, enveloped
her
criminals, about
deserted, forsaken, is
devils, sees
taken by the devil, he will be
divided into two parts
dogs, sees
black
doomed, being
double, of being
eyes, of big
fancy, illusions of
sleep, on going to ●
fire, visions of
world is on
hearing, illusions of
home, away from, is
images, phantoms, sees
night
black
closing eyes, on
dark, in the
frightful
insects, sees
insulted, he is
man, naked m. in bed ●
mortification, after
music, he hears
delightful
neglected his duty, he has
he is
people, sees
noise, making ●
pregnant, she is
pursued by enemies
religious
scream, obliging to
small, things appear

Delusions,
 smell, of
 spectres, ghosts, spirits, sees
  black forms when dreaming
 strange, familiar things seem
 strangers, he sees
  surrounded by
 visions, has
  evening
  closing the eyes, on
  horrible
   dark, in the
   strikes at them and hold up the
    cross •
 vivid
 well, he is
 women are evil and will injure his
  soul •
 wrong, he has done
Dementia senilis, talking, with foolish,
  night •
Desires, full of
 indefinite
 present, things not
 this and that
Despair
 heat, during
 religious despair of salvation
 social position, of
Dipsomania, alcoholism
 weakness of character, from
Discontented, displeased, dissatisfied
  morning
  evening
   amel.
 everything, with
 himself, with
Discouraged
  morning, bed, in •
  evening
 anxiety, with
 business, aversion to
 irresolution •
 praying, with •
 waking, on
Disgust
 everything, with

Dishonest
Doubtful, recovery, of
 soul's welfare, of
Dream, as if in a
Dullness, sluggishness, difficulty
 of thinking and compre-
 hending, torpor
 morning
  waking, on
 afternoon
 evening
  amel.
 damp air, from
 heat, during
 mental exertion, from
 waking, on
 warm room, on entering a
Eat, refuses to
Eccentricity, religious
Ecstasy, heat, during
Effeminate ★
Embittered, exasperated
Emptiness, sensation of ★
Envy
 avidity, and
 hate, and
 qualities of other's at
Escape, attempts to
Estranged, being kind with strangers,
 but not with his family and
 entourage
Exacting, too ★
Exaltation, religious ★
Excitement, excitable
 evening
  bed, in
 night
 bad news, after
 chill, during
 joy, from
 menses, during
 weakness, with
Exertion, agg. from mental
Express herself, cannot ★
Fanaticism

Fancies, exaltation of
      evening, bed, in
      night
      heat, during
      sleeplessness, with
    vivid, lively, midnight, after •
    waking, on
Fastidious
Fear, apprehensions, dread
      morning
        waking, on •
      evening
        twilight
      night
    alone, of being
      evening
    apoplexy, of
      evening •
    crossing a bridge or place, of
    crowd, in a
      public places, of; agoraphobia
    dark, of
    death, of
    diarrhoea with fear
    disaster, of
    disease, of impending
    dogs, of ★
    eating, of
    escape, with desire to
    everything, constant of
    evil, of
    fit, of having a
    get talked about, to
    ghosts, of
      evening
      night
    high places, of
    humiliated, of being
    insanity, losing his reason, of
    life long
    men, dread, fear of
    misfortune, of
    **narrow place, in; claustropho-
      bia**
    vaults, churches and cellars, of

Fear,
    neglected, of being •
    opinions of others, of
    overpowering
    palpitation, with
    people, of; anthropophobia
    position, to lose his lucrative
    poverty, of
    rail, of going by
    suffocation, of, night
    tremulous
    waking, on
    women, of
    work, dread of
Finance, aptitude for
    inaptitude for
Flatterer
Flattery, gives everything, when flat-
    tered
Forgetful
    drunkards, forgetfulness in
    mental exertion, from
    words while speaking, of; word
      hunting
Forsaken feeling
    evening
Frightened easily
Frivolous
Gamble (*see* **Play**)
Gestures
    hands, involuntary motions of
      the
      folding hands •
    talking, gesticulates, while, head,
      with
    wringing the hands
Greed, cupidity
Grief
    morning
    *business in morning, when think-
      ing of his* •
    headache from grief
    silent
    submissiveness, with •
Grunting
Hatred
    women, of •
Haughty
Heedless

Hide, desire to
High places agg.
Homesickness
*Horrible things, sad stories, affect her
    profoundly*
Hurry, haste
    occupation, in
Hypochondriasis
    evening
    morose
    weeping, with
Hypocrisy
Hysteria
    changing symptoms •
    fainting, hysterical
    menses, before
        during
        after
Ideas abundant, clearness of mind
    evening
        bed, in
    night
Imbecility
Impatience
    heat, with
Impulsive
Inconsolable
Indifference, apathy
    business affairs, to
    chill, during
    everything, to
    fever, during
    joy and suffering, to
    joyless
    opposite sex, to ★
    pleasure, to
Indiscretion
Indolence, aversion to work
    evening
    physical
Inquisitive
Insanity, madness .
    black insanity with despair and
        weary of life from fear of
        mortification or of loss of po-
        sition
    climacteric period, during

Insanity,
    drunkards, in
    erotic
    fortune, after gaining
    melancholy
    menses, during
        suppressed, with
    mortification, from
    position, from fear to lose the
    puerperal
    religious
    restlessness, with
    travel, with desire to
Introspection
Irresolution, indecision
    evening
    indolence, with
Irritability
    daytime
        morning, waking, on
        evening
    air, in open
    children, in
    chill, during
    eating, after
    heat, during
    menses, during
        before ★
    questioned, when
    sadness, with
    taciturn
    takes everything in bad part
    waking, on
    warm room, in
Jealousy
    drunkenness, during
    men, between
Jesting, aversion to
    joke, cannot take a
    roguish •
Joy, headache from excessive
Jumping, bed, out of
    mania, in
Kisses everyone (affectionate) •
Kleptomania
    steals money ★

Lamenting, bemoaning, wailing
    anxious
    fever, during
    heat of whole body except hands, with •
    sadness, in •
Lascivious, lustful
Late, always too
Laughing
    easily
    eating, after ★
    involuntarily
        eating, after •
    weeping or laughing on all occasions
Liar
    charlatan and
Libertinism
Loathing, general
Loathing, life, at
    work, at
Looked at, agg. mental symptoms
    cannot bear to be ★
Loquacity, night
Love with one of the own sex, homosex-
    uality, tribadism
Malicious, spiteful, vindictive
Mania
    menses, suppressed, after •
Marriage seemed unendurable, idea of
Memory, active
Memory, weakness of
    expressing oneself, for
        pains, from, suddenly ★
    labor, fatigue, from mental
    names, for proper
    verses, to learn
    words, of
Mildness
Misanthropy
Mischievous
Mistakes, localities, in
    speaking, in
        misplacing words
    writing, in
        omitting letters

Moaning, groaning, whining
    child, if it desires to be carried
    children, carried, while being •
    heat, during
        with anxious breathing ★
    sleep, during
    stool, before •
Monomania
Mood, alternating
    changeable, variable
    repulsive
Morose, cross, fretful, ill-humor, peevish
    morning, bed, in
    afternoon
    evening
    amel.
    children, in
    chill, during
    eating, after
    hypochondriasis, in
    walking in open air, after •
Morphinism
Music agg.
Naked, wants to be, sleep, in
Narrating her symptoms agg.
Nymphomania
Obscene, lewd
Obstinate, headstrong
Offended, easily; takes everything in bad part
Optimistic
Play, passion for gambling, to make money
Praying
Pregnancy, mental affections in
Prostration of mind, mental exhaustion, brain-fag
Quarrelsome, scolding
Quiet disposition
    clasped, with hands •
    hypochondriasis, in
Rage, fury
    evening
    night
    headache, with
    paroxysms, in

Rashness
Reading, aversion *to* read
    passion to read medical books
Rebels against poultice
Religious affections
    fanaticism
    horror of the opposite sex
    melancholia
    narrow-minded in religious questions
    very religious ★
Remorse
    evening •
    night •
    waking, on •
Reproaches himself
Repugnance, everything, to ★
Reserved
Restlessness
    morning, rising, after •
    night
    anxious
    bed, in
    driving out of
    tossing about in
    conscience, of
    driving about
    heat, during
    after
    menses, before
    · *during*
    motion amel. •
    moving constantly amel.
    walking, air amel., in open
    warm bed agg.
Reverence for those around him
Rocking amel.
Roving, senseless, insane
Runs, street at night, in •
Sadness, despondency, dejection,
    mental depression, gloom,
    melancholy
    morning
    evening
    air, in open, amel.
    anger, after
    from

Sadness,
    bad news, after
    business, when thinking of
    · *chill, during*
    climaxis, during
    drunkards, in
    drunkenness, during
    eating, after
    epistaxis, after •
    heat, during
    injuries, head, of the.
    labor, from
    menses, before
        during
        suppressed
    misfortune, as if from
    mortification, after
    periodical
    perspiration, during
    pollutions, from
    puerperal
    quiet
    talk, indisposed to
    vexation, after
    walking, air, in open, amel.
    warm room, in
Selfishness, egoism
Selflessness
Senses, dull, blunted
    vanishing of
Sensitive, oversensitive
    children
    heat, during
    moral impressions, to
    music, to
    noise, to·
    puberty, in
Sentimental
Serious, earnest
Servile, obsequious, submissive
Shrieking, screaming, shouting
    anger, in
    children, in
    sleep, during
    delusions, from
    pain, with the
    sleep, during

Sighing
> heat, during
> sleep, in
> waking, on •

Sit, inclination to
Sits, erect
> stiff, quite
> **still**
> *wrapped in deep, sad thoughts*
> *and notices nothing, as if*

Slowness
Speech, hesitating
> *wandering*

Spying everything
Squanders, boasting, from
Staring, thoughtless
Starting, startled
> *evening*
> *dreams, in*
>> from a dream
> *sleep, during*
>> *from*
> *sleepiness with*

Strange crank
Stupefaction, as if intoxicated
> *afternoon*
> injury to head, after

Suicidal disposition
> anxiety, from
> *drowning, by*
> heat, during
> poison, by
> shooting, by
> *thoughts*

Suspicious, mistrustful
> *enemy, considering everybody his* •

Sympathy, compassion
Talk, indisposed to, desire to be silent, taciturn
> *heat, during*
> *sadness, in*
Talking, sleep, in
Theorizing
Thoughts, control of thoughts lost
> *persistent*
>> **night**
> desires, of
> **music, in night about** •

Thoughts,
> *rush, flow of*
>> *evening*
>>> *in bed*
>> *night*
>> *sleeplessness from*
> *thoughtful*
> *vanishing of*
> *wandering*

Timidity
> awkward, and
> **bashful**

Torpor
Twilight agg. mental symptoms
Unconsciousness, coma, stupor
> morning
> evening
> *apoplexy, in*
> chill, during
> **crowded room, in a**
> dream, does not know where he
>> is, waking, on
> *fever, during*
> menses, during
> *parturition, during*
> **transient**
>> **afternoon in warm room** •
> **warm room, in**

Ungrateful, avarice, from
Unsympathetic
Usurer
Vanity
Walk, walking in open air amel. mental
> symptoms
Wearisome
> evening
Weary of life
> *mortification, after* •
Weeping, tearful mood
> morning
> afternoon, 16h. •
> *night*
> agg.
> **air, in open, amel.**
> aloud, wobbing

Weeping,
  alternating with laughter
  amel.
  anger, after
  answering a question, at •
  anxiety, after
  causeless
  children, in
  chill, during
  consolation amel.
  coryza, during
  desire to weep, all the time
  disturbed at work, when •
  easily
  eating, after
  heat, during
  interrupted, when •
  involuntary
  joyful or sad thing, at
  menses, before
    during
  mortification, after
  nursing, while
  pain, with the
  perspiration, during
  pregnancy, during
  sleep, in
  stool, before
  telling of her sickness, when
  trifles, at
    laughing or weeping on
    every occasion
  waking, on
  walking in open air amel.
Well, says he is, when very sick
Will, weakness of
Work, aversion to mental
  desire for, evening
Yielding disposition

PULSATILLA NUTALLIANA

Anger, irascibility
Anxiety
Discomfort, night

Dullness, sluggishness, difficulty of think-
  ing and comprehending, torpor
    morning
Homesickness
Irritability
  noise, from
Restlessness
  night
Sadness, despondency, dejection, mental
  depression, gloom, melancholy
    afternoon
Spoken to, averse to being
Weeping, trifles, at

PYRETHRUM
PARTHENIUM

Delirium
Excitement, excitable
Loquacity
Restlessness
Stupefaction, as if intoxicated

PYROGENIUM

Ailments from :
  excitement, emotional ★
  work, mental
Anxiety
Confusion of mind
  identity: duality, sense of
Delirium
  closing the eyes, on
  sepsis, from
Delusions, imaginations, hallucinations,
  illusions
  bed, too hard
  body covers the whole bed •
  scattered about bed tossed
    about to get the pieces to-
    gether
  crowded with arms and legs
  double, of being
  identity, errors of personal
    someone else, she is

Delusions,
  large, himself seems too
  rich, as if he is ★
  wealth, of
Duality, sense of ★
Excitement, excitable
Fear, apprehension, dread
Irritability
Loquacity
Prostration of mind, mental exhaus-
  tion, brain-fag
Restlessness
  anxious
  bed, tossing about in
Rocking amel.
Sadness, despondency, dejection, men-
  tal depression, gloom, melan-
  choly
Senses, acute ★
Sensitive, oversensitive
Speech, faster than ever before, espe-
  cially during fever ●
Talks, himself, to
Thinking, faster than ever before, espe-
  cially during fever ●
Weeping, causeless, without knowing
  why

PYRUS AMERICANUS

Clairvoyance
Confusion of mind, identity, as to his
Delusions, body, able to go out of body
  and walk around, looking down
  upon ●
  crowded with arms and legs
  identity, errors of personal
Determination, gloomy ●
Discouraged
Fear, happen, something will
Foolish behavior
Gestures, convulsive
Hysteria
Moaning, groaning, whining
Reading, averison to read

Restlessness
Sadness, despondency, dejection, mental
  depression, gloom, melancholy
Selfishness, egoism
Unconciousness, coma, stupor
Weeping, tearful mood

QUASSIA AMARA

Absent-minded unobserving
Anxiety, night amel. ●
  midnight, after
  reading, preventing ●
  sleep, on going to
Dipsomania, alcoholism
Discomfort

QUERCUS E GLANDIBUS

Dipsomania, alcoholism

RADIUM METALLICUM

Company, aversion to; alternating with
    bursts of pleasantry and sar-
    casm
Company, desire for; aversion to soli-
    tude, company amel.
Fear, ghosts, of
Irritability
Morose, cross, fretful, ill-humor, peevish
Restlessness
Sadness, despondency, dejection, mental
    depression, gloom, melancholy

RAJANIA SUBSAMARAJA

Abusive, insulting
Answers, incoherently
Confusion of mind, heat, during
Delirium, muttering
Dullness, sluggishness, difficulty of think-
    ing and comprehending, torpor
Eccentricity
Gestures, grasping or reaching at some-
    thing, at flocks; carphologia
Indifference, surroundings, to the
Lascivious, lustful
Obscene, lewd songs
Rage, fury
Religious, songs •
Sighing
Speech, incoherent
Weeping, tearful mood

RANUNCULUS ACRIS

Anxiety
Restlessness

RANUNCULUS BULBOSUS

Absent-minded, unobserving

Absorbed, buried in thought
Abstraction of mind
Abusive, insulting
    forenoon •
Ailments from :
    anger vexation
Anger, irascibility
    alternating with cares •
    alternating with discontentment •
        discouragement
        timidity
    easily
    trembling, with
Anguish, forenoon
Anxiety
    morning, waking, on
    forenoon
    evening
    night
    eating, before
    after
    future, about
Capriciousness, daytime
    evening
Carefulness
Cares, alternating with quarrelsome-
    ness •
Censorious, critical
Cheerful, evening, bed, in
Company, desire for; aversion to soli-
    tude, company amel.
    evening
    alone agg., while
Concentration, difficult
    on attempting to concentrate has
    a vacant feeling
Confidence, want of self
Confusion of mind
    morning
    concentrate the mind, on attempt-
    ing to
    loses his way in well-known
    streets
    mental exertion, from
Cowardice
Death, desires

553

Delirium
    look fixed on one point, staring
Delirium tremens, mania-a-potu
    loquacity, with
Delusions, imaginations, hallucinations,
    illusions
    spectres, ghosts, spirits, sees
    strange, familiar things seem
    war, being at
    water, of
Dipsomania, alcoholism
Discomfort, heat, during •
Discontented, displeased, dissatisfied
    evening
Discouraged
    alternating with anger
    quarrelsomeness •
Dullness, sluggishness, difficulty of
    thinking and comprehending,
    torpor
    mental exertion, from
    pollution, after
Escape, attempts to
Excitement, evening, bed, in
Exertion, agg. from mental
Fear, apprehension, dread
    evening
    alone, of being
    evening
    ghosts, of
    evening
    night
    solitude, of
    tremulous
    work, dread of
Forgetful
Imbecility
Indifference, apathy
Indolence, aversion to work
    morning
Irritability
    forenoon
    evening
    alternating with cowardice •
    timidity
Lamenting, bemoaning, wailing
Laughing, sardonic

Loathing, work, at
Malicious, spiteful, vindictive
Meditation
Mood, changeable, variable
Morose, cross, fretful, ill-humor, peevish
Offended, easily; takes everything in
    bad part
Prostration of mind, mental exhaus-
    tion, brain-fag
Quarrelsome, scolding
    morning
    forenoon
    alternating with care and discon-
    tentment •
Restlessness
    night
    feverish
    headache, during
    internal
    walking, while
Sadness, despondency, dejection, mental
    depression, gloom, melancholy
    evening
    suicidal disposition, with
Senses, dull, blunted
    vanishing of
Sensitive, oversensitive
    evening
    want of sensitiveness
Sit, inclination to
Staring, thoughtless
Stupefaction, as if intoxicated
    knows not where he is
    vertigo, during
Suicidal disposition, sadness, from
Talks, himself, to
Thinking, complaints agg., of
Thoughts, thoughtful
    vanishing of
    mental exertion, on
Timidity
    afternoon
    alternating with quarrelsome-
    ness •
    vexation
Unconsciousness, coma, stupor, morning
    dream, does not know where he is

Violent, vehement
Wearisome
Weeping, tearful mood
> *evening*
> headache, with

RANUNCULUS SCELERATUS

Absent-minded, unobserving
Anxiety
> night
> waking, on
Cheerful, evening, bed, in
Concentration, difficult
Confusion of mind
> morning
Delirium
Delusions, dead person, sees
> vermin, sees crawl about
> worms, creeping of
Discouraged, evening
Dullness, sluggishness, difficulty of thinking and comprehending, torpor
> evening
> sleeplessness, with
Excitement, evening, bed, in
Fear, apprehension, dread
Grief
Hydrophobia
Ideas, deficiency of
Indolence, aversion to work
> morning
> evening
Irritability
Laughing
> immoderately
> sardonic
> violent
Memory, weakness of
> thought, for what has just
Morose, cross, fretful, ill-humor, peevish
Prostration of mind, morning
Restlessness, night
> *bed, tossing about in*

Sadness, despondency, dejection, mental depression, gloom, melancholy
> evening
Senses, dull, blunted
Shrieking, screaming, shouting
> anxiety, from
Sighing
Sit, inclination to
Thoughts, vanishing of
Unconsciousness, coma, stupor, vertigo, during
Work, aversion to mental

RAPHANUS SATIVUS

Activity, mental
Anxiety
> *hypochondriacal*
> stool, during
Aversion, children, to
> little girls (a woman) •
> men, to
> sex, to her own •
> women, to
Capriciousness
Concentration, difficult
Confusion of mind
> morning, rising and after, on
> night
Death, presentiment of
> alternating with rage •
Delusions, disease, unrecognized, has an •
> places at a time, of being in different
> talking, she is •
Dipsomania, alcoholism
Dullness, sluggishness, difficulty of thinking and comprehending, torpor
Excitement, excitable
Fear, apprehension, dread
> burden, of becoming a •
> death, of
> men, dread, fear of
> women of

555

Forgetful
 menses, during •
Hatred, woman, from a ★
Hopeful, alternating with sadness
Hysteria
 menses, during first day of •
Indifference, apathy
Insanity, madness
 capricious •
Jealousy
Lascivious, lustful
Loathing, general
 evening
Mania
Memory, active
Memory, weakness of
Murmuring in sleep
Muttering, sleep, in
Nymphomania
Prostration of mind, mental exhaustion, brain-fag
Quarrelsome
 sleep, in
Rage, fury
Sadness, despondency, dejection, mental depression, gloom, melancholy
 waking, on
Sensitive: noise, aversion to
Stupefaction, as if intoxicated
Talking, sleep, in
 comatose sleep, in
Weeping, alternating with hopefulness •
 waking, on
Work, aversion to mental

RATANHIA PERUVIANA

Anger, irascibility
Anxiety
 night
  waking, on
  midnight, after
 alone, when
 fear, with
 waking, on

Company, desire for; aversion to solitude, company amel.
 alone agg., while
Confusion of mind, air, amel. in open
Death, desires
 pains, during •
Fear, night
 midnight, after
 alone, of being
 happen, something will, alone, when, amel. by conversation •
 tremulous
 waking, on
Indifference, sleepiness, with
Indolence, sleepiness, with
Irritability
Loathing, general
Mood, changeable, variable
Morose, cross, fretful, ill-humor, peevish
Quarrelsome, scolding
Restlessness
Starting, sleep, falling, on
 during
 from
Stupefaction, as if intoxicated
Wearisome

RAUWOLFIA SERPENTINA

Abrupt, rough
Anguish
Anxiety
Catatonia
Company aversion to, alone, amel. when
Concentration, difficult
Confusion of mind
Death, thoughts of
Delusion unreal everything seems
Excitement, excitable
 alternating with sadness
Exertion, agg. from mental
 amel.
Fear, apprehension, dread
 evil, of
Indifference, apathy
Irresolution, indecision
Irritatability

Kill herself, sudden impulse to
Memory, weakness of
       done, for what has just
Mistakes, spelling in speaking
       writing, in
Morose, cross, fretful, ill-humor, peevish
Prostration of mind, mental exhaus-
       tion, brain-fag
Restlessness
       night
       bed, in
Rudeness
Sadness, despondency, dejection, men-
       tal depression, gloom, melan-
       choly
Schizophrenia, catatonic
              paranoid
Suicidal disposition
Thoughts, wandering

RESERPINUM

Activity, mental
Anxiety
Excitement, excitable
Loathing, work, at, evening •
Quarrelsome, scolding
Sadness, despondency, dejection, mental
       depression, gloom, melancholy
Schizophrenia, catatonic
       hebephrenia
Suicidal, disposition

RHAMNUS FRANGULA

Sadness, despondency, dejection, mental
       depression, gloom, melancholy

RHEUM PALMATUM

Absorbed, buried, in thought
Anger, irascibility
Anxiety
       conscience, as if guilty of a crime
       fever, during
       motion, from
       stooping, when

Asks for nothing
Attitude, assumes strange ★
Avarice
Aversion, everything, to
Brooding
Capriciousness
Confusion of mind
       morning, waking on
       intoxicated, as after being
       waking, on
Delirium
       night
       raging, raving
       sleep, during
Delusions, imaginations, hallucinations,
       illusions
       night
       fancy, illusions of
       people, sees
Desires, full of
       **impatiently many things, dis-
       likes its favourite play-
       things, child •**
       present, things not
Discomfort
Discontented, displeased, dissatisfied
       everything, with
Dream, as if in a
Dullness, sluggishness, difficulty of think-
       ing and comprehending, torpor
       says, nothing
       waking, on
Excitement, excitable
Fear, apprehension, dread
       death, of
Forgetful
Frown, disposed to
Gestures, strange attitudes and posi-
       tions
Ideas, deficiency of
Imbecility
Impatience
Impetuous
Indifference, apathy
       everything, to
Indolence, aversion to work
       morning
Introspepction
Irresolution, indecision

Irritability
> night ★
> children, in
> **chill, during**
> **dentition, during**
> *heat, during*
> **perspiration, during**

Lamenting, bemoaning, wailing
> **stool, if children urging**
> **before ●**

Moaning, groaning, whining
> sleep, during

Mood, changeable, variable

Morose, cross, fretful, ill-humor, peevish
> night
> children, in

Play, aversion to p. in children

Quarrelsome, scolding
> sleep, in

Quiet, disposition

Remorse

Reserved

Restlessness
> bed, tossing about in
> children, in
> > **dentition, during ●**
> heat, during
> internal

Rudeness, naughty children, of

Sadness, despondency, dejection, mental
> depression, gloom, melancholy

Sensitive: want of sensitiveness

Shrieking, screaming, shouting
> *children, in*
> > night
> > **stool, on urging to ●**
> > **during**
> *dentition, during*
> *sleep, during*

Sit, inclination to

Somnambulism

Speech, delirious
> night
> sleep before midnight, in
> wandering
> night

Starting, sleep, during

Stupefaction, as if intoxicated

Talk, indisposed to, desire to be silent,
> taciturn

Talking, sleep, in

Unconsciousness, coma, stupor
> dream, as in a
> *screaming, interrupted by*

Wearisome

Weeping, tearful mood
> night
> **children, in**
> > *night*
> perspiration, during
> sleep, in
> whimpering
> > sleep, during

Whining, whimpering, sleep, in ★

Will, weakness of

RHODODENDRON CHRUSANTHUM

Absent-minded, unobserving

Answers, slowly

Anxiety
> fever, during
> house, on entering

Aversion, everything, to

Business, averse to

Capriciousness

Chaotic, confused behavior

Cheerful, gay, mirthful

Concentration, difficult

Confusion of mind
> *morning*
> > rising and after, on
> > waking, on
> air, in open
> bed, while in
> coition, after
> rising, after
> waking, on
> walking, air amel., in open

Delirium
> frightful
> maniacal

Delirium tremens, mania-a-potu

Delusions, imaginations, hallucinations,
    illusions
        calls him, someone
        fancy, illusions of
        fire, visions of
        images, phatons, sees
            frightful
        visions, has
            horrible
Dipsomania, alcoholism
Discontented, displeased, dissatisfied
*Dullness, sluggishness, difficulty of think-
    ing and comprehending, torpor*
        morning
Excitement, feverish, menses, during
        menses, during
Fear, apprehension, dread
        insanity, losing his reason, of
        thunderstorm, of
Forgetful
        words while speaking, of; word
            hunting
Heedless
Ideas, deficiency of
Indifference, apathy
        agreeable things, to
        company, society, to •
        irritating, disagreeable things, to
        work, with aversion to
Indolence, aversion to work
        morning ★
Insanity, madness
Irritability
Mania
Memory, weakness of
        said, for what has
        say, for what is about to
        write, for what is about to
Mistakes, speaking, in
        misplacing words
        writing, in
            omitting words
Mood, changeable, variable
Morose, cross, fretful, ill-humor, peevish
Prostration of mind, fever, in
Restlessness
        eating, after

Sadness, despondency, dejection, mental
        depression, gloom, melancholy
Senses, dull, blunted
        vanishing of
Sensitive: want of sensitiveness
Sit, inclination to
Starting, sleep, during
Stupefaction, as if intoxicated
        morning, rising, after
Thoughts, vanishing of
**Thunderstorm, mind symptoms
        before**
        during, mind symptoms
Unconsciousness, coma, stupor
        transient, morning on rising
        drowsiness in head •
Weeping, children, babies, in
Work, aversion to mental

RHODIUM METALLICUM

Cheerful, gay, mirthful

RHODIUM OXYDATUM
NITRICUM

Delusions, hearing, illusions of

RHUS GLABRA

Delusions, imaginations, hallucinations,
    illusions
Dullness, sluggishness, difficulty of
    thinking and comprehending,
    torpor
Fear, people, of; anthropophobia
Indifference, apathy
Indolence, aversion to work
Memory, weakness of
Restlessness

RHUS RADICANS

Company, aversion to
        alternating with bursts of pleas-
            antry and sacrasm
Concentration, difficult

Confusion of mind, night, lying down,
    on lying, when
Delusions, criticised, she is
    strange, places seemed
Dullness, afternoon
Irresolution, indecision
    projects, in
Jesting
Mistakes, speaking, in
Sadness, afternoon
Unconsciousness, standing, while
    transient

RHUS TOXICODENDRON

Absent-minded, unobserving
Absorbed, buried in thought
Activity, mental, evening
    sleeplessness, with
Ailments from :
    anger, vexation
        anxiety, with
    anticipation, foreboding, presen-
        timent
    business failure
    fright
    hurry
    mortification
    pecuniary loss
    work, mental
Anger, irascibility
    night
    talking of others, from
    trifles, at
    waking, on
Anguish
        afternoon
    driving from place to place
Anorexia mentalis
Answers abruptly, shortly, curtly
    aversion to answer
    hastily
    slowly
Anxiety
        morning
            rising, on and after
            amel.
        waking, on
        afternoon

Anxiety,
        evening
            twilight, in the
            night
            midnight, after
                3h., after
        air amel., in open
        alone, when
        bed, in
            driving out of
        breathing deeply amel.
        business, about
        children, about his
        chill, during
        conscience, as if guilty of a crime
        dark, in
        fear, with
        fever, during
        future, about
        house, in
        hypochondriacal
        mental exertion, from
        rising, after
        sitting bent ●
        sleep, on going to
            during
        stool, before
            after
        suicidal disposition, with
        thought, from sad ●
        waking, on
        walking, air amel., in open
        weary of life, with
Business, averse to
Busy
Calculating, inability for
Cares, business, about his
    relatives, about
Carried, desires to be
            fast
Censorious, critical
        evening
Chaotic, confused behavior
Cheerful, gay, mirthful
        evening, bed, in
        chill, during
Childish behavior

*Company, aversion to; presence of other
    people agg. the symptoms; de-
    sire for solitude*
    weeping, with •
Complaining
Comprehension, easy
Concentration, active
Concentration, difficult
Confidence, want of self
Confusion of mind
    morning
        rising and after, on
            after, amel.
    evening
    chill, during
    dream, as if in
    intoxicated, as if
    sitting, while
    waking, on
    walking, while
Conscientious about trifles
Contradictory to speech, intentions are
Conversation agg.
Cowardice
Darkness agg.
Death, agony before
    desires
    presentiment of
    thoughts of
Delirium
    night
    bed and escapes, springs up sud-
        denly from
    business, talks of
    busy
    loquacious
    mild
    murmuring
    muttering
        himself, to
    persecution in d., delusions of
    quiet
    sepsis, from
    sleep, falling asleep, on
    sleeplessness, and ★
    trembling, with

Delirium tremens, mania-a-potu
*Delusions, imaginations, hallucina-
    tions, illusions*
    evening, bed, in
    bed, drives him out of, someone •
        sinking, is
        someone is in bed with him
    business, is doing •
    calls him, on waking, someone
    clouds, sees
    die, he was about to
    dirty, he is
    dying, he is
    engaged in some occupation, is
    fancy, illusions of
    figures, sees
    fire, vision of
    glass, wood etc., being made of
    home, away from, is
    images, phantoms, sees
        frightful
    injured, is being
    looking at her, everyone is
    murdered, he will be
    people looking at him
    persecuted, he is
    poisoned, he is about to be
    pursued by enemies
        he was
    roaming in the fields •
    strange, familiar things seem
    swimming, is
    visions, has
    watched, she is being
    work: hard at work, is
Desires, full of
Despair
    chill, during
    heat, during
    social position, of
Dipsomania, alcoholism
Discontented, displeased, dissatisfied
    evening
Discouraged
    evening

*Dullness, sluggishness, difficulty of think-
    ing and comprehending, torpor*
    evening
    chill, during
    damp air, from
    eating, after
    injuries of head, after
    motion amel. •
    walking, while
    writing, while
Dwells on past disagreeable occur-
    rences
    night
    midnight, after •
Ennui, tedium
Envy, avidity, and
Escape, attempts to
    run away, to
    springs up suddenly from bed
Excitement, excitable
    evening, bed, in
    heat, during
Exertion, agg. from mental
Fancies, exaltation of
    evening, bed, in
    sleeplessness, with
Fear, apprehension, dread
    morning
    evening
      twilight
    night
    breath away, takes
    crowd, in a
    dark, of
    death, of
    evil, of
    ghosts, of
    hurt, of being ★
    killing, of
    men, dread, fear of
    misfortune, of
    murdered, of being
    overpowering
    people, of; anthropophobia
    poisoned, of being

Fear,
    position, to lose his lucrative
    sadness, with
    sighing, with
    sleep, before
      go to sleep, fear to
    suicide, of
    superstitious •
    thinking, sad things, of •
    tremulous
    weary of life, with
Forgetful
    evening
    chill, during
    drunkards, forgetfulness in
    eating, after
    heat, during
    (-ness) old people, of
    walking after eating, while •
Forsaken feeling
    air, amel. in open •
    friends, by his, sensation as if ★
Frightened easily
    trifles, at
Gestures, grasping or reaching at some-
    thing, at flocks; carphologia
    picks at bedclothes
    plays with his fingers
Greed, cupidity
Hatred
Heedless
Home, desire to go
Hurry, haste
    eating, while ★
Hypochondriasis
Hysteria
Ideas, abundant, clearness of mind
    evening in bed
    deficiency of
Imbecility
Impatience
Impulsive
Inconsolable
Indifference, apathy
    company, society, while in
Indolence, aversion to work
    morning

Industrious, mania for work
    menses, before
Initiative, lack of
Insanity, madness
    black insanity with despair and
        weary of life from fear of
        mortification or loss of position
    fortune, losing, after
    melancholy
    position, from fear to lose the
Irritability
    morning, waking, on
    night
    air, in open
    amel.
    chill, during
    spoken to, when
    waking, on
    walking in open air amel.
Lamenting, bemoaning, wailing
Languages, unable for
Loathing, life, at
    evening
Looked at, cannot bear to be
Loquacity
Mania
Meditation
Memory, active
    alternating with dullness •
Memory, loss of, injuries of head, after
Memory, weakness of
    done, for what has just
    happened, for what has
    names, for proper
    occurrences of the day, for
    say, for what is about to
    words, of
    write, for what is about to
Mildness
Misanthropy
Mistakes, calculating, in
    writing, in
Moaning, groaning, whining
    sleep, during

Morose, cross, fretful, ill-humor,
    peevish
    morning, bed, in
    evening, bed, in
    night
    air, in open
    house, agg. in, amel. walking
    in open air
    sleep, in
    waking, on
Muttering
    sleep, in
Nibble, desire to ★
Occupation, desire for
Play, with fingers, during sleep ★
Praying
Prostration of mind, mental exhaus-
    tion, brain-fag
Quarrelsome, scolding
Rebels against poultice
Religious affections
Reproaches others
Restlessness
    daytime
    night
    midnight, after
    anxious
    bed, driving out of
    go from one bed to another,
    wants to
    tossing about in
    children, in
    chill, during
    eating, after
    heat, during
    internal
    menses, during
    suppressed, during
    move, must constantly
    sleepiness, with
Rocking amel.
Sadness, despondency, dejection, men-
    tal depression, gloom, melan-
    choly
    morning
    afternoon, twilight, in

Sadness,
    evening
    night
        bed, in
        midnight, after
    air amel., in open
    anxious
    causeless
    children, in
    chill, during
    darkness, in
    heat, during
    house, in
    injuries, head, of the
    labor, during
    menses, suppressed, from
    misfortune, as if from
    perspiration, during
    puberty, in
    sleepiness, with
    sleeplessness from sadness
    walking, air, in open
        amel.
    warm room, in
    wet weather, during
Selflessness
Senses, dull, blunted
    vanishing of
Sensitive, oversensitive
    noise, to
Serious, earnest
Shrieking, aid, in sleep, for
        springs up from bed, and
    brain, cry
Sighing
    heat, during
    perspiration, during
Sit, inclination to
Slowness
Speech, incoherent
    slow
    wandering
Spit, desire to
Spoken to, averse to being

Starting, startled
    noise, from
    paroxysmal
    sleep, falling, on
        during
Striking, knocking his head against
        wall and things
Stupefaction, as if intoxicated
    morning
    restlessness, with
Suicidal, disposition
    evening
        twilight, in •
    courage, but lacks
    drowning, by
    fear of death, with
    heat, during
    thoughts
Superstitious
Suspicious, mistrustful
Talk, indisposed to, desires to be silent,
        taciturn
    others agg., talk of
Talking, sleep, in
    business, of
Talks, himself, to
Thinking, sad things agg., of •
Thoughts, disagreeable
    midnight, after •
    frightful
    persistent
    unpleasant subjects, haunted
        by
    rush, flow of
        evening in bed
    thoughtful
    tormenting
    vanishing of
        chill, during
        standing, while •
        turning head, on •
        writing, while
Timidity
    night
Twilight agg. mental symptoms

Unconsciousness, coma, stupor
    head, on moving
      turning, on •
    meningitis, in
    muttering
Unfortunate, feels
Walk, walking in open air amel. mental
    symptoms
Wearisome
Weary of life
    evening
    fear of death, but
Weeping, tearful mood
    morning
    evening
    night
    **causeless, without knowing
      why**
    easily
    involuntary
    perspiration, during
    sleep, in
    stool, before
      during
    walking in open air amel.
    whimpering
Work, aversion to mental
    desire for
    impossible
Writing agg. mind symptoms

RHUS VENENATA

Absent-minded, unobserving
Cheerful, gay, mirthful
Concentration, difficult
Dullness, sluggishness, difficulty of
    thinking and comprehending,
    torpor
Fear, apprehension, dread
Forgetful
Irritability
Loathing, life, at
Morose, cross, fretfull, ill-humor, peevish

Restlessness
    night
      midnight, after
    heat, during
*Sadness, despondency, dejection, mental
    depression, gloom, melancholy*
Stupefaction, as if intoxicated
Thoughts, disconnected
Weary of life

RIBONUCLEINICUM
ACIDUM

Concentration, difficult
    studying, learns with difficulty
Escape, attempts to
Heedless
Indifference
Optimistic
Quarrelsome, scolding
Sadness, despondency, dejection, men-
    tal depression, gloom, melancholy
Shrieking, trifles, at
Weary of life
Weeping, tearful mood

ROBINIA PSEUDACACIA

Ambition, loss of
Anxiety, fright, after
Bed, remain in, desires to
Black and sombre, aversion to every-
    thing that is
Dancing
Death, desires
    thoughts of
Discontented, displeased, dissatisfied
Excitement, menses, before
Fanaticism
Fear, night
    black, of everything
    death, of
    suffocation, of
Haughty
Indolence, aversion to work
Insanity, erotic

Lamenting, bemoaning, wailing
Laughing
Memory, weakness of, thought, for
    what has just
Nymphomania
Obscene, lewd
Religious affection
    fanaticism
Sadness, despondency, dejection, mental
    depression, gloom, melancholy
Thoughts, vanishing of
Weeping, sleep, in

ROSMARINUS OFFICINALIS

Anxiety

RUMEX CRISPUS

Dipsomania, alcoholism
Excitement, excitable
Fancies, unpleasant
Fear, misfortune, of
Gestures, covers mouth with hand
Indifference, apathy
    external things, to
    surroundings, to
Indolence, aversion to work
    morning
Irritability
    noon
Jumping, bed, out of
Restlessness
    evening
    night
Sadness, despondency, dejection, men-
    tal depression, gloom, melan-
    choly
    suicidal disposition, with
Somnambulism
Suicidal, disposition
    sadness, from
Thinking, aversion to
Thoughts, stagnation of, evening •
Work, aversion to mental

RUMEX ACETOSA

Moaning, groaning, whining
Unconsciousness, coma, stupor

RUSSULA FOETENS

Delusions, imaginations, hallucinations,
    illusions
Unconsciousness, coma, stupor

RUTA GRAVEOLENS

Absent-minded, unobserving
Anger, irascibility
Anxiety
    daytime
    afternoon
    evening
    midnight, before, 23 h. •
    chest, from stitching in •
    conscience, as if guilty of a crime
    fear, with
    fever, during
    headache, with
    stitching in spine, from •
    sudden
Aversion, everything, to
Cheerful, gay, mirthful
Confidence, want of self
Confusion of mind
    morning
      waking, on
    evening
    night
    abortion, after •
    chill, during
    waking, on
Contradict, disposition to
Contradictory, action are c. to intention
Contrary
Cowardice
Death, desires, afternoon •
    evening
Deceived, always being ★
Delirium, abortion, after •

Delirium tremens, mania-a-potu
Delusions, imaginations, hallucinations,
    illusions
    bed, hard, too
    calls, someone
    crime, committed a, he had
    criminals, about
    deceived, being ★
    images, phantoms, sees
    people, sees, someone is behind
      him
Despair
Dipsomania, alcoholism
Discontented, displeased, dissatisfied
    himself, with
    others, with ★
Discouraged, anxiety, with ★
Dullnes, sluggishness, difficulty of
    thinking and comprehending,
    torpor
    morning, waking, on
    evening
Fear, apprehension, dread
    death, of, during heat
    evil, of
    hurt, of being
    water, of
Forgetful
Frightened, touch, from
Heedless
Ideas, deficiency of
Imbecility
Indifference, apathy
Indolence, aversion to work
    sitting, while
Irresolution, indecision
Irritability
    afternoon
Light, desire for
Loathing, life, at
Mania
Memory, weakness of
Mood, changeable, variable
Morose, cross, fretful, ill-humor, peevish
    afternoon

Prostration of mind, mental exhaus-
    tion, brain-fag
Quarrelsome, scolding
Rage, fury
Religious affections
Remorse
Restlessness
    afternoon
    evening
    night
    anxious
    dinner, after
    feverish
    headache, during
    heat, during
    pressing in liver, from ●
*Sadness, despondency, dejection, men
    tal depression, gloom, melan-
    choly*
    afternoon
    evening
    anxious
Shrieking, touched, when
    waking, on
Sit, inclination to
Slowness
Starting, fright, from and as from
    sleep, during
      from
      touch, from slightest ●
    touched, when
Stupefaction, as if intoxicated
Suspicious, mistrustful
Unconsciousness, coma, stupor
Weary of life
    afternoon
    evening
Weeping, tearful mood
    night
    waking, on

S

SABADILLA

Absorbed, buried in thought
Abstraction of mind
Ailments from :
    fright
    work, mental
Anger, irascibility
    trifles, at
Animation agg. ★
Answers, aversion to a.
    refuses to answer
Anxiety
        night
    causeless
    conscience, as if guilty of a crime
    eating, while
    fever, during
    pressure on the chest, from
Bed, jumps out of, and runs recklessly
        about •
Chaotic, confused behavior
Cheerful, gay, mirthful
    heat, during
Comprehension easy
Concentration, difficult
Confusion of mind
        morning on rising and after
    eating, after
    intoxicated, as if
    sitting, while
    walking, while
Consolation, kind words agg.
    sympathy agg.
Delirium
    fever, during
    sleeplessness, and ★
    trembling, with

Delusions, imagination, hallucinations, illusions
    abdomen is fallen in, his stomach devoured, his scrotum swollen •
    body are deformed, some parts of ★
    body, shrunken, like the dead, is •
    state of his body, to the •
    withering, is •
    crime, committed a, he had
    die, time has come to
    diminished, all is
        abdomen has fallen in •
        shrunken, parts are
    disease, has incurable
    emaciation, of
    enlarged
        chin is
        scrotum is swollen •
    fancy, illusions of
    limbs are crooked •
    pregnant, she is
    scrotum is swollen, his •
    separated from the world, thoughts
        are •
    sick, being
    small; of being smaller
    soul, body was too small for soul
        or separated from
    stomach, has corrosion of; an
        ulcer
    thoughts being outside of body •
    withering, body is •
Dipsomania, alcoholism
Discomfort
    evening
Dream, as if in a
Dullness, sluggishness, difficulty of thinking and comprehending, torpor
    perspiration, during
    pollutions, after
Ecstasy, heat, during
Excitement, excitable
Exertion, agg. from mental
Exhilaration

Fancies, exaltation of
      evening in bed
      heat, during
      sleeplessness, with
Fear, apprehension, dread
    causeless
    death, of
    disease, of impending
    evil, of
    noise, from
    stomach, of ulcer in
    water, of
Feigning, sick
Frightened easily
    fever, during
Haughty
Hydrophobia
Hypochondriasis
    imaginary illness
Ideas abundant, clearness of mind
      evening
      night
      erroneous ★
      fixed ★
      imaginary disease, of ★
Imbecility
Indifference, apathy
    alternating with excitement
    jesting, to ●
    others, towards
Indolence, aversion to work
Insanity, madness
    alternating mental with physical
      symptoms
    alternating with metrorrhagia,
      other mental symptoms
Introspection
Irritability
      morning
      night
      chill, during
Jumping, bed, out of
Laughing
    ludicrous, everything seems
Mania

Meditation
Memory, weakness of
Mental symptoms alternating with
    physical
Mood, changeable, variable
Moral feeling, want of
Morose, cross, fretful, ill-humor, peevish
    night
    sleepiness, with
    waking, on
Nervous, alternations with physical ★
Nymphomania
Passionate
Prostration of mind, mental exhaus-
    tion, brain-fag
Quiet disposition
Rage, fury
    cold applications to head amel. ●
Religious affections
Remorse
Reserved
Rest, desire for
Restlessness
      night
    anxious
Raving, senseless, insane
Sadness, despondency, dejection, mental
      depression, gloom, melancholy
    criminal, as if being the greatest ●
Senses, dull, blunted
Sensitive, oversensitive
    noise, to
Sentimental
Starting, startled
      morning, after waking
    fright, from and as from
    noise, from
    perspiration, during
    sleep, during
      from
    trifles, at
Stupefaction, as if intoxicated
      morning after rising
Talk, indisposed to, desire to be silent,
      taciturn

Thinking, complaints agg., of
Thoughts, erroneous
    persistent
        separated, mind and body are
    rapid, quick
    rush, flow of
        evening in bed
        sleeplessness from
    thoughtful
Unconsciousness, coma, stupor
    mental insensibility
Unfeeling, hard hearted
Violent, vehement
Vivacious
Weeping, waking, on
Work, aversion to mental
    impossible

SABAL SERRULATUM

Anger, consoled, when
    sympathy agg. ●
    wakes in ★
Consolation, kind words agg.
Irritability, consolation agg.
    sexual appetite, loss of, from ★
Sympathy agg.
Symptoms, broods over his own ★

SABINA

Anger, irascibility
Anxiety
      evening
        bed, in
      night
        midnight, before
      bed, in
      fear, with
      fever, during
      future, about
      stool, before
Confusion of mind
      afternoon
      eating, after
      intoxicated, as after being

Consolation, kind words agg.
Cowardice
Delirium
Discouraged
Dullness, sluggishness, difficulty of think-
      ing and comprehending, torpor
Fear, apprehension, dread
    abortion from f., threatening
    evil, of
    misfortune, of
    music, from
Forgetful
Forsaken feeling
Hypochondriasis
    morose
Hysteria
Imbecility
Indifference, apathy
    joyless
Indolence, aversion to work
    morning
    walking, while
Irritability
Jesting, aversion to
Lascivious, lustful
Magnetized, discuss to be, mesmerism
    amel.
Memory, weakness of
    business, for
    done, for what has just
Mood, changeable, variable
Morose, cross, fretful, ill-humor, peevish
Music agg.
    aversion to
Nymphomania
Quiet, repose and tranquillity, desires,
    walking in open air, on
Reserved
    walking in open air, while
Restlessness
    evening
      bed, in
    heat, during
Sadness, despondency, dejection, mental
    depression, gloom, melancholy
    air, in open
    music, from

Sensitive, oversensitive
    music, to
    noise, to slightest
    want of sensitiveness
Sentimental
Shamelessness
Speech, wandering
Starting, noise, from
    sleep, from
Stupefaction, as if intoxicated
    vertigo, during
Talk, indisposed to, desire to be silent,
    taciturn
    morning
        walking, while
Talking, sleep, in
Unconsciousness, coma, stupor
Walk, walking in open air agg. mental
    symptoms
Wearisome
    air, in open
Weeping, tearful mood
    aloud, wobbing
    anger, after
    music, from
    sleep, in
    waking, on

SACCHARUM OFFICINALE

Ailments from :
    anger, vexation
    excitement, emotional
Anxiety
Capriciousness
Delusions, bed, sinking, is
Dullness, sluggishness, difficulty of
    thinking and comprehending,
    torpor
Homesickness
Indifference, apathy
Insolence, children, in ●
Irritability
Mistakes, writing, in
    omitting words
Moaning, children, in

Modesty, increased ●
Morose, cross, fretful, ill-humor, peevish
    children, in
Quarrelsome, scolding
Rocking amel.
Sadness, despondency, dejection, mental
    depression gloom, melancholy
    evening, 21h ●
    chill, during
Starting, sleep, during
Talk, indisposed to, desire to be silent,
    taciturn
Violent, vehement

SACCHARUM LACTIS

Delusions, imaginations, hallucinations,
    illusions
    people: behind him, someone is
Homesickness
Hysteria
Sighing

SALICYLICUM ACIDUM

Absent-minded, unobserving
Anxiety
Cares, worries, full of
Confusion of mind
Delirium
    fever, during
Delusions, imaginations, hallucinations,
    illusions
    music, he hears
Dullness, sluggishness, difficulty of think-
    ing and comprehending, torpor
Excitement, excitable
Forgetful
Grief, silent
Irritability, sadness, with
Loquacity
Quiet, wants to be
Sadness, despondency, dejection, men-
    tal depression, gloom, melancholy
Speech, incoherent
Stupefaction, as if intoxicated
Unconsciousness, coma, stupor

SALIX NIGRA

Dullness, sluggishness, difficulty of think-
ing and comprehending, torpor
Insanity, erotic
Nymphomania
Satyriasis

SALIX PURPUREA

Dullness, sluggishness, difficulty of thinking and comprehending, torpor
Irritability

SALAMANDRA MACULATA

Unconsciousness, looking downward,
on •

SAMBUCUS NIGRA

Ailments from :
    anger, vexation
      anxiety, with
        fright, with
    anxiety
    excitement, emotional
    fright
    grief
Anger, irascibility
Anxiety
    night
    fear, with
    heart ★
    sleep, during
      on starting from
    waking, on
Confusion of mind
    morning
      rising and after, on
    perspiration, during
Contrary
Delirium
    periodic
    sleeplessness, and ★
    trembling, with

Delusions, imaginations, hallucinations,
    illusions
    faces, sees
      closing eyes, on
    fancy, illusions of
      heat, during
    images, phantoms, sees
      closing eyes, on
      in bed
      frightful
      wall, on the
    room walls, sees horrible things
      on the
    spectres, ghosts on closing eyes,
      sees
    visions, has, closing the eyes, on
      horrible
      monsters, of
Dipsomania, alcoholism
Discontented, displeased, dissatisfied
    everything, with
Disgust
    everything, with
Dullness, sluggishness, difficulty of
    thinking and comprehending,
    torpor
Escape, attempts to
Excitement, excitable
Fancies, exaltation of
Fear, apprehension, dread
    night after waking
    suffocation, of
    unaccountable, vague
Frightened, easily
    night
Fussy ★
Hysteria, fainting, hysterical
Irritability
Moaning, chill, during
    sleep, during
      eyelids half closed, rolling of
      head, with
Mood, repulsive
Morose, cross, fretful, ill-humor, peevish
Restlessness
    perspiration, during

Sadness, heat, during
Sensitive, oversensitive
Shrieking, screaming, shouting
Starting, startled
    anxious
    perspiration, during
    sleep, during
        from
Stupefaction, as if intoxicated
Unconsciousness, fever, during
    perspiration, during •
Wearisome
Weeping, tearful mood
    alternating with laughter
    coughing, during
    desire to weep, all the time
    sleep, in

SAMBUCUS CANADENSIS

Restlessness

SANGUINARIA CANADENSIS

Anger, irascibility
Anxiety
    fear, with
Borrows trouble ★
Clinging, held, wants to be
        amel., being
Concentration, difficult
        afternoon
Confusion of mind
        eructations amel.
Delirium
Delusions, journey, he is on a
    railway train, she is in a r. car,
      begs others to hold her •
    talking rapidly, all around her
      are •
Desires, indefinite
Dipsomania, alcoholism
Dullness, sluggishness, difficulty of think-
    ing and comprehending, torpor

Eccentricity
Excitement, excitable
Fancies, lascivious
Fear, apprehension, dread
Frightened easily, night
Gestures, hands, motion, involuntary,
    of the
Grumbling ★
Hopeful
    recovery, of •
Hysteria
Impatience
    afternoon
Indifference, apathy
Indolence, aversion to work
    damp weather, in •
Irritability
    morning
    afternoon
    headache, during
    pollutions, after
Mood, changeable, variable
Morose, cross, fretful, ill-humor, peevish
    afternoon
Muttering
Rage, insults, after
Reclining, half ★
Recognizes everything, but cannot move
    (catalepsy)
Restlessness, night
Sadness, despondency, dejection, mental
    depression, gloom, melancholy
    pollutions, from
Senses, acute
Sensitive, oversensitive
    light, to
    noise, to
        painful sensitiveness to
        stepping, of
    odors, to
Singing
Starting, sleep, from
Thoughts: disgusting thoughts with
        nausea •
Torpor
Unconsciousness, coma, stupor

SANICULA AQUA

Anger, waking, on
Anxiety, motion, from downward
Carried, desires to be
Darkness agg.
     aversion to •
Delusions, people, sees: dark, someone
     is behind him when walking
     in the
Fear, dark, of
     downward motion, of
     falling, of
     riding in a carriage, when
     robbers, of
     touch, of
     work, dread of
Fishy ★
Forgetful
Irresolution, indecision
Irritability
     alternating with cheerfulness
     children, in
Laughing, alternating with vexation,
     ill-humor
Light, desire for
Memory, weakness of
Mood, changeable, variable
Morose, cross, fretful, ill-humor, peevish
Obstinate, headstrong
Occupation, changing constantly •
Restlessness
     anxious
Sadness, despondency, dejection, mental
     depression, gloom, melancholy
Sensitive, oversensitive
Shrieking, urinating, before ★
Suspicious, mistrustful
Talk, slow learning to
Thoughts, wandering
Touched, aversion to being
Touchy ★
Travel, desire to
Wander, desire to
Work, aversion to mental

SANTONINUM

Absent-minded, unobserving
Concentration, difficult
Confidence, want of self
Dancing
Delirium
     sleep, during
Delusions, imaginations, hallucinations,
     illusions
     animals, of
     cherries, sees •
     figures, sees
Desire, everything, for •
Dullness, sluggishness, diffiiculty of
     thinking and comprehending,
     torpor
Excitement, excitable
Irresolution, indecision
Irritability
Laughing
     hysterical
Restlessness
Sadness, despondency, dejection, men-
     tal depression, gloom, melan-
     choly
Unconsciousness, coma, stupor

SAPONINUM

Censorious, unoccupied, when; close ap-
     plication amel. •
Company, aversion to; presence of
     other people agg. the symp-
     toms; desire for solitude
     menses, during
Delirium
Dullness, sluggishness, difficulty of think-
     ing and comprehending, torpor
Irritability
     exertion, from mental
Loathing, general
Memory, weakness of
Mood, changeable, variable
Morose, cross, fretful, ill-humor, peevish
Quiet, wants to be, afternoon •
Restlessness
     afternoon
     night

Sadness, despondency, dejection, mental
    depression, gloom, melancholy
      menses, after
Unconsciousness, coma, stupor
Work, aversion to mental

SARCOLACTICUM ACIDUM

Anger, trifles, at
Anxiety, exercise, from •
Discouraged
Irritability
Sadness, despondency, dejection, mental
    depression, gloom, melancholy

SAROTHAMNUS SCOPARIUS

Absent-minded, unobserving
Anger, irascibility
Anguish
Concentration, difficult
Dullness, sluggishness, difficulty of think-
    ing and comprehending, torpor
Excitement, excitable
    night
Indifference, apathy
Indolence, aversion to work
Initiative, lack of
Irritability
    trifles, from
Restlessness
Sadness, despondency, dejection, mental
    depression, gloom, melancholy
      trifles, about
Satyriasis
Thoughts, vanishing of

SARRACENIA PURPUREA

Activity, mental, alternating with in-
    difference •
Anxiety, everything, about •
Buoyancy
Capriciousness
Cheerful, gay, mirthful
Concentration, difficult

Conscientious about trifles
Delirium
Delusions, criminal, he is a
    disgraced, she is
Dullness, sluggishness, difficulty of think-
    ing and com-prehending, torpor
      morning
Envy
Forgetful
Frightened easily
Indifference, apathy
    alternating with activity •
Indolence, aversion to work
Laughing
Memory, weakness of
Reproaches himself
Restlessness
Sadness, despondency, dejection, mental
    depression, gloom, melancholy
      morning
      noon
      headache, during
Suicidal disposition
Suspicious, mistrustful
Weeping, sleep, in

SARSAPARILLA

Absent-minded, unobserving
Absorbed, buried in thought
Abstraction of mind
Anger, irascibility
    former vexations, about
    past events, about
Anguish
Anxiety
    forenoon
Aversion, everything, to
    forenoon •
Bad temper, morning ★
Capriciousness
    afternoon
Cheerful, gay, mirthful •
    daytime
    afternoon
    evening

Concentration, difficult
Confusion of mind
    morning
    evening
       amel. •
    sitting, while
Contradiction, is intolerant of
Contrary
Conversation agg.
Delusions, body, brittle, is
    dead persons, sees
    friendless, he is
    images, sees frightful
    spectres, ghosts, spirits, sees
Dipsomania, alcoholism
Discontented, displeased, dissatisfied
    everything, with
Disgust
    everything, with
Doubtful, recovery during climacteric
    period, of •
Dullness, sluggishness, difficulty of thinking and comprehending, torpor
    forenoon
Dwells, recalls old grievances
Emptiness, sensation of ★
Excitement, heat, during
Exertion, agg. from mental
Fear, apprehension, dread
    recover, during climacteric period
    she will not •
    sleep, before
    tremulous
Forgetful
Forsaken feeling
Gestures, hands, motions, involuntary
    of the, spinning and weaving
      scratching thighs •
Idiocy
Imitation, mimicry
Impatience
    itching, from
Indifference, apathy
    forenoon
    pleasure, to
    sleepiness, with
Indolence, aversion to work
    sleepiness, with

Industrious, mania for work
    afternoon •
    heat, during
Introspection
Irritability
    daytime
    morning
    afternoon
    menses, during
Jesting
Memory, weakness of
Mistakes, writing, in, wrong words,
Moaning, groaning, whining
Mood, alternating
    changeable, variable
    repulsive
Morose, cross, fretful, ill-humor, peevish
    morning
    forenoon
    afternoon
    fly on wall, by •
    work, with inclination to •
Offended, easily; takes everything in bad part
Prostration of mind, mental exhaustion, brain-fag
Quiet, disposition
Restlessness, night
    midnight, before
Sadness, despondency, dejection, mental
    depression, gloom, melancholy
    morning
    forenoon
      amel.
    masturbation, from
    pain, from •
    pollutions, from
Sensitive, oversensitive
    pain, to
Shrieking, screaming, shouting
    urinating, before
Singing
Starting, evening on falling asleep
    dreams, from a dream
    fright, from and as from
    sleep, on falling
      during
      from
    sleepiness, with

Stupefaction, as if intoxicated
    morning
Sulky
Talk, indisposed to, desire to be silent,
    taciturn
Thinking, complaints agg., of
Unconsciousness, coma, stupor
    menses, during
    standing, while
    vertigo, during
Unfortunate, feels
Wearisome
Weeping, tearful mood
    morning
    forenoon
    urination, before
    during
Work, mental, impossible

SCROPHULARIA NODOSA

Ailments from:
    anger, vexation
Anger, irascibility
Anxiety, future, about
Delusions, objects appear on closing
    eyes •
Unconsciousness, coma, stupor

SCUTELLARIA LATERIFOLIA

Ailments from:
    excitement, emotional
    work, mental
Cheerful, gay, mirthful
Concentration, difficult
    studying, reading etc., while
Confusion of mind, mental exertion,
    from
Delirium tremens, mania-a-potu
Dullness, morning on rising
Excitement, excitable
Fear,
    happen, something will ★
Hydrophobia
Hysteria
Joy: headache from excessive joy

Restlessness
    evening
Sadness, despondency, dejection, mental
    depression, gloom, melancholy
Sensitive, pain, to
Starting, startled
    sleep, from
Striking, himself, knocking his head
    against wall and things ★
Work, aversion to mental

SECALE CORNUTUM

Abstraction of mind
Ailments, from:
    anger, vexation
    fright
    sexual excesses
Anguish
Answers abruptly, shortly, curtly
    aversion to answer
    hesitating
    refuses to answer
Anxiety
    chill, during
    fear, with
    fever, during
    menses, during
    after
    mental exertion, from
    stool, during
Beside oneself, being
Bite, desire to
Capriciousness
Chaotic, confused behavior
Cheerful, gay, mirthful
Child bed agg.
Clothed inproperly ★
Company, aversion to; presence of
    other people agg. the symp-
    toms; desire for solitude
Concentration, difficult
Confusion of mind
    night
    identity, duality, sense of
Conscientious about trifles

Contemptuous
  relations, for •
Cowardice
Darkness agg. ★
Death, desires
Defiant
Delirium
  night
  abandons her relatives •
  absurd things, does •
  aroused, on being
  convulsion, after
  erotic
  exaltation of strength, with ★
  fever, during
  frightful
  headache, during
  laughing
  maniacal
  mild
  muttering
  naked in delirium, wants to be
  quiet
  raging, raving
  rambling
  sepsis, from
  silent
  sleep, comatose, during
  sleepiness, with
  violent
  water, jumping into
Delusions, imaginations, hallucina-
  tions, illusions
  night
  animals, of
  bed, someone is in bed with him
  double, of being
  fancy, illusions of
  figures, sees
  images, sees, frightful
  room: sea, room is like the form of
    a troubled •
  sick, two sick people were in bed,
    one of whom got well and the
    other did not •
  violent
  visions, has
    closing the eyes, on
Dementia, senilis

Despair
Destructiveness
Dipsomania, alcoholism
Discomfort
Discouraged
Dresses, indecency ★
Dullness, sluggishness, difficulty of
  thinking and comprehending,
  torpor
Excitement, excitable
  feverish
Exhilaration
Fancies, exaltation of
Fear, apprehension, dread
  death, of
    menses, before
  evil, of
    menses, before
      during
Fight, wants to
Foolish behavior
  spasm, during •
Forgetful
  coition, after
  sexual excesses, after
Forsaken feeling
Forsakes relations •
Gestures, clapping overhead •
  convulsive
  fingers spread apart ★
  grasping, genitals during spasms
Haughty
hysteria
Idiocy
Imbecility
Indifference, apathy
  everything, to
  exposure of her person, to
Indolence, aversion to work
  physical
Insanity, madness
  behaves like a crazy person
  laughing, with
  puerperal
Irritability
Jesting
Jumping: river, impulse to j. into the ★
Kill, desire to

Lamenting, bemoaning, wailing
Laughing
    beside herself, claps hands over
      head (after abortion) •
    sardonic
    spasmodic
Loathing, general
Loathing, life, at
Loquacity
Malicious, spiteful, vindictive
Mania
    rage, with
    violence, with deeds of
Memory, weakness of
    names, for proper
Mistakes, speaking, in
Moaning, groaning, whining
    night
Mocking, relatives, at his •
    sarcasm
Muttering
Naked, wants to be
    delirium, in
Nymphomania, menses, during
    metrorrhagia, during
Obstinate, headstrong
    children
Pleasure, sleeplessness, during •
Prostration of mind, mental exhaustion, brain-fag
    convulsions, from
Rage, fury
    biting, with
    chained, had to be
    kill people, tries to
    malicious
    shrieking, with
    sleep, rage followed by continuous deep •
    suicidal disposition, with
Remorse
Restlessness
    heat, during
    menses, during
    women, in
Rocking amel.

Sadness, despondency, dejection, mental depression, gloom, melancholy
Senses, dull, blunted
    vanishing of
Sensitive, noise, to
Shamelessness
    exposes the person
Shrieking, screaming, shouting
Sighing
Sit, inclination to
Speech, confused
    hesitating
    low
    slow
    unintelligible
    wandering
Spit, desire to
Starting, sleep, during
    from comatose sleep
Stupefaction, as if intoxicated
    convulsions, between
    vertigo, during
Suicidal disposition
    drowning, by
    throwing himself from a height
Suspicious, mistrustful
Talk, indisposed to, desire to be silent, taciturn
Tastlessness in dressing
Tears her genitals •
    himself
Thoughts, disagreeable
    persistent
Timidity
Unconsciousness, coma, stupor
    convulsions, after
    incomplete
    mental insensibility
    parturition, during
    pregnancy, during
    transient
    vertigo, during
Weary of life
Weeping, tearful mood
    menses, during

SEDUM ACRE

Delirium,
  exaltation of strength, with

SELENIUM

Absent-minded, unobserving
Absorbed, buried in thought
Ailments from:
  anger, vexation
  debauchery
  sexual excesses
  work, mental
Amorous
Anger, irascibility
  trifles, at
Anxiety
  health, about
  study, during ★
Aversion, persons, to certain
Business, incapacity for
Company, aversion to; presence of other
  people agg. the symptoms;
  desire for solitude
  friends, of intimate
Comprehension, easy
Concentration, difficult
Confusion of mind
  coition, after
  pollutions, from
Cruelty, inhumanity
Delirium
  sleeplessness, and ★
Delirium tremens, mania-a-potu
Delusions, imaginations, hallucinations,
  illusions
Despair
Dipsomania, alcoholism
  menses, before •
Discontented, displeased, dissatisfied
  coition, after
Doubtful, soul's welfare, of
Dullness, sluggishness, difficulty of think-
  ing and comprehending, torpor
  mental exertion, from
  sexual excesses, after •

Ecstasy
Excitement, excitable
  agg.
Exertion, agg. from mental
Fanaticism
Fancies, lascivious
  impotency, with
  repulsive, when alone
Fear, apoplexy, of
  crowd, in a
  disease, of impending
  men, dread, fear of
  occupation, of •
  people, of; anthropophobia
  work, dread of
Forgetful
  sleep, he remembers all he had
    forgotten, during
Forgotten things come to mind in sleep
Fussy ★
Hypochondriasis
Ideas, deficiency of
Imbecility
Indifference, apathy
  surroundings, to
Irritability
  climacteric period, during
  coition, after
  pollutions, after
Lascivious, lustful
  impotence, with
Laughing, spasmodic
Loquacity
  evening
  excited
  perspiration, during
  rambling ★
Memory confused
Memory, weakness of
  business, for
  labor, for mental
Mistakes, speaking, in
  wrong syllables, gives
Moaning, groaning, whining
Morose, cross, fretful, ill-humor, peevish
  coition, after

Prostration of mind, mental exhaus-
    tion, brain-fag pollutions, af-
    ter
Reading aloud agg. ★
Religious affections
    fanaticism
    melancholia
Remorse
Revelry, feasting
Sadness, despondency, dejection, mental
    depression, gloom, melancholy
      forenoon
      evening
    chill, during
    coition, after
    periodical
    perspiration, during
Senses, dull, blunted
Sensitive, certain persons, to
Speech, babbling
Starting, evening on falling asleep
    sleep, on falling
Stupefaction, as if intoxicated
    rouses with difficulty
Suspicious, mistrustful
Talking, sleep, in
Theorizing
Thoughts, intrude, sexual
    sexual ●
      impotency, with ●
Unconsciousness, coma, stupor
    waking, after
Weeping, chill, during
Work, aversion to mental
    fatigues
    impossible
    sexual excesses, after

SENECIO AUREUS

Ailments from:
    homesickness
Amorous ★
Aversion, his own mind, to ★
    members of family, to
Cheerful, alternating with sadness
Concentration, difficult

Confusion of mind
Ecstasy, alternating with sadness ●
Elated, alternating with sadness ●
Excitement, excitable
    menses, during
Exhilaration
Homesickness
Hysteria
    night ●
    sleeplessness, with
Insanity, puerperal
Irritability
Mania
Memory, active
Mood changeable ★
Restlessness, night
    midnight, before
    women, in
Sadness despondency, dejection, men-
    tal depression, gloom, melan-
    choly
      evening
    menses, during
Self centred ★
Selfishness, egoism
Talk, indisposed to, menses, during
Thoughts, future, of the
    past, of the, evening ●
    thoughtful, evening
Unconsciousness, exertion, after
Weeping, tearful mood

SENECIO JACOBAEA

Sadness, despondency, dejection, mental
    depression, gloom, melancholy

SENEGA

Abusive, insulting
Affectionate
Ailments from:
    mortification
Anger, irascibility
    alternating with cheerfulness
      exhilaration
    trifles, at ·
    violent

Anxiety
 motion amel., from
 rest, during
Chaotic, confused behavior
Cheerful, gay, mirthful
 alternating with anger
  burst of passion
 followed by irritability
 foolish, and
Childish behavior
Concentration, difficult
Confusion of mind
 morning
Discomfort, eating, supper, after
Dullness, sluggishness, difficulty of thinking and comprehending, torpor
Excitement, excitable
 feverish
Fancies, exaltation of
Fear, apprehension, dread
Foolish behavior
Hopeful
Hypochondriasis
Imbecility
Indifference, apathy
Indolence, aversion to work
 morning ★
Industrious, mania for work
Insanity, madness
Irresolution, indecision
Irritability
 morning
 forenoon
Loathing, general
Mania
Memory, active
 past events, for
Memory, weakness of
Mood, alternating
 changeable, variable
Morose, forenoon
Passionate
Playful
Prostration of mind, mental exhaustion, brain-fag

Quarrelsome, scolding
Rage, fury
 alternating with cheerfulness
Restlessness
Sadness, despondency, dejection, mental depression, gloom, melancholy
 evening
Sensitive, oversensitive
 noise, to
  painful sensitiveness to
Serious, earnest
 evening
Shrieking, screaming, shouting
Starting, sleep, during
 sleeplessness, with
Stupefaction, as if intoxicated
Thoughts, stagnation of
Tranquillity, serenity, calmness
Unconsciousness, coma, stupor
 eyes, pressure in e. and obstruction of sight ●
Violent, vehement
Vivacious
Weeping, children, in
Work, desire for mental

SENNA

Anger, wakes in ★
Restlessness
 night
  bed, tossing about in
Shrieking, children, in
Weeping, children, babies, in

SEPIA SUCCUS

Abrupt, harsh
Absent-minded, unobserving
 dreamy
Absorbed, buried in thought
Abusive, insulting
Activity
 amel.
Affection, stifled ★

Affections, in general ★
Ailments from:
    anger, vexation
        anxiety, with
        fright, with
        suppressed
    anticipation, foreboding, presen-
        timent
    business-failure
    debauchery
    disappointment
    embarrassment
    excitement, emotional
    fright
    love, disappointed
    mortification
    scorn, being scorned
    sexual excesses
    work, mental
Ambition, loss of
Amorous
Anger, irascibility
    morning
    contradiction, from
    former vexations, about
    menses, before ●
    past events, about
    trembling, with
    trifles, at
        agg. ★
    violent
Anguish
    eating, while ●
    after
Answers, monosyllable
    rapidly
    slowly
Antagonism with herself
Anxiety
    morning
        perspiration, during
        rising, amel. on and after
        waking, on
    evening
        twilight, in the
            bed, in
    night
        waking, on
    alone, when
    anger, during

Anxiety,
    bed, in
    chill, during
    climacteric period, during
    coition, after ●
    congestion to chest, from
    eating, while
        after
    exertion of eyes, from ●
    fear, with
    fever, during
    flushes of heat, during
    future, about
    head: perspiration on forehead,
        with
        perspiration on forehead, with
        cold
    headache, with
    health, about
    hypochondriacal
    looking steadily ●
    moaning, with ●
    others, for ★
    paroxysms, in
    periodical
    perspiration, with cold
    reading, while
    riding, while
    sewing ●
    stool, during
        as for stool
    thoughts, from disagreeable
    thunderstorm, during
    tobacco, from smoking
    urination, before
        when the desire is resisted ●
    vexation, after
    waking, on
    walking rapidly, when, which
        makes him walk faster
Avarice
    squandering on oneself, but
Aversion, everything, to
    his own mind, to ★
    husband, to
    members of family, to
    men (females), to ★

Bed, desires to remain in, morning
Beside oneself, being
Business, averse to
Busy
Capriciousness
Cares, worries, full of
    domestic affairs, about
Censorious, critical
Change, desire for
Cheerful, gay, mirthful
    evening, bed, in
    night
        alternating with lachrymose mood
        sadness
    thunders and at lightening, when
    it
Climacteric period agg.
Clinging, held, wants to be
    amel., being
Company, aversion to; presence of other
    people agg. the symptoms;
    desire for solitude
    alone, amel. when
    avoids the sight of people
        lies with closed eyes, and ●
    fear of being alone, yet
    loathing at company
    menses, during
    perspiration, during
    presence of strangers, aversion to
Company, desire for; aversion to soli-
    tude, company amel.
    alone agg., while
Complaining
    others, of ●
Concentration, difficult
Confusion of mind
    morning
        rising and after, on
    forenoon
    afternoon
    evening
        night
    coition, after
    dream, as if in
    eating, after
    heat, during

Confusion of mind
    lying, when
    menses, before
    mental exertion, from
    sitting, while
    spoken to, when ●
    stitching in chest, from ●
    talking, while
    waking, on
    walking, while
        air, in open
    weeping amel. ●
Conscientious about trifles
Consolation, kind words agg.
Contradict, disposition to
Contradiction, is intolerant of
Contradictory to speech, intentions are
    actions are contradictory to inten-
    tions
Contrary
Conversation agg.
Country, desire for ★
Cowardice
Dancing
    amel.
Death, desires
        convalescence, during
    dying, feels as if
    presentiment of
Deceitful, sly
Deception causes grief and mortifica-
    tion ★
Defiant
Delirium, at night
    arms, extends
    chill, during
    delusions, with
    fantastic
    haemorrhage, after
    laughing
    waking, on
Delirium tremens, mania-a-potu
Delusions, imaginations, hallucination,
    illusions
        night
        alone, graveyard, she is a. in a
        anxious

Delusions,
  body: fibre in her right side, feels
    every •
  calls him, someone
    during sleep •
  dead, multilated corpse
  doctors come, three
  fancy, illusions of
    eyes, on closing
  images, phantoms, sees
    night
    closing eyes, on
  sleep, before
  laughed at, mocked, being
  laughter, with
  mutilated bodies, sees
  people, sees
  poor, he is
  robbed, is going to be
  sick, being
    work, and for this reason will
    not
  side, she can feel every muscle,
    and fibre of her right •
  something comes from above
    which presses chest
  spectres, ghosts, spirits, sees •
    closing eyes, on
  starve, family will
  talking, persons as though near,
    of (about midnight) •
  unfortunate, he is
  visions, has
    closing the eyes, on
  water, of
    talking of, with •
Dementia, senilis
Despair
  chill, during
  existence, about miserable •
  heat, during
  perspiration, during
  recovery, of
  social position, of
Dipsomania, alcoholism

*Dirtiness, urinating and defecating
  everywhere,*
    children
Discontented, displeased, dissatisfied
  everything, with
Discouraged
  morning
  coition, after •
Doubtful
  recovery, of
Dream, as if in a
**Dullness, sluggishness, difficulty of
  thinking and comprehend-
  ing, torpor**
  morning
  forenoon
  afternoon
  evening
  coition, after •
  eating amel.
  heat, after •
  paroxysmal
  pollution, after
  sleepiness, with
*Dwells on past disagreeable occur-
  rences*
  recalls disagreeable memories
Eat, refuses to
Eccentricity
  metrorrhagia, after •
**Emptiness, sensation of ★
  faintness, sensation of, with ★**
Envy
  avidity, and
Escape, family, children, from her
Estranged from her family
Excitement, excitable
  morning
  evening in bed
  night
  agg.
  company, in
  feverish, dinner, after •
  perspiration, during
  waking, on
Exertion, agg. from mental

Fancies, anxious, night, during fever •
    exaltation of
        night
        closing the eyes in bed, on
        sleeplessness, with
    lascivious
    waking, on
Fastidious, occasionally ★
Fear, apprehension, dread
    morning
    alone, of being
    apoplexy, of
    approaching him, of others
    consumption, of
    death, of
        impending d., of
        soon, that she will die
    disease, of impending
    evil, of
    ghosts, of
    going out, of
    humiliated, of being
    insanity, losing his reason, of
    joints are weak, that •
    men, dread, fear of
    narrow places, vaults, churches
        and cellars, of
    people, of; anthrophobia
        yet agg. if alone ★
    physician, of ★
    position, to lose his lucrative
    poverty, of
    recurrent
    riding in a carriage, when
    society, of his position in
    solitude, of
    speak, to
    spoken to, when
    starving, of
    stool, of involuntary •
    suicide, of
    thunderstorm, of
    touch, of
    tremulous
Feces, urinating and going to stool
    everywhere, children
Feigning, sick, sleep ★
Foolish behavior

Forgetful
    afternoon
    evening
Forsaken feeling
    beloved by his parents, wife,
        friends, feels is not being
Frightened easily
    night
        waking, on
    trifles, at
Frown, disposed to ★
Gestures, makes
    furious
    grasping genitals, delirium, dur-
        ing ★
    ridiculous or foolish
    strange attitudes and positions
        arms, of
        gait, in
    talking, gesticulates while
Greed, cupidity
Grief
Hatred, persons who had offended him,
    of
    male and female, each other for ★
Heedless
Homesickness
Horrible things, sad stories, affect her
    profoundly
Hurry, hasty
    occupation, in
    walking, while
    work, in
Hypochondriasis
    imaginary illness
    suicide, driving to
Hypocrisy
Hysteria
    menses, before
    sexual excesses, after
Ideas abundant, clearness of mind
    night
    deficiency of
Imbecility
Impatience
    sitting, while •
    working, in

Impetuous
    heat, with •
Impulse, walk, to ★
Inconsolable
Indifference, apathy
    forenoon
    business affairs, to
    children, to her
    everything, to
    family, to his
    fever, during
    his own, to ★
    lies with eyes closed
    life, to
    loved ones, to
    money-making, to
    opposite sex, to ★
    pleasure, to
    reactions, to
    welfare of others, to
Indolence, aversion to work
    afternoon
    physical
    pollutions, after
Industrious, mania for work
    menses, before
Injure himself, fears to be left alone, lest
    he should
    feels as if she could easily injure
        herself •
Inquisitive
Insanity, madness
    climacteric period, during
    haemorrhage, after
    menses, with copious •
Introspection
Irresolution, indecision
Irritability
    daytime
    morning
        7h.
    alternating with indifference
    children, in
    chill, during
    coition, after
    consolation agg.
    exertion, from

Irritability,
    menses, before
        during
    music, during
        piano, of
    perspiration, during
    sadness, with
    spoken to, when
    waking, on
Jealousy, children, between
    women, between
Kleptomania
Lamenting, bemoaning, wailing
Lascivious, lustful
Laughing
    night
    involuntarily
    sleep, during
    waking, on •
    weeping or laughing on all occa-
        sions
Libertinism
Loathing, general, smoking, when •
Loathing, life, at
Magnetized, diseres to be easy to
    magnetize
    mesmerism amel.
Malicious, spiteful, vindictive
    loved ones, to •
Mania
    menses, before •
Meditation
Memory, weakness of
    expressing oneself, for
    labor, for mental
        fatigue, from
Menses, mental symptoms agg. before
        during
Mildness
Misanthropy
Mistakes, speaking, in
    misplacing words
    words, using wrong
        name of object seen instead
            of one desired
        names, calls things by wrong
    work, in
    writing
        wrong words

Moaning, groaning, whining
    colic, during ★
    sleep, during
Mocking: others are mocking at him,
    thinks
    sarcasm
Mood, alternating
    changeable, variable
    repulsive
Moral feeling, want of
Morose, cross, fretful, ill-humor, peevish
    morning
    sleepiness, with
    waking, on
Morphinism
Music agg.
    piano playing, from
    aversion to
Obstinate, headstrong
Occupation, diversion amel.
Offended, easily; takes everything in
    bad part
Passionate
Pessimist
Plans, making many
Positiveness
Praying
    fervent
Prostration of mind, mental ex-
    haustion, brain-fag
    afternoon
    coition, after
Quarrelsome, scolding
Quiet, disposition
Rage, fury
Reading, unable, to read
Rebels against poultice
Religious affections
Reproaches others
Restlessness
    evening
      bed, in
    night
      closing eyes agg., on
    anxious
    bed, driving out of
      go from one bed to another,
      wants to

Restlessness,
    tossing about in
    chest, from congestion in •
    closing eyes at night agg.
    coition, after
    driving about
    heat, during
      after
    internal
      morning on waking •
    menses, during
      suppressed, during
    sitting, while
    sleepiness, with
    strangers agg., presence of •
    waking, on
Sadness, despondency, dejection,
    mental depression, gloom,
    melancholy
    morning
      rising, amel. after •
      waking, on
    evening
    air, in open
    anger, after
    anxious
    causeless
    chill, during
    climaxis, during
    coition, after
    coughing, after
    eating, while •
    headache, during
    health, about
    heat, during
    menses, before
      during
      suppressed
    music, from
    perspiration, during
    pollutions, from
    respiration, with impeded
    suicidal disposition, with
    sultry weather, in •
    thunderstorm amel. •
    waking, on
    walking in open air, while and
      after

Secretive
Sensitive, oversensitive
   menses, before
   mental impressions, to
   music, to
      a very strong sense of rhythm ★
      piano, to
   noise, to
     slightest, to
   odors, to
   sensual impressions, to
Serious, earnest
Shrieking, screaming, shouting
   hold on to something, shrieking unless she ●
   menses, before ●
   must shriek, feels as though she
   pain, with the
   sleep, during
      menses, before
   waking, on
Sighing
   heat, during
   perspiration, during
Singing
Sit, inclination to
Sits, stiff, quite
      delirium, in ●
     still
Slander, disposition to
   hypocritical, and
Slowness
   motion, in
Somnambulism
   do mental work, to
Speech, confused
   hasty
   slow
   wandering, night
Spoken to, averse to being
Spying everything
Starting, startled
      noon
         sleep, in
      coition, after ●
     easily

Starting,
   fright, from and as from
   sleep, on falling
      during
     from
      menses, before ●
Strange, everything seems
Strangers: presence of strangers agg.
Stupefaction, as if intoxicated
   heat, during
   vertigo, during
Suicidal disposition
   despair about his miserable existence ●
   hypochondriasis, by
   pains, from
   sadness, from
   shooting, by
Suppressed or receding skin diseases or haemorrhoids, mental symptoms agg. after
Suspicious, mistrustful
Sympathetic ★
Talk, indisposed to, desire to be silent, taciturn
      afternoon
   others agg., t. of
Talking, sleep, in
   loud
Theorizing
Thinking, complaints agg., of
Thoughts, disagreeable
   disease, of
   future, of the
   persistent
   rush, flow of
      night
       sleeplessness from
   sexual
   thoughtful
   tormenting
   vanishing of, spoken to, when ●
Thunderstorm, mind symptoms during amel.
      loves ★
Timidity
Tranquillity, serenity, calmness

Unconsciousness, coma, stupor
kneeling in church, while •
menses, during
riding, while
trifles, at •
vertigo, during
Undertakes things opposed to his intentions
Unfortunate, feels
Unsympathetic, unscrupulos
Violent, vehement
Vivacious
Wearisome
Weary of life
Weeping, tearful mood
  night
  agg.
  aloud, sobbing
  alternating with laughter
  amel.
  causeless
    without knowing why
  consolation agg.
  coughing, during
  headache, with
  involuntary
  irritable
  menses, before
    during
  nervous, feels so, she would scream unless she held on to something •
  perspiration, during
  sleep, in
  spells of ★
  telling of her sickness, when
  toothache, with •
  trifles, at, laughing or weeping on every occasion
  waking, on
  walking in open air, when
Well, before an attack, feels w. ★
Will, contradiction of
Work, aversion to mental
  impossible
    headache, during •
Writing, difficulty in expressing ideas when

SERPENTARIA ARISTOLOCHIA

Dullness, sluggishness, difficulty of thinking and comprehending, torpor
Memory, weakness of
Morose, cross, fretful, ill-humor, peevish
Restlessness, bed, tossing about in

SIEGESBECKIA ORIENTALIS

Anger, irascibility
Company, aversion to; presence of other people. agg. the symptoms; desire for solitude
Discontented, everything, with
Fear, touch, of
Indifference, apathy
Indolence, aversion to work
Rudeness
Sadness, despondency, dejection, mental depression, gloom, melancholy
Striking
Thoughts, disconnected
Time passes too quickly, appears shorter
Work, mental, impossible

SILICEA TERRA (SILICA)

Abrupt, rough
Absent-minded, unobserving
Abstraction of mind
Abusive, insulting
Activity, mental
Affectionate
Ailments from:
  anger, vexation
  anticipation, foreboding, presentiment
  contradiction
  egotism
  fear
  friendship, deceived
  fright
  sexual excesses
  work, mental

Amorous

Anger, irascibility
> evening
> aroused, when
> *contradiction, from*
> violent

Anticipation, examination, before

Anxiety
> evening
>> bed, in
> night
>> waking, on
> midnight, before
>> on waking, amel. on rising ●
> midnight, after, 3h.
> *anticipation, from, an engagement* ★
> bed, in
> *conscience, as if guilty of a crime*
> dinner, after
> dreams, on waking from frightful
> eating, after
> fear, with
> *fright, after*
> *future, about*
> health, about
>> climacteric period, during
> *himself, about* ●
> *lying, while*
> **menses, during**
> motion, amel. from
> **noise, from**
>> in ear ●
> sitting, while
> sleep, before
>> during
> standing, while
> *trifles, about*
> waking, on
> walking amel., while
> weary of life, with

Audacity

Avarice

Awkward ★

Bargaining

Bed, remain in, desires to

Bite: objects, bites ★

Beside oneself, being

Capriciousness

Carefulness

Cares, worries, full of

Cautious, anxious

Censorious, critical

Cheerful, gay, mirthful
> evening, bed, in
> night
> sleep, during

Character, lack of ★

Clairvoyance

Clinging, held amel., being

Company, desire for; aversion to solitude, company amel.
> alone agg., while

Complaining

Concentration, difficult
> forenoon
> *attention, cannot fix* ★
> **studying, reading etc., while** ★

Confidence, want of self

Confusion of mind
> morning
>> rising and after, on
>> *waking, on*
> evening
> night on waking
> conversation agg. ●
> *eating, after*
> epileptic attack, before
>>> after
> headache, with
> identity, duality, sense of
> *intoxicated, as if*
> *mental exertion, from*
> riding, while
> sitting, while
> *talking, while*
> vertigo, with
> *waking, on*

Conscientious about trifles
> eating, during

Consolation, kind words agg.

Contemptuous

Contradiction, is intolerant of
> restrain himself to keep from violence, has to

Contrary
Conversation agg.
Counting continually
Cowardice
Dancing
    amel.
Darkness agg. ★
Death, desires
    dying, feels as if
    sensation of
Deceitful, sly
Defiant
Delirium
        night
    anxious
    delusions, with
    fantastic
    frightful
    throwing from window
Delirium tremens, mania-a-potu
Delusions, imaginations, hallucina-
      tions, illusions
    animals, of
    body, divided, is
    criminals, about
    dead persons, sees
    divided into two parts
    dogs, sees
    double, of being
    fail, everything will
    fancy, illusions of
    half, left h. does not belong
      to her •
    head, large, seems too
    house is full of people
    images, phantoms, sees
        night
      all over, sees
      closing eyes, on
      dwells upon
      frightful
         night ★
    injury, is about to receive
    journey, he is on a
    lascivious
    needles, sees
    people: behind him, someone is
    pins, about
    places, two, at the same time, of
      being in

Delusions,
    possessed by enemies
      he was
    side, she does not own her left
    spectres, ghosts, spirits, sees
    thieves, sees
      house, in
    vermin, sees crawl about
    visions, has
      horrible
    walks beside him, someone
    water, of
    worms, creeping of
    wrong, he has done
Dementia, epileptics, of
Desires, indefinite
Despair
    recovery, of
Dipsomania, alcoholism
Dirtiness
    urinating and defecating every-
      where, children
Discomfort, afternoon
Discontented, displeased, dissatisfied
Discouraged
Disgust
Dishonest
Dream, as if in a
Dullness, slugishness, difficulty of
      thinking and comprehend-
      ing, torpor
      morning
        waking, on
      forenoon
      afternoon
      evening amel.
    children, in
    conversation, from
    damp air, from
    dreams, after
    eating amel.
    heat, during
    mental exertion, from
    possessed, being
    pursued by enemies
    reading, while
    waking, on
    writing, while

Duty, no sense of duty
    stimulate sense of, to ★
Ecstasy
Effeminate
Egotism, self-esteem
Elegance, want of
Excitement, excitable
    evening in bed
    agg.
Exertion, agg. from mental
Fancies, absorbed in
    exaltation of
        evening in bed
        night
    frightful
    sleeplessness, with
    lascivious
    waking, on
Fear, apprehension, dread
    night
    appearing in public, of
    dark, of
    evil, of
    examination, before
    failure, of
    falling, of
    life long
    lightning, of
    lying in bed, while
    noise, from
    people, of; anthropophobia
    pins, pointed things, of
    robbers, of
        waking, on
    suffocation, of, night
    thunderstorm, of
    undertaking anything
        new enterprise, a ●
    waking, on
        dream, from a
    work, dread of
        literary, of
Feces, urinating and going to stool
    everywhere, children
Feigning sick
Finance, inaptitude for

Flatterer
Forgetful
    morning
    night
    eating amel., after ●
    mental exertion, from
    waking, on
    words while speaking, of; word
        hunting
Forsaken, beloved by his parents, wife,
    friends, feels is not being
Frightened easily
    waking, on
Frivolous
Gestures, awkward in
    confused
    grasping, evening on falling
        asleep ●
        fingers in the mouth, chil
        dren put
    hands, motions, involuntary,
        of the
        throwing about
    uncertain
Godless, want of religious feeling
Grief
Gristly ★
Guilt, sense of, trifles, about ★
Haughty
Heedless
Homesickness
Horrible things, sad stories, affect her
    profoundly
House-keeping, women unable to
Hurry, haste
    always in
Hypochondriasis, pollutions, after
Hypocrisy
Hysteria
    pollutions, after
Ideas abundant, clearness of mind
    evening
        bed, in
    night
    deficiency of
Imbecility

Impatience
    always
Inconsolable
Inconstancy
Indifference, apathy
    chill, during
    duties, to
    external things, to
Indolence, aversion to work
    afternoon
Insanity, madness
Irresolution, indecision
    changeable
    marry, to
Irritability
    morning
    forenoon
    evening
    aroused, when
    children, in
    chill, during
    coition, after
    consolation agg.
    headache, during
    spoken to, when
    trifles, from
Jesting, aversion to
Jumping : river, impulse of j. into the
        ★
Kill, desire to
Kleptomania
Lamenting, bemoaning, wailing
    night on waking •
    waking, on
Lascivious, lustful
    morning, in bed •
    dreaming, after •
Late, always too
Laughing
    night
    midnight
    sleep, during
    spasmodic
Liar
Loathing, life, at
    work, at

Looked at, cannot bear to be
Magnetized, desires to be
    mesmerism amel.
Mania
    demoniac
Mathematics, horror of mathematics
Memory, active
    short, but
Memory, wearkness of
    colours, for
    labor, for mental
        fatigue, from
    orthography, for
    places, for
    words, of
Menses, mental symptoms agg. during
Mildness
Mistakes, lotalities, in
    reading, in
    speaking, in
        misplacing words
        words, using wrong
    writing, in
Moaning, convulsions, in
    pain, with ★
    sleep, during
Monomania
Mood, changeable, variable
    repulsive
Morose, cross, fretful, ill-humor,
    peevish
    forenoon
    children, in
    coition, after
    trifles, about
    women, in
Muttering
    evening in bed •
    night on waking
Nymphomania
    menses, after suppressed
Objective, reasonable
Obstinate, headstrong
    children
        cry when kindly spoken to, yet •

Occupation, diversion amel.
Offended, easily; takes everything in bad part
Optimistic
Persevere, cannot ★
Postponing everything to next day
Prostration of mind, mental exhaustion, brain-fag
    afternoon
    reading, from
    writing, after
Quarrelsome, scolding
    evening
Quiet, disposition
Reading, aversion to read
    agg. ★
Recognizes, relatives, does not recognize his
Religious affections
    melancholia
Remorse
    trifles, about ●
Reproaches himself
Reserved
Restlessness
    forenoon
    night
        midnight, after
    anxious
    bed, driving out of
        tossing about in
    headache, during
    internal
    pain, from
    sitting, while
    waking, on
Reverence for those around him
Sadness, despondency, dejection, mental depression, gloom, melancholy
    morning
    alone, when
    heat, during
    masturbation, from
    menses, during
        after
        suppressed
    sleepiness, with
Self-control, want of

Selfishness, egoism
Senses, acute
    dull, blunted
Sensitive, oversensitive
    mental impressions, to
    noise, to
        painful sensitiveness to
        slightest, to
    voices, to
    sensual impressions, to
    steel points directed toward her
Servile, obsequious, submissive
Shrieking, screaming, shouting
    children, in
        spoken to, when ●
    convulsions, before
        after
    must shriek, feels as though she
    sleep, during
    waking, on
Sighing
Sit, inclination to
Sluggishness, processes, in ★
Somnambulism
    do day labor, to
    new and full moon, at ●
Speech, delirious, night
    facile
    fluent
    loud, sleep, in
    unintelligible
Spoken to, averse to being
Squanders, order, from want of
Starting, startled
    noon
        sleep, in
    night
    dream, from a
    easily
    fright, from and as from
    noise, from
    sleep, on falling
        during
        from
    sleepiness, with, afternoon ●
    touched, when
    tremulous
    trifles, at

Strange, crank, in dressing
Stupefaction, as if intoxicated
    rising, on •
    vertigo, during
Suicidal disposition
    drowning, by
    menses, during
    perspiration, during
    throwing himself from a height
Suspicious, mistrustful
Talk, indisposed to, desire to be silent,
    taciturn
      loud •
    others agg., talk of
    slow learning to
Talking, sleep, in
      loud
Theorizing
Thinking, aversion to
Thoughts, persistent
    unpleasant subjects, haunted
    by,
      on waking
    rush, flow of
      evening in bed
      night
      sleeplessness from
      walking, on
    sexual
    two trains of thoughts
Thunderstorm, mind symptoms during
Timidity
    alone, when •
    appearing in public, about
      talk in public, to
    awkward, and
    bashful ★
Touched, aversion to being
Tranquillity, serenity, calmness
Trifles seem important
Unconsciousness, coma, stupor
    cold, after taking •
    conduct, automatic
    riding, while
    sitting, while
    transient
    vertigo, during
Undertakes nothing, lest he fail

Ungrateful, avarice, from
Unreliable, promises, in his
Violent, vehement
    crossed, when •
Washing, cleanliness, mania for
Weary of life
    perspiration, during
Weeping, tearful mood
    morning
    afternoon
    evening
    night
      waking, on
    carried, child cries piteously if taken
      hold of or c.
    children, in
    chill, during
    consolation agg.
    convulsions, during
    coughing, during
    despair, from
    sleep, in
    spoken to, when
      kindly (children)
    stool, during
    touched, when ★
    trifles, at
    waking, on
    walking in open air, when
    whimpering, sleep, during
Will, loss of
    weakness of
Work, aversion to mental
    fatigues
    impossible
    afternoon
Writing, difficulty in expressing ideas
    when
    fatigues •
    inability for
      learning to write in children
Yielding disposition

SINAPIS ALBA

Concentration, difficult
    studying, reading etc., while

SINAPIS NIGRA

Activity, mental, night
Answers, abruptly, shortly, curtly
    snappishly
Anxiety
**Concentration difficult, attention,
    cannot fix ★**
Delirium
    fever, during
Discontented, displeased, dissatisfied
Dullness, sluggishness, difficulty of think-
    ing and comprehending, torpor
Fancies, lascivious
*Fear, coition, impotency from fear
    during* ●
    heart, of disease of
Hypochondriasis
Irritability
Lascivious, erections, with
Morose, cross, fretful, ill-humor, peevish
Sadness, disease, about
Spoken to, aversion to being

SIUM LATIFOLIUM

Fear, death, of
Prostration of mind, mental exhaus-
    tion, brain-fag

SOLANUM ARREBENTA

Impatience, trifles, about
Starting, sleep, from

SOLANUM CAROLINENSE

Dementia, epileptics, of
Sadness, despondency, dejection, men-
    tal depression, gloom, melan-
    choly

SOLANUM MAMMOSUM

Anger, irascibility
    happen, at what he thinks may
Delirium, bed and escapes, springs up
    suddenly from

Dullness, waking, on
Irritability
Jumping, bed, out of
Malicious, spiteful, vindictive
Restlessness
    driving about
Thoughts, wandering
Work, mental, impossible

SOLANUM NIGRUM

Beside oneself, being
Delirium
    raging, raving
Delusions, night
    voices, hears
Escape, attempts to
Frightened, waking, on
Gestures, convulsive
    *grasping or reaching at some-
        thing, at flocks; carphologia
        night
    chewing and swallowing, on* ●
    picks at bed clothes
Imbecility
Insanity, madness
Laughing, sardonic
Mania
    rage, with
Memory, weakness of,
    labor, for mental
Moaning, night
Rage, fury
    shrieking, with
Restlessness
Shrieking, screaming, shouting
    brain cry
Starting, startled
Stupefaction, as if intoxicated
Unconsciousness, coma, stupor
    apoplexy, in
    fever, during
Weeping, tearful mood
Work, aversion to mental

SOLANUM OLERACEUM

Ailments from:
grief
Sadness, despondency, dejection, mental
depression, gloom, melancholy

SOLANUM TUBEROSUM

Restlessness
bed, tossing about in
Unconsciousness, incomplete

SOLANUM TUBEROSUM AEGROTANS

Anxiety, future, about
waking, on
Break things, desire to
Censorious, critical
Delusions, thieves, sees
house, in
Destructiveness
Fear, robbers, of
Irritability
expressions, from unintelligible •
Loquacity, evening
Morose, cross, fretful, ill-humor, peevish
Restlessness, night
Sadness, despondency, dejection, mental
depression, gloom, melancholy
Starting, sleep, during
Thoughts, past journeys, of the •
rush, flow of, afternoon, 17h. •
wandering, listening, while •
work, at •

SOLANIUM ACETICUM

Touched, ticklishness

SPHINGURUS (SPIGGURUS)

Unconsciousness, coma, stupor

SPIGELIA ANTHELMIA

Absent minded, unobserving
Absorbed, buried in thought
future, about •
Activity, mental
Ailments from:
anticipation, foreboding, presentiment
quarrels
sexual excesses
Anger, irascibility
face, with red
Anxiety
evening
air, in open
alternating with exhilaration
breathing deeply, on
conscience, as if guilty of a crime
fear, with
fever, during
future, about
pains, from the abdomen
eyes •
Beside oneself, being
Blasphemy
cursing, and
Capriciousness
Cares, worries, full of
relatives, about
Chaotic, confused behavior
Cheerful, gay, mirthful
morning
evening, bed, in
alternating with anxiety
palpitation •
sadness
pain, with all •
Concentration, difficult
studying, reading, etc., while
Confiding
Confusion of mind
evening
air, in open
dream, as if in
sitting, while
stooping, when
walking in open air, while

Conscientious about trifles
Contented
Conversation agg.
Cowardice
Cursing, swearing
Death, during chill, desires
Delirium
Delirium tremens, mania-a-potu
Delusions, fire, visions of
    feet, higher than head ★
    floating in air ★
    pins, about
    spectres, ghosts, spirits, sees
Desires, full of
Despair
Dipsomania, alcoholism
Discouraged
Disobedience
Dullness, sluggishness, difficulty of thinking and comprehending, torpor
Eccentricity
Ennui, tedium
Envy
Excitement, excitable
    evening in bed
    chill, during
    sadness, after
    trembling, with
Exertion, agg. from mental
Fear, apprehension, dread
    evil, of
    hurt, of being
    pins, pointed things, of
    suffering, of
    suffocation, of
    touch, of
Forgetful
Forsaken feeling
Heedless
High-spirited
Ideas abundant, clearness of mind
    chill-during
    deficiency of
Imbecility
Impatience
Inconstancy
Indifference, pleasure, to
Indignation

Indolence, aversion to work
    evening
Industrious, mania for work
Irresolution, indecision
Irritability
    evening
    alternating with cheerfulness
    chill, during
Jesting, aversion to
Lascivious, lustful
Loathing, life, at
    evening
Meditation
Memory, active
Memory, weakness of
    labor, for mental
    names, for proper
Mood, changeable, variable
Morose, cross. fretful, ill-humor, peevish
    evening
Occupation, diversion amel.
Offended, easily; takes everything in bad part
Overactive
Prostration of mind, mental exhaustion, brain-fag
Rebels against poultice
Restlessness
    night
    anxious
    chill, during
    driving about
Sadness, despondency, dejection, mental depression, gloom, melancholy
    evening
    anger, from
    anxious
    chill, during
    perspiration, during
    suicidal disposition, with
Sensitive, oversensitive
    noise, to
    painful sensitiveness to
    steel points directed towards her

Serious earnest
Shrieking, pain with the, feet •
Slander, disposition to
Somnambulism
Speech, incoherent
Starting, sleep, during
Stupefaction, as if intoxicated
Suicidal disposition
        evening
    sadness, from
Suspicious, mistrustful
Talk, indisposed to, desire to be silent,
        taciturn
Talking, sleep, in
Thinking, complaints agg., of
Thoughts, future, of the
        profound, future, about his
        rush, flow of
        thoughtful
Timidity
Tranquillity, serenity, calmness
Unconsciousness, coma, stupor
        morning
Violent, vehement
Vivacious
Walk: walking in open air agg. mental
        symptoms
Weary of life
        evening
Weeping, tearful mood
    coryza, during
    heat, during
Work, aversion to mental
    impossible
Writing, desire for

SPIGELIA MARYLANDICA

Mania
Runs about
Speech, incoherent
        wild
Weeping, alternating with laughter

SPIRANTHES AUTUMNALIS

Anxiety, conscience, as if guilty of a
        crime

Complaining
Confusion of mind
Discomfort
Ennui, tedium
Hysteria
Restlessness, night
Sadness, despondency, dejection, mental
        depression, gloom, melancholy

SPIRAEA ULMARIA

Ennui, tedium
Hydrophobia
Indolence, aversion to work
Loathing, oneself, at
Morose, cross, fretful, ill-humor, peevish
Remorse, indiscretion, over past •
Restlessness, night

SPONGIA TOSTA

Absent minded, unobserving
Abstraction of mind
Abusive, insulting
Anger, irascibility
        alternating with cheerfulness
Anguish, cardiac
Answers: aversion to answer
Anxiety
        morning, waking, on ★
        night
        midnight, after
        air, amel. in open
        alternating with exhilaration
        bed, passing off on sitting up in •
        **dreams, on waking from
          frightful**
        faintness, with
        fear, with
        fever, during
        flushes of heat, during
        future, about
        house, in
        lying, while
        paroxysms
        periodical

Anxiety,
   sleep, during
   waking, on
   walking, while
      air, in open
   weary of life, with
Aversion, everything, to
Barking
Capriciousness
Cheerful, gay, mirthful
   alternating with absence of mind
      aversion to work •
      distraction •
      irritability
      lachrymose mood
      quarrelsomeness
      seriousness
      vexation
      weeping
   destruction, with ★
   followed by prostration
Concentration, difficult
Confusion of mind
   intoxicated, as if
   walking, while
Contemptuous
Contrary
Dancing agg.
Death, desires
   thoughts of
Defiant
Delirium, delusions, with
   fantastic
   fever, during
   sleep, during
      falling asleep, on
   sleeplessness, and ★
Delusions, imaginations, hallucinations,
      illusions
   falling asleep, on
   fancy, illusions of
   figures, sees
   fire, visions of
   images, phantoms, sees
      night
      frightful

Delusions,
   motion, up and down, of
   persecuted, he is
   pursued, tormented by a frightful
      scene mournful event of the
      past, and •
   spectres, ghosts on closing eyes,
      sees
   visions, has
      night
      closing the eyes, on
      horrible, events, of past •
      vivid
Desires, sing, to ★
Despair, heat, during
Dipsomania, alcoholism
Discontented, displeased, dissatisfied
   everything, with
Disgust
   everything, with
Dullness, sluggishness, difficulty of think-
      ing and comprehending, torpor
   alternating with hilarity and
   mirth
      singing •
   says nothing
Dwells on past disagreeable occur-
      rences
Excitement, excitable
   morning
   agg.
Exertion, agg. from mental
Fancies, exaltation of
      night
      sleeplessness, with
   sleep, on falling asleep
Fear, apprehension, dread
      night
         waking, after
   death, of
   disease, of impending
   evil, of
   ghosts, of
   happen, something will
   heart, of disease of
   heat, during

Fear,
>insanity, losing his reason, of
>misfortune, of
>palpitation, with •
>*perspiration, with* •
>recurrent
>*suffocation, of*
>>*night*
>>heart disease, in
>>*waking, on*

Frightened, easily
>*night*
>waking, on

Frivolous
High-spirited
Hypochondriasis
Ideas, abundant, clearness of mind
>closing the eyes, on

Imbecility
Impatience
Impertinence
Inconsolable
Indifference, apathy
Indiscretion
Indolence, aversion to work
Insolence
Irritability
>morning
>alternating with cheerfulness
>headache, during

Jesting
Laughing
Loathing, life, at
Mania
Memory, weakness of
>labor, for mental

Mildness
Mischievous
Mood, changeable, variable
>repulsive

Morose, cross, fretful, ill-humor, peevish
Obstinate, headstrong
Overactive
Prostration of mind, mental exhaustion, brain-fag
Quarrelsome, scolding
>alternating with gaiety and laughter

Reserved
Restlessness
>night
>anxious
>heat, during

Rudeness
Sadness, despondency, dejection, mental depression, gloom, melancholy
>anxious
>*heat, during*
>impotence, with

Senses, dull, blunted
Shrieking, sleep, during
Sighing
Singing
>alternating with distraction •
>>hatred of work •
>involuntarily

Sit, inclination to
Somnambulism
Speech, loud, in sleep
>wandering

Starting, startled
>morning after waking
>night
>easily
>*fright, from and as from*
>noise, from
>perspiration, during
>sleep, during
>**from**
>*trifles, at*

Stupefaction, as if intoxicated
Suicidal disposition, intermittent fever, during
>*perspiration, during*

Sulky
Talk, indisposed to, desire to be silent, taciturn
Talking, sleep, in
>loud

Terror ★
Thinking, complaints agg., of
Thoughts, intrude, closing eyes, on •
>rush, flow of
>>*night*
>tormenting, past disagreeable events, about

Timidity

Unconsciousness, chill, during
Wearisome
Weary of life
Weeping, tearful mood
    morning
    night
    alternating with cheerfulness
    anger, after
    anxiety, after
    coughing, during
    heat, during
    perspiration, during
    sleep, in
Witty
Work, aversion to mental
    impossible ·

SQUILLA (SCILLA) MARITIMA

Amorous ★
Anger, irascibility
    easily
Anxiety
    morning on waking
    night
    midnight, after
    fever, during
    hypochondriacal
    waking, on
Audacity
Bed, aversion to, shuns bed
Chaotic, confused behavior
Cheerful, gay, mirthful
Concentration, difficult
Confusion of mind
    morning
    dream, as if in
    intoxicated, as after being
    sleeping, after
    waking, on
Courageous
Delirium, haemorrhage, after
Dream, as if in a
Dullness, sluggishness, difficulty of thinking and comprehending, torpor
    morning

Fear, apprehension, dread
    bed, of the
    death, of
    evil, of
Firmness
Haughty
Indifference, apathy
    work, with aversion to
Indolence, aversion to work
    morning
Insanity, madness
Irritability
Malicious, spiteful, vindictive
Moaning, groaning, whining
Moral feeling, want of
Morose, cross, fretful, ill-humor, peevish
Prostration of mind, mental exhaustion, brain fag
Restlessness, bed, tossing about in
    waking, on
Sadness, despondency, dejection, mental depression, gloom, melancholy
Sit, inclination to
Stupefaction, as if intoxicated
    morning
Talk, indisposed to, desire to be silent, taciturn
Thinking, aversion to
Timidity, evening about going to bed
Unconsciousness, coma, stupor
Unfeeling, hardhearted
Wearisome
Weeping, tearful mood
    whimpering
Work, aversion to mental
Writing, aversion to

STANNUM METALLICUM

Absent-minded, unobserving
Absorbed, buried in thought
Abstraction of mind
Activity, fruitless ●
Admonition, kindly agg.
Ailments from:
    anger, vexation
        anxiety, with
    excitement, emotional

Ailments from:
>> fright
>> reverses of fortune

Anger, irascibility
>> talk, indisposed to
>> *violent*

Anguish
>> daytime
>> menses, during

Answers, abruptly, shortly, curtly
>> *aversion to answer*

Anxiety
>>> *evening*
>> constriction of chest, from •
>> *domestic affairs, during pregnancy, about*
>> fever, during
>> *future, about*
>> knows not, what to do with himself ★
>> lying, while
>> *menses, before*
>>> during
>>>> amel.
>> motion, from
>> pregnancy, in
>> sleep, during

Avarice, anxiety about future, from

Aversion, men, to
>> persons, to certain
>> society, to ★

Barking

Begging, sleep, in •

Beside oneself, being

Blank ★

Business, averse to

Busy, fruitlessly

Cares, worries, full of

Carried, desires to be, shoulder, over

Cheerful, gay, mirthful

Clairvoyance

Company, aversion to; presence of other people agg. the symptoms; desire for solitude
>> alone, amel. when

Company, desire for; aversion to solitude, company amel.
>> alone agg., while

Concentration, difficult

Confusion of mind
>> morning
>> evening
>> vertigo, with
>> waking, on

Conversation agg.

Cowardice

Dancing amel.

Delusions, imaginations, hallucinations, illusions
>> afternoon, it is always
>> *disease, has incurable*
>> enlarged, distances are
>> fancy, illusions of
>> fire, visions of

Despair
>> heat, during
>> perspiration, during

Discontented, displeased, dissatisfied
>> everything, with

Discouraged

Distances, inaccurate judgement of

Doubtful, recovery, of

Dullness, sluggishness, difficulty of thinking and comprehending, torpor
>>> morning on waking
>>> evening
>> chill, during
>> waking, on

Ecstasy

Emptiness, sensation of ★

Envy, avidity, and

Excitement, excitable
>>> agg.
>> palpitation, with violent

Exertion, agg. from mental

Exuberance

Fancies, exaltation of

Fear, apprehension, dread
>>> night
>> crowd, in a
>> death, of
>> disease, of impending
>>> incurable, of being
>> *evil, of*
>> jumps out of bed from f.

Fear,
> lifelong
> men, dread, fear of
> people, of; anthropophobia
> poverty, of, spending in order to
> > not being short of money in
> > future
> pregnancy, during

Forgetful
> morning
> > waking, on
> waking, on

Greed, cupidity

Grief, future, for the

Hatred
> men, of
> revenge, hatred and

Howling

Hypochondriasis

Hysteria

Ideas, deficiency of
> fixed ★

Idleness

Imbecility

Impatience

Inconsolable

Inconstancy

Indifference, apathy
> everything, to
> external things, to
> pleasure, to

Indolence, aversion to work

Industrious, mania for work
> menses, before

Insanity, madness

Introspection

Irresolution, indecision

Irritability
> daytime
> air, amel. in open
> headache, during

Jesting

Lamenting, bemoaning, wailing
> asleep, while

Laughing agg.

Looks down, before him ★

Loquacity

Malicious, spiteful, vindictive

Memory, weakness of

Menses, mental symptoms agg. before
> during

Mildness

Misanthropy

Mischievous

Mistakes, reading, in
> time, in; afternoon, always imag-
> > ines it is

Moaning, sleep, during

Mocking

Mood, alternating
> *changeable, variable*

Morose, cross, fretful, ill-humor, peevish
> air amel., in open
> *talk, indisposed to*

Music agg.
> sleepiness from ●

Muttering

Nymphomania

Offended, easily; takes everything in
> bad part

Passionate

Pessimist

Praying, timidity ●

Prostration of mind, mental exhaus-
> tion, brain fag
> trembling, with

Quarrelsome, scolding

Quiet disposition

Reading, mental symptoms agg. from

Religious affections

Repeated ★

Reserved

Rest, desire for

Restlessness
> night
> midnight, after, 1h.
> busy
> driving about
> waking, on

Sadness, despondency, dejection, men-
> *tal depression, gloom, melan-*
> *choly*
> daytime
> anxious
> headache, during

Sadness,
    heat, during
    menses, before
      during
        amel.
    talk, indisposed to
Self, knows not what do with her ★
Senses, dull, blunted
    vanishing of
Sensitive, oversensitive
    certain persons, to
    music, to
    noise, to
    odors, to
    pain, to
Shrieking, convulsions, during epilep-
    tic
    must shriek, feels as though she
Sighing
Sit, inclination to
Sociability
Somnambulism
Speech, affected
    hasty
    nonsensical
Starting, fright, from and as from
    sleep, during
Stupefaction, as if intoxicated
    vertigo, during
Sulky
Suspicious, mistrustful
Talk, indisposed to, desire to be silent,
    taciturn
      sadness, in
Talking agg. all complaints
    sleep, in
    supplicates timidly •
Thinking, complaints agg., of
Thoughts, persistent
    vanishing of
Time, fritters away his
Tranquillity, serenity, calmness
Unconsciousness, coma, stupor
    pain, from
    vertigo, during
Undertakes many things, perseveres in
    nothing

Violent, vehement
Walk, walking in open air amel. mental
    symptoms
Weeping, tearful mood
    night
    agg.
    involuntary
    nervous all day, feels so, feels like
      crying all the time, but it
      makes her worse •
    pregnancy, during
    sleep, in
    whimpering, sleep, during
Work, mental, impossible
Writing agg. mind symptoms

STANNUM IODATUM

Sadness, despondency, dejection, mental
    depression, gloom, melancholy

STAPHYSAGRIA

Abrupt, harsh
Absent-minded, unobserving
    dreamy
    inadvertance
Absorbed, buried in thought
Abusive, insulting
Adulterous
Affectionate
Ailments from :
    anger, vexation
      indignation, with
      silent, grief, with
      suppressed
    anticipation, foreboding, presen-
      timent
    cares, worries
    death of a child
      parents or friends, of
    disappointment
    embarrassment
    excitement, emotional
      moral ★
      sexual
    grief
    honor, wounded

Ailments from :
   indignation
   jealousy
   love, disappointed
   unhappy
   mortification
      indignation, with •
   position, loss of
   reproaches
   reverses of fortune
   rudeness of others
   scorn, being scorned
   sexual excesses
   work, mental
Ambition
Amorous
Anger, irascibility
   morning
   always ★
   cough from anger
   face, with pale, livid
      red
   himself, with
   mistakes, about his
   throws things away
   trembling, with
   trifles, at
   violent
   weeping from pain, with
Anguish,
      afternoon ★
   nap, after ★
Anxiety
      morning
      afternoon, sleep, after ★
   conscience, as if guilty of a crime
   exaggerated ★
   fear, with
   future, about
   health, about
   hypochondriacal
      mania to read medical books
   menses, anger and anxiety **dur**ing
   others, for
   salvation, about
      faith, about loss of his

Anxiety,
      scruples, excessive religious
      scrupulous as to their
         religious practices, too
   sitting, while
   suicidal disposition, with
      thinking about it, from
   vexation, after
   walking, while
      amel.
      rapidly, when
   weary of life, with
Audacity
Avarice
Aversion, persons, to all
   wife, to his ★
   sex, to opposite
Blasphemy
   cursing, and
Blood, wounds, cannot look at
Break things, desire to
Busy, himself, with
Calculating, inability for
Capriciousness
   morning
Cares, worries, full of
   morning
Carried, desires to be
Censorious, critical
Chaotic, confused behavior
Cheerful, gay, mirthful
      afternoon
      evening, bed, in
      alternating with anxiety
         quarrelsomeness
         sadness
      drunkenness, during
      quarrelsome, and
Company, aversion to; presence of
      other people agg. the symp-
      toms; desire for solitude
   alone, amel. when
   bear anybody, cannot
   loathing at company
Concentration, active

Concentration, difficult
  aversion to ★
  on attempting to concentrate, has
    a vacant feeling
  studying, reading etc., while
Confidence, want of self
Confusion of mind
  morning
  concentrate the mind, on attempt-
    ing to
  mental exertion, from
  periodical ●
  standing, while
  talking, while
  waking, on
Conscientious about trifles
Consolation, kind words agg.
Contented
Contradict, disposition to
Contradiction, is intolerant of
Coquettish, not enough
Courageous, alternating with discour-
    agement
Cowardice
Credulous
Cruelty, inhumanity
Cursing, swearing
Death, desires
  presentiment of
Delusions, imagination, hallucinations,
    illusions
  body, greatness of, as to
  crime, committed a, he had
  criticised, she is
  fancy, illusions of
  fortune, he was going to lose his
  happened anything, of having
  humility and lowness of others,
    while he is great
  insults, of ★
  large, himself seems too
  low down, everything beneath him
    seems too ●
  murdered, he will be
  past anxious thoughts and things
    are present ●

Delusions,
  people, behind him, someone is
    walking, when ●
  persecuted, he is
  pursued, he was
  rain, he hears
  small, things appear
  something else, objects appear as
    if ●
  starve, family will
  strange, everything is
    familiar things seem
  taste, of
  unfortunate, he is
  unreal, everything seems
  walks behind him, someone
  wife, run away from him, will ●
Desire, uncontrollable, itching, for ★
Despair
  health, of
  social position, of
Destructiveness
Dipsomania, alcoholism
Dirtiness
Discontented, displeased, dissatisfied
  everything, with
  himself, with
Discouraged, alternating with courage
                hope
Disobedience
Doubtful
Dream, future, about the ●
Dullness, sluggishness, difficulty of
    thinking and comprehending,
    torpor
  morning
    waking, on
  conversation, from
  emotions, from
  masturbation, after
  mortification, after ●
  sleepiness, with
  waking, on
Dwells on past disagreeable occur-
    rences
  grief from past offences

Ecstasy

Egotism, self-esteem

    speaking about themselves in company, always

Envy

    avidity, and

Escape, family, children, from her

    children, on waking •

Estranged from her family

    wife, from his

Excitement, excitable

    evening in bed

    agg.

    moral, ailments from ★

    nervous

    palpitation, with violent

    swallows continually while talking •

Exertion, agg. from mental

Fancies, exaltation of

    evening in bed

    happened, thinks they had •

    sleeplessness, with

    lascivious

    sleep, preventing

Fear, apprehension, dread

    apoplexy, of

    death, of

        impending d., of

    disease, of impending

    evil, of

    faith, to lose his religious ★

    family, to bring up his ★

    heights, of

    high places, of

    insanity, losing his reason, of

    murdered, of being

    narrow places, in; claustrophobia

    people, of; anthropophobia

    position, to lose his lucrative

    rags, of ★

    rage, to fly into a

    self-control, of losing

    society, of his position in

    suffocation, of

    walking, while

        rapidly •

Fire, wants to set things on

    throws things into •

Flatterer

Forgetful

    emotions, after

    pollutions, after •

    sexual excesses, after

    words while speaking, of; word hunting

Fright, menses, during ★

Frightened, easily

Gamble (*see* Play)

Generous, too much

Gestures, plays with his fingers, counting money, as if

Greed, cupidity

Grief

    daytime •

    evening amel.

    condition, about his •

    headache from grief

    offenses, grief from long past

Hatred, persons who had offended him, of

Haughty

Heedless

Hide, desires to

High places agg.

Homesickness

Honor, wounded

Horrible things, sad stories, affect her profoundly

Hurry, haste

    always in

Hypochondriasis

    pollutions, after

    sexual excesses, from

    suicide, driving to

Hysteria

    pollutions, after

Ideas abundant, clearness of mind

    evening

    night

    deficiency of

Imbecility

    sexual excitement, with

Impatience

Impertinence
Impetuous
    morning •
Impulse, morbid, rash
Impulsive
Indifference, apathy
    morning on waking
    agreeable things, to
    eating, to
    everything, to
    external things, to
    masturbation, after •
    pleasure, to
    taciturn
    work, with aversion to
Indignation
Indiscretion
Indolence, aversion to work
Industrious, mania for work
Injustice, cannot support
Insanity, anger, from
    black insanity with despair and
        weary of life from fear of
        mortification or of loss of
        position
    haemorrhage, after
    melancholy
    mortification, from
    position, from fear to lose
    sexual excesses, from
Insolence
Interruption agg. mental symptoms
Introspection
Irresolution, indecision
    marry, to
Irritability
    daytime
    morning
    children, in
    chill, during
    coition, after
    consolation agg.
    heat, during
    pollutions, after
    spoken to, when
    talking, while

Jealousy
    drunkenness, during
Jesting
    aversion to
Jumping, height from a, impulse to j. ★
Kill, desire to
Kleptomania
Lamenting, bemoaning, wailing
Lascivious, lustful
Laughing, weeping or laughing on all
    occasions
Liar
Libertinism
Loathing, life, at
Looking backwards, as if fol-
    lowed •
Loquacity
    insane
    precocious ★
Malicious, spiteful, vindictive
Mania
    night, midnight, agg. about •
    alternating with depression
Marriage seemed unendurable, idea of
Mathematics, inapt for algebra
    horror of mathematics
Meditation
Memory, active, short, but
Memory, weakness of
    colors, for
    dates, for
    forms, for
    labor, for mental
    music, for
    names, for proper
    persons, for
    places, for
    read, for what has
    say, for what is about to
    thought, for what has just
    words, of
Misanthropy
Mistakes, speaking, in
    words, using wrong
    time, in: confounds future with
        the past, present with the past
    writing, in

Mood, alternating
    changeable, variable
Morose, cross, fretful, ill-humor, peevish
    daytime
    morning
    children, morning early in •
Music agg.
    palpitation when listening to
Nymphomania
Obscene, lewd
Obstinate, headstrong
**Offended, easily takes everything
    in bad part**
    offences, from past
Pities herself
Play, passion for gambling to make
    money
Presumptuous
*Prostration of mind, mental exhaus-
    tion, brain-fag*
    convulsions, from
    vexation, from •
Quarrelsome, scolding
    morning
    *alternating with gaiety and
      laughter*
    anger, without
Rage, fury
Reading: passion to read medical books
Rebels against poultice
Religious affections
    very religious ★
Reproaches others
Reserved
Restlessness
    daytime
    afternoon
    air amel., in open
    anxious
    bed, tossing about in
    coition, after
    company, in ★
    driving about
    heat, during
    sexual excitement, in •
    sitting, while

Rudeness, naughty children, of
*Sadness, despondency, dejection, mental
    depression, gloom, melancholy*
    daytime
    night
    chill, during
    coition, after
    drunkards, in
    drunkenness, during
    health, about
    heat, during
    masturbation, from
    menses, suppressed, from
    mercury, after abuse of
    misfortune, as if from
    suicidal disposition, with
Senses, dull, blunted
    vanishing of
Sensitive, oversensitive
    children
    external impressions, to all
    moral impressions, to
    noise, to
    odors, to
    puberty, in
    reprimands, to
    rudeness, to
    touch, to
    want of sensitiveness
Sentimental
Serious, earnest
Singing, trilling
Smaller, things appear
Snappish ★
Speech, bombast, worthless
    low
Spoken to, averse to being
Starting, night
    dream, from a
    fright, from and as from
    sleep, during
Striking
    desires to strike
Stupefaction, as if intoxicated
    motion, from
    vertigo, during

Suicidal, disposition
    drowning, by
    fear of death, with
    hypochondriasis, by
    love, from disappointed ★
    sadness, from
    shooting, by
    throwing himself from a height
Suspicious, mistrustful
Talk, indisposed to, desire to be silent,
    taciturn
    sexual excesses, after •
Talks, humming
Tastelessness in dressing
Temerity
Thinking, complaints agg., of
Thoughts, intrude, sexual
    persistent
    rush, flow of
        evening in bed
        sleeplessness from
    thoughtful
    tormenting, sexual
    vanishing of
        interrupted, when
        mental exertion, on
        speaking, while
        wandering
Throws things away
    morning
    persons who offend, at •
Time, fritters away his
Timidity
    bashful
    company, in
Tranquillity, serenity, calmness
Unfortunate, feels
Ungrateful
Verses, makes
Violent, vehement
Wearisome
Weary of life
Weeping, tearful mood
    admonition, from
    aloud, sobbing
    anger, after

Weeping, tearful mood
    causeless
    consolation agg.
    easily
    eating, while, in children
    offence, about former
    pains, with the
    pretends, without actual tears ★
    remonstrated, when
    spoken to, when
    trifles, at, laughing or weeping on
        every occasion
    vexation, from old
Will, weakness of
Work, aversion to mental
    fatigues
    impossible
Yielding disposition

STICTA PULMONARIA

Absent-minded, unobserving
Concentration, difficult
Dancing
Delusions, floating in air
    bed, resting in, is not
    light, incorporeal, he is
Hysteria
    fainting, hysterical
    lie down, must
    light and noise agg. •
    loss of blood, after •
    sleeplessness, with
Jumping
Loquacity
Restlessness
    sleeplessness, from
Talk: desire to t. to someone ★
    must
    listens, does not care whether
    anyone •

STIGMATA MAYDIS

Delirium

STILLINGIA SILVATICA

Ailments from:
    anticipation, foreboding, presen-
        timent
Anxiety
Dullness, sluggishness, difficulty of think-
        ing and comprehending, torpor
Fear, death, of
Sadness, despondency, dejection, mental
        depression, gloom, melancholy
Suspicious, mistrustful

STRAMONIUM

Absent-minded, unobserving
Absorbed, buried in thought
Abstraction of mind
Abusive, insulting
Affectation
Affections, in general ★
Ailments from:
    anger, vexation
        anxiety, with
        fright, with
    anticipation, foreboding, presen-
        timent
    bad news
    fright
    injuries, accidents, mental symp-
        toms from
    mortification
    reproaches
Amorous
    menses, before ★
Anger, irascibility
    alternating with cheerfulness
        laughing
    contradiction, from
    face, with red
    trifles, at
    violent
Anguish
Answers, aversion to answer
    disconnected
    imaginary questions
    incorrectly
    refuses to answer

Antics, plays
    delirium, during
    drunkenness, during
Anxiety
    night, children, in
    coffee, after
    company, when in
    for ★
    conscience, as if guilty of a crime
    conversation, from
    cough, during whooping
    coughing, from
    crowd, in a
    dark, in
    fever, during
    future, about
    motion, from
    noise of rushing water, from
    salvation, about
    sleep, during
    speaking, when
    stool, during
    strangers, in the presence of
    tunnel in a train, in •
    waking, on
Astonished
Automatism, motion (automatic) ★
Barking
Begging, entreating, supplicating
Beside oneself, being
Bite, desire to
    delirium, during
    objects, bites ★
    people, bites
Black and sombre, aversion to every-
    thing that is
Boaster, braggart
Break things, desire to
Brooding
Business, talks of
Busy
Capriciousness
Cautious
Chases imaginary objects •
Cheerful, gay, mirthful
    night
    alternating with anger

Cheerful, alternating with
    burst of passion
    irritability
    moaning
    sadness
    violence
    dancing, laughing, singing, with
    menses, during
Childbed, agg.
Childish behavior
Clairvoyance
Climb, desire to
Clinging to persons or furniture etc.
    child awakens terrified, knows no
    one, screams, clings to those
    near
    held, wants to be
    amel. being
Clothed, improperly ★
Company, aversion to; presence of
    other people agg. the symp-
    toms; desire for solitude
    alone, amel. when
    fear of being alone, yet
    presence of strangers, aversion to
Company, desire for; aversion to soli-
    tude, company
    amel.
    night
    alone agg., while
    menses, during •
Concentration, difficult
Confidence, want of self
Confusion of mind
    night, on walking about after
    midnight •
    bed, makes him jump out of
    chill, during
    identity, as to his
    duality, sense of
    perspiration, during
    vertigo, with
    waking, on
    walking about after midnight, on
    •
Conscientious about trifles
Contemptuous

Contradiction, is intolerant of
Cowardice
Crawling, bed, around in •
Cruelty, inhumanity
Cursing, swearing
Dancing
Darkness agg.
Death, desires
    presentiment of
    alternating with rage •
    thoughts of
Delirium
    day and night
    noon, 16-24 h. •
    night
    addresses objects •
    alternating with coma
    tetanic convulsions, lies on his
    back, knees and thighs flexed,
    hands joined •
    answers abruptly
    anxious
    arms, extends
    bed and escapes, springs up sud-
    denly from
    creeps about in •
    busy
    chill, during
    comical
    crying, with

    help, for
    dark, in
    delusions, with
    erotic
    exaltation of strength, with
    face muscles constantly in play •
    fantastic
    fever, during
    fierce
    foolish, silly
    foreign language, talks in a •
    frightful
    gay, cheerful
    alternating with laughing, sing-
    ing
    whistling, crying •
    headache, during
    heat agg.

Delirium,

    horses, talks about •
    injuries to head, after
    intermittent
    laughing
    look fixed on one point, staring
       staring with wrinkled face •
    loquacious
    maniacal
    menses, during
    mild
    moves, queer •
    murmuring
    muttering
    naked in delirium, wants to be
    noisy
    nonsense, with eyes open
    persecution in delirium, delusions
       of
    rabid
    raging, raving
    recognizes no one
    restless
    scolding
    shy, hides himself •
    singing
    sleep, during
    stupid •
    trembling, with
    violent
    vivid
    waking, on
    wild

Delirium tremens, mania-a-potu

    delusions, with
    escape, attempts to
    face, with red, bloated
    praying, with •
    trembling, with

**Delusions, imaginations, halluci-
nations, illusions**

    activity, with
    alone, she is always
       wilderness, being alone in a •
    angels, seeing
    animals, of
       bed, on

Delusions,

  .   *beetles, worms etc.*
      creeping in her
      frightful
      jump out of the ground •
      persons are
      rats, mice, insects etc.
    **assembled things, swarms,
crowds, etc.**
    beautiful, she is beautiful and
      wants to be •
    bed, creases, is full of •
      drawn from under her •
      someone is in bed with him
    bitten, will be
    black objects and people, sees
    body, alive on one side, buried on
      the other •
      divided, is
      scattered about bed, tossed
        about to get the pieces
        together
    bugs and cockroaches, of •
    business, they are pursuing ordi-
      nary
    **catches at imaginary appear-
ances**
      people, at •
    cats, sees
    changed, everything is
    churchyard, visits a
      dancing in, he is
    conversing, d. with
    corners, animals and figures com-
      ing out of, sees •
      people coming out of, sees •
      seems something coming out
        of, and towards him ★
    creeping things, full of •
    cut through, he is •
      in two
    danger, impression of
    dead, he himself was
      persons, sees
    deserted, forsaken, is
    devils, sees
      he is a devil
      possessed of a devil, is

Delusions,

devoured by animals, of being •
die, he was about to
disease, he has every
distinguished, is
divided into two parts
   cuts in two parts, or
divine, being
dogs, sees
   attack him •
   biting his chest •
   others are, barks at them to be
     understood
   swarm about him
doomed, being
double, of being
dying, he is
engaged in some occupation, is
   ordinary occupation, in
enlarged
   body, parts of
   tall, is very
executioner, visions of an •
   elongated •
faces, sees, elongated •
fall, things will
falling, he is
fancy, illusions of
   heat, during
feet, separated from body, are •
fighting, peoples are
figures, sees
fire, visions of
   house, on
   room is on •
fishes, flies etc., sees
floating, bed, swimming in
fowls, sees •
friends, he had never seen them
   (after waking) •
God, he is, then he is devil •
   communication with, he is in
grave, he is in his
grimaces, sees
hand, separated from body, is
hat is a pair of trousers which he
   tries to put on •

Delusions,

head, disease will break out of •
hearing, illusions of
honest, he is not •
house is full of people
   surrounded, is •
husband, neglects her ★
identity, errors of personal
images, phantoms, sees
   black
   dark, in the
   frightful
   rising out of the earth •
   side, at his •
inanimate objects are persons
influence, is under a powerful
injury, is about to receive
   injured, is being
insects, sees
jealousy, with
   lovers concealed behind stove,
     wife has •
large, himself seems too
   parts of body seem too
lascivious
laughter, with
legs, cut off, are
   three, has
light, incorporeal, he is
limbs are separated
loquacity, with
lying crosswise •
mice, sees
murdered, roasted and eaten, he
   was •
   he will be
music, he hears
naked, he is •
new, everything is
objects, delusions from bright
   flight from o. •
obscene
people, sees
   converses with absent
   seize them, sees a number of
     strangers and tries to •
persecuted, he is

Delusions,
    pleasing
    poor, he is
    position, she is not fitted for
        her •
    possessed, being
    power over all disease, has •
    proud
    pure, she is •
    pursued by enemies
        ghosts, by
        he was
    rabbits, sees •
    rats, sees
    religious
    scream, obliging to
        with
    see, cannot
    sick, being
    side, he is alive on one and buried
        on the other •
    small, things appear
        things grow smaller
    snakes in and around her
    spectres, ghosts, spirits, sees
        closing eyes, on
        pursued by, is
    spinning, is
    statue, poses as, to be admired ★
    strange, everything is
        familiar things seem
    strangers, he sees
        friends appears as
    tactile hallucinations
    talking, dead people, with
        inanimate objects with names,
    talking to; but observes no one
        standing by him •
        spirits, with
    tall, he is
        she is very
    violent
    visions, has
        daytime
        night
        closing the eyes, on

Delusions,
    horrible
        beside him •
        dark, in the
        monsters, of
    vivid
    voices, hears
        dead people, of
        distant
    walk, he cannot
    weeping, with
    whistling, with
    wife is faithless
    wolves, of
Dementia, epileptics, of
Despair
    heat, during
    pains, with the
    religious despair of salvation
Destructiveness
    clothes, of
Dipsomania, alcoholism
    excitement from
Discontented, displeased, dissatisfied
Discouraged
Disgust ★
Disorderly ★
Distances, inaccurate judgement of
        exaggerated, are
        runs against things which
            appear to him distant •
Doubtful, soul's welfare, of
Dream, as if in a
Dresses, indecently; improperly
Drinking, mental symptoms after
Dullness, sluggishness, difficulty of think-
    ing and comprehending, torpor
        morning on rising
        drunkenness, during
        think long, unable to
        waking, on
Eccentricity
    alternating with sadness
    religious
Ecstasy

Egotism, self-esteem
Escape, attempts to
   mania puerperalis, in •
   restrained with difficulty, is
   shrieking, with •
Exaltation, religious ★
Excitement, excitable
  alternating with convulsions •
  bad news, after
  heat, during
  **water poured out, from hear-
   ing**
Exertion, agg. from mental
Exhilaration
Extravagance
Exuberance
Eyes, evades look of other persons •
Fancies, absorbed in
  confused
  exaltation of
   frightful
  lascivious
  pleasant
  strange •
  vivid, lively
Fear, apprehension, dread
  night
  alone, of being
  night
  animals, of
  approaching him, of others
  delirium, in
  black, of everything
  brilliant objects, looking glass, or,
   cannot endure sight of
  cemetries ★
  dark, of
  death, of
  delusions, fear from •
  devoured by animals, of being •
  dogs, of
  escape, with desire to
  evil, of
  falling, of
   everything is falling on her •
  fire, things will catch

Fear,
  ghosts, of
  imaginary things, of
  imbecile, to become •
  injured, of being
  insanity, losing his reason, of
  mirrors in room, of
  misfortune, of
  murdered, of being
  narrow places, in; claustrophobia
   vaults, churches and cellars, of
  noise, rushing water, of
  people, of, yet agg. if alone ★
  *physician, will not see her; he
   seems to terrify her*
  strangers, of
  suffocation, of
  touch, of
  tunnel, of •
  waking, on
  water, of
Fills pockets with anything •
Fire, wants to set things on
Foolish behavior
Forgetful
  morning
Forsaken feeling
  isolation, sensation of
Frightened easily
  animals, from ★
  delusions, from •
  *wakens terrified, knows no one,
   screams, clings to those near* •
  waking, on
Frown, disposed to
Gestures, makes
  clapping of the hands
  extravagant •
  **grasping or reaching at some-
   thing, at flocks; carphologia**
  genitals during spasms, at
  picks at bed clothes
  quickly •
  hands, motions, involuntary, of
  the

Gestures,
  head, to the
  spinning and weaving
  throwing about
    overhead
  waving in the air
  winding a ball, as if
  indicated his desires by •
  ridiculous or foolish
  spinning, imitates ★
  stamps the feet
  strange attitudes and positions
    arms, of
  usual vocation, of his
  violent
  wringing the hands
Gossiping
Grief
Grimaces
Haughty
  stupid and haughty
Heedless
Helplessness, feeling of
Hide, desire to
Howling
Hurry, haste
  drinking, on
  movements, in
  walking, while
Hydrophobia
  prophylactic ★
  screams or howls in a high voice •
Hypochondriasis
  weeping, with
Hysteria
  menses, during
Ideas abundant, clearness of mind
    headache, during heat after
  deficiency of
Idiocy
  bite, desire to
Imbecility
  laughing for nothing
  sexual excitement, with
Imitation, mimicry
  voices and motions of animals,
    of •

Impertinence
  acts, in his
Impetuous, perspiration, with
Impulse, rash
  fire, to set on ★
Inconsolable
  alone and darkness agg. •
Inconstancy
Indifference, apathy
  agreeable things, to
  alternating with timidity
  business affairs, to
  complain, does not
  exposure of her person, to
  fever, during
  pleasure, to
  suffering, to
Indiscretion
Indolence, aversion to work
Industrious, mania for work
Insanity, madness
  anxiety, with
  behaves like a crazy person
  burrows in ground with his mouth,
    like a pig •
  cheerful, gay
  company, with desire for light
    and •
  convulsions, with
  crazy things, does all sorts of ★
  drunkards, in
  erotic
  escape, desire to
  face, with pale
  fortune, after gaining
  gluttony, alternating with refusal
    to eat
  haughty
  heat, with
  insensibility, painlessness, with
    general
  lamenting, moaning, only
  laughing, with
  loquacious
  megalomania
  menses, during
  paroxysmal

Insanity,
> *pregnancy, in*
> *puerperal*
> **religious**
> restlessness, with
> *sleeplessness, with*
> stamps the feet
> staring of eyes
> *strength increased, with*
> suppressed eruptions, after
> travel, with desire to
> wantonness, with
> weeping, with

Insolence
Intemperance, agg. ★
Introspection
Irritability
> morning
> *alternating with cheerfulness*
> menses, during
> spoken to, when

Jealousy
> *accuses wife of being faithless* ●
> *neglect, accuses husband of*

Jesting
> *ridiculous or foolish*

Jumping
> **bed, out of**

Kicks
Kill, desire to
> *knife, with a*

Killed, desires to be
Kisses everyone
Kleptomania
Lamenting, bemoaning, wailing
> night
> asleep, while
> *waking, on*

Lascivious, lustful
Laughing
> actions, at his own
> alternating with groaning
> rage, frenzy
> sadness
> vexation, ill-humor
> violence
> convulsions, before, during or after
> delirious ●

Laughing,
> ill humor, with ●
> imbecility, in
> immoderately
> *loudly*
> paroxysmal
> *rage, with* ●
> *sardonic*
> silly
> *sleep, during*
> *spasmodic*
> speechlessness, with ●
> trifles, at
> violent

Libertinism
Light, aversion to
> **desire for**

Loathing, general
Loathing, life, at
Longing, sunshine, light and society,
> for

Looked at, cannot bear to be
Loquacity
> alternating with rage ●
> heat, during
> *insane*
> *menses, during*

Ludicrous, things seem
Malicious, spiteful, vindictive
Mania
> cold perpspiration, with
> erotic ★
> *hands, claps* ●
> *rage, with*
> shrieking in
> tears own hair
> himself to pieces with nails
> violence, with deeds of

Memory, confused
Memory, loss of:
> *insanity, in*

Memory, weakness of
> *expressing oneself, for*
> names, for proper
> persons, for
> said, for what has
> say, for what is about to
> thought, for what has just

Menses, mental symptoms agg. during
    after
Mental symptoms alternating with
    physical ★
Mildness
Misanthropy
Mischievous
Mistakes, localities, in
    names, in
    speaking, in
        misplacing words
        reverses words
        spelling, in
        words, using wrong
            names, calls thing by wrong
            says plums, when he
            means pears
    writing, in
        omitting letters
        transposing letters
Moaning, groaning, whining
    alternating with laughing
    loud
    menses, after •
    perspiration, during
    restlessness, with
Mobility ★
Monomania
Mood, alternating
    changeable, variable
    perspiration, during
Moral feeling, want of
Morose, cross, fretful, ill-humor, peevish
    laughing, followed by loud •
Morphinism
Multilating his body
Muttering
Naive
    intelligent, but very
Naked, wants to be
    constantly, wants to be •
    delirium, in
Nymphomania
    menses, before
        suppressed, after
Obscene, lewd
    songs
    talk

Obstinate, headstrong
Occupation, diversion amel.
Offended, easily; takes everything in
    bad part
Passionate
Pathetic •
Pertinacity
Piety nocturnal (*see* praying) ★
Praying
    night
    kneeling and
    menses, during •
    piety, nocturnal •
Profanity ★
Prophesying
Proportion, sense of, disturbed ★
Prostration of mind, mental ex-
    haustion, brain-fag •
Quarrelsome, scolding
    causeless •
Rage, fury
    alternating with convulsions •
        consciousness ★
        presentiment of death •
    biting, with
    convulsions, rage with
    delusions put him into rage •
    drinking, while
    hallucinations, from •
    headache, with
    insults, after
    kill people, tries to
    laughing, with •
    paroxysms, in
    shining objects, from
    shrieking, with
    stand, unable to •
    suicidal disposition, with
    taken up, child on being •
    tossing about in bed, making
        unintelligible signs •
    touch, renewed by
    violent
    water, at sight of
Recognize: relatives, does not recognize
    his
    speaking, does not recognize the
        one to whom he i •

Refuses to take the medicine
Religious affections
> bible, want to read all day the
> *children, in*
> *melancholia*
> *narrow-minded in religious questions*

Remorse
Reproaches himself
Reserved, air, in open
Restlessness
> night
> bed, go from one b. to another, wants to
>> *tossing about in*
> heat, during
> internal
> *menses, during*
> metrorrhagia, during
> *sleepiness, with*

Rhythmic ★
Roving, senseless, insane
Rudeness
Runs about
Sadness, despondency, dejection, mental depression, gloom, melancholy
> evening
>> bed, in
>> night, bed, in
> *alone, when*
> *clear weather* •
> company, desire for •
> continence, from
> darkness, in
> heat, during
> menses, before
> *sunshine, in* •

Satyriasis
Scratches with hands
Searching on floor
Self, accusation ★
> reproaches ★
Senses, dull, blunted
> vanishing of

Sensitive, oversensitive
> light, to
> noise, to
>> water splashing, to
> pain, to
> want of sensitiveness

Shamelessness
Shining objects agg.
> *amel.*
Shrieking, screaming, shouting
> day and night •
> brain-cry
> *cannot, but wants to scream* •
> children, in
> *chorea, in*
> *convulsions, before*
>> epileptic, before
>> during epileptic
> delusions, from
>> *with*
> drunkenness, during
> fever, during
> hoarse
> sleep, during
> sudden
> touched, when ★
> waking, on

Sighing
> menses, after
> perspiration, during
> **throat, with grasping at** •

Singing
> alternating with weeping
>> and laughing •
> fever, during
> *latin paternoster* •
> sleep, in

Sits, erect
> *stiff, quite*
> still
> *wrapped in deep, sad thoughts and notices nothing, as if*

Size, incorrect judge of
Slander, disposition to
Smaller, things appear
Somnambulism

Speech, affected
  babbling
  confused
  extravagant
  foolish
  foreign tongue, in a
  hasty
  incoherent
    sleep, during
  loud
  nonsensical
  prattling
  unintelligible
  violent
  voice, in a shrill
  wandering
Spit, desire to, faces of people, in
Spoken to, averse to being
Squanders
Staring, thoughtless
Starting, startled
  night
  fright, from and as from
  sleep, during
  from
Strange, crank
Stranger, presence of strangers agg.
Striking
  about him at imaginary objects
  boy clawing his father's face
  ●
Striking himself, head, his
Stupefaction, as if intoxicated
  chill, during
  heat, during
  perspiration, during ●
  sits motionless like a statue
Suicidal disposition
  heat, during
  intermittent fever, during
  knife, with
    razor, with a
  throwing himself from a height
Superstitious
Suspicious, mistrustful
Talk, indisposed to, desire to be silent,
  taciturn
    sits, does not move

  others agg., talk of
Talking, pleasure in his own
  sleep, in
    confess themselves loud, they
Talks, when alone
  absent persons, with ●
  dead people, with
  himself, to
    only when alone
  one subject, of nothing but
Tastelessness in dressing
Tears things
  himself
  pillow with teeth
Terror ★
Thinking, aversion to
Thoughts, persistent
  homicide
  repetition, of
  ridiculous
  sexual
  strange
    pregnancy, in
  vanishing of
Threatening
Throws things away
Timidity
  bashful
  delirium, during
Torpor
Touched, aversion to being
Trance, alternating with spasms every
  summer ●
Unconsciousness, coma, stupor
  morning
  alcoholic
  apoplexy, in
  chill, during
  dream, as in a
  eyes, with fixed
  fever, during
  incomplete
  mental insensibility
  remains fixed in one spot, motion-
    less like a statue

Unconsciousness,
   semi-consciousness
   sexual excitement, with
   sitting upright, while
   starts up in a wild manner, but could not keep the eyes open •
   twitching of limbs, with
   vertigo, during
   waking, after
Verses, makes
violent, vehement
   alternating with laughing •
   deeds of violence, rage leading to
Walks, circle, in
Wanders, restlessly, about
Weary of life
   heat, during
Weeping, tearful mood
   morning
   evening
   night
      weeps all night, laughs all day •
   aloud, sobbing
   alternating with cheerfulness
   laughter
      and singing •
   singing
   chill, during
   contradiction, from
   dark, in •
   day, during ★
   desire to weep, all the time
   heat, during
   involuntary
      amel. by vinegar •
   menses, during
      after
   nervous all day, feels so
   offence, from •
   pains, with the
   perspiration, during
   piteous
   sad thoughts, at
   sexual excitement, with ★
   sleep, in

Weeping,
   spasmodic
   touched, when
   trifles, at
   violent
   waking, on
   whimpering
Whistling
Wildness
Writing, indistinctly, writes

STRONTIUM METALLICUM

Anger, stabbed anyone, so that he could have
   violent, fit of ★
Busy
Confusion of mind
Darkness agg.
Destructiveness
Fear, evil, of
Light, desire for ★
Sadness, evening in bed
Starting, night, midnight in sleep, before
   anxious
Striking, about him at imaginary objects

STRONTIUM CARBONICUM

Absorbed, buried in thought
Ailments from:
   anger, vexation
   anticipation, foreboding, presentiment
   scorn, being scorned
Anger, irascibility
   violent
Anxiety
   afternoon
   evening
      bed, in
   night
      midnight, before
   bed, in
   conscience, as if guilty of a crime
   fear, with

waking, on
Confusion of mind, spirituous liquors,
    from
Delusions, criminals, about
Dipsomania, alcoholism
Discontented, displeased, dissatisfied
Dullness, sluggishness, difficulty of think-
    ing and comprehending, torpor
Excitement, palpitation, with violent
Fear, apprehension, dread
    afternoon
    evening
    dark, of
Forgetful
Frightened easily
Grief
Haughty
Impetuous
Indolence, aversion to work
Irritability
Malicious, spiteful, vindictive
Memory, weakness of
Morose, cross, fretful, ill-humor, peevish
Quarrelsome, scolding
Remorse
Restlessness
Sadness, despondency, dejection, men-
    tal depression, gloom, melan-
    choly
    waking, on
Shrieking, sleep, during
Sit, inclination to
Starting, startled
    evening on falling asleep
    fright, from and as from
    sleep, on falling
      during
Striking
Sulky
Talk, indisposed to, desire to be silent,
    taciturn
Thoughts, thoughtful
Violent, vehement
    deeds of violence, rage leading to
Wearisome

STROPHANTUS HISPIDUS

Dipsomania, alcoholism
Fear, ordeals, of

STROPHANTUS SARMENTOSUS

Anxiety
    heart ★
Fear, apprehension, dread
    touch on chest wall, of ●

STRYCHNINUM PURUM

Activity, mental
Answers: aversion to answer
    disconnected
    hastily
    rapidly
Anxiety
Approach of persons agg.
Company, desire for; aversion to soli-
    tude
Confusion of mind
    morning
Delirium
Delirium tremens, mania-a-potu
Delusions, dead person, sees
    faces, sees
      hideous
    pursued by enemies
Dullness, sluggishness, difficulty of think-
    ing and comprehending, torpor
Excitement, excitable
    nervous
Fear, apprehension, dread
    approaching him, of others
    happen, something will
    injured, of being
Frightened easily
Gestures, hands, motions, involuntary,
    of the, face, to the ●
Ideas abundant, clearness of mind
Idiocy, giggling ●
Imbecility

Irritability
Kicks
Lamenting, bemoaning, wailing
Laughing
    immoderately
    sardonic
    silly
    spasmodic ★
Memory, active
Memory, weakness of
Moaning, groaning, whining
    loud
Morose, cross, fretful, ill-humor, peevish
Rage, fury
Restlessness, night
    bed, tossing about in
**Sadness, despondency, dejection,
    mental depres sion, gloom,
    melancholy**
Senses, acute
Sensitive, oversensitive
    noise, to
Shrieking, screaming, shouting
    convulsions, before
    sleep, during
Speech, hasty
    incoherent
Starting, startled
    convulsive
    sleep, on falling
    touched, when
Striking
Stupefaction, as if intoxicated
Unconsciousness, coma, stupor
    morning
        10 h.
    evening
        20 h. ●
Weeping, tearful mood
    paroxysmal

STRYCHININUM NITRICUM

Delirium tremens, mania-a-potu
Dipsomania, alcoholism

STRYCHNINUM PHOSPHORICUM

Hysteria
Laughing, immoderately
Moral feeling, want of
Prostration of mind, mental exhaustion, brain-fag

STRYCHNOS GAULTHERIANA

Hydrophobia

SUCCINUM

Fear, apprehension, dread
    narrow places, in: claustrophobia
        trains and closed places, of ●
Hysteria

SULPHURICUM ACIDUM

Absent-minded, unobserving
Abstraction of mind
Ailments from :
    debauchery ★
Anger, irascibility
    morning on waking
    talk, indisposed to
    trifles, at
    waking, on
Answers: aversion to answer
    difficult
    inappropriate
    irrelevantly
    refuses to answer
    slowly
Anxiety
    daytime
    morning
    evening amel.
    future, about
Bilious disposition
Capriciousness
Cheerful, gay, mirthful
    evening, bed, in
Clinging, held amel., being

Company, aversion to; presence of other people agg. the symptoms; desire for solitude
Concentration, difficult
Confidence, want of self
Confusion of mind
    morning
    evening
    scratching of the right side of head in •
    sitting, while
Cowardice
Death, desires
    presentiment of
Delirium
    night
    bed and escapes, springs up suddenly from
    fever, during
    raging, raving
Delirium tremens, mania-a-potu
Delusions, animals, of
    dead persons, sees
Despair
Dipsomania, alcoholism
Discontented, everything, with
Discouraged
    alternating with exaltation
Dullness, sluggishness, difficulty of thinking and comprehending, torpor
    morning
    diabetes, in
Eccentricity
    alternating with timidity •
Escape, attempts to
Excitement, excitable
    evening in bed
    alternating with sadness
    nervous
    trifles, over
Exhilaration
Fear, apprehension, dread
    daytime, only
    morning
        until evening •
    evil, of
Frightened easily

Grief
Hurry, haste
    eating, while
    mental work, in
    movements, in
        fast enough, cannot do things
    occupation, in
    walking, while
    work, in
    writing, in
Hypochondriasis
Hysteria
Imbecility
Impatience
    perspiration, during
    trifles, about
Indifference, apathy
Industrious, mania for work
    menses, before
Irresolution, indecision
Irritability
    daytime
    morning
        waking, on
    sadness, with
    talking, while
    waking, on
Jesting
Jumping, bed, out of
Loathing, life, at
Mental symptoms alternating with physical ★
Memory, active
Memory, weakness of
Mistakes, speaking, in
Moaning, groaning, whining
    lifting, when •
Mood, agreeable
    alternating
    changeable, variable
    perspiration, during
Morose, cross, fretful, ill-humor, peevish
    day time
    morning
        waking, on

Music amel.
Muttering
    sleep, in
Nymphomania, menses, after •
Offended, easily; takes everything in
    bad part
Praying
Prostration of mind, mental exhaustion, brain-fag
    injuries, from
Quarrelsome, scolding
Rage, fury
Recognize, relatives, does not r. his
Restlessness
    night
    anxious, compelling rapid walking
    bed, tossing about in
    busy
Sadness, despondency, dejection, mental depression, gloom, melancholy
    daytime
    morning
    air, in open
Serious, earnest
Shrieking, screaming, shouting
    sleep, during
    menses, before
Singing
Speech, abrupt
    monosyllabic
    unintelligible
Starting, startled
    sleep, during
    from
    trifles, at
Stupefaction, as if intoxicated
    rouses with difficulty
Sulky
Suspicious, mistrustful
Talk, indisposed to, desire to be silent,
    taciturn
Timidity
    alternating with exaltation
Tranquillity, serenity, calmness

Unconsciousness, coma, stupor
    diphtheria, in
    incomplete
Vivacious
Wearisome
Weary of life
Weeping, tearful mood
    night
    anxiety, after
    sleep, in
Writing agg. mind symptoms ★

SULPHUR HYDROGENISATUM

Delirium
    convulsions, before
Mania
Unconsciousness, coma, stupor

SULPHUR IODATUM

Absent minded, reading, while
Anxiety
    driving from place to place
Business, incapacity for
Cheerful, gay, mirthful
Company, aversion to; presence of other people agg. the symptoms; desire for solitude
Concentration, difficult, studying, reading etc., while
Confidence, want of self
Confusion of mind, morning
    evening
    mental exertion, from
Conscientious about trifles
Cowardice
Delirium, night
Delusions, dead persons, sees
    fancy, illusions of
Despair
Discontented, displeased, dissatisfied
Discouraged
Dullness, sluggishness, difficulty of thinking and comprehending, torpor

Duty, aversion to domestic
Excitement, excitable
    feverish
Exertion, agg. from mental
Fear, exertion, of
    happen, something will
    insanity, losing his reason, of
    misfortune, of
    people, of; anthropophobia
Frightened, waking, on
Hurry, haste
    walking, while
    work, in
Hysteria
Impatience
Indifference, apathy
    duties, to
        domestic, to
    surroundings, to the
Indolence, aversion to work
Irritability
    alternating with cheerfulness
Mood, changeable, variable
Neglects, household, the
Prostration of mind, mental exhaus-
    tion, brain-fag
Restlessness
    night
    move, must constantly
*Sadness, despondency, dejection, mental
    depression, gloom, melancholy*
Senses, dull, blunted
Sensitive, oversensitive
Starting, sleep, during
    waking, on
Stupefaction, as if intoxicated
Suspicious, mistrustful
Thoughts, persistent
    tormenting
    wandering
Timidity
Weeping, evening

SULFANILAMIDUM

Cheerful, alternating with sadness
Confusion of mind
Delirium

Dullness, sluggishness, difficulty of
    thinking and comprehending,
    torpor
Exhilaration
Indifference, apathy
Indolence, aversion to work
Infantile behavior
Irritability
Mania, alternating with depression
Memory, weakness of
    forms, for
    music, for
    words, of
Restlessness
Sadness, despondency, dejection, mental
    depression, gloom, melancholy
Schizophrenia
Stupefaction, as if intoxicated
Thoughts, disconnected

SULFONALUM

Delusions, arms, she has four •
    double, head and pair of limbs
        are •
    head, two heads, having
    legs, has four •
    limbs, has four, eight ★
Irritability
Morose, cross, fretful, ill-humor, peevish

SULFONAMIDUM

Anguish
Company, aversion to; presence of
    other people agg. the symp-
    toms; desire for solitude
Contradict, disposition to
Delusions, imaginations, hallucinations,
    illusions
Disobedience
Exertion, agg. from mental
Indolence, evening
Insanity, persecution mania
Irritability
    lying, amel. on •
Quarrelsome, scolding

Sadness, despondency, dejection, mental
    depression, gloom, melancholy
    alternating with quarrelsomeness
Sensitive, noise, to
Work, aversion to mental

SULPHUROSUM ACIDUM

Anxiety
Rage, fury
Singing

SULPHUR (LOTUM SUBLIMATUM)

Abrupt, rough
Absent-minded, unobserving
    starts when spoken to
Absorbed buried in thought
    evening
Abstraction of mind
Abusive, insulting ★
Affections, in general ★
Ailments from:
    anger, vexation
      anxiety, with
      fright, with
    bad news
    business failure
    death of a child
    dipsomania
    discords between chief and sub-
      ordinates
      parents, friends, between ★
    egotism
    embarrassment
    friendship, deceived
    fright
    hurry
    literary, scientific failure
    love, disappointed
    mortification
    scorn, being scorned ·
    sexual excesses
Air, castles (plans), builds, in ★
Amativeness
    want of amativeness in women
Amorous
Amusement, averse to

Anger, irascibility
    morning
      waking, on ★
    forenoon, 11h.
    alternating with quick repentance
    former vexations, about
    himself, with
    mistakes, about his
    past events, about
    tear himself to pieces, could ●
    violent
Anguish
Anorexia mentalis
Answers abruptly, shortly, curtly
    aversion to answer
    difficult
    refuses to answer
    repeats the question first
    slowly
Anxiety
    morning
      perspiration, during
    forenoon
    evening
      bed, in
    night
      waking, on
    midnight, before
    air amel., in open
    bed, in
    business, about
    clothes and open windows, must
      loosen
    cold drinks amel.
    conscience, as if guilty of a
      crime
    dinner, amel. after ●
    drinking cold water amel.
    eating amel., after
    exaggerated ★
    fear, with
    fever, during
    flatus, with obstructed ●
    friends at home, about
    future, about
    head, with heat of
    and cold feet ●

Anxiety,
    health, about
    hypochondriacal
        mania to read medical books
    menses, before
      during
    oppression, with •
    others, for
    pains, from the stomach
    paroxysms, in
    periodical
    pressure on the chest, from
    salvation, about
      faith, about loss of his
      scruples, excessive reli-
      gious
      scrupulous as to their religious
        practices, too
    stool, during
    waking, on
Ardent
Audacity
Avarice
    alternating with squandering
Aversion to being approached
    education, to ★
    everything, to
    persons, to all
      literary, to ★
    sex, religious aversion to opposite
    women, to
Bargaining
Beside oneself, being
Break things, desire to
Brooding
Brutality, drunknness, during
Business, averse to
    neglects his
    talks of
Busy
    fruitlessly
Capriciousness
Carefulness
Cares, worries, full of
    others, about
Carried, desires to be
Cautious, anxious
Censorious, critical

Charlatan
Cheerful, gay, mirthful
    morning
    evening
      ill-humor during the day
      bed, in
    night
    convulsions, after •
    foolish, and
    sleep, during
    waking, on
Child bed, mental symptoms during
Clinging, held amel., being
Company, aversion to; presence of other
    people agg. the symptoms;
    desire for solitude
    alone, amel. when
    bear anybody, cannot
Company, desire for; aversion to soli-
    tude,
    company amel.
Complaining
    sleep, in
Comprehension, easy
    drunkenness, during
Concentration, active
Concentration, difficult
    studying, reading, etc., while
Confidence, want of self
    failure, feels himself a
Confounding objects and ideas
Confusion of mind
    morning
      rising and after, on
      waking, on
    forenoon
    afternoon
    evening
    night
      waking, on
    air, in open
      amel.
    arouse himself, compelled to
    ascending agg.
    dream, as if in
    eating, after
    identity, as to his
    mental exertion, from

Confusion of mind
　　mixes subjective and objective
　　motion of the head, from
　　sleeping, after
　　waking, on
　　walking, while
　　　　amel.
　　　　air, in open
　　　　　　amel.
　　warm room, in
Conscientious about trifles
Consolation, kind words agg.
　　sympathy agg.
Contrary
Conversation agg.
Coquettish, too much
Corrupt, venal
Courageous
Cowardice
　　sadness, with •
Crawling, rolling on the floor
Death, desires
　　presentiment of
Deceitful, sly
Defiant
Delirium
　　　　evening
　　　　night
　　　answers correctly when spoken
　　　　to, but delirium and uncon-
　　　　sciousness return at once
　　　anxious
　　　busy
　　　chill, during
　　　closing the eyes, on
　　　delusions, with
　　　fantastic
　　　fever, during
　　　foolish, silly
　　　gay, cheerful
　　　haemorrhage, after
　　　laughing
　　　loquacious
　　　meningitis, cerebrospinalis
　　　muttering
　　　　sleep, in
　　　raging, raving
　　　rambling

Delirium,
　　restless
　　sleep, falling asleep, on
　　sleeplessness, and ★
　　trembling, with
Delirium tremens, mania-a-potu
**Delusions, imaginations, halluci-
　　nations, illusions**
　　　evening
　　　　bed, in
　　　night
　　animals, of
　　assembled things, swarms, crowds
　　　etc.
　　beautiful
　　　rags seem, even •
　　　things look
　　black, she is •
　　body, black, is •
　　calls him, someone
　　ciphers, sees
　　clothes are beautiful
　　criminals, about
　　dead persons, sees
　　devils, sees
　　diminished, all is
　　disgraced, she is
　　dogs, sees
　　doomed, being
　　emaciation, of
　　faces, sees
　　　closing eyes, on
　　　hideous
　　falling asleep, on
　　fancy, illusions of
　　　chill, during
　　figures, sees
　　fire, visions of
　　great person, is a
　　grimaces, sees
　　　falling asleep, on •
　　grotesque
　　happened anything, of having
　　images, phantoms, sees
　　　closing eyes, on
　　　　in bed
　　　frightful

Delusions,
    injury, is about to receive
      injured, is being
    longer, things seem
    ludicrous
    noise, hears
    numeral, appeared nine inches
      long (night on waking, amel.
      lying on other side)
    old rags are as fine as silk •
    people, sees
      morning on waking •
    persecuted, he is
    possessed, being
    pregnant, she is
    rain, he hears
    religious
    rich, as if he is ★
    smell, of
    spectres, ghosts, spirits, sees
      closing eyes, on
    strange, familiar things seem
    tall: things grow taller
      she is very ★
    thin, is getting •
    time seems earlier, passes too
      quickly
    tumbling of everything on him (at
      night, when only half awake) •
    vermin, sees crawl about
    visions, has

      closing the eyes, on
      horrible
    voices, hears, calling him (at
      night) •
    want, he will come to
    wealth, of
    wrong, he has done
Dementia
    senilis
    syphilitics, of
Desires, beautiful things, finery ★
Despair
    heat, during
    religious despair of salvation
    social position, of

Destructiveness
    clothes, of
Dipsomania, alcoholism
    drinking on the sly •
    idleness, from
Dirtiness
    urination and defecating every-
      where, children
Discomfort
    evening
**Discontented, displeased, dissatis-
    fied**
    everything, with
    himself, with
Discouraged
    morning
Disgust
    **nausea, from her own effluvia
      leading to** •
Dishonest
Disobedience
Distances, exaggerated, are
Doubtful, recovery, of
    soul's welfare, of
Dream, as if in a
**Dullness, sluggishness, difficulty
    of thinking and compre-
    hending, torpor**
    morning
    forenoon
    afternoon
    evening
    amel.
    children, in
    dinner, during •
    heat, during
    loss of fluids, after
    mental exertion, from
    perspiration, during
    reading, while
    stooping, on •
    *understands questions only after
      repetition*
    walking rapidly, after
Duty, no sense of duty
    stimulate sense of, to ★

Dwells on past disagreeable occurrences
    night
    recalls old grievances
        disagreeable memories
Eccentricity
Ecstasy
    perspiration, during
Egotism, self-esteem
Elegance, want of
Embittered, exasperated
Emptiness, sensation of ★
Envy
    avidity, and
    qualities of others, at
Escape, attempts to
Excitement, excitable
        noon
        evening in bed
        night
        bad news, after
        chill, during
        coffee, as after
        exertion, after ●
        feverish, night ●
        heat, during
        tea, after ●
        walking: air, on w. in open
Exertion, agg. from mental
Failure, feels himself a ★
Fanaticism
Fancies, exaltation of
        evening
            bed, in
            night
        closing the eyes in bed
        sleeplessness, with
        walking in open air
    laughable, before falling asleep ●
    perspiration, during
    sleep, falling asleep, on
    waking, on
Fear, apprehension, dread
        afternoon
        night

Fear,
    blind, of going
    cold, of taking
        heat, during ●
    crowd, in a
    death, of
        menses, before
    disease, of impending
    dreams, of terrible
    evil, of
        evening
    failure, of
    faith, to lose his religious ★
    fever, of (while chilly)
    ghosts, of
        night
            waking, on
    high places, of
    insanity, losing his reason, of
    killing, of
    lifelong
    looking before her, when ●
    men, dread, fear of
    menses, before
    misfortune, of
    narrow places, in; claustrophobia
    noise, from
    overpowering
    people, of; anthropophobia
    position, to lose his lucrative
    poverty, of
    recurrent
    robbers, of
        midnight on waking
    starving, of
    suffocation, of
        night
    thunderstorm, of
    touch, of
    urinating, after ●
    waking, on
    water, of
    work, dread of
        literary, of

Feces passed on the floor
    urinating and going to stool every where, (children)
Flatterer
Flattery, gives everything, when flattered
Foolish behavior, happiness and pride
Forgetfulness
    night
    loss of fluids, from
    mental exertion, from
    name, his own
    old people, of
    words while speaking, of; word hunting
Forsaken beloved by his parents, wife, friends, feels is not being
Frightened easily
    evening
    pains, from •
    waking, on
    dream, from a
Frivolous
Frown, disposed to ★
Gamble (*see* **Play**)
Gestures, awkward in
    grasping or reaching at something, at flocks; carphologia
    children put everything in mouth
    picks at bed clothes
    hands, motions, involuntary, of the
    hands restlessly busy ★
    put everything in mouth (children) •
    strange attitudes and positions head, of
    talking, gesticulates with head while
    wringing the hands
Godless, want of religious feeling
Greed, cupidity
Grief
Hatred
    persons who had offended him, of
    revenge, hatred and

Haughty
Heedless
High places agg.
Hopeful
Horrible things, sad stories, affect her profoundly
House-keeping, women unable to
Hurry, haste
    awkward from
    eating, while
    movements, in
        involuntary hurry in movements •
    walking, while
Hydrophobia
Hypochondriasis
    daytime and merry in evening •
    morose
    suicide, driving to
    suppression of eruptions, after •
Hypocrisy
Hysteria
    menses, before
        during
    moon agg., increasing •
Ideas abundant, clearness of mind
    evening in bed
        night
    deficiency of
    fixed ★
Idiocy
Idleness
Imbecility
    old rags are as fine as silk •
Impatience
    morning
        forenoon, 11 h. •
    dinner, during •
    headache, during
    trifles, about
    urinating, before •
Impetuous
    perspiration, with
    urination, before •
Inconsolable
Inconstancy
Independent ★

Indifference, apathy
　　business affairs, to
　　duties, to
　　everything, to
　　external things, to
　　life, to
　　others, toward
　　personal appearance, to •
　　pleasure, to
　　welfare of others, to
Indolence, aversion to work
　　morning
　　evening
　　　amel.
　　physical
Industrious, mania for work
Initiative, lack of
Inquisitive
Insanity, madness
　　black insanity with despair and
　　　weary of life from fear of
　　　mortification or of loss of
　　　position
　　climacteric period, during
　　drunkards, in
　　eats filth •
　　erotic
　　megalomania
　　melancholy
　　position, from fear to lose the
　　puerperal
　　religious
　　suppressed eruptions, after
Introspection
Irresolution, indecision
　　ideas, in
Irritability
　　daytime
　　morning
　　　rising, after
　　　waking, on
　　evening
　　alternating with hypochondriac
　　　mood during day, merry in
　　　evening
　　chill, during
　　exertion, from

Irritability,
　　heat, during
　　menses, during
　　perspiration, during
　　remorse, with easy and quick •
　　sadness, with
　　spoken to, when
　　taciturn
　　trifles, from
　　waking, on
Jealousy, brutal from, gentle husband
　　becoming
　　saying and doing what he wouldn't
　　　say and do
　　strike his wife, driving to
Jesting, aversion to
　　joke, cannot take a
Kicks, sleep, in
Kleptomania
Lamenting, bemoaning, wailing
　　asleep, while
Languages, unable for
Lascivious, lustful
Laughing
　　evening
　　night
　　agg.
　　dream, laughing during comic d.
　　　continues after waking •
　　serious matters, over
　　sleep, during
　　　on going to •
　　spasmodic
Liar
Libertinism
Loathing, general, evening
Loathing, life, at
　　work, at
Longing, repose and tranquillity, for
Looked at, cannot bear to be
Loquacity
　　evening
　　drunkenness, during
Love with one of own sex, homosexu-
　　ality, tribadism

Loves, animals, cats ★
Magnetized, desires to be, mesmerism
　　amel.
Malicious, spiteful, vindictive
　　night
Mania
　　demoniac
Mathematics, horror of
Mean ★
Meditation
Memory, active
　　short, but
Memory, weakness of
　　business, for
　　do, for what was about to
　　facts, for past
　　　recent, for
　　　　old people, in
　　forms, for
　　happened, for what has
　　heard, for what has
　　names, for proper
　　orthography, for
　　persons, for
　　places, for
　　said, for what has
　　say, for what is about to
　　thought, for what has just
　　verses, to learn
　　words, for
Mildness
Misanthropy
Mistakes, differentiating of objects, in
　　localities, in
　　speaking, in
　　　misplacing words
　　　reverses words
　　　spelling, in
　　　words, using wrong, name of
　　　　object seen of instead of one
　　　　desired
　　　　names, calls things by wrong
　　time, in
　　writing, in
　　　repeating words

Moaning, groaning, whining
　　sleep, during
Monomania
Mood, alternating
　　changeable, variable
　　repulsive
Morose, cross, fretful, ill-humor, peevish
　　daytime
　　morning
　　evening
　　fever, during
Murmuring in sleep
Music agg.
　　palpitation when listening to
Muttering, sleep, in
Naive, intelligent, but very
Naked, wants to be, sleep, in
Neglects business
Nymphomania
　　menses, after suppressed
Obscene, lewd
Obstinate, headstrong
　　stool, during ●
Offended, easily; takes every thing in
　　bad part
Optimistic
Passionate
Perseverance
Philosophy, ability for
Plans, making many
Play. aversion to p. in children
　　inability to
　　passion for gambling
　　　to make money
Praying
Prostration of mind, mental ex-
　　haustion, brain-fag
Prying ★
Qualmishness ★
Quarrelsome, scolding
Quiet, wants to be, repose and tranquil-
　　lity, desires
Rage, fury
Reading, passion to read medical books
Rebels against poultice

Religious affections
> *children, in*
> fanaticism
> horror of the opposite sex
> mania
> *melancholia*
> puberty, in
> **speculations, dwells on** •
> **very religious** ★

Remorse
> quickly, repents

Reproaches himself
> others

Resignation

Restlessness
> daytime
> day and night
> morning
> noon
> evening
> **night**
> midnight, after
> *anxious*
> *bed, tossing about in*
> children, in
> coughing, with •
> eating, after
> headache, during
> *heat, during*
> internal
> **menses, before**
> > during
> *perspiration, amel. during* •
> sitting, while

Revelry, feasting

Reverence for those around him

Rolling on the floor

Runs about

Sadness, despondency, dejection,
> **mental depression, gloom,**
> **melancholy**
> daytime
> day and night
> morning
> afternoon
> *evening*
> > *amel.*

Sadness, evening
> *bed, in*
> > night, bed, in
> air, in open
> causeless
> children, in
> **climaxis, during**
> *disease, about*
> *dwelling constantly on her condition* •
> eating: hasty eating from sadness •
> **eruptions, suppressed, with**
> heat, during
> injuries of the head, from
> labor, during
> masturbation, from
> menses, from suppressed
> misfortune, as if from
> periodical
> *perspiration, during*
> pollutions, from
> puberty, in
> sleeplessness from sadness
> suicidal disposition, with
> walking in open air, while and after
> wringing the hands

Satyriasis

Selfishness, egoism

Senses, acute
> dull, blunted

Sensitive, oversensitive
> afternoon
> music, to
> noise, to
> odors, to

Sentimental

Serious, earnest

Servile, obsequious, submissive

Shrieking, screaming, shouting
> brain cry
> **children, during sleep, in**
> *convulsions, before*
> > during epileptic
> *sleep, during*
> waking, on

Sighing
  sleep, in
Singing
  sleep, in
  waking, on •
Sit, inclination to
  supporting body, hands, with ★
Slowness
Somnambulism
  climbing the roofs, the railing of
    bridge or balcony
  do day-labor, to
Speech, anxious, in sleep
  delirious, in sleep, before mid-
    night
  incoherent
  loud, in sleep
  nonsensical
  vivacious
  wandering
    night
Spit, desire to
Spoiled, children
Spoken to, averse to being
  alone, wants to be let
  called agg. mental symptoms,
    being •
Squanders
Starting, startled
    noon
      sleep, in
    afternoon
    evening, asleep, on falling
    night
    anxious
  called by name, when •
  dreams, in
    from a dream
    easily
    fright, from and as from
    noise, from
    pain, from •
  sleep, on falling
    during
    from
  spoken to, when
  trifles, at

Strange, crank in dressing
    opinions and acts, in
Strength increased, mental, drunken-
    nes, more intelligent during
Stupefaction, as if intoxicated
    morning, 11 h. •
    evening
    vertigo, during
    walking in open air, when
Suicidal disposition
    courage, but lacks
    drowning, by
    hypochondriasis
    sadness, from
    shooting, by
    throwing himself, window, from
Sulky
Suppressed or receding skin diseases
    or haemorrhoids, mental symp-
    toms agg. after
Suspicious, mistrustful
Sympathy, agg.
Talk, indisposed to, desire to be
    silent, taciturn
    slow learning to
Talking agg. all complaints
    sleep, in
    business, of
    excited
    loud
Tastelessness in dressing
Tears things
Theorizing
Thoughts, business at evening in bed, of
    control of thoughts lost
    disagreeable
    disconnected
    disease, of
    intrude and crowd around each
      other
      work, while at
    persistent
      expressions and words
        heard recur to his mind
    rush, flow of
      evening in bed
      night

Thoughts,
>business accomplished, of,
>>evening •
>sleeplessness from
>walking in open air, on
>sexual
>stagnation of
>strange
>*thoughtful*
>tormenting
>vagueness of
>vanishing of

Time, fritters away his
>passes too quickly, appears shorter

Timidity
>awkward, and
>**bashful**

Touch everything, impelled to
>does not know if objects are real
>>until she has touched them •

Tranquillity, serenity, calmness

Unconciousness, coma, stupor
>morning
>answers correctly when spoken
>to, but delirium and uncon-
>sciousness return at once
>crowded room, in a
>fever, during
>*jaw dropping*
>*meningitis, in*
>menses, during
>perspiration, with cold •
>*scarlatina, in*
>*stool, during*
>walking in open air, while

Undertakes many things, perseveres in
>nothing •

Unfeeling, hardhearted
Unfortunate, feels
Ungrateful
>avarice, from
Unreliable, promises, in his
Unsuccessful, thinks himself ★
Untidy
Usurer
Vanity
Violent, vehement

Walk, walking in open air agg. mental
>symptoms
Washing, aversion to w. in childen •
>cleanliness, mania for
Wearisome
Weary of life
Weeping, tearful mood
>morning
>**forenoon, 11h** •
>evening
>night
>aloud, wobbing
>alternating with laughter
>anger, with ★
>anxiety, after
>causeless
>chill, during
>**climacteric period, at** •
>consolation agg.
>convulsions, during
>coughing, during
>heat, during
>perspiration, during
>sleep, in
>stool, during
>trifles, at
>vexation, from
>waking, on
>whimpering
>>sleep, during
Whistling
Will, loss of
>weakness of
Work, aversion to mental
>desire for
>fatigues

SUMBULUS MOSCHATUS

Activity, mental
Anger, irascibility
>alternating with sadness
Anxiety
Cheerful, gay, mirthful
>evening
>alternating with lachrymose mood

Concentration, difficult
Confidence, want of self
Confusion of mind, morning
    pollutions, from
Delirium tremens, mania-a-potu
Delusions, legs don't belong to her
    melting away, sensation of, agg.
       from change, amel. in recum-
       bent position ●
Despair
Dullness, sluggishness, difficulty of
    thinking and comprehending,
    torpor
      morning
Eccentricity
    chorea, with
Ecstasy
Emotions, easily excited ★
Excitement, excitable
    evening
    music, from
    trifles, over
Exhilaration
Exuberance
Fear, insanity, losing his reason, of
    vertigo, of ●
Frightened easily
    trifles, at
Hurry, haste
Hypochondriasis
Hysteria
    fainting, hysterical
Ideas abundant, clearness of mind
    evening
Indolence, aversion to work
Insecurity mental
Irritability
    afternoon
    evening
    music, from harsh ●
    walking, when
Laughing
    hysterical
    spasmodic
Loathing, general
Memory, weak, words, for
Mildness

Mistakes, calculating, in
    writing, in
Morose, cross, fretful, ill-humor, peevish
Music amel.
    faintness on hearing
Nymphomania
Occupation, desire for
Passionate
    trifle, at every
Prostration of mind, mental exhaus-
    tion, brain-fag
Restlessness
    reading, while
Sadness, despondency, dejection, mental
    depression, gloom, melancholy
Smiling
Starting, startled
    easily
Summing-up difficult
Unconsciousness, music, from
Unfeeling, hardhearted
Vivacious
Weeping, alternating with laughter
    hysterical
Witty
Work, desire for mental
    impossible

(BACILLUS) SYCOCCUS

Fear
    animals, of
    dogs, of

SYMPHYTUM OFFICINALE

Ailments from :
    sexual excesses
Indolence, morning ★

SYPHILINUM

Absent-minded, unobserving
Abusive, insulting
Anger, irascibility
Anti-social ★
Aversion, society, to ★

Business, averse to
Calculating, inability for
*Company, aversion to; presence of other
        people agg. the symptoms;
        desire for solitude*
Company, desire for; aversion to soli-
        tude, company amel.
Concentration, active
Concentration, difficult
        calculating, while
        studying, reading etc., while ★
Confusion of mind   .
        calculating, when
Consolation, kind words agg.
        sympathy agg.
Contradiction, is intolerant of
Delirium
        night
Delusions, imaginations, hallucinations,
        illusions
        insane, she will become
        ditry, he is ★
        washing, of
Despair
        recovery, of
Dipsomania, alcoholism
Discontented, displeased, dissatisfied
Disgust
Disobedience ★
Doubtful, recovery, of
*Dullness, sluggishness, difficulty of think-
        ing and comprehending, torpor
        children, in*
Dwells on past disagreeable occur-
        rences
Fear, death, of
        insanity, losing his reason, of
        paralysis, of
        waking, aggravation on •
Forgetful
        words while speaking, of; word
        hunting
Imbecility
Impulses, wash, to ★

Inconstancy
Indifference, apathy
        everything, to
        future, to •
        loved ones, to
        relations, to
Indolence, aversion to work
Insanity, madness
        megalomania
Irritability
        headache, during
Jumping, bed, out of
Kill, desire to
Lamenting, bemoaning, wailing
Laughing, causeless
Liar
        *lies, never speaks the truth, does
                not know what she is saying*
Malicious, spiteful, vindictive
Mathematics, inapt for
Memory, weakness of
        dates, for
        happened, for what has
        names, for proper
        persons, for
        places, for
        read, for what has
        sudden and periodical
Mistakes, calculating, in
Morose, cross, fretful, ill-humor, peevish
Obstinate, headstrong
        children
Offended, easily; takes everything in
        bad part
Prostration of mind, mental exhaus-
        tion, brain-fag
        waking, on
Restlessness
        night
        headache, during
*Sadness, despondency, dejection, mental
        depression, gloom, melancholy*
        business, when thinking of
        disease, about

Secretive
Sensitive, noise, to
Shrieking, screaming, shouting
    children, in
Speech, slow
Squanders
Striking, fists, with •
Suspicious, mistrustful
Sympathy, agg.
        resents ★
Thoughts, disconnected
Unsocial ★
Violent, beats the head ★
Washing always her hands
Weeping, tearful mood
    causeless
       crying from birth ★

T

TABACUM

Anguish, walking in open air
Answers: aversion to answer
    refuses to answer
Anxiety
    afternoon
      16h.
       amel. •
    evening
    night
    air, in open
    alone, when
    causeless
    fear, with
    paroxysms, in ★
    perspiration, with cold
    pressure on the chest, from
    shuddering, with
    stool, during
    sudden
    thinking about it, from
    waking, on
    walking, while
      air, in open
    weeping amel.
Business, incapacity for
Cheerful, gay, mirthful
    dancing, laughing, singing, with
Childish behavior, epilepsy, after ★
Climacteric period agg.
Company, desire for; aversion to soli-
    tude, company amel.
      evening
      night
    alone agg., while
Comprehension, easy
Concentration, difficult
    studying, reading, etc., while
Confidence, want of self

Confusion of mind
 dinner, after
 eating, after
 heat, during
 motion, from
 vomiting amel.
Courageous
Cowardice
Dancing
Death, presentiment of
Delirium
 murmuring
  himself, to
 muttering
  himself, to
 quiet
 raging, raving
 recognizes no one
Delusions, assembled things, swarms,
  crowds, etc.
 beautiful, things look
 images, phantoms, sees
  night
 frightful
 sleep, preventing
 small, things grow smaller
 visions, has horrible, night
Despair
Discontented, displeased, dissatisfied
Discouraged
 anxiety, with ★
Dullness, sluggishness, difficulty of think-
  ing and comprehending, torpor
 eating, after
Excitement, excitable
Fear, apprehension, dread
  afternoon
   16 h. ●
  evening
  night
 alone, of being
  evening
 crowd, in a
 death, of
 disaster, of
 disease, of impending
 eating food, after

Fear,
 exertion, of
 falling, of
 happen, something will
 misfortune, of
  afternoon
 narrow places, in; claustrophobia
 nausea, after ●
 noise, from
 people, of; anthropophobia
 solitude, of
 weeping amel.
 work, dread of
Forgetful
Gestures, makes, automatic
 hands, motions, involuntary,
  of the
Hypochondriasis
Ideas abundant, clearness of mind
  night
Idiocy
Inconsolable, dream, in his
Indifference, apathy
  life, to
  pleasure, to
Indolence, aversion to work
Irresolution, indecision
Irritability
Jesting
Laughing
 causeless
Loathing, life, at
 work, at
Loquacity
 cheerful, exuberant
Memory, weakness of
 expressing oneself, for
 names, for proper
 orthography, for
Misanthropy
Mistakes, writing, in
Moaning, groaning, whining
Mood, changeable, variable
Morose, cross, fretful, ill-humor, peevish
Music, earache from

Muttering
Plans, making many
Prostration of mind, mental exhaustion, brain-fag
Rage, fury
Recognize: relatives, does not recognize his
Resignation
Restlessness
    afternoon
    night
    anxious
       driving from place to place •
    bed, tossing about in
    driving about
    headache, during
Sadness, despondency, dejection, mental depression, gloom, melancholy
    anxious
    climaxis, during
    complaining amel. •
    menses, during
    respiration, with impeded
    walking, while and after
       air, in open
Senses, dull, blunted
Sensitive, oversensitive
    music, to
Sighing
Singing
Speech, delirious
    embarrassed
    foolish
    low
    unintelligible
Starting, startled
    bed, in
    easily
    noise, from
    sleep, on falling
       during
Stupefaction, as if intoxicated
Suicidal disposition
    courage, but lacks
    fear of death, with

Talk, indisposed to, desire to be silent, taciturn
Talks, himself, to
Thoughts, persistent
    rush, flow of
    night
    vanishing of
    wandering
Time, fritters away his
Timidity
    bashful
Unconsciousness, coma, stupor
    cold water, head amel., poured over •
    trance, as in a
    uraemic coma
    vertigo, during
    vomiting amel.
    warm room, in
Unfortunate, feels
Weeping, tearful mood
    afternoon
    night
    amel.
    sleep, in
Work, mental, impossible
Wretched ★

TANACETUM VULGARE

Anxiety
Concentration, difficult
Confusion of mind
Delusions, insane, she will become
Exhilaration
Fear, noise, from
Foolish behavior
Hydrophobia
Indifference, interrogatories, to •
Jesting, ridiculous or foolish
Moaning, groaning, whining
Prostration of mind, mental exhaustion, brain-fag
Sensitive, noise, to
Shrieking, screaming, shouting
Speech, incoherent
Unconsciousness, coma, stupor
    vomiting amel.

TANGHINIA VENENIFERA

Delirium

TANNICUM ACIDUM

Hydrophobia

TARAXACUM OFFICINALE

Anxiety
    motion amel.
    sitting, while
    standing, amel. while
Audacity
Besides oneself, being
Cheerful, gay, mirthful
    followed by irritability
Concentration, difficult
Confusion of mind
    headache, with
    walking, while
Contented
Courageous
Delirium
    muttering
Dipsomania, alcoholism
Dullness, sluggishness, difficulty of think-
    ing and comprehending, torpor
Exertion, agg. from mental
Fear, death, of
    work, dread of
Forgetful
Heedless
Impatience
Indifference, apathy
Indolence, aversion to work
    morning
    works well after beginning, but •
Irresolution, indecision
    indolence, with
Irritability
    morning
Laughing
Loathing, work, at
Loquacity
    perspiration, during
Memory, weakness of
Mood, changeable, variable

Morose, cross, fretful, ill-humor, peevish
    morning
Muttering
Prostration of mind, mental exhaus-
    tion, brain-fag
Reading, mental symptoms agg. from
Religious affections
Restlessness
    night
    anxious
    bed, tossing about in
    driving, about
    waking, on
Sadness, despondency, dejection, men-
    tal depression, gloom, melan-
    choly
    morning
        waking, on
    unoccupied, when •
Sensitive, noise, crackling of paper, to
Sit, inclination to
Speech, prattling
Stupefaction, as if intoxicated
Talk, desire to talk to someone
    indisposed to, desire to be silent,
    taciturn
    morning
Talks, himself, to
Tranquillity, serenity, calmness
Unconsciousness, coma, stupor
    air amel., in open •
    reading, from
    semi-consciousness
    sitting, while
Walk, walking in open air agg. mental
    symptoms

TARENTULA HISPANICA

Abrupt, rough
Absent-minded, unobserving
Abusive ★
Activity, fruitless ★
    mental ★
Ailments from;
    anger, vexation
    bad news
    excitement, emotional

Ailments from;
  grief
  love, disappointed
    unhappy
  punishment
  reproaches
Anger, irascibility
  contradiction, from
  conversation, from
  touched, when
  violent
Anguish
  lamenting, moaning •
Anorexia mentalis
Answers: abruptly, shortly, curtly
  aversion to answer
  imaginary questions
  questioned, does not answer,
    when •
  refuses to answer
Anxiety
  causeless
  exercise, amel.
  future, about
Bilious disposition, difficulty with someone, after •
    grief, after •
Bite, convulsions, with
  himself, bites
Black and sombre, aversion to every-
  thing that is
Business, desire for
Busy
  fruitlessly
Censorious, critical
Cheerful, gay, mirthful
  morning on waking
  air, in open
  alternating with sadness
  room amel., in the •
  waking, on
  walking in open air and after, on
Clairvoyance
Colors, aversion to red, yellow, green
  and black •
  blue, aversion to •
  charmed by blue, green, red •

Company, aversion to; presence of other
  people agg. the symptoms; de-
  sire for solitude
  fear of being alone, yet
  presence of strangers agg.* ★
Company, desire for; aversion to solitude company amel.
  alone, yet fear of people while
Complaining
  threatening, and •
Concentration during conversation,
  difficult
Consolation, kind words agg.
Contradiction, is intolerant of
Contrary
Crafty ★
Cruelty, inhumanity
Cursing, swearing
Cynical ★
Dancing
  wild
Darkness, lie down in the dark and not
  be talked to, desire to •
Death, agony before
  thoughts of
    afternoon
Deceitful, sly
Delirium
  headache, during
  hysterical, almost
  maniacal
  nonsense, with eyes open
  raging, raving
Delusions, imagination, hallucination,
  illusions
  absurd, ludricous figures are
    present
  animals, of
    frightful
  assaulted, is going to be
  faces, sees
    closing eyes, on
    diabolical, crowd upon him
    hideous
  fancy, illusions of
  figures, sees

Delusions,
> *images, phantoms, sees*
>> *closing eyes, on*
>> frightful
> insane, she will become
> insects, sees
> insulted, he is
> legs are cut off
> *sick, being*
> small: smaller, of being
> spectres, ghosts, spirits, sees
> *strangers, room, seem to be in the*
> unseen things, of •
> visions, has
>> closing the eyes, on
>> horrible
>> monsters, of

Dementia
> sadness, with •

Despair, alternating with anger ★
> *chill, during*

Destructiveness
> **clothes, of**
> *cunning* •

Discontented, displeased, dissatisfied
> himself, with
> menses, during

Discouraged
> evening, eating amel. •

Disgust
> consciousness of his unnatural
> state of mind •

Disobedience

Dullness, sluggishness, difficulty of thinking and comprehending, torpor

Eat, refuses to

Eating, amel. after
> evening amel. •

Eccentricity

Ennui, tedium

Excitement, excitable
> *night*
> dancing, singing and weeping, with •
> heat, during
> *menses, during*
> *music, from*
> nervous

Exhilaration

Fancies, lascivious
> repulsive, when alone

Fear, apprehension, dread
> alone, of being
> approaching him, of others
> causeless
> consumption, of
> death, of
> disease, of impending
> eating, of
> evil, of
> fever, of typhus •
> groundless ★
> happen, something will
> insanity, losing his reason, of
> misfortune, of
> music, from
> noise, from
> *touch, of*
> waking from a dream, on
> *walking rapidly, of* ★
> water, of

Feigning sick
> *paroxysms, faintness* •

Foolish behavior

Forgetful: profession, forgets her •

Frightened easily, waking from a dream, on

Gestures, makes
> grasping or reaching at something, at flocks; carphologia
> fingers in the mouth, children put
> hands, motions, involuntary, knitting, as if •
>> restlessly busy ★
> nervous
> plays with his fingers
> *ridiculous or foolish*
> *wringing the hands*

Grief
> *afternoon* •

Hatred

Hide, desire to
> fear of being assaulted •

Hurry, haste
   everybody must hurry
   movements, in
   walking, while
Hypochondriasis
   masturbation, after •
Hysteria
   lascivious
   ludicrous •
   moaning agg., sighing amel. •
   music amel. •
   touch and pressure, intolerance of •
Ideas, deficiency of
Impatience
Impulsive ★
Impressionable
Impulse, run, to; dromomania
Indifference, apathy
      morning till 15 h. •
      evening
   alternating with cheerfulness
   external things, to
Indolence, aversion to work
Industrious, mania for work
Insanity, madness
   erotic
   laughing, with
   love, from disappointed •
   paroxysmal
   periodical
   restlessness of legs, with •
   sleeplessness, with
   strength increased, with
   threatens destruction and
   death •
Irresolution, indecision
   acts, in
   ideas, in
Irritability
   coition, amel. after •
   menses, during
   touched, when ★
Jesting
   waking, on
Jumping
Kicks

Kill, threatens to
Kleptomania
Lamenting, bemoaning, wailing
Lascivious, lustful
Laughing
   company, in •
   desire to laugh
   immoderately
   involuntarily
   mocking •
   nervous ★
   sardonic
   screams, then ★
   stupid expression, with
Light, aversion to
   shuns
Loathing, general
Looked at, cannot bear to be
Looking others in distress agg. ★
Loquacity
Ludicrous, things seem
Malicious, spiteful, vindictive
Mania
   abuses everyone
   destruction, followed by laughter
      and apologies, of •
   paroxysmal •
   periodical
   sexual mania in men
      women, in
   singing, with
   tears, clothes
      hair, own
Memory, weakness of
Mischievous
Moaning, groaning, whining
   night
   contradicted, when
Mocking
   old age, in •
Mood, alternating
   changeable, variable
Moral feeling, want of
Morose, cross, fretful, ill-humor, peevish
   contradiction, by
   menses, during
   waking, on

Music agg.
    agreeable, is
    amel.
        music amel. restlessness of
        extremities •
Naked, wants to be ★
Nymphomania
    chorea, with •
    coition agg. •
Obscene, lewd
Obstinate, headstrong
Occupation, diversion amel.
Pains, sympathetic ★
Passionate
Pities, sick, desire to show being •
Play, desire to
Playful
Profanity ★
Pull one's hair, desires to
    she presses her head and pulls
    her hair ★
Quarrelsome, scolding
Rage, fury
    pulls hair ★
Relaxation amel. ★
Restlessness
        night, midnight, 5h. after •
    anxious
        compelling rapid walking
    bed, go from one bed to another,
    wants to
        tossing about in
    driving about
    menses, during
    music, from
Runs about
Sadness, despondency, dejection, men-
    tal depression, gloom, melan-
    choly
        morning on waking
        afternoon
        evening amel. when eating •
        night amel.
    air, amel. in open
    alternating with vivacity
    causeless
    eating, amel. after

Sadness,
    fault, as if in •
    heat, during
    house, on entering
    music, from
    sexual excitement, after •
    supper, amel. after
    waking, on
    warm room, in
Scratches with hand
Self - control, loss of ★
Self-torture
Senses, acute
Sensitive, oversensitive
    mental impressions, to
    music, to
    noise, to
        music amel.
Shamelessness
    exposes the person
Shining objects amel.
Shrieking, screaming, shouting
    laughter, after •
Singing
    hoarse, until very
        exhausted, and •
    involuntarily
    singing, dancing and weeping •
Somnambulism
Speech, abrupt
    threatening •
Spoken to, averse to being
Starting, startled
    sleep, during
    from
    sleepiness, with
Steals money, without necessity ★
Strangers: presence of strangers agg.
Striking
    anger, his friends from
    himself
        head, his
        strikes her head with her
        hands, her body and others •
Stupefaction, as if intoxicated
    convulsions, between
    waking, on

Suicidal disposition
Sympathy, compassion
Talk, indisposed to, desire to be silent,
    taciturn
        heat, during
Tears things
    hair, her
        and pressed her head •
Terror ★
Thoughts, persistent
Threatening
    destroy, threatens to •
    kill, threatens to
Throws things away
Timidity, bashful
Torments himself
Touched, aversion to being
Unconsciousness, coma, stupor
Understands questions addressed to
        her, does not •
Violent, vehement
    deeds of violence, rage leading to
Vivacious
    alternating with sorrow •
Weeping, tearful mood
        morning
        afternoon
        night
    alternating with laughter
    causeless
    consolation agg.
        from c. •
    contradiction, from
    hysterical
    looked at, when
    refused, when anything
    sleep, in
    vexation, from
Work, desire for mental

TARENTULA CUBENSIS

Delirium
    pains, with the
    sepsis, from
Sympathy, compassion

TAXUS BACCATA

Anxiety
Delirium
Helplessness, feeling of
Imbecility
Impatience
Restlessness
    bed, in
Sighing
Unconsciousness, coma, stupor

TELA ARANEA

Absent-minded, unobserving

TELLURIUM METALLICUM

Anger, irascibility
    violent
Cheerful, alternating with impatience
Dullness, morning
Excitement, excitable
Fear, apprehension, dread
    touch, of
Fishy ★
Forgetful
Indifference, apathy
Irritability
    alternating with cheerfulness
Laughing agg.
Memory, weakness of
    business, for
Neglects, everything
Restlessness
    bed, in
Retention, sense of ★
Sadness, despondency, dejection, mental
        depression, gloom, melancholy
Sensitive, oversensitive
    touch, to
Tranquillity, serenity, calmness
Work, mental, impossible

TEPLITZ AQUA

Anxiety

Company, aversion to; presence of
    other people agg. the symp-
    toms; desire for solitude

Irritability
    spoken to, when

Memory, weakness of
    business, for
    read, for what has
    said, for what has

Morose, cross, fretful, ill-humor, peevish

Restlessness, bed, tossing about in

Spoken to, averse to being

Weeping, tearful mood

TEREBINTHINIAE OLEUM

Anxiety
    evening in bed
    bed, in

Concentration, difficult

Confusion of mind
    urination amel. •

Courageous

Delirium
    answers correctly when spoken to,
      but delirium and unconscious-
      ness return at once
    maniacal
    muttering
    sepsis, from

Delusions, imaginations, hallucinations,
    illusions
    floating in air

Dullness, sluggishness, difficulty of
    thinking and comprehending,
    torpor
    urine amel., copious flow of

Excitement, excitable

Fear, apoplexy, of
    waking, on

Hydrophobia

Hypochondriasis

Hysteria, fainting, hysterical
    move any part of body, cannot •

Ideas abundant, clearness of mind

Insanity, madness

Loathing, life, at

Mania

Memory, active

Restlessness, bed, tossing about in

Sadness, despondency, dejection, men-
    tal depression, gloom, melan-
    choly
    headache, during

Sensitive, oversensitive

Shrieking, dentition, during

Starting, sleep, from

Stupefaction, as if intoxicated
    sleepiness, with

Suicidal disposition
    hanging, by

Thoughts, rush, flow of

Trance

Unconsciousness, coma, stupor
    answers correctly when spoken to,
      but delirium and u. return at
      once
    fever, during
    restlessness, with •
    stool, after
    uraemic coma

Weary of life

Work, mental, impossible

TEREBINTHINA CHIOS

Delusions, imaginations, hallucinations,
    illusions

Excitement, excitable

Fear, apprehension, dread

Lascivious, lustful

Sadness, despondency, dejection, men-
    tal depression, gloom, melancholy

Unconsciousness, coma, stupor

TETRADYMITUM

Delusions, fire, visions of

TEUCRIUM MARUM VERUM
(MARUM VERUM)

Anger, irascibility
    easily
    voices of people
Cheerful, gay, mirthful
    evening
    air, in open
    walking in open air and after, on
Confusion of mind
Delirium tremens, mania-a-potu
Desire, exercise in open air, for •
Discontented, displeased, dissatisfied
Dullness, sluggishness, difficulty of think-
    ing and comprehending, torpor
Eccentricity
    evening
Excitement, excitable
    evening
    hearing horrible things, after
    nervous
    perspiration, during
    trembling, with
Exhilaration
    evening
Horrible things, sad stories, affect her
    profoundly
Indolence, aversion to work
Irritability
    noon
    chill, during
    dinner, during •
    after
    eating, during
    after
    headache, during
    talking, while
Loquacity
    evening
    chill, during
    heat, during
Magnetized desire to be, mesmerism
    amel.

Morose, cross, fretful, ill-humor, peevish
Narrating her symptoms agg.
Prostration of mind, mental exhaus-
    tion, brain-fag
Restlessness
    night
Sadness, cold, from becoming
Sensitive, oversensitive
    children
    eating, during •
    after
    heat, during
    noise: voices, to
    puberty, in
Singing
    involuntarily
Sit, inclination to
Somnabulism
Spoken to, averse to being
Starting, midnight in sleep, after
    dream, from a
    sleep, during
Talk, others agg., of
Talking, unpleasant things agg., of
Thoughts, rush, flow of
Violent, vehement
Walk, walking in open air amel. mental
    symptoms
Wearisome
Weeping agg.
Work, aversion to mental

THALLIUM METALLICUM AUT ACETICUM

Excitement, excitable
Hysteria
Impatience
Indifference, apathy
Irritability
Lamenting, bemoaning, wailing
Restlessness
Sadness, despondency, dejection, mental
    depression, gloom, melancholy
Shrieking, screaming, shouting
Weeping, tearful mood
Work, mental, impossible

THALAMUS

Anguish
Anxiety, causeless
Company, aversion to; presence of other people agg. the symptoms; desire for solitude
Dullness, sluggishness, difficulty of thinking and comprehending, torpor
Indifference, anosognosia (real or pretended ignorance of the disease, especially paralysis) •
Laughing, spasmodic
Schizophrenia, catatonic
    hebephrenia
Sits, still
Weeping, spasmodic

THEA CHINENSIS

Activity, sleeplessness, with
Affectionate
Anger, irascibility
Anguish
Anxiety
Aversion, everything, to
Cheerful, gay, mirthful
Concentration, active
Confidence, want of self, beer amel. •
Confusion of mind, walking, while
Conversation, aversion to
Death, presentiment of
    predicts the time
Delirium
    laughing
    loquacious, rhyme, in •
Delirium tremens, mania-a-potu
Delusions, imaginations, hallucinations, illusions
    bells, hears ringing of
    door bell •
    dragged from the lowest abyss of darkness (at night, on waking) •
    hearing, illusions of
Discontented, everything, with

Disgust
    everything, with
Eccentricity
Ecstasy
    amorous
Excitement, excitable
    night on waking
    nervous
Exhilaration
Fear, night
    death, of sudden
    exertion, of
    happen, something will
    killing, of
Frightened easily
    night
Ideas abundant, clearness of mind
Impulsive
Indolence, aversion to work
Irritability
    night, 22-2h •
Kill, desire to
    herself, sudden impulse to
    sudden impulse to kill
    throw child into fire, sudden impulse to
Loathing, general
Loquacity
Mania
Morose, cross, fretful, ill-humor, peevish
Pleasure, waking from a dream of murder, on •
Phophesying, predicts the time of death
Quarrelsome, scolding
Restlessness, night
    bed, tossing about in
    waking, on
Sadness, despondency, dejection, mental depression, gloom, melancholy
Senses, acute
Sensitive, oversensitive
Speech, fluent
    interesting •
Starting, sleep, from
Strength increased, mental

Suicidal disposition
    throwing himself, window, from
Talk, indisposed to, desire to be silent,
    taciturn
Thinking, aversion to
Thoughts, frightful
    persistent
    rush, flow of
    thoughtful
    tormenting
Throws things away
Travel, desire to
Unconsciousness, evening
Verses, makes
Vivacious
Weeping, tearful mood
Witty
Work, aversion to mental
Writing, aversion to

THERIDION CURASSAVICUM

Activity, fruitless ★
Anxiety
    hysterical
Beside oneself, being
Business, averse to
Busy
    fruitlessly
Cheerful, gay, mirthful
    headache, with ●
    hysterical ●
Climacteric period agg.
Confidence, want of self
Confusion of mind
    identity: duality, sense of
        head separated from body, as
        if
    laughing agg. ●
Cowardice
Death: dying, feels as if
Delusions, imaginations, hallucinations,
    illusions
    double, of being
    head belongs to another

Delusions, head,
    lift it off, can ●
    separated from body, is
    time seem earlier, passes too
    quickly
Desires, indefinite
Despair
    recovery, of
Discontented, displeased, dissaftisfied
    himself, with
Discouraged
Distances, exaggerated, are
Duality, Sense of ★
Dullness, sluggishness, difficulty of think-
    ing and comprehending, torpor
Excitement, excitable
    evening
    climacteric period, during
Fear, apprehension, dread
    noise, from
    tremulous
Frightened easily
Gestures, makes, plays with his fingers
    wringing the hand ★
Hysteria
    climacteric period, at
    lie down, must
    puberty, at
Imbecility
Indifference, apathy
    pleasure, to
Indolence, aversion to work
    morning
    sleepiness, with
Industrious, mania for work
Insanity, climacteric period, during
Joyous, headache, during ★
Loquacity
    busy
    excited
    hilarity, with ★
Memory, weakness of, labor, for mental
Mistakes, time, in
Occupation, desire for
Restlessness
    bed, driving out of
    busy

Sadness, despondency, dejection, mental
    depression, gloom, melancholy
       evening
    headache, during
    walking, while and after
Senses, dull, blunted
Sensitive, oversensitive
    noise, to
       shrill sounds, to
       slightest, to
       striking of clocks, ringing
       of bells, to
    odors, to
    pain, to
Sighing
Singing
    headache, with ●
    trilling
Starting, startled
    easily
    noise, from
Thoughts, vanishing of, closing eyes,
    on ●
Time passes too quickly, appears shorter
Unconsciousness, exertion, after
Work, desire for mental

THIOPROPERAZINUM

Absent-minded, unobserving
Anguish, evening
Anxiety
Company, aversion to; presence of
    other people agg. the symp-
    toms; desire for solitude
       evening
Comprehension, easy
Confusion of mind
Delusions, separated from the world,
    he is
Excitement, afternoon
    evening
    alternating with taciturnity, af-
    ternoon ●
Impatience
Indifference, apathy
Love with one of own sex, homosexual-
    ity, tribadism

Memory, weakness of, words, for
Restlessness
Sadness, despondency, dejection, men-
    tal depression, gloom, melan-
    choly
Schizophrenia
    catatonic
    hebephrenia

THUJA OCCIDENTALIS

Absent-minded, unobserving
Absorbed, buried in thought
Abstraction of mind
Abusive, husband, to ★
    mother, to ★
Ailments from :
    anticipation, foreboding, presen-
       timent
    quarrels
    sexual excesses
Anger, irascibility
    contradiction, from
    easily
    trifles, at
    violent, when things don't go
       after his will ●
Answers, irrelevantly, parturition, after ●
    slowly
Anxiety
    afternoon, 16-17 h. ●
    night
    anticipation, from, an engage-
       ment ★
    coldness of feet at night, during ●
    conscience, as if guilty of a crime
    eating, after
    fear, with
    future, about
    paroxysms, in ★
    salvation, about
    sudden
    vaccination, after ●
    waking, on
Aversion, everything, to
    husband, to ★
    mother, to ★
Beside oneself, being
    trifles, from

Capriciousness
Cares, worries, full of
Chaotic, confused behavior
Cheerful, gay, mirthful
> afternoon
> heat, during

Company, aversion to; presence of other people agg. the symptoms; desire for solitude
> *avoids the sight of people*
> *parturition, after* •
> *presence of strangers, aversion to*

Concentration, difficult

Confusion of mind
> morning
>> waking, on
> evening
> dinner, after
> dream, as if in
> eating, after
> heat, during
> identity, as to his
>> duality, sense of
> intoxicated, as if
> loses his way in well-known streets
> mental exertion, from
> sitting, while
> smoking, after
> standing, while
> *talking, while*
> walking, while

Conscientious about trifles
> trifles, occupied with

Consolation, kind words agg.
Contemptuous, self, of
Contradiction, is intolerant of
Contradictory, actions are contradictory to intention
Contrary
Conversation agg.
Cowardice
Death, conviction of
> *desires*
Deceitful, sly

Delirium tremens, mania-a-potu
Delusions, imaginations, hallucinations, illusions
> animals, of
>> *abdomen, are in* •
>> passing before her •
> body, brittle, is
>> *delicate, is* •
>> lighter than air, is
>> pieces, in danger of coming in •
>> thin, is •
> building stones, appearance of •
> calls, someone
> criminal, he is a
> dead persons, sees
> *die, he was about to*
>> time has come to
> diminished, thin, he is too •
> divided into two parts
>> cut in two parts, or, which part he has possession on waking, and could not tell of •
> double, of being
> emaciation, of
> fancy, illusions of
> floating in air ★
> glass, she is made of
>> *wood, glass, etc., being made of*
> head belongs to another
> head, standing, on ★
> heavy, is
> higher power ★
> identity, errors of personal
> *images, phantoms, sees*
>> *night*
>> *closing eyes, on*
> light, incorporeal, he is
> mind and body are separated
> music, he hears
> over-powered, as if ★
> people, sees
>> beside him, are
>> converses with absent
> pregnant, she is
> present, someone is
> pursued by enemies, he was
> small, things appear

Delusions,
   soul, body was too small for soul or
      separated from
   spectres, ghosts, spirits, sees
      closing eyes, on
   strange, familiar things seem
   strangers, he sees ●
      room, seem to be in the
   superhuman, control, is under
   thin, body is ●
   visions, has, night
      closing the eyes, on
   voices, abdomen, are in his ●
      hears, abdomen, in his ●
   walks beside him, someone
   war, being at
   wrong, he has done
Despair
   religious despair of salvation
Dipsomania, alcoholism
Discomfort
Discontented, displeased, dissatisfied
Discouraged
Disgust
   everything, with
Distraction ★
Dream, as if in a
*Dullness, sluggishness, difficulty of think-
   ing and comprehending, torpor*
      morning
         waking, on
      perspiration, during
      waking, on
Dwells on past disagreeable occur-
   rences
Excitement, excitable
   night
      waking, on
   menses, before
   waking, on
Exhilaration
Fanaticism
Fancies, exaltation of
   sleeplessness, with
   lascivious
      lying down, while ●

Fastidious ★
Fear, apprehension, dread
   apoplexy, of
   *approaching him, of others
      delirium*
   disease, of impending
   eating, food after
   evil, of
   insanity, losing his reason, of
   music, from
   physician, will not see her, he
      seems to terrify her
   stomach, arising from
   strangers, of
   touch, of
   wind, of
Fishy ★
Forgetful
   morning
      waking, on
   waking, on
   *words while speaking, of; word
      hunting*
Frail, sensation of being ●
Gestures, makes, covers mouth with
   hands ★
Haughty
Heedless
Hurry, haste
   mental work, in
   movements, in
   occupation, in
   walking, while
Hypochondriasis
Hysteria
Ideas abundant, clearness of mind
      heat, during
   deficiency of
   fixed ★
   wander ★
Idiocy
Imbecility
Impatience
Impetuous, perspiration, with
Inconstancy
   thoughts, of

Indifference, apathy
    external things, to
    opposite sex, to •
Indolence, aversion to work
    eating, after
Industrious, heat, during
Insanity, madness
    touched, will not be •
Irresolution, indecision
    changeable
Irritability
    morning
        waking, on
    afternoon
    chill, during
    coition, after
    eating, after
    family, to her •
    headache, during
    perspiration, during
    sleep, when roused by noise during
    waking, on
    walking, when
Jealousy
Jesting, aversion to
Kill herself, sudden impulse to
Laughing, spasmodic
Loathing, life, at
Loquacity
Meditation
Memory, active
Memory, weakness of
    done, for what has just
    expressing oneself, for
    labor, for mental
    persons, for
    say, for what is about to
    words, of
Mildness
Mistakes, calculating, in, cannot calculate after childbirth •
    speaking in
        misplacing, words
        words, using wrong

Mistakes,
    writing, in
        omitting letters
        syllables
        words
        wrong words
Moaning, heat, during
    sleep, during
Monomania
Mood, changeable, variable
    repulsive
Moonlight, mental symptoms from
Morose, cross, fretful, ill-humor, peevish
    morning, in bed
        waking, on
    eating, after
    hurry, with •
    pollutions, after
    waking, on
Music agg.
    organ agg., of
    amel.
    trembling from
        feet, of •
Obstinate, headstrong
    children
Occupation, diversion amel.
Offended, easily; takes everything in bad part
Passionate
Prostration of mind, mental exhaustion, brain-fag
Quarrelsome, scolding
Quiet disposition
    parturition, after •
Religious affections
    fanaticism
Reproaches himself
Restlessness
    morning
    forenoon
    afternoon
    17 h.
    evening
        bed, in
    night

Restlessness
   anxious
   bed, tossing about in
   dinner, after
     amel. after •
   heat, during
   menses, during
   sleep, before
   walking, while

Sadness, despondency, dejection, mental depression, gloom, melancholy
   morning after waking
   forenoon
   afternoon
   evening in bed
   menses, during
   music, from
   perspiration, during
   sleeplessness from sadness
     with
   walking, while and after
   wine amel. •

Sensitive, oversensitive
   morning
   music, to
     sacred music, to
   sensual impressions, to

Serious, earnest
   evening

Shrieking, screaming, shouting
   sleep, during

Sighing, heat, during
   perspiration, during

Slowness

Speech, confused
   finish sentence, cannot
   hasty
   hesitating
   monosyllable
   slow

Starting, sleep, during
   from

Strangers presence of, agg.

Strength increased, mental

Stupefaction, as if intoxicated
   morning
     rising, after
   knows not where he is
   motion, from

Suicidal disposition
   thoughts
   throwing himself, window, from

Suspicious, mistrustful

Talk, indisposed to, desire to be silent, taciturn
     morning on waking
       walking, while

Talks, fast ★

Talking, sleep, in

Thinking, complaints agg., of

Thoughts as if from abdomen •
   disagreeable
   persistent
     separated, mind and body are
   stagnation of
   thoughtful
   vanishing of, speaking, while
   wandering

Time passes too quickly, appears shorter

Touch everything, impelled to

Touched, aversion to being

Trifles seem important

Ugly (in behavior) ★

Walks, circle, in a
   walking in open air agg. mental symptoms

Wearisome

Weary of life

Weeping, tearful mood
   night
     sleep, in
   consolation agg.
   desires to weep, all the time
   menses, during
   music, from
   sleep, in
   spoken to, when

Work, aversion to mental
   impossible

Wrong, cannot tell, what is ★

THUJA LOBII

Anguish
Inifference, apathy
    himself, to •
    surroundings, to the
Sadness, anxious
Schizophrenia, hebephrenia
Suicidal disposition
    thoughts
Weeping, tearful mood
Will, loss of

THYMOLUM

Company, desire for; aversion to soli-
    tude, company amel.
Confusion of mind
Despair
Exertion, agg. from mental
Irritability
Loquacity
Morose, cross, fretful, ill-humor, pee-
    vish
Restlessness
Sadness, despondency, dejection, men-
    tal depression, gloom, melan-
    choly
    headache, during
Satyriasis

THYROIDINUM

Anger, irascibility
Anguish
Capriciousness
Contradiction, is intolerant of
Delusions, persecuted, he is
Despair, recovery, of ★
Euphoria
    alternating with quarrelsomeness •
Gestures, makes, grasping ★
    hands, restlessly busy ★
Grumbling ★
Hysteria
Idiocy
Imbecility
Indifference, everything, to ★
Insanity, puerperal

Irritability
    menses, before
Laughing, peculiar, to herself ★
Mania
Memory, weakness of
Quarrelsome, family, with her
Rage, evening
Restlessness
Sadness, waking, on
Thinking, complaints agg., of
Tranquillity, serenity, calmness
Weeping, undresses and ★
Work, aversion to mental ★

THYREOTROPINUM

Anxiety
Excitement, excitable
    alternating with sadness
Sadness, despondency, dejection, men-
    tal depression, gloom, melan-
    choly
Weeping, tearful mood

TILIA EUROPAEA

Anger, contradiction, from
Anxiety, air amel., in open
    fear, with
    house, in
Censorious, critical
Company, aversion to; presence of
    other people agg. the symp-
    toms; desire for solitude
Concentration, difficult
    forenoon
Confusion of mind, morning
    waking, on
    night
    waking, on
Contradiction, is intolerant of
Discontented, displeased, dissatisfied
Dullness, sluggishness, difficulty of think-
    ing and comprehending, torpor
Fear, apprehension, dread
    crowd, in a
    people, of; anthropophobia
    room, on entering

Irritability
    morning
    dinner, after
Lamenting, bemoaning, wailing
    fever, during
Love with one of the own sex homosex-
    uality, tribadism, love-sick
Morose, cross, fretful, ill-humor, pee-
    vish
Pleasure
    morning
Quarrelsome, scolding
    evening
Sadness, despondency, dejection, men-
    tal depression, gloom, melan-
    choly
    dinner, after
    eating, after
Serious, earnest
Sighing
Speech, delirious, during fever
Thoughts, thoughtful
Unconsciousness, dinner, after
Weeping, tearful mood
    heat, during

TONGO

Anxiety
Cheerful, gay, mirthful
Confusion of mind, intoxicated, as if
Fear: work, dread of
Indifference, sleepiness, with
Indolence, aversion to work
    dinner, after
    sleepiness, with
Loathing, general, forenoon •
Restlessness
Sadness, despondency, dejection, men-
    tal depression, gloom, melan-
    choly
Talk, indisposed to, desire to be silent,
    taciturn

TRACHINUS DRACO

Anxiety
Delirium, raging, raving
Fear, death, of
Hydrophobia

TRADESCANTIA DIURETICA

Sighing

TRIFOLIUM PRATENSE

Confusion of mind, morning
Dullness, sluggishness, difficulty of
    thinking and comprehending,
    torpor

TRILLIUM PENDULUM

Anger, irascibility
Anguish
Anxiety, climacteric period, during
Confusion of mind, identity, duality,
    sense of
Delusions, double, of being
Excitement, excitable
Fear, death, of
    disease, of impending
Irritability
Restlessness, bed, tossing about in
Sadness, despondency, dejection, men-
    tal depression, gloom, melan-
    choly

TRIOSTEUM PERFOLIATUM

Cheerful, gay, mirthful
Company, aversion to; alone, amel.
    when
Concentration, difficult
Discuss, desire to •
Irritability
    evening
    noise, from
Prostration of mind, mental exhaus-
    tion, brain-fag
Rage, evening
Sadness, despondency, dejection, mental
    depression, gloom, melancholy

TROMBIDIUM MUSCAE DOMESTICAE (ACARUS)

Confusion of mind
Contradict, disposition to

Contrary
Forgetful
Ideas, deficiency of
Loquacity
Restlessness
      midnight, 2h. after
      move, must constantly
Thoughts, disconnected

TUBERCULINUM BOVINUM KENT

Abstraction of mind
Abusive, insulting
Ailments from:
    excitement, emotional
    work, mental
Anger, irascibility
    throws things away
    violent, fit of ★
    waking, on
Answers monosyllable, "no" to all questions
Anticipation, dentist, physician, before
    going to
Anxiety, evening
    night in children
        midnight, before
    exaggerated ★
    fever, during
    headache, with
Audacity ★
Break things, desire to
Change, desire for
Cheerful, gay, mirthful
Confusion of mind
    walking in open air, while
Cursing, swearing
Delirium
Delusions, imaginations, hallucinations,
    illusions
    large, people seem too (during
      vertigo)
    snakes in and around her
    strange, familiar things seem

Delusions,
    places seemed
    surroundings strange ★
Despair
Destructiveness
Dipsomania, alcoholism
Discontented, displeased dissatisfied
**Dullness, sluggishness, difficulty
    of thinking and compre-
    hending, torpor**
    children, in
Escape, attempts to
Excitement, excitable
Exertion, agg. from mental
Fear, apprehension, dread
    animals, of
    cats, of ●
    dogs, of
    happen, somthing will
    waking, on
Forgetful
Heedless
Hopeful
Horror, awakes in ★
Hysteria
Ideas abundant, clearness of mind
Idiocy
    shrill shrieking, with
Impulse, run, to; dromomania
Indifference, apathy
Indolence, aversion to work
    morning ★
Industrious, mania for work
Insanity, madness
    alternating mental with physical
      symptoms
    travel, with desire to
Irritability
    morning on waking
    children, in
    waking, on
Lascivious, lustful ★
Looked at, cannot bear to be
Loquacity, changing quickly from one
    subject to another
    heat, during
    rambling ★

Malicious, spiteful, vindictive
Memory, weakness of
Mental symptoms alternating with physical
Mistakes, speaking, using wrong words in, name of object seen instead of one desired
Moaning, groaning, whining
    convulsions, in
Mood, alternating
    changeable, variable
Morose, cross, fretful, ill-humor, peevish
Music amel.
Obstinate, headstrong
    children
    excessively obstinate ★
Offended, easily; takes everything in bad part
Precocity ★
Pull one's hair, desires to
Quarrelsome, scolding
Rage, pulls hair ★
Reckless, rashness ★
Restlessness
    night
    children, in
Sadness, despondency, dejection, mental depression, gloom, melancholy
Self-torture
Sensitive, oversensitive
    noise, to
Shamelessness, children, in ●
Shrieking, screaming, shouting
    children, in
      sleep, during
    menses, before ★
    sleep, during
Speech, nonsensical
Starting, startled
    sleep, on falling
Strange, everything seems
Striking himself, knocking his head against wall and things
Suicidal disposition
Talk, indisposed to, desire to be silent, taciturn

Talking, sleep, in
Thoughts, intrude, night ●
    persistent
      night
      tormenting, night
Threatening
Throws things away
    persons, at
Torments himself
Touched, aversion to being ★
Travel, desire to
Trifles, seem important
Unconsciousness, shrieking, with ●
Violent, beats the head ★
Wander, desires to
Weary of life
Weeping, spoken to, when
    trifles, at, children at the least worry
Whining, whimpering, ailment, with little ★
Work, aversion to mental

TUBERCULINUM KOCH

Mania
Sensitive, music, to

TUBERCULINUM RESIDUUM

Discouraged
Sadness, despondency, dejection, mental depression, gloom, melancholy
Weary of life

TUSSILAGO FRAGANS

Censorious, critical
Complaining
Contented, 10-23 h.
Malicious, spiteful, vindictive
Speech, benevolent ●
Tranquillity, serenity, calmness

TUSSILAGO PETASITES

Delirium tremens, mania-a-potu

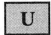

UPAS TIEUTE

Ailments from:
    sexual excesses
Anger, irascibility
Concentration, difficult
Dullness, sluggishness, difficulty of think-
    ing and comprehending, torpor
Irritability
    evening, in bed •
Memory, weakness of
Morose, cross, fretful, ill-humor, peevish
    evening in bed
Restlessness
    morning
    afternoon
    coition, during •
Sadness, despondency, dejection, mental
    depression, gloom, melancholy

URANIUM METALLICUM

Irritability

URANIUM NITRICUM

Confusion of mind, sleeping, after
Dullness, sluggishness, difficulty of think-
    ing and comprehending, torpor
Indolence, aversion to work
Morose, cross, fretful, ill-humor, peevish
Restlessness
    night
Sadness, despondency, dejection, mental
    depression, gloom, melancholy
Stupefaction, as if intoxicated
Unconsciousness, coma, stupor

URTICA URENS

Restlessness

USTILAGO MAYDIS

Amativeness
Company, aversion to; presence of
    other people agg. the symp-
    toms; desire for solitude
    desires solitude to practise mas-
    turbation
Confusion of mind, morning
Dullness, sluggishness, difficulty of think-
    ing and comprehending, torpor
Fancies, lascivious
Hysteria
Irritability
    heat, during
    pollutions, after
    questioned, when
    spoken to, when
Lascivious, lustful
Mania
Morose, cross, fretful, ill-humor, peevish
Restlessness
    night
    bed, tossing about in
Sadness, despondency, dejection, men-
    tal depression, gloom, melan-
    choly
    menses, after
    pollutions, from
Satyriasis
Suicidal disposition
Talk, indisposed to, desire to be silent,
    taciturn
Thoughts, sexual
    masturbation, with •
Weeping, tearful mood
    pollutions, after

UVA URSI

Morose, cross, fretful, ill-humor, pee-
    vish

VACCIN ATTÉNUÉ BILIÉ

Anger, irascibility
Anguish
Anxiety
Cares, worries, full of
Death, sensation of
Excitement, excitable
    reading in foreign language, while •
Fear, death, of impending
Forgetful, words while speaking, of; word hunting
Hypochondriasis
Inconstancy
Sadness, despondency, dejection, mental depression, gloom, melancholy
Sensitive, noise, to
Work, mental, fatigues

VACCININUM

Cares, worries, full of
Carried, desires to be
Fear, smallpox, of
Impatience
Irritability
Morose, cross, fretful, ill-humor, peevish
Restlessness
Shrieking, screaming, shouting
Weeping, tearful mood
    heat, during

VALERIANA OFFICINALIS

Absent-minded, unobserving
Activity, mental ★
Affections, in general ★
Anger, irascibility
    easily
Animation agg. ★
Answers, incoherently
    irrelevantly

Anxiety
    air amel., in open
    fear, with
    fever, during
    house, in
    hypochondriacal
Beside oneself, being
Busy
Capriciousness
Cheerful, gay, mirthful
    evening
Clairvoyance
Climacteric period agg.
Comprehension, easy
Confusion of mind
    evening
    heat, during
    identity, as to his
    intoxicated, as after being
    sitting, while
    standing, while
    stooping, when
Courageous
Darkness agg.
Delirium
    mild
    quiet
    trembling, with
    wild
Delusions, imaginations, hallucinations, illusions
    animals, of
     bed, on
    bed, someone is in bed with him
    danger, impression of
    double, of being
    fancy, illusions of
    figures, sees
    floating in air
    home, is away from
    identity, errors of personal
        someone else, she is
    images, phantoms, sees
        night
    light, incorporeal, he is

Delusions,
>   people, sees
>   beside him, are
>   person, she is some other
>   poor, he is
>   strange, familiar thing seem
>   visions, has

Desolate, room appears •
Despair
Dipsomania, alcoholism
Discomfort
Discouraged
Dream, as if in a
Dullness, sluggishness, difficulty of think-
>   ing and comprehending, torpor
Eccentricity
Ecstasy
Embittered, exasperated
Emotions predominated by the intel-
>   lect
Escape, attempts to
>   window, from
Excitement, excitable
>   evening
>   climacteric period, during
>   coffee, as after
>   heat, during
>   nervous
>   *trembling, with*
>   wine, as from
Exhilaration
Extremes, goes to ★
Fancies, exaltation of
>   vivid, lively
Fear, apprehension, dread
>   evening
>   *air amel., in open*
>   dark, of
>   misfortune, of
>   narrow places, in; claustrophobia
>   *room, on entering*
>   warm room, of •
Forgetful, name, his own
Forsaken feeling
Grumbling ★
Heedless
Homesickness
Hypochondriasis

Hysteria
>   climacteric period, at
Ideas abundant, clearness of mind
>   *evening*
>   perspiration, during
>   deficiency of
>   erroneous ★
Inconstancy
Indolence, aversion to work
Industrious, mania for work
Irritability
Laughing
>   evening
>   spasmodic
Light, desire for
Loathing, life, at
Loquacity
Memory, active
Memory, weakness of
Mental symptoms alternating with
>   *physical* ★
Mistakes, localities, in
Mood, alternating
>   *changeable, variable*
Morose, cross, fretful, ill-humor, peevish
Prostration of mind, mental exhaus-
>   tion, brain-fag
Quiet disposition
>   hypochondriasis, in
Recognize: relatives, does not recog-
>   nizes his
Restlessness
>   *night*
>   air amel., in open
>   anxious
>   bed, tossing about in
>   driving about, in open air
>   heat, during
>   hypochondriacal
>   tremulous
Sadness, despondency, dejection, mental
>   depression, gloom, melancholy
>   alone, when
Selfishness, egoism
Senses, acute
Sensitive, oversensitive
>   heat, during
Serious, earnest

Shrieking, screaming, shouting
      stool, during ★
Strange, everything seems
Stranger, sensation as if one were a
Stupefaction, as if intoxicated
      stooping, on
Suicidal disposition, intermittent fever,
      during
Thoughts, rapid, quick
      rush, flow of
            drunkenness, as in ●
      wandering
Threatening
Twilight agg. mental symptoms
Unconsciousness, coma, stupor
      chill, during
      dream, as in a
      pain, from
Vivacious
Wander, house, desires to w. about ●
Weary of life
      heat, during
Weeping, alternating with laughter
Work, aversion to mental
Wriggles (squirms) ★

VARIOLINUM

Delirium
      fever, during
      mild
      wild
Fear, death, of, sleep, followed by
      deep ●
      smallpox, of
Restlessness, bed, tossing about in
Sensitive, odor, to

VENUS MERCENARIA

Concentration, difficult
Delusions, separated from the world,
      he is
Ennui, tedium
Indifference, apathy
Irritability, noise, from
Sadness, despondency, dejection, mental
      depression, gloom, melancholy

Schizophrenia
Thoughts, disconnected
Weeping, trifles, at

VERATRUM ALBUM

Absent-minded, unobserving
Absorbed, buried in thought
Abusive, insulting
      husband insulting wife before
            children or vice versa
Activity, restless ★
Adulterous
Affectation ★
      gestures and acts, in
      words, in
Affections, in general ★
Affectionate
Ailments from :
      ambition, deceived
      anger, vexation
          anxiety, with
          silent grief, with
      anticipation, foreboding, presen-
          timent
      business failure
      disappointment
      excitement, emotional
      fear
      fright
      grief
      honor, wounded
      injuries, accidents; mental symp-
          toms from
      joy, excessive
      love, disappointed
      mortification
      pecuniary loss
      scorn, being scorned
      surprises, pleasant
Amativeness
Ambition
      means, employed every possible
Amorous
Anger, irascibility
      contradiction, from
      cough from anger
      violent

Anguish
>   morning
>   opression, with
>   > *desire to sit up or jump out of bed* •
>   > *palpitation, with*
>   > **perspiration, cold perspiration on forehead, with** •
>   stool, before
>   > during
Anorexia mentalis
Answers, aversion to answer
>   difficult
>   *incorrectly*
>   **monosyllable**
>   *refuses to answer*
Antics, plays
Anxiety
>   morning
>   evening
>   > bed, in
>   *night*
>   midnight, before
>   > waking, after
>   midnight, after, 3h.
>   air amel., in open
>   anger, during
>   bed, in
>   *chill, during*
>   *conscience, as if guilty of a crime*
>   dinner, after
>   eating, after
>   eructations, ending with •
>   *fear, with*
>   fever, during
>   *fright, about*
>   *future, about*
>   menses, during
>   > anger and anxiety
>   mental exertion, from
>   perspiration, with cold
>   rising from lying, after •
>   > from a seat, on
>   **salvation, about**
>   shuddering, with

Anxiety,
>   sleep, during
>   *standing, while*
>   stool, before
>   > *during*
>   vexation, after
>   waking, on
Audacity
Aversion, children, to her own
>   husband, to
>   > *and children*
Bed, remain in, desires to, sexual excitement, from •
Beside oneself, being
Bite, desire to
>   shoe and swallowing the pieces, bites his •
>   spoon etc., bites
Blindness pretended •
Boaster, rich, wishes to be considered as
Break things, desire to
Brooding
>   evening •
>   **corner or moping, brooding in a**
Busy
Capriciousness
Carried, desires to be
>   fast
Cautious
Censorious, critical
>   *find fault or is silent, disposed to* •
Cheerful, gay, mirthful
>   night
>   chill, during
>   clapping one's hand
Childbed, mental symptoms during
Climacteric period agg.
Company, aversion to; presence of other people agg. the symptoms; desire for solitude
Company, desire for; aversion to solitude, company amel.
Complaining
>   pain on waking, of

Comprehension, easy
Concentration, difficult
Confidence, want of self
Confusion of mind
   morning
  chill, during
  heat, during
  paroxysms of pain, during
  sitting, while
  standing, while
  stooping, amel. when
Conscientious about trifles
Contemptuous
  hard for subordinate and agreeable pleasant to superiors or
   people he has to fear
Contradiction, is intolerant of
Courageous
Cowardice
Cruelty, inhumanity
Cursing, swearing
   night •
  all night and complaints of stupid
   feeling •
  rage, in
Deafness, pretended •
Death, agony before
  presentiment of
  sensation of
  thoughts of
Deceitful, sly
Deception causes grief and mortification ★
Delirium
  night
  answers abruptly
  anxious
  apathetic
  bed and escapes, spring up sud-
   denly from
  chill, during
  coldness, with •
  comical
  erotic
  fever, during
  frightful
  furious ★
  gay, cheerful

Delirium,
  haemorrhage, after
  headache, during
  hysterical, almost
  injuries to head, after
  laughing
  lochia, during •
  loquacious
  maniacal
  meningitis, cerebrospinalis
  menses, before
   during
  mild
  muttering
  noisy
  nonsense, with eyes open
  pains, with the
   from
  persecution in delirium, delusions
   of
  perspiration, with cold •
  quiet
  raging, raving
  recognizes no one
  religious
  restless
  sepsis, from
  sleep, during
  sleeplessness, and ★
  \ *sopor, with*
  thirst, with
  trembling, with
  violent
  wild
Delirium tremens, mania-a-potu
Delusions, imaginations, hallucinations,
  illusions
  abroad, being •
  animals, of
  anxious
  blind, he is
  Cancer, has a •
  Christ, himself to be
  crime, committed a, he had
  criminals, about
  cursing, with
  deaf and dumb •
  dirt, eating •
  disease : deaf, dumb and has

Delusions,

    cancer, is •

distinguished, is

dogs, sees

doomed, being

dumb, he is •

engaged in some occupation, is

fancy, illusions of

fire, world is on

God, communication with, he is

    in

great person, is a

hear, he cannot

heaven, is in

    talking with God

home, is away from

hunter, he is a

images, phantoms, sees

labor, pretends to be in, or thinks

    she has pains •

laughter, with

loquacity, with

misfortune, inconsolable over fan-

    cied •

murdered, he will be

noise, hears

    making a, d. •

nose seems longer

people, sees

    converses with absent

persecuted, he is

possessed, being

pregnant, she is

prince, is a •

proud

rain, he hears (at night)

rank, he is a person of

religious

rich, as if he is ★

ruined, he is

scream, with obliging to

squanders, money •

strange, familiar things seem

    land, as if in a

suicide, driving to

Delusions,

    thieves, sees

        dreams of robbers, is fright-

        ened on waking, and thinks

        dream is true •

unfortunate,, he is

voices, hears

vow, keep it, must •

wealth, of

work, is hard at

Dementia

Despair

    chill, during

    heat, during

    menses, before •

    pains, with the

    perspiration, during

    recovery, of

    religious despair of salvation

        suppressed menses, dur-

        ing •

    social position, of

Destructiveness

    clothes, of

        cuts them up •

    drunkenness, during

Dictatorial, domineering, dogmatical,

    despotic

Dipsomania, alcoholism

Dirtiness

Discouraged

    moaning, with

Doubtful, soul's welfare, of

Dream, as if in a

Dullness, sluggishness, difficulty of think-

    ing and comprehending, torpor

    night on waking

    damp air, from

    waking, on

Dwells on past disagreeable occur-

    rences

Eat, refuses to

Eccentricity

    religious

Ecstasy

Egotism, self-esteem

Embraces, inanimate objects, even •
Erroneous, notions ★
Escape, attempts to
    meningitis cerebrospinalis, in •
    run away, to
    springs up suddenly from bed
Estranged, being kind with strangers,
        but not with his family
        and entourage
    ignores his relatives
Excitement, excitable
    chill, during
    heat, during
    menses, during
    religious
Exertion, agg. from mental
    amel.
Extravagance
Exuberance
Fancies, exaltation of
Fear, apprehension, dread
    morning
    evening
    alone, of being
    apoplexy, of
        stool, during •
    breath away, takes
    cholera, of
    death, of
        menses, during
    diarrhoea from
    escape, with desire to
    evil, of
    imaginary things, of
    insanity, losing his reason, of
    misfortune, of
    overpowering
    poisoned, of being
    position, to lose his lucrative
    robbers, of
    society, of his position in
    starting, with
    tremulous
Feces, swallows his own
Feigning sick
    pregnancy •
Foolish behavior

Foppish
Forgetful
    words while speaking, of; word
        hunting
Forsaken feeling
Fright, menses, during ★
Frightened easily
    chill, during •
    fever, during
    waking, on
Frown, disposed to ★
Gestures, makes
    clapping of the hands
    grasping or reaching at some-
        thing, at flocks; carphologia
    hands, motions, involuntary, of
        the
        head, to the
    ridiculous or foolish
    slow
    stamps the feet
    uncertain
Gossiping
Gourmand
Greed, cupidity
Grief
Hard for inferiors and kind for superi-
    ors
Haughty
    pregnancy, during •
    stupid and haughty
Heedless
High-spirited
Home, desires to go
    desires to leave home
Homesickness
Honor, wounded
    sense of honor, no
Hopeful
Howling
    all night •
Hurry, haste
Hydrophobia
Hypochondriasis
Hysteria
    menses, during

Ideas abundant, clearness of mind
    deficiency of
    imaginary disease, of ★
    vanish ★
Idiocy
Imbecility
    rage, stamps the feet
Imitation, mimicry
Impertinence
    acts, in his
Impulsive, rash
Inconsolable
    fancied misfortune, over ●
Inconstancy
Indifference, apathy
    daytime
    chill, during
    desire, has no, no action of the
      will
    everything, to
    exposure of her person, to
    external things, to
    fever, during
    notices nothing ●
    typhoid, in
Indignation
Indiscretion
Indolence, aversion to work
    morning ★
Industrious, mania for work
    menses, before
Inquisitive
Insanity, madness
    anxiety, with
    behaves like a crazy person
    black insanity with despair and
      weary of life from fear of
      mortification or of loss of posi-
      tion
    cheerful, gay
    climacteric period, during
    eat, refuses to
    erotic
    escape, desire to
    face, with pale
      red, with

Insanity,
    fortune, after gaining
      losing, after
    gluttony, with
      alternating with refusal to eat
    haemorrhage, after
    haughty
    heat, with
    laughing, with
    megalomania
    melancholy
    menses, during
    mild
    noisy
    pain, from intolerable
    persecution mania
    position, from fear to lose
    puerperal
    religious
    restlessness, with
    silent
    stamps the feet
    suicidal disposition, with
    travel, with desire to
    wantonness, with
Insolence
Interruption agg. mental symptoms
Intriguer
Introspection
Irresolution, marry, to
Irritability
    morning
    forenoon
    chill, during
    spoken to, when
    trifles, from
Jealousy
    men, between
Jesting, ridiculous or foolish
Kisses everyone
    menses, before
Lamenting, bemoaning, wailing
    evening ●
    night
Lascivious, lustful

Laughing
> night
> alternating with groaning
>> whining, moaning
> constant
> sardonic
> spasmodic

Liar
> *lies, never speaks the truth, does not know what she is saying*

Libertinism

Loathing, life, at

Looks down, before him ★

Loquacity
> cheerful, exuberant
> *religious subjects, about* •

Malicious, spiteful, vindictive

Mania
> demoniac
> lochia, from suppressed
> *rage, with*
> *singing, with*
> *tears, clothes*
>> hair, own
>> himself to pieces with nails

Marriage, obsessed by idea of m. excited sexual girls are

Memory, active

Memory, weakness of
> facts, for
>> recent, for
> persons, for
> said, for what has
> say, for what is about to

Menses, mental symptoms agg. during

Mental symptoms alternating with physical ★

Mildness

Mischievous

Mistakes, localities, in

Moaning, groaning, whining
> alternating with laughing
> heat, during
> perspiration, during

Mocking
> ridicule, passion to

Mood, changeable, variable

Moral feeling, want of

Morose, cross, fretful, ill-humor, peevish
> forenoon
> *contradiction, by*

Muttering

Naive, intelligent, but very

Naked, wants to be

Noise, inclined to make a

Nymphomania
> *loquacity, with* •
> *menses, before*
>> *during*
>> suppressed, after
> puerperal

Obscene, lewd
> man searching for little girls
> songs
> talk

Obstinate, headstrong
> simpleton, as a

Occupation, diversion amel.

Offended, easily; takes everything in bad part

Overactive

Play, passion for gambling

Pompous, important

Praying
> kneeling and

Prejudices, traditional

Profanity ★

Prostration of mind, mental exhaustion, brain-fag
> injuries, from

Quarrelsome, scolding
> night •

Rage, fury
> *night*
> *biting, with*
> *constant*
> cursing, with
> *headache, with*
> *heat on body, with* •
> *paroxysms, in*
> *shrieking, with*
> *violent*

Recognize anyone, does not
  relatives, does not recognize his
Religious affections
  melancholia
Remorse
Reproaches, himself
  others
Reserved
Restlessness
  evening
  night
  anxious
  bed, go from one bed to another,
    wants to
    tossing about in
  busy
  driving about
  eating, after
  pregnancy, during
Reverence, lack of
Roving, senseless, insane
Rudeness
Runs about
  in paroxysms, agg. evening ●
Sadness, despondency, dejection,
    mental depression, gloom,
    melancholy
    morning on waking
    evening
  chill, during
  climaxis, during
  labor, during
  menses, before
  puerperal
  talk, indisposed to
Satyriasis
Senses, acute
  dull, blunted
  vanishing of
Sensitive, oversensitive
  chill, during
Serious, earnest
Shamelessness
  childbed, during lying - in, in ●
  exposes the person

Shrieking, screaming, shouting
  evening agg. ●
  delusions, with
  sleep, during
Sighing, perspiration, during
Singing
  night
  fever, during
  hilarious, jealousy, night ●
  trilling
Sit, inclination to
Sits still
  wrapped in deep, sad thoughts
    and notices nothing, as if
Slander, disposition to
Slowness
Smiling
  foolish
  never
Sombambulism
Speech, hasty
  nonsensical
  wandering
Spit, desire to
  faces of people, in
Spoken to, averse to being
Spying everything
Squanders, money ●
Starting, startled
  easily
  fright, from and as from
  sleep, on falling
    during
    from
  sleepiness with
Strange, crank
  opinions and acts, in
Strength increased, mental
Striking
  drunkenness, during
Stupefaction, as if intoxicated
Suicidal disposition
  delusions, from
  despair, from religious ●
  drowning, by
  throwing himself, window, from

Suppressed or receding skin diseases
    or haemorrhoids, mental symp-
    toms agg. after
Suspicious, mistrustful
**Talk, indisposed to, desire to be
    silent, taciturn**
        pregnancy, during •
        sadness, in
        others agg., talk of
Tears things
Theorizing
Thinking, aversion to
Thoughts, disagreeable
    disconnected
    erroneous
    persistent
    rapid, quick
    rush, flow of
    strange
    vanishing of
Timidity
Touched, aversion to being
Tranquillity, serenity, calmness
Truth, tell the plain
Unconsciousness, coma, stupor
      morning
    dream, as in a
    emotion, after
    exertion, after
    fever, during
    meningitis, in
    menses, during
      suppression of
    motion, on least
    pain, from
    rising up, on
    semi-consciousness
    stool, after
Undertakes many things, perseveres in
    nothing
Unfortunate, feels
Violent, vehement
    chases family out of house •
    deeds of violence, rage leading to
Vivacious

Wander, desire to
    pregnancy, during •
    restlessly, wanders about
Weary of life
Weeping, tearful mood
      evening
      night
    agg.
    alternating with laughter
    chill, during
    coughing, during
    heat, during
    involuntary
    menses, during
    pains, with the
    perspiration, during
    sleep, in
    whimpering
      sleep, during
Wildness
Work, mental, impossible

VERATRUM VIRIDE

Answers: refuses to answer
Anxiety
Bed, remain in, desires to
Clairvoyance
Confusion of mind, afternoon
Death, desires
    thoughts, of
      fear, without
Delirium
    fever, during
    meningitis cerebrospinalis
    raging, raving
    scolding
    sepsis, from
    trembling, with
    violent
Delusions, imaginations, hallucinations,
    illusions
    poisoned, he is about to be
    pursued by enemies, he was
Dementia, epileptics, of
Eccentricity
    fancies, in

Excitement, excitable
Fear, death, of
    physician, will not see her; he
        seems to terrify her
    poisoned, of being
Forgetful
Gestures, grasping, picks at bed clothes
Grimaces
Howling
Insanity, madness
    convulsions, with
    laughing, with
    megalomania
    puerperal
    silent
Irritability
Jumping, bed, out of
Kicks
Lamenting, bemoaning, wailing
Laughing, constant
Loquacity ★
    evening
    insane
Mania
    rage, with
Memory, weakness of
Mistakes, speaking, in, omitting words
Morose, cross, fretful, ill-humor, peevish
Prostration of mind, mental exhaus-
    tion, brain-fag
Quarrelsome, scolding
Refuses to take the medicine
Restlessness
    night
Sadness, despondency, dejection, men-
    tal depression, gloom, melan-
    choly
Shrieking, screaming, shouting
    convulsions, before
        during epileptic
Sighing
Speech, unintelligible
    wild
Spit, desire to
Striking himself
    chest, his
Stupefaction, as if intoxicated

Suspicious, mistrustful
Unconsciousness, coma, stupor
    semi-consciousness
Violent, vehement
Wander, desire to
Weeping, hysterical

VERBASCUM THAPSUS AUT THAPSIFORME

Absent-minded, unobserving
Abstraction of mind
Anger, irascibility
    evening, amel.
Anxiety
    evening amel.
    daily
Beside oneself, being
Chaotic, confused behavior
Cheerful, gay, mirthful
    afternoon
    evening
Company, desire for; aversion to soli-
    tude, company amel.
Concentration, difficult
Confidence, want of self
Confusion of mind
Cowardice
Delusions, imaginations, hallucinations,
    illusions
    dead persons, sees
    fancy, illusions of
    lascivious
    spectres, ghosts, spirits, sees
        throng upon him
    war, being at
Despair
Discouraged
Dullness, sluggishness, difficulty of think-
    ing and comprehending, torpor
Eccentricity
Excitement, excitable
Exertion, agg. from mental
Fancies, exaltation of
    lascivious
Foolish behavior
Forgetful
High-spirited

Howling
Ideas abundant, clearness of mind
Imbecility
Indifference, apathy
    sleepiness, with
Indolence, aversion to work
    morning
        rising, on
    sleepiness, with
Industrious, mania for work
    heat, during
Irritability
    daytime
    evening amel.
Joy, fits of joy with bursts of laughter
Laughing
    immoderately
    joy, with excessive
Memory, active
Memory, weakness of
    thought, for what has just
Mood, alternating
    changeable, variable
Morose, cross, fretful, ill-humor, peevish
Overactive
Prostration of mind, mental exhaus-
    tion, brain-fag
Reading aloud agg. ★
Restlessness, night
Sadness, despondency, dejection, mental
    depression, gloom, melancholy
Sit, inclination to
Stupefaction, as if intoxicated
Thoughts, intrude and crowd around
    each other
    persistent
    rush, flow of
Timidity
    daytime
Unconsciousness, coma, stupor
Wearisome

VERATRINUM

Anxiety
Delirium
Delusions, imaginations, hallucinations,
    illusions
Unconsciousness, coma, stupor

VESPA CRABRO

Abstraction of mind
Anxiety
    fear, with
Death, dying, feels as if
Delirium
Muttering
Rest, desire for
Restlessness, night
Sadness, despondency, dejection, mental
    depression, gloom, melancholy
    menses, before
Unconsciousness, coma, stupor
    conduct, automatic
    waking, while

VIBURNUM OPULUS

Answers: aversion to answer
Hysteria
Irritability
Restlessness
    menses, during
Sadness, despondency, dejection, mental
    depression, gloom, melancholy
Work, mental, impossible

VIBURNUM TINUS

Hypochondriasis
    anxiety, future, about
    fear, misfortune, of
    sadness, morning

VINCA MINOR

Ailments from:
    anger, vexation
    work, mental
Anger, irascibility
    alternating with quick repentance
    face, red tip of nose, with
Confusion of mind, stooping, when
    writing, while
Death, thoughts of
Exertion, agg. from mental

Fear, death, of
> sadness, with
> misfortune, of
> sadness, with

Irritability

Morose, cross, fretful, ill-humor, peevish
> repentance, followed by •

Restlessness

Sadness, despondency, dejection, mental depression, gloom, melancholy

Starting, startled

Weeping, tearful mood
> *involuntary, weakness, from*

VIOLA ODORATA

Absent-minded, unobserving

Absorbed, buried in thought

Activity, emotional •
> mental

Anxiety

Chaotic, confused behavior

Cheerful, gay, mirthful

Childish behavior

Comprehension, easy

Concentration,, difficult

Confusion of mind

Delusions, imaginations, hallucinations, illusions
> fancy, illusions of
> snakes in and around her

Disobedience

Dullness, sluggishness, difficulty of thinking and comprehending, torpor

Eat, refuses to

Emotions predominated by the intellect

Excitement, excitable

Fancies, exaltation of
> capricious

Forgetful

Hypochondriasis
> weeping, with

Hysteria

Ideas abundant, clearness of mind
> perspiration, during

Imbecility

Impressionable

Industrious, mania for work

Introspection

Irritability
> music, during
> violin, of •

Loquacity

Magnatized, desires to be, mesmerism amel.

Memory, active

Memory, weakness of
> read, for what has
> for what has just

Mildness

Mood, changeable, variable

Morose, cross, fretful, ill-humor, peevish

Music, agg.
> *violin playing agg.*
> aversion to
> violin, of •
> headache from

Obstinate, headstrong

Offended, easily; takes everything in bad part

Prostration of mind, mental exhaustion, brain-fag

Quarrelsome, scolding

Restlessness

Sadness, despondency, dejection, mental depression, gloom, melancholy

Sensitive, music, to
> violin, to •

Speech, voice, in a low soft •

Talk, indisposed to, desire to be silent, taciturn

Thoughts, disconnected
> persistent
> rapid, quick
> rush, flow of
> thoughtful
> vanishing of
> speaking, while
> wandering

Unconsciousness, coma, stupor

Weeping, tearful mood
> causeless
> **chill, during**
> involuntary
> refused, when anything is

Work, aversion to mental

VIOLA TRICOLOR

Absent-minded, unobserving
Abusive, insulting
Anxiety
    eating, after
    fever, during
    future, about
Capriciousness
Chaotic, confused behavior
Cheerful, evening
       ill-humor during the day
Confidence, want of self
Confusion of mind
    chill, during
    walking, while
Cowardice
Discontented, displeased, dissatisfied
      himself, with
Discouraged
Disobedience
Dullness, sluggishness, difficulty of think-
      ing and comprehending, torpor
Fancies, exaltation of, evening in bed
         sleeplessness, with
    sleep, preventing
Fear, apprehension, dread
    eating food, after
Howling
Hurry, haste
    movements, in
    occupation, in
Ideas, abundant, clearness of mind
      evening
      night
Impatience
    heat, with
Indifference, apathy
    fever, during
Indolence, aversion to work
    afternoon
    evening
Introspection
Irritability
      daytime
      evening amel.
    alternating with hypochondriac
    mood during day, merry in
    evening

Lamenting, bemoaning, wailing
Loquacity
    evening
Memory, weakness of
Morose, cross, fretful, ill-humor, peevish
    daytime
    talk, indisposed to
Obstinate, headstrong
Prostration of mind, pollutions, after
Quarrelsome, scolding
Quiet, disposition
Restlessness
    internal
Sadness, despondency, dejection, mental
      depression, gloom, melancholy
        evening amel.
Sensitive, oversensitive
Shrieking, screaming, shouting
Sit, inclination to
Stupefaction, as if intoxicated
Suspicious, mistrustful
Talk, indisposed to, desire to be silent,
    taciturn
Thoughts, rush, flow of
        evening in bed
        sleeplessness, from
        vanishing of
Tranquillity, serenity, calmness
Wearisome
Weeping, tearful mood
Work, aversion to mental

VIPERA BERUS

Absorbed, buried in thought
Anguish
Anxiety
Confusion of mind
Death, desires
    presentiment of
Delirium
    alternating with sopor
    intoxicated, as if
    raging, raving
    sepsis, from
Delusions, night
    home, is away from

Despair
 pains, with the
Development of children arrested
Discouraged
Dullness, sluggishness, difficulty of think-
 ing and comprehending, torpor
Excitement, excitable
Exertion, agg. from mental
Home, desires to go
Indifference, apathy
 external things, to
Irritability
 headache, during
Mania
Morose, cross, fretful, ill-humor, peevish
Muttering
Poisoned, feeling ★
Rage, fury
Restlessness
  night
  anxious
  headache, during
Sadness, despondency, dejection, mental
 depression, gloom, melancholy
 heat, during
Senses, dull, blunted
Shrieking, screaming, shouting
Sighing
Speech, delirious
 hesitating
 incoherent
 intoxicated, as if
Stupefaction, as if intoxicated
Talks, himself, to
Torpor
Unconsciousness, coma, stupor
Weeping, convulsions, during

VIPERA ASPIS

Anguish
Contradict, disposition to
Delirium
Impatience
Irritability
Pessimist
Restlessness

Sadness, despondency, dejection, mental
 depression, gloom, melancholy
  menses, before
Unconsciousness, coma, stupor

VISCUM ALBUM

Abstraction of mind
Activity
Ailments from:
 fright
Anxiety
Cheerful, gay, mirthful
Company, aversion to; alone, amel.
 when
Confusion of mind, intoxicated, as if
Consolation, kind words agg.
Cowardice
Delusions, imaginations, hallucinations,
 illusions
  body, lighter than air, is
  fancy, illusions of
  floating in air
  spectres, ghosts, spirits, sees
Discouraged
Disgust, medicine bottle, at sight of
 the •
Dream, as if in a
Dwells on past disagreeable occur-
 rences
Exhilaration
Fear, apprehension, dread
 crowd, public places, of; agora-
  phobia
 death, of
 places, buildings etc. ★
 telephone, of •
Feces, swallows his own
Forgetful
Ground gives way ★
Hysteria
Indifference, apathy
Indolence, aversion to work
Irritability
Memory, weakness of
Mistakes, speaking, in

writing, in
Morose, cross, fretful, ill-humor, peevish
Optimistic
Plans, making many
Prostration of mind, mental exhaus-
        tion, brain-fag
Refuses to take the medicine
Restlessness
        night
*Sadness, despondency, dejection, mental
        depression, gloom, melancholy*
Sensitive, noise, to
Speech, incoherent
Strength increased, mental
Stupefaction, as if intoxicated
Thoughts, frightful
        night on waking
        persistent
Time passes too quickly, appears shorter
Unconsciousness, coma, stupor
        conduct, automatic
Violent, vehement
Weeping, tearful mood
        trifles, at
Work, mental, impossible

VOESLAU AQUA

Excitement, excitable
Inconstancy
Irritability
Morose, cross, fretful, ill-humor, peevish
Restlessness
        working, while

WIESBADEN AQUA

Activity
Anxiety
        future, about
cheerful, gay, mirthful
Gestures, makes, light
Impatience
Morose, cross, fretful, ill-humor, pee-
        vish
Restlessness
        anxious
Thinking, aversion to
Unconsciousness, coma, stupor
Weeping, tearful mood

WILDBAD AQUA

Anxiety
Indolence, aversion to work
Memory, weakness of
Restlessness, midnight, 4h. after
Sadness, despondency, dejection, men-
        tal depression, gloom, melan-
        choly
Weeping, sleep, in

WYETHIA HELENOIDES

Fear, apprehension, dread
Restlessness
Sadness, despondency, dejection, men-
        tal depression, gloom, melan-
        choly

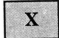

X-RAY

Company, aversion to; presence of
other people agg. the symptoms; desire for solitude
Irritability
Kill, desire to
menses, before •
during
Sadness, despondency, dejection, mental depression, gloom, melancholy
waking, on

XANTHOXYLUM
FRAXINEUM
(AMERICANUM)

Anguish, menses, during
Anxiety
future, about
Confusion of mind
identity, duality, sense of
Delirium
Delusions, imaginations, hallucinations,
illusions
die, he was about to
double, of being
Fear, apprehension, dread
death, before menses, of
happen, something will
menses, before
Frightened easily
Hysteria
amenorrhoea, in •
Indifference, apathy
daytime
life, to

Restlessness, women, in
Sadness, despondency, dejection, mental depression, gloom, melancholy
morning on waking
menses, before

XEROPHYLLUM

Concentration, difficult
Dullness, sluggishness, difficulty of
thinking and comprehending,
torpor
Memory, weak, names, for proper
words, for
Unconsciousness, coma, stupor

YUCCA FILAMENTOSA

Fancies, lascivious
Irritability
Memory, weakness of
Mistakes, speaking, using wrong words
    in
      writing, in
        wrong words, figures
Mood, changeable, variable
Restlessness
    night
Sadness, despondency, dejection, men-
    tal depression, gloom, melan-
    choly
Sensitive, noise, to
Thoughts, wandering
Work, aversion to mental

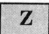

ZEA ITALICA

Washing, bathing, mania for •

ZINCUM METALLICUM

Absent-minded, unobserving
Activity, sleeplessness, with
Ailments from:
    anger, vexation
      fright, with
      silent grief, with
    excitement, emotional
    fright
    grief
    mortification ★
    sexual excesses
Anger, irascibility
    noon
    evening
    alternating with cheerfulness
        discouragement
        sadness
        timidity
    aroused, when
    delusions during climaxis, with
    easily
    stabbed anyone, so that he could
    have
    trembling, with
    violent
    voices of people
Answers, repeats the question first
    slowly
Anxiety
    daytime
    morning
    afternoon
    evening amel.

Anxiety
>   night
>>   waking, on
>   air amel., in open
>   alone, when
>   alternating with contentment •
>   apparitions while awake, from
>   horrible
>   *conscience, as if guilty of a crime*
>   dark, in
>   dreams, on waking from frightful
>   fear, with
>   *fever, during*
>   menses, before
>>   during
>>   amel.
>   sleep, during
>>   menses, after
>   waking, on

Automatism ★

Busy

Capriciousness
>   noon •
>   evening

Cares, others, about
>   relatives, for

Chaotic, confused behavior

Cheerful, gay, mirthful
>   morning
>   forenoon
>   *evening*
>>   *bed, in*
>   alternating with irritability
>>   sadness
>   melancholy, with ★

Childbed, mental symptoms during

Climacteric period agg.

Closing eyes amel.

Company, desire for; aversion to soli-
>   tude, company amel.
>   alone agg., while

Concentration, difficult
>   children, in

Confidence, want of self

Confusion of mind
>   morning
>>   waking, on
>   afternoon
>   evening
>   dinner, after
>   dream, as if in
>   eating, after
>   headache, with
>   *waking, on*
>   *wine, after*

Contented

Darkness agg.

Death, desires
>   presentiment of
>>   calmly, thinks of death •
>   *sensation of*
>   *thoughts of*
>>   afternoon
>>   *evening* •

Delirium
>   *bed and escapes, springs up sud-*
>>   *denly from*
>   frightful
>   laughing
>   maniacal
>   *murmuring*
>   raging, raving
>   violent
>>   restrained and calmed with
>>   great difficulty, is •
>   waking, on

Delirium tremens, mania-a-potu
>   *excitement, with*

Delusions, imaginations, hallucina-
>   *tions, illusions*
>   night
>   accused, she is
>   animals, of
>   *arrested, is about to be*
>   crime, committed a, he had
>   dead persons, sees
>   *devils, sees*
>>   *after her, devil is* •

Delusions,
> dogs, sees
> double, objects are
> enlarged
>> head is
> fancy, illusions of
> fire, visions of
> goitre, one has, which he cannot
>> see over when sitting down •
> *grief and anger, from*
> horses, sees
> *images, phantoms, sees*
>> night
>>> moving up and down, sees •
> light, incorporeal, he is
> longer, things seem
> money, he is counting
> murdered, he will be
> *persecuted, he is*
> pursued by enemies
>> police, by
> spectres, ghost, spirits, sees
>> waking, on
> thieves, sees
> visions, has horrible, waking, on •
> *voices, abusive and filthy lan*
>> *guage, voices from within him*
>> *speaking in* •

Despair, recovery, of
Dipsomania, alcoholism
> *excitement from*
Discomfort
> eating, after
>> dinner, after
Discontented, displeased, dissatisfied
> afternoon
Discouraged
> alternating with anger
>> irritability •
Dream, as if in a
Dullness, sluggishness, difficulty of
thinking and comprehend-
ing, torpor
> noon
> afternoon
> children, in
> closing eyes, on •
> dinner, after

Dullness,
> headache, with •
> lying amel. •
> paroxysmal
> sleepiness, with
> *understands questions only after*
>> *repetition*
> wine, after
Emptiness, sensation of ★
Ennui, tedium
Envy
Escape, attempts to
> restrained with difficulty, is
Excitement, excitable
>> evening
>>> bed, in
>> night
> climacteric period, during
> *hearing horrible things, after*
> trifles, over
Exertion, agg. from mental
> amel.
Exhilaration
Fancies, exaltation of
>> *night*
> *lascivious*
> vivid, lively
Fear, apprehension, dread
>> noon •
>> *evening*
>>> amel.
>> night
> alone, of being
> alternating with sadness •
> *apoplexy, of*
> dark, of
> death, of
> falling, of
> ghosts, of
> *hydrocephalus, in* •
> imaginary things, to
> lifelong
> misfortune, of
> noise, from
> *robbers, of*
> waking, on
> work, dread of

Forgetful
    headache, during
Frightened easily
        noon •
        waking, on
Fussy ★
Gestures, makes, automatic
        *grasping or reaching at some-
            thing, at flocks; carphologia*
        genitals, delirium, during ★
        picks at bed clothes
        strange attitudes and positions
Grief, delusions from •
Heedless
*Horrible things, sad stories, affect her
        profoundly*
Hurry, drinking, on
        eating, while
Horror ★
Hypochondriasis
        afternoon
        eating, after
Hysteria
        menses, amel. during •
Ideas abundant, clearness of mind
        deficiency of
Imbecility
Impatience
        headache, during
        perspiration, during
        talk of others, during •
Impetuous
Inconstancy
Indifference, apathy
        enuui, with
        sleepiness, with
Indolence, aversion to work
        dinner, after
        eating, after
        sadness, from
        sleepiness, with
Industrious, mania for work
Insanity, madness
        convulsions, with
        erotic
        puerperal
        suppressed eruptions, after

Irresolution, indecision
Irritability
        daytime
        morning
        noon
        afternoon
        evening
            amel.
        alternating with cheerfulness
                        sadness
                        timidity
                        wrath ★
        children, in
        headache, during
        menses, during
        music, during
            piano, of
        talking, while
Kisses everyone, menses, before
Lamenting, bemoaning, wailing
Lascivious, lustful
Laughing
        evening
        alternating with sadness
        constant
        convulsions, before, during or af-
            ter
        immoderately
        sardonic
        spasmodic
        trifles, at
Light, shuns
Loathing, life, at
Loquacity
        alternating with chill and heat ★
        chill, during ★
Malicious, spiteful, vindictive
        anger, with
Mania
        erotic ★
        rage, with
        suppressed eruptions, after
Memory, active
Memory, loss of :
        epileptic fits, after
Memory, weakness of
        done, for what has just
Menses, mental symptoms agg. during

Mental symptoms alternating with physical ★
Mildness
Mistakes, speaking in
       words, using wrong
       writing, omitting letters in
Moaning, groaning, whining
       daytime ●
       night
Mood, alternating
       changeable, variable
              perspiration, during
Morose, cross, fretful, ill-humor, peevish
       morning
       noon ●
       afternoon
       evening
       convulsions, before
       talking of others, on ●
Morphinism
Music agg.
       piano playing, from
Nymphomania
       menses, after suppressed
       pregnancy, during
       puerperal
Obstinate, headstrong
Offended, easily; takes everything in bad part
Play, desire to dirty trick on others or their teachers, school boys play a
Prostration of mind, mental exhaus tion, brain-fag nursing, after
Quarrelsome, scolding
Quiet disposition
Rage, fury
              evening
Recognize, relatives, does not r. his
Religious affections
Remorse
Repeated ★
Restlessness
       morning
       evening
       night

Restlessness,
       midnight, after
       anxious
       bed, tossing about in
       menses, during suppressed
       waking, on
Runs, fright, as if in ●
Sadness, despondency, dejection, mental depression, gloom, melancholy
       daytime
       morning
       noon
       noon, lively, and in evening sad, or vice versa ●
       afternoon
       evening
              amel.
       alone, when
       alternating with anger ●
              contentment ●
              fear ●
              irritability
       climaxis, during
       dinner, after
       eating, after
       epilepsy, before attack of
       labor, during
       menses, during
              amel.
       work - shy, in
Secretive
Senses, acute
       dull, blunted
Sensitive, oversensitive
       noon ●
       mental impressions, to
       music, to
              piano, to
       noise, to
              aversion to
              talking, of
              voices, of
       sensual impressions, to

Shrieking, screaming, shouting
    anger, from ★
    brain cry
    children, in, evening
       when moved ★
    chorea, in
    convulsions, before
    hydrocephalus, in
    sleep, during
       menses, before
    waking, on
Sit, inclination to
Slowness
    old people, of
Somnambulism
    disappearance of old eruptions,
       after •
    suppressed emotions, after •
Speech, angry •
    incoherent
    slow
    unintelligible, evening after lying
       down •
Spoken to, averse to being
Starting, startled
    noon
    night, during menses •
    easily
    menses, during
    sleep, during
    from
       menses, during •
    trifles, at
Stupefaction, as if intoxicated
    noon •
    afternoon
    evening
    epistaxis, after •
    paroxysms, in •
    vertigo, during
Suicidal disposition
Sulky
Superstitious
Suppressed or receding skin diseases
    or haemorrhoids, mental symp-
    toms agg. after

Talk, indisposed to, desire to be
    silent, taciturn
       evening
    others agg., talk of
Talks, troubles, of her ★
Talking, sleep, in
Thinking, complaints agg., of
Thoughts, disconnected
    persistent, alone, when
    rush, flow of
       night
    vanishing of
    wandering
Thunderstorm, mind symptoms before
Timidity
    alternating with anger •
       irritability •
       sadness •
       vexation
    bashful
Torments everyone with his com-
    plaints
Touched, ticklishness
Tranquillity, serenity, calmness
Unconsciousness, coma, stupor
    morning
    noon
    evening
    exanthema slow to appear,
       when •
    semi-consciousness
    suppression of eruptions, after •
    transient
    vertigo, during
Violent, vehement
    deeds of violence, rage leading to
Vivacious
Walk, aversion to •
Wearisome
    evening
Weary of life
Weeping, tearful mood
    evening amel.
    night
    anger, with ★
    anxiety, after
    causeless

Weeping,
- *menses, before*
  - during
- sleep, in
- *vexation, from*
- whimpering
  - anger, with •
Work, aversion to mental
- *impossible*
Writing, difficulty in expressing ideas
- when

ZINCUM ACETICUM

Anxiety
Delirium
- maniacal
Delirium tremens, mania-a-potu
Eat, refuses to ★
Restlessness
Work, aversion to mental ★

ZINCUM CYANATUM

Hysteria

ZINCUM MURIATICUM

Anxiety
Delusions, imaginations, hallucinations,
- illusions
  - smell, of
Fear, apprehension, dread
Gestures, makes, grasping or reaching at
- something, at flocks; carphologia
- picks at bed clothes
Irritability
Memory, weakness of
Starting, trifles, at

ZINCUM OXYDATUM

Anxiety, conscience, as if guilty of a
- crime
Hypochondriasis
Laughing, immoderately
- involuntarily
- sardonic
- spasmodic

Morose, cross, fretful, ill-humor, peevish
Restlessness
- conscience, of

ZINCUM PHOSPHORICUM

Ailments from:
- fright
- sexual excesses
Anger, agg.
- trifles, at
- violent
Anxiety, morning
- afternoon
- night
- fever, during
- menses, during
- waking, on
Cheerful, evening
Company, desire for; aversion to solitude; company
- amel.
Concentration, difficult
- studying, reading etc., while ★
Confusion of mind ★
- morning
  - waking, on
- evening
- eating, after
Death, presentiment of
Delirium, frightful
- raging, raving
- violent
Delusions, dead persons, sees
- fancy, illusions of
- fire, visions of
- flatus, that everybody notices his ★
- images, phantoms, sees, night
Desires, more than she needs
Dullness, sluggishness, difficulty of thinking and comprehending, torpor
Escape, attempts to
Excitement, excitable
Exertion, agg. from mental
Fancies, exaltation of

Fear, apprehension, dread
>   evening
>   night
>   death, of
>   ghosts, of
>   robbers, of
>   waking, on

Forgetful

Gestures, makes, grasping or reaching at something, at flocks; car- phologia
>   picks at bed clothes

Heedless

Imbecility

Impatience

Impetuous

Indifference, apathy

Indolence, aversion to work

Insanity, madness

Irresolution, indecision

Irritability
>   morning
>   **evening**
>   headache, during
>   menses, during

Laughing, sardonic
>   silly
>   spasmodic

Loathing, life, at

Loquacity

Malicious, spiteful, vindictive

Memory, weakness of

Mood, changeable, variable

Morose, cross, fretful, ill-humor, peevish

Obstinate, headstrong

Offended, easily; takes everything in bad part

Prostration of mind, mental ex- haustion, brain-fag

Restlessness, morning
>   evening
>   night
>   anxious

Sadness, despondency, dejection, mental depression, gloom, melancholy
>   morning
>   afternoon
>   evening

Senses, dull, blunted

Sensitive, music, to
>   **noise, to**

Shrieking, sleep, during

Sits, still

Speech, incoherent

Starting, sleep, during

Stupefaction, as if intoxicated

Suicidal, thoughts

Talk, indisposed to, desire to be silent, taciturn

Talking, sleep, in

Thoughts, vanishing of
>   wandering

Timidity

Unconsciousness, coma, stupor
>   menses, during

Weeping, tearful mood
>   menses, during

Work, aversion to mental

ZINCUM PICRICUM

Memory, weakness of

Nymphomania

Prostration of mind, mental exhaus- tion, brain-fag

Satyriasis

ZINCUM SULPHURICUM

Anxiety

Delirium

Laughing
>   involuntarily

Talking, sleep, in ★

ZINCUM VALERIANICUM

Ailments from:
>   excitement, emotional ★

Anguish

Busy

Excitement, excitable

Hurry, haste

Hypochondriasis

Hysteria
>   climacteric period, at

Irritability
Morose, convulsions, before
Restlessness
Sadness, epilepsy, before attack of

ZINGIBER OFFICINALE

Activity, mental
Cheerful, gay, mirthful
Emptiness, sensation of ★
Forgetful
Hypochondriasis
Ideas abundant, clearness of mind
Indolence, aversion to work
Irritability, evening
        menses, during
Memory, active
Memory, weakness of
Mood, agreeable
Restlessness
        evening
        midnight, 2h. after
Sadness, despondency, dejection, mental
        depression, gloom, melancholy
Unconsciousness, coma, stupor
        fever, during

ZIZIA AUREA

Cheerful, alternating with sadness
        followed by melancholy
Conversation, aversion to
Desires, exercise, for
Discontented, himself, with
        weeping amel.
Dream, as if in a
Excitement, excitable
Exhilaration
        sadness, after ●
Fancies, exaltation of
Hypochondriasis
Hysteria
Indifference, apathy
        everything, to
        irritability, with ●

Indolence, aversion to work
        contented, with ●
Irritability
        alternating with indifference
        sadness, with
Loathing, life, at
Memory, active
Sadness, despondency, dejection, men-
        tal depression, gloom, melan-
        choly
        exhilaration, after
        quiet
Suicidal disposition
Weary of life
Weeping, tearful mood
        alternating with laughter